PLUMER'S
PRINCIPLES & PRACTICE OF
INTRAVENOUS THERAPY

SEVENTH EDITION

Sharon M. Weinstein, RN, CRNI, MS
Executive Director, The Premier Foundation
Director, Office of International Affairs
Premier, Inc.
Oak Brook, Illinois

Infusion Therapy Consultant
Former Faculty, Department of Surgery
Finch University of Health Sciences/The Chicago Medical School
North Chicago, Illinois

Chair, Intravenous Nurses Certification Corporation,
Board of Directors

Past President, The Intravenous Nurses Society, Inc.

Leader, Intravenous Therapy Delegations
  to People's Republic of China, Austria, Germany
Commonwealth of Independent States, and Egypt

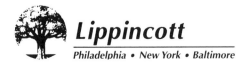
Lippincott
Philadelphia • New York • Baltimore

Acquisitions Editor: Margaret B. Zuccarini
Developmental Editor: Deedie McMahon
Senior Project Editor: Sandra Cherrey Scheinin
Senior Production Manager: Helen Ewan
Production Coordinator: Patricia McCloskey

Art Director: Doug Smock
Manufacturing Manager: William Alberti
Indexer: Ann Cassar
Compositor: The PRD Group
Printer: R. R. Donnelley & Sons Company/Crawfordsville

Edition 7th

9 8 7 6 5 4 3 2 1

Library of Congress Cataloging-in-Publication Data

Weinstein, Sharon.
    Plumer's principles & practice of intravenous therapy / Sharon M. Weinstein.—7th ed.
        p. cm.
    Includes bibliographical references and index.
    ISBN 0-7817-1988-7 (alk. paper)
    1. Intravenous therapy.   I. Title: Plumer's principles and practice of intravenous
therapy.   II. Title: Principles & practice of intravenous therapy.

RM170.P57 2000
615'.6—dc21   00-044395

Care has been taken to confirm the accuracy of the information presented and
to describe generally accepted practices. However, the authors, editors, and
publisher are not responsible for errors or omissions or for any consequences from
application of the information in this book and make no warranty, express or
implied, with respect to the content of the publication.

The authors, editors, and publisher have exerted every effort to ensure that
drug selection and dosage set forth in this text are in accordance with the current
recommendations and practice at the time of publication. However, in view of
ongoing research, changes in government regulations, and the constant flow of
information relating to drug therapy and drug reactions, the reader is urged to
check the package insert for each drug for any change in indications and dosage
and for added warnings and precautions. This is particularly important when the
recommended agent is a new or infrequently employed drug.

Some drugs and medical devices presented in this publication have Food and
Drug Administration (FDA) clearance for limited use in restricted research settings.
It is the responsibility of the health care provider to ascertain the FDA status of
each drug or device planned for use in his or her clinical practice.

Contributors

Mary Ann Daehler, RN, OCN, CRNI, MS
Oncology Nurse Clinician
Holy Family Hospital
Des Plaines, Illinois

Carole DeCicco, RN, MSN, CRNP, CS
Nurse Practitioner
Willowcrest Division
Albert Einstein Healthcare Network
Philadelphia, Pennsylvania

Anne Marie Frey, RN, BSN, CRNI
IV Nurse Clinician
Children's Hospital of Philadelphia
Philadelphia, Pennsylvania

Dorothy Jackson, RN, CRNI
IV Nursing Consultant
Flint, Michigan

Susan Y. Pauley, RN, CRNI
IV Supervisor
Massachusetts General Hospital
Boston, Massachusetts

Barbara St. Marie, RN, CNP
Pain Specialist
University of Minnesota/Fairview Health
   System
Minneapolis, Minnesota

Reviewers

Judith A. Ackeret, RN,C, MS
Assistant Professor
Baker University, School of Nursing
Stormont-Vail Campus
Topeka, Kansas

Helene Hakim, RN, MSN
Clinical Nursing Instructor and Lecturer
University of Texas at Tyler
School of Nursing
Tyler, Texas

Mary Rebecca Harry, RN, BSN, MEd
Clinical Instructor
Crowder College, School of Nursing
Neosho, Missouri

Linda E. McCuistion, RN, BSN, PHd
Associate Professor
Our Lady of Holy Cross College
New Orleans, Louisiana

Acknowledgments

Plumer's Principles & Practice of Intravenous Therapy, Seventh Edition, is the result of the collaborative efforts of its original authors, Ada Lawrence Plumer and Faye Cosentino; the contribution of Margaret M. McCluskey, RN, OCN, MPH, MA, CHES; and the outstanding contributors to this edition: Mary Ann Daehler, Carole DeCicco, Anne Marie Frey, Dorothy Jackson, Susan Y. Pauley, and Barbara St. Marie, and myself. I am so grateful to them for their valuable contributions to this text, and for the contributions that they have individually and collectively made to our professional practice. I would also like to thank the manufacturers of infusion products and equipment for their information and assistance, as well as the authors and publishers who permitted use of their copyrighted materials in producing this text.

A special thank you to Margaret Belcher Zuccarini, Senior Editor, at Lippincott Williams & Wilkins and Deedie McMahon, Sandra Cherrey Scheinin, and Doug Smock for their encouragement, support, and technical assistance in developing a superior manuscript—one that readily supports the Plumer name.

Thanks are extended to William Eudailey, PharmD, and to the late David Blaess, RPh, who served as my mentors, and who taught me to apply the principles gleaned from Plumer's book to my daily practice. Men of vision, they gave me the opportunity to explore the world of infusion therapy.

There are professionals in the infusion specialty whose names are synonymous with quality. Two such individuals are the late Cheryl Gardner, CRNI, and Jaclyn Tropp, CRNI. As a fellow board member, Cheryl demonstrated a passion for quality IV patient care. I have had the privilege of knowing and working with Jackie for over 15 years. An inspiration to many IV nurses nationwide, her zest for our practice continues to inspire me. In the face of great adversity, she has constantly striven to expand her educational base, to educate others, and to share our specialty practice.

Finally, thanks to my husband Steve, and to Heidi, Jason, Marla, and Rob, for delighting in and acknowledging my continuing passion for infusion therapy.

SMW

Special Acknowledgment

As Plumer's celebrates its 30th year as the *premier* source of information in infusion therapy, it is appropriate to recognize the woman who first penned this text. The name Ada Plumer is synonymous with infusion therapy. A leader, pacesetter, and co-founder of the professional society, Plumer set the tone for our professional practice, served as a mentor to many nurses, and encouraged excellence in the delivery of intravenous nursing care.

From my first entry into this rapidly changing field to today, I have used Plumer's book as a reference, a guide, and a bible for professional practice. The "original" IV reference manual retains its position today as the only complete source of information available to the practicing clinician, student, and educator. The success of the current edition is attributed to Plumer . . . the growth of our practice is likewise a result of her initial efforts. Many thanks from all of us in whom you have instilled a passion for excellence in intravenous nursing practice.

Preface

For 30 years, *Plumer's Principles & Practice of Intravenous Therapy* has retained its position as the most reliable, complete source of information addressing intravenous therapy for practicing clinicians, educators, and students. Completely updated and revised to meet the changing needs of our professional practice, this seventh edition, like its predecessors, provides the most current base of knowledge available to those who share the responsibility of ensuring high-quality infusion care to patients in a diversity of clinical settings.

The practice of infusion therapy is a multifaceted one. Infusion therapy is at the core of patient care. Our practice continually changes as a result of changing patient care delivery systems, the impact of managed care, reengineering of the health care system, and the impact of integrated health care delivery systems. These changes have had a dramatic impact on our professional practice as we move on the continuum, from care delivered in the acute care environment to care delivered in alternative sites. One thing remains unchanged, however, and that is the continuous need for an unprecedented high level of expertise for delivering infusion therapy.

Plumer's Principles & Practice of Intravenous Therapy, Seventh Edition, has been updated and reorganized to create a resource that clearly exceeds these needs. The addition of boxes, tables, legal issues, step-by-step directions, nursing alerts, tables, and reference to evidence-based practice creates an easy-to-use format and easy-to-access references. A more integrated approach to content results in a streamlined five-section organization. Part I reviews the history, legal implications, nursing role and responsibilities, and application of the Intravenous Nurses Society Standards of Practice. Managing risk and improving quality round out Part I.

Part II has undergone dramatic change. Now addressing assessment and monitoring, this section has been expanded to encompass fluid and electrolyte balance, principles of parenteral fluid administration, as well as relevant anatomy and physiology, laboratory data, ongoing monitoring, and potential complications. A new chapter on defining and documenting evidence-based practice has been added.

Part III, Principles of Equipment Selection and Clinical Applications, presents safety principles, state-of-the-art equipment, methods for assessing product and equipment needs, peripheral intravenous therapy, central venous catheterization, and advanced vascular access. This area has been completely updated, consistent with our practice. Intraarterial therapy has been updated with new content and new art.

Patient-specific therapies are addressed in the revamped Part IV. With a plethora of talented contributing authors creating the most current and complete source of information available today, I know that you will be pleased. Carole DeCicco has again revised the chapter on parenteral nutrition. I have known and worked with Carole since 1962; she has over 30 years of experience in this intensive field, and is an active educator and nurse practitioner. Susan Pauley completely revised the section on transfusion therapy, consistent with the dramatic changes in practice and revised Standards. A new author, Mary Ann Daehler, has updated material on antineoplastics previously prepared by Margaret McCluskey. Barbara St. Marie, a renowned expert in pain management, has written the chapter on Pain, emphasizing practical aspects of care, IV conscious sedation, and continuous local anesthesia. The chapter on drug administration has been rewritten with an emphasis on therapeutic monitoring and drug level ranges.

Part V addresses special applications. Ann Marie Frey has updated the information on pediatric infusion therapy. Dorothy Jackson, another new author and recognized expert, has edited the section on alternate site settings and cost factors, bringing the voice of experience to home care, longterm and subacute environments. Intravenous therapy in the older adult patient has been added.

The seventh edition includes new appendices and extensive reference to the use of the World Wide Web and evidence-based practice. Revised to meet the needs of the clinician responsible for delivering high-quality infusion care, regardless of the clinical setting in which care is provided, *Plumer's Principles & Practice of Intravenous Therapy*, Seventh Edition, retains its place as the most essential tool available in intravenous practice today. May you enjoy it and gain value from it.

Sharon M. Weinstein, RN, CRNI, MS

Contents

List of Tables

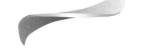

OVERVIEW
OF
INTRAVENOUS
THERAPY

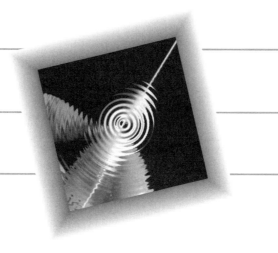

C H A P T E R   1

History of

Intravenous Therapy

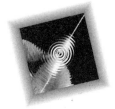

K E Y   T E R M S

Hypotonicity
Parenteral
Pyrogens
Quill and Bladder
Standards of Practice

■ EARLY HISTORY AND METHODOLOGY

Almost 400 years have passed since the discovery of blood circulation. William Harvey's 1628 research stimulated increased experimentation, and he found that the heart is both a muscle and a pump.

Renaissance Period

In 1656, Sir Christopher Wren, the famed architect of St. Paul's Cathedral in London, injected opium intravenously into dogs. Wren, known as the father of modern intravenous (IV) therapy, used a **quill and bladder.** In 1662, Johann Majors made the first successful injection of unpurified compounds into human beings, although death resulted from infection at the injection site.

In 1665, an animal near death from loss of blood was saved by the infusion of blood from another animal. In 1667, a 15-year-old Parisian boy was the first human to receive a transfusion successfully; lamb's blood was administered directly into the boy's circulation by Jean Baptiste Denis, physician to Louis XIV (Cosnett, 1989). The enthusiasm aroused by this success led to promiscuous transfusions of blood from animals to humans with fatal results, and in 1687, by an edict of church and parliament, animal-to-human transfusions were prohibited in Europe. Nearly 150 years passed before serious attempts were again made to inject blood into people.

The 19th Century

James Blundell, an English obstetrician, revived the idea of blood transfusion. In 1834, saving the lives of many women threatened by hemorrhage during childbirth, he proved that animal blood was unfit to inject into humans and that only human blood was safe. Nevertheless, complications persisted, with infections developing in donors and recipients. With the discovery of the principles of antisepsis by Pasteur and Lister, another obstacle was overcome, although reactions and deaths continued.

The first recorded attempt to prevent coagulation during transfusion was in 1821 by Jean Louis Prévost, a French physician who, with Jean B. A. Dumas, used defibrinated blood in animal transfusions (Cosnett, 1989).

In the middle to late 19th century, increased knowledge of bacteriology, pharmacology, and pathology led to new approaches. Ignaz Semmelweis, a Viennese obstetrician, was the first to correlate the effect of hand washing on prevention of infection. Semmelweis is credited with a 90% reduction of maternal deaths between 1846 and 1848. Meanwhile, chemist Louis Pasteur was proving that bacteria were living microorganisms, although his ideas were challenged by many researchers and practitioners.

In 1889, William Halsted of the Johns Hopkins Hospital, in cooperation with Goodyear Rubber Company, introduced the use of surgical gloves in the operating theater. Ten years later, the use of rubber gloves was widely accepted as a means of protecting patients and physicians (Sutcliff, 1992).

French physiologist Claude Bernard is credited with experimental injection of sugar solutions into dogs. The precursor to modern nutritional support, Bernard's experiments were followed by the subcutaneous injection of fat, milk, and camphor by Menzel and Perco in Vienna. Work in nutritional support remained at a standstill for many years.

20th Century Advances

In the 20th century, IV therapy advanced rapidly. Blood transfusions and **parenteral** fluids, which bypass the intestines, were administered, and parenteral nutrition became possible as well. Moreover, nurses became skilled both in administering and monitoring infusions.

Transfusion Therapy

In 1900, Karl Landsteiner proved that not all human blood is alike when he identified four main classifications. In 1914, sodium citrate was found to prevent blood from clotting (Cosnett, 1989), and since then, rapid advances have been made (Table 1-1).

T A B L E   1 – 1
20TH CENTURY PROGRESS IN INFUSION THERAPY

Year	Significant Advancement
1900	Karl Landsteiner discovered three of four main blood groups.
1914	Sodium citrate was first used to preserve blood.
1914	Hydrolyzed protein and fats were administered to animals.
1925	Dextrose was used as an infusate.
1935	Marriot and Kekwick introduced slow-drip method of transfusion.
1937	Rose identified amino acids essential for growth.
1940	Disposable plastic administration sets were developed.
1945	Flexible intravenous (IV) cutdown catheter was introduced.
1950	Rochester needle was introduced.
1960	Peripherally inserted catheter lines introduced in intensive care areas.
1963–65	First success with hyperalimentation at the University of Pennsylvania.
1970	Centers for Disease Control (CDC) guidelines for IV therapy were published.
	First edition of *Plumer's Principles and Practice of Intravenous Therapy* published.
1972	Access of implanted ports introduced.
1973	The National Intravenous Therapy Association (NITA) was founded.
	Broviac tunneled catheter was introduced.
1976	Fat emulsions were used for nutritional support.
1980	NITA Standards of Practice were published.
	NITA National Office opened.
	IV Nurse Day was recognized by U.S. House of Representatives.
1981	CDC Guidelines were revised and published.
1982	Implantable ports were used for long-term access.
	First IV teaching program in People's Republic of China.
1983	Home blood transfusion initiated.
	Osteoport™ was developed.
1984	First edition of *Core Curriculum for Intravenous Nursing* published.
1985	Intravenous Nurses Certification Corporation offered its first credentialing examination (CRNI).
1986	Use of patient-controlled analgesia increased.
1987	NITA changed its name to the Intravenous Nurses Society (INS).
1990	Safe Medical Device Act and Food and Drug Administration Device Reporting regulations published.
	INS Revised Standards of Practice published.
1992	U. S. Food and Drug Administration issued alert concerning needlestick injuries.
1995	Occupational Safety and Health guidelines for handling cytotoxic drugs published.
1996	LPNI examination offered to LPN/LVNs by INS.
	CDC Guidelines revised and published.
1998	INS celebrated its 25th Anniversary (Houston, TX).
1999	*Journal of Intravenous Nursing* offered CE/recertification units.

(continued)

<table>
<tr><td colspan="2" align="center">**T A B L E   1 – 1**</td></tr>
<tr><td colspan="2" align="center">20TH CENTURY PROGRESS IN INFUSION THERAPY *(Continued)*</td></tr>
</table>

Year	Significant Advancement
2000	*Core Curriculum for Intravenous Nursing,* 2nd edition, published.
	Publication of Revised Standards of Practice.
	Publication of INS Policies and Procedures Manual.
	CRNI Exam Preparation Guide & Practice Questions published.
	First public member added to the INS board of directors.
2000	*Plumer's* 7th edition is published—30 years of IV therapy.

In 1911, Dr. Ottenberg of New York demonstrated the use of donor blood; his theory that safe transfusion was possible from a donor whose serum agglutinated the recipient's red blood cells was readily accepted. Dr. Ottenberg further suggested that it was unsafe to use a donor whose red blood cells were acted on by the recipient's serum. These research findings evolved into the universal donor concept still valid today.

Hugh Leslie Marriot and Alan Kekwick, English physicians, introduced the continuous slow-drip method of blood transfusion; their findings were published in 1935 (Cosnett, 1989).

The Rh factor was discovered in 1940, and the American Association of Blood Banks was formed in 1947. The invention of the first cell separator in 1951 introduced component therapy (for more information, see Chap. 19).

Parenteral Fluids

Administration of parenteral fluids by the IV route has been widely used only since the late 1950s. The difficulty in accepting this procedure resulted from the lack of safe fluids. The fluids then in use contained substances called **pyrogens,** proteins that are foreign to the body and not destroyed by sterilization. These caused chills and fever when injected into the circulation. The 1923 discovery and elimination of pyrogens led to safer and more frequent IV administration of parenteral fluids. In 1925, the most frequently used parenteral fluid was normal saline (0.9% sodium chloride). Because of its **hypotonicity,** water could not be administered IV and had to be made isotonic. A certain percentage of sodium chloride added to water achieved this effect (Cosnett, 1989). After 1925, dextrose was used extensively to make isotonic fluids and provide a source of calories.

Infusion Nursing

Massachusetts General Hospital is credited with many firsts in medical history. The first nurse to hold the title "IV nurse" is known to have practiced at this Boston hospital. Early on, IV nurses were responsible for phlebotomy, transfusion therapy, venipuncture, and maintaining equipment. Emphasis was placed on the technical responsibility of maintaining the infusion and keeping the needle and tubing apparatus patent. The sole requisite for being an IV nurse was the ability to perform a venipuncture skillfully.

At the time, IV therapy was limited to use in surgery and treating dehydration. Infusates were administered through rubber administration sets and 16- to 18-gauge steel needles strategically placed in the antecubital fossa and secured with an arm board.

As knowledge of electrolyte and fluid therapy grew, more parenteral fluids became available, and additional knowledge was then needed to monitor the fluid and electrolyte status of the patient. The nurse assigned to the patient in need of IV therapy was expected to have a working knowledge of fluid and electrolyte balance and to assess the "whole" patient in terms of fluid needs. Normal saline was no longer the only electrolyte fluid. Today, more than 200 commercially prepared IV fluids are available to meet patients' needs.

Parenteral Nutrition

W. C. Rose identified amino acids in 1937, leading to the development of protein hydrolysates for human infusion. A whole new approach to IV therapy and a respite to the starving patient evolved between 1963 and 1965, when members of the Harrison Department of Surgical Research at the University of Pennsylvania showed that sufficient nutrients could be given to juvenile beagles to support normal growth and development (Cosnett, 1989). This led to what is known today as *total parenteral nutrition* (TPN).

In the mid-1960s, as a result of animal TPN research, Stanley Dudrick developed the first formula for parenteral nutrition, a method by which sufficient nutrients are administered into the central vein to support life and maintain growth and development. Home TPN was introduced in 1983. Research into the use of antioxidants, the role of amino acids, and indications for medium-, short-, and long-chain triglycerides in TPN continues today (Grant, 1992).

Early Intravenous Devices and Equipment

Cutdown procedures were performed frequently until 1950, with the introduction of the Rochester needle, a resinous catheter on the outside of a steel introducer needle. On successful insertion, the catheter was slipped off the needle into the vein and the needle was removed. Desert Pharmaceutical Co. introduced the Intracath in 1958, minimizing the need for surgical cutdown. McGaw Laboratories introduced the first small vein set with foldable wings in 1957; this product is known today as a winged infusion needle.

Since the 1980s, tunneled catheters have enhanced central venous access. Totally implanted access devices are now used routinely (for more information, see Chaps. 12 through 14).

The first IV fluid containers were made of glass. Plastic bags were introduced in the 1970s. Because they do not require air venting, these containers reduced the risks of air embolism and airborne contamination. Today, plastic is the primary container for IV fluids, whereas glass containers are used when the fluid stability in plastic is a concern.

In the mid-1940s, disposable plastic IV administration sets became available and eventually replaced the reusable rubber tubings. Manufacturers have continued to keep pace with demands for technologically advanced products that ensure patient safety and reliability in the delivery of infusion therapy.

Progress in Clinical Practice

In the 1970s, tremendous scientific, technologic, and medical advances occurred, and IV therapy gained recognition as a highly specialized field. Nurses performed many of the functions formerly reserved for the medical staff—intra-arterial therapy, neonatal therapy, and antineoplastic therapy. Professional societies were established to provide a forum for the exchange of ideas, knowledge, and experiences, with the ultimate goal of raising standards and increasing the level of patient care.

On October 1, 1980, the United States House of Representatives recognized the profession and declared an official day of honor for IV nurses: "Resolved, that IV Nurse Day be nationally celebrated in honor of the National Intravenous Therapy Association, Inc., on January 25 of each year." The proclamation was presented by the Honorable Edward J. Mackey from the Fifth Congressional District of the Commonwealth of Massachusetts (Gardner, 1982).

■ THE INTRAVENOUS NURSES SOCIETY, INC.

The Intravenous Nurses Society, Inc. has continued to grow worldwide. Educational offerings have expanded to include advanced studies in an effort to meet the needs of the advanced practitioner.

Credentialing

The Intravenous Nurses Certification Corporation likewise expanded to include the National Board of IV Nurse Examiners, the Licensed practical/vocational nurse (LP/VN) Board of Nurse Examiners, and an Executive Committee. The first examination to become a Certified LPN or LVN in IV therapy was offered on September 7, 1996. Certified LP/VNs continue to recertify by continuing education at this time. A basic entry-level examination is in development for the generalist nurse.

Professional IV nurses are encouraged to prepare for the credentialing process through video and audio tapes, a revised core curriculum, educational programs, the society's professional journal, clinical textbooks, and published **Standards of Practice.**

Because delivery of IV therapy permeates all clinical settings, the role of the IV nurse is now well established as integral to multidisciplinary, high-quality care in all practice settings (Baranowski, 1995). The growth of this specialty practice has expanded the roles of IV nurses nationally and internationally. IV nurses are constantly striving to find new and more efficient ways to perform their services in an integrated health care environment.

■ INFUSION NURSING IN THE 21ST CENTURY

Nurses continue to lead the labor sector throughout the United States, and advanced-practice nursing has grown dramatically (Kalisch & Kalisch, 1995). In one study (Coffman and Spetz, 1999), the authors demonstrated the need for 43,000 additional registered nurses by the year 2010 to keep pace with the local population growth. Data on national trends in nursing school enrollment indicate that nurse educators are in general quicker than educators in other fields to adjust enrollment in response to market signals (Salsberg, Wing, & Brewer, 1998). With new graduates producing a relatively new workforce in many institutions, there will be an increasing need for IV resource experts.

The challenge for nurses is to effect health policy through use of their knowledge and skills. Wakefield (1999) stated that the value assigned to nursing will be based on a standard that measures how the profession effects access and achieves the highest-quality care at the lowest cost.

References and Selected Readings

Asterisks indicate references cited in text.

*Baranowski, L. (1995). Presidential address: Take ownership. *Journal of Intravenous Nursing, 18*(4), 163.

*Coffman, J., & Spetz, J. (1999). Maintaining an adequate supply of RNs in California. *Image: Journal of Nursing Scholarship, 31*, 389–391.

*Cosnett, J.E . (1989). Before our time: The origins of intravenous fluid therapy. *Lancet, 4,* 768–771.

*Gardner, C. (1982). United States House of Representatives honors the National Intravenous Therapy Association, Inc. *Journal of the National Intravenous Therapy Association, 5*(1), 14.

*Grant, J.P. (1992). *Handbook of total parenteral nutrition* (3rd ed., pp. 21–29). Philadelphia: W.B. Saunders.

*Griffith, J.M., Thomas, N., & Griffith, L. (1991). MDs bill for these routine nursing tasks. *American Journal of Nursing, 90*(10), 65–73.

*Kalisch, P.A., & Kalisch, B.J. (1995). *The advance of American nursing* (3rd ed.). Philadelphia: J.B. Lippincott.

*Salsberg, E., Wing, P., & Brewer, C. (1998). Projecting the future supply and demand for registered nurses. In: E. O'Neil & J. Coffman (Eds.), *Strategies for the future of nursing.* San Francisco: Jossey-Bass.

*Sutcliff, J. (1992). *A history of medicine.* New York: Barnes & Noble.

*Wakefield, M. (1999). Nursing's future in health care policy. In: E. Sullivan (Ed.), *Creating nursing's future* (pp. 41–49). St. Louis: Mosby.

Review Questions

Note: Questions below may have more than one right answer

1. The clinical use of amino acids led to the development of which of the following?

   a. Antioxidants

   b. Home total parenteral nutrition

   c. Protein hydrolysates

   d. Triple-mix fluid

2. The initial role of the IV specialist included which of the following?

   a. Phlebotomy

   b. Crossmatching of blood

   c. Maintaining equipment

   d. Maintaining IV lines

3. Three of the four main blood groups were discovered by:

    a. Karl Landsteiner

    b. Florence Seibert

    c. William Halsted

    d. W. C. Rose

4. The first national certification examination for nurses was offered in:

    a. 1983

    b. 1985

    c. 1988

    d. 1991

5. Primary fluids in use in the mid-1950s included:

    a. Lactated Ringer's injection

    b. 5% Dextrose in water

    c. 0.9% Sodium chloride (normal saline)

    d. 0.45% Sodium chloride (half-normal saline)

Minimizing Risk and

Improving Quality in

Intravenous Therapy

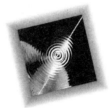

K E Y   T E R M S

Assault	Malpractice
Battery	Plan of Corrective Action
Benchmarking	Quality Improvement
Civil Law	Tort
Criminal Law	Unusual Occurrence Report
Flow Charting	

■ PROFESSIONAL NURSING AND LEGAL SAFEGUARDS

The law and its interpretation lead to doubts and questions regarding the legal rights and obligations of nurses to administer intravenous (IV) therapy. As IV therapy becomes more complex and specialized, and as IV clinicians gain national acceptance, nurses are becoming more involved in procedures formerly performed solely by physicians. Because violation of the Medical Practice Act is a criminal offense, IV nurses need to be well versed on the subject and the law, not only to protect themselves but to ensure safe, high-quality care for their patients.

To clarify the roles of nurses and physicians in various aspects of health care, joint policy statements have been issued by the medical societies and nursing associations on a number of procedures, including IV therapy.

Policy Statements and State Laws

Joint statements are written when questions arise regarding the nurse's professional responsibility or obligation to perform specific therapeutic measures and these questions are not answered in existing statutes (ie, nurse practice acts and medical practice acts). This is considered the most useful way to deal with procedures performed by members of both professions. Sponsors of joint statements include the following:

- State nurses' associations, which are concerned with specific areas of nursing practice
- State medical societies, which are concerned with therapeutic measures that were formerly solely within the realm of medical practice and that legally must be prescribed by a physician
- State hospital associations, which are concerned with institutional liability for therapeutic measures performed in member health care facilities

Rulings on proposed laws, amendments to laws, or even issues raised by joint statements may also be made by attorneys general and state boards of nursing. In some states, the nurse practice acts relating to the definition of nursing are global. They usually do not refer to specific procedures because, with the frequent changes in professional practice, it would be impractical for state legislators to review proposed changes before implementation in a practice setting.

With regard to IV therapy, state boards of nursing have sought the input of IV nursing professionals and professional societies to ensure high levels of care. Moreover, professional nursing societies are taking an expanded role in decision making as it pertains to this specialty practice. Standards of practice that provide criteria for judgment and ensure maximal safety for the patient as well as protection for the physician, nurse, and health care organization are widely recognized and used. Some strategies for minimizing risks related to IV nursing practice are outlined in Box 2–1.

BOX 2–1 Strategies for Reducing Risks Related to IV Therapy

- Keep abreast of laws and regulations governing practice.
- Stay up to date on defined standards of practice and their clinical application.
- File incident reports and record sentinel events (unforeseen outcomes resulting in a negative response to treatment) as appropriate.
- Ensure that informed consent is obtained and on file as needed.
- Participate in product evaluation processes and ensure safe use by providing internal product education.
- Maintain continued competency in your professional practice; ensure that you meet credentialing criteria.
- Monitor patients' responses and unforeseen reactions to treatment; document these events appropriately and in a timely manner.
- Ensure that safety standards are maintained; be aware of Occupational Safety and Health Administration (OSHA) regulations; practice risk management.
- Participate in the quality improvement process in your institution.

Federal Statutes

Federal statutes are laws enacted by Congress and published in the *Federal Register*. Such laws relevant to IV nursing include those addressing occupational health and safety, infection control, environmental hazards, medical device safety, control of drug abuse, federally funded insurance programs, and patient self-determination acts (Table 2–1).

Professional Standards of Care

In 1912, the Third Clinical Congress of Surgeons of North America resolved to address the need to standardize hospital work and equipment, referring to the minimum level considered essential to proper care and treatment of hospitalized patients. Later in the 20th century, the American Nurses Association (ANA) and the Joint Commission on Accreditation of Hospitals and Healthcare Organizations (JCAHO), in consort with various specialty societies, developed practice standards (see Chap. 4).

TABLE 2 – 1
SOURCES OF STANDARDS OF CARE RELATED TO IV THERAPY

Source	Agency	Examples of Standard
Federal statutes	Occupational Safety and Health Administration (OSHA)	• Hazard Communication Standard • Practice Guidelines for Handling Cytotoxic Drugs • Occupational Safe Exposure to Bloodborne Pathogens
	United States Food and Drug Administration (FDA)	Safe Medical Device Act of 1990
	Drug Enforcement Agency (DEA)	Controlled Substances Act
State statutes	Department of Health	Licensure of health care facilities
	Board of Nursing	Nurse Practice Act
	Board of Regents	
Private/professional bodies	Joint Commission for the Accreditation of Hospitals and Healthcare Organizations (JCAHO)	• Accreditation manual for hospitals • Accreditation manual for home health care
	American Nurses Association	Standards of Nursing Practice
	Intravenous Nurses Society (INS)	Intravenous Nursing Standards of Practice
	American Association of Blood Banks (AABB)	Technical manual
	ECRI	Health devices standard nomenclature
Institutional bodies	Intravenous Therapy or Nursing Department	Job descriptions; nursing policies and procedures

Applying Law to Practice

In hospitals and states in which no written opinion relevant to IV therapy exists, nurses are legally required to perform any nursing or medical procedure they are directed to carry out by a duly licensed physician unless they have reason to believe harm will result to the patient from doing so. To meet their legal responsibilities to patients, nurses must be qualified by knowledge and experience to execute the procedure; otherwise, they may properly refuse to perform it.

In cases in which the nurse finds no medical reason to question a physician's order, the nurse's failure to carry out such an order subjects him or her to liability for any consequent harm to the patient. It has been established by law that in a question of negligence, individuals are not protected because they have "carried out the physician's orders." Rather, they are held liable in relation to their knowledge, skill, and judgment.

Currently, several states recommend that schools of professional nursing include an IV therapy course in the curriculum. The course should provide the student nurse with clinical instruction and experience in IV therapy. IV nursing specialists have been instrumental in developing the content for such programs.

Roles of Contracted Personnel

Among the dramatic changes in today's health care environment are the decreasing numbers of private duty nurses and contracted (agency) personnel. However, cyclic staff shortages continue to create a market niche for these patient care providers. Thus, nurses working in institutions that use private duty and contracted nurses as well as nurses whose employers are contracted agencies must be aware of their own accountability for their actions and practice in addition to their accountability to their employers, patients, and colleagues.

Private Duty Nurse

A private duty nurse, who works under the direction, supervision, and control of a hospital and private physician, is subject to the rules and regulations of the hospital concerning all matters relating to nursing care. The institution's joint policy statement may note that the private duty nurse who has complied with the criteria applicable to the administration of IV therapy may give an IV infusion.

Agency Nurse

Nationwide, temporary staffing agencies provide valuable assistance during shortages of licensed professional personnel. When given responsibility for the administration of intravascular therapies, agency personnel must be oriented to the health care facility's policies and procedures and the functions performed by specialized department personnel. When the facility must use agency staff, every effort should be made to ensure patient safety, public protection, and viability of the IV therapy program.

Guarding Against Malpractice

The IV nurse's risk of involvement in **malpractice** suits is increasing with the increasing complexity of therapy and delegation of responsibility for infusion therapy in some institutions to less qualified paraprofessionals. In many cases, the professional nurse is legally responsible for the work performed by nonlicensed assistive personnel. Therefore, many of the functions performed by the nurse have important legal consequences. An understanding of the legal principles and guidelines involved is necessary if daily professional actions are not to result in unwanted malpractice suits. Terminology related to potential litigation is presented in Box 2–2.

If the hospital or involved professional person (or both) is to be charged with malpractice resulting from injury to a patient, the patient's representative should be able to demonstrate that

1. A standard of care or duty can be established.
2. The standard of care or duty was not met.
3. The patient was harmed or injured because the standard was not met.
4. It was possible to foresee that injury or harm would result from not meeting the standards (depending on state law).

Personal Liability and Protective Measures

The rule of personal liability states that "every person is liable for his [or her] own tortious conduct" (his own wrongdoing). No physician can protect a nurse from an act of negligence by bypassing this rule with verbal reassurances. The nurse cannot

---

BOX 2–2 **Legal Terms**

- **Criminal law**—Actions judged under criminal law include violation of the Nurse Practice Act, which is prosecuted by a government authority and punishable by fine or imprisonment, or both. An example of a criminal act is unlawful administration of IV therapy.
- **Civil law**—Actions judged under civil law relate to conduct affecting the legal rights of the private person. According to civil law, the guilty party is responsible for damages (*compensation*).
- **Tort**—A private wrongful act (of omission or commission) for which relief may be obtained by injunction or damages. Examples of a **tort** include assault, battery, negligence, slander, libel, false imprisonment, and invasion of privacy. Assault includes anticipation of harm; battery is the actual infliction of harm.
- **Malpractice**—Negligent conduct of professionals characterized by not acting in a prudent manner and resulting in damage to another person or property.

avoid legal liability even though another person may be sued and held liable. For example, the physician who orders placement of a peripherally inserted central catheter (PICC) cannot assume responsibility for the nurse who is negligent in implementing the action. If harm occurs as a result of the action, the nurse is held liable for this wrongdoing.

The rule of personal liability is relevant to medication errors as well. Medication errors are a common cause of malpractice claims against nurses. Negligence results from the administration of a drug to the wrong patient, at the wrong time, in an incorrect dosage, or in an improperly prescribed manner. If the physician writes an incomplete or partially illegible order and the nurse fails to clarify it before administration and harm results, the nurse is liable for negligence. The same applies to the administration of IV fluids. Nurses have a legal and professional responsibility to know the purpose and effect of the IV fluids and medications they administer. They must ensure that patients receive the prescribed volume of fluid at the prescribed rate of flow.

The rule of personal liability applies to directors of nursing and to nurses under their supervision. Although directors/nurse managers usually are not held liable for the negligence of nurses under their supervision (because every person is liable for his or her own wrongdoing), a director is expected to know if the nurse is competent to perform assigned duties without supervision.

On the other hand, directors who are negligent in the assignment of an inexperienced nurse or a nurse who requires supervision may be held liable for the acts of the nurse. Floating nurses to units to provide direct patient care when they are not experienced at the assigned level is a good example. Some institutions float nurses only to like intensive care units.

Observe Carefully

Nursing today requires a strong knowledge base and good observation skills. The act of observation is the legal and professional responsibility of the nurse. Frequent observation is imperative for the early detection and prevention of complications. Undetected complications that are allowed to increase in severity because of failure to observe the patient constitute an act of negligence on the part of the nurse (see Chap. 10).

Establish Therapeutic Relationships

Nurse–patient relationships play a significant role in influencing patients to initiate legal liability against nurses. Nurses performing IV therapy must be particularly aware of and attentive to the emotional needs of their patients, particularly when patients experience pain and apprehension during such procedures as catheter insertion. Clearly, specialists must foster appropriate interpersonal relationships. Nurses who are impersonal, aloof, and so busy with the technical process of starting an IV infusion that they have no time for establishing kindly relationships are the suit-prone nurses whose personalities may initiate resentment and later malpractice suits.

Patients most likely to sue are those who are resentful, frequently hostile, uncooperative, and dissatisfied with the nursing care. By demonstrating respect, care, and concern for all patients, as well as rendering skilled, efficient nursing care, nurses may avoid malpractice claims.

Review and Clarify Current Policies and Procedures

Policies and procedures should be detailed, and all nurses practicing infusion therapy should be required to know them and review them periodically. Policies and procedures should follow national guidelines established by the Centers for Disease Control and Prevention (CDC) and Standards of Practice established by the Intravenous Nurses Society (INS). These guidelines provide a model for IV nurses and foster optimal care for the patient receiving IV therapy.

Keep Credentials Up to Date

Credentialing of IV nurses nationwide began with the first certification examination in 1985. The credentialing process consists of three components: licensure, accreditation, and certification.

Licensure represents the entry into practice level afforded to all professional nurses who successfully complete the registered nurse examination. Accreditation establishes that a program or service meets established guidelines.

Accreditation is offered to facilities, agencies, and other health care providers by such groups as JCAHO, which is an accrediting body that evaluates (rates) the programs of hospitals and home care agencies.

Certification is the highest level attainable by the professional IV nurse. It is the process by which society attests to the professional and clinical competence of the person who successfully completes the process.

Preserve Confidentiality

Confidentiality of patient information consists of three related components: privacy, confidentiality, and security (Conner, 1999). With current advances in communication, such as electronic mail (e-mail) and other communication systems, including fax machines, cellular or cordless telephones, answering machines, and voice mail, nurses need to be aware and vigilant in preventing the misdirection, printing, interception, rerouting, or reading of information by unintended recipients.

Technology alone cannot ensure the legal and ethical use of e-mail and other communications in the health care environment. The e-mail message, for example, accurately documents communication and, as such, is part of the medical record and a legal document.

Expert security sources recommend the use of multilevel, individual passwords for all e-mail users, as opposed to generic group sign-ons and systems that require a single pass code (Dorodny, 1998). Monitored audit trails and increased accountability of caregivers to their patients should be established (Connor, 1999). Health information has become a commodity over the Internet and every precaution should be taken to maintain the confidentiality of electronic additions to the clinical record.

Use Performance Evaluations

A standard must be carefully defined for the health care institution or the nurse to evaluate adequate performance. Tools useful in guiding this process include the following:

- INS Standards of Practice (INS, 1998, 2000)
- State Board of Nursing regulations for registered nurses and licensed practical/vocational nurses
- American Nurses Association Standards of Nursing Practice
- Policies and procedures of the employing health care institution or agency

■ PROFESSIONAL NURSING AND QUALITY IMPROVEMENT

The complexity of infusion therapy practice today mandates a higher level of expertise and training than ever before. An illustration of this point involves the issues associated with placement of a long-term catheter, such as the PICC.

Qualified Personnel

The placement of a PICC requires special training and demonstrated competency on the part of the professional registered nurse. Each state sets its own practice guidelines, and not all states consider the placement of PICC catheters to be within the scope of professional nursing practice. The INS assembled a task force to standardize the usage, terminology, and adjunctive guidelines for the insertion of PICCs. A teaching program has also been developed (see Chaps. 12 through 14). Still, the institution or facility should contact the respective state Board of Nursing to determine policy. Each health care facility must establish criteria that qualify nurses to insert a PICC. The criteria should be within the institution's own legal guidelines. Such a program should address

- Indications
- Care and maintenance
- Advantages
- Legal issues
- Placement technique
- Product education
- Complications

Minimal standards for successful completion of an educational program include

- Satisfactory performance during initial probationary/review period
- Successful completion of in-house IV certification course
- Clinical competency evidenced by actual practice
- Successful completion of in-house requirements for PICC insertion

Risk Reduction

Given the continued growth of infusion therapy practice and the shift to alternative care settings, the potential for associated risks is higher than ever before. The institution is responsible for the quality of care delivered by its agents.

Report Product Problems

Because risk may be enhanced as a result of inappropriate use of medical devices, the U.S. Food and Drug Administration evaluates approximately 2000 medical devices monthly. The evaluation assesses

- Good manufacturing controls
- Application for a device existing before 1976 (in current use)
- Implantable or hazardous devices

Nurses and other health care providers are encouraged to report problems with equipment and other medical devices (see Chap. 12) directly to: Medical Device and Laboratory Product Problem Reporting Program (PRP), United States Pharmacopeia, 12601 Twinbrook Parkway, Rockville, MD 20853; (800) 638-6725.

File Unusual Occurrence Reports

A report is required for any accident or error resulting in actual or potential injury or harm. The report should contain only factual statements regarding the incident. Each report must be immediately followed by a full investigation into all possible causes, and corrective action must be taken immediately to prevent its recurrence.

Unusual occurrence reports should be routinely filed when there is a deviation from the standards. These reports are used as an internal reporting mechanism for a facility's quality assurance program. Components of the report may be found in Box 2-3. This type of a report may also be used to help identify problem patterns and institute corrective actions. Surveillance programs documented by such reports can be effective in preventing unsafe or insecure environments that can result in injuries to the patient.

> **BOX 2–3 Components of an Unusual Occurrence Report**
>
> - Admitting diagnosis
> - Date of occurrence
> - Patient's room number/location
> - Patient's age
> - Location of occurrence
> - Type of occurrence (medication error, policy and procedure)
> - Factual description
> - Patient's prior clinical condition
> - Results/interventions

Safety

Leape (Buerhaus, 1999), a health policy analyst, suggests in a study in the *Harvard Medical Practice Journal* that nearly 4% of people who are hospitalized have an adverse event. The study further states that at least two thirds of the events are preventable, meaning that approximately 1 million preventable injuries and 120,000 preventable deaths from injury occur annually. Based on the findings, Leape asserts that the cost of adverse events to health care facilities in 1998 was approximately $100 billion. Much of the increase in adverse events is attributed to a more complex health care system and to the acuity of the patient population at the turn of the century.

The National Patient Safety Foundation, established in 1997 by the American Medical Association, brought together representatives from nursing, pharmacy, medicine, and patient advocacy groups to examine ways to improve safety in health care across the health care continuum. On a hospital-wide level, organizations have continued to emphasize quality improvement processes.

Quality Assurance Process

The JCAHO previously mandated an ongoing program for monitoring quality-based outcomes. The trend continues to be toward process improvement, which involves pursuing opportunities to improve the quality of care and to ensure positive patient outcomes. Typically, quality assurance has focused on

- Identification of deficiencies or problem areas
- Analysis and interpretation
- Plans for corrective action
- Evaluation of the outcome of corrective action
- Resolution

This assessment process has typically been useful in improving the quality of care to patients receiving IV therapies (see Chap. 10).

Identify Deficiencies or Problem Areas

Problems and deficiencies may be readily identified through incident reports, patient complaints, employee complaints, questionnaires, patient satisfaction surveys, and suggestions from patients, visitors, or other staff. In assessing the need for further investigation, the facility should determine the character of the problem or deficiency, which in most cases involves noncompliance with standards of care. Examples of questions to ask include the following:

- Does the deficiency/problem relate to the quality of patient care?
- Does the deficiency/problem occur frequently enough to require correction?
- Can the deficiency/problem be solved?
- Do the potential benefits to patient care warrant the cost of investigation and resolution?

Methods and instruments used for evaluation may include criterion-based studies, interviews with patients and staff members, surveys, and observations. Experimental research designs can be an excellent method for assessing and collecting meaningful data about the problem, although such designs can be complex and costly. First, however, study methodology and criteria must be established before data can be collected, analyzed, and interpreted. The Standards of Practice of the INS and guidelines of the CDC, American Association of Blood Banks (AABB), and JCAHO may all be beneficial in developing criteria for IV practice standards by which to assess problems and measure performance (INS, 1998, 2000; AABB, 1999; CDC, 1998; JCAHO, 1999).

Analyze and Interpret

In collecting, analyzing, and interpreting data related to meeting the standards of practice and care, *compliance* refers to those situations in which the criteria are met. *Noncompliance* refers to the situations in which the criteria are not met. Both compliance and noncompliance are usually expressed in percentages. The expected compliance rate should be reasonable and achievable.

In most studies, findings are compiled statistically. These statistics provide a meaningful and concise description of the deficiency or problem. The data can then be used to calculate the average result, the difference between individual results and the average, and the relationship between the average result on one part of the study and the average result on another part.

Plan Corrective Action

Once the findings are compiled, analyzed, and interpreted, a **plan of corrective action** can be developed. Components of the plan may address

- Changes that the environment can best accommodate
- Potential barriers or constraints
- Areas of potential support
- Needed resources

The best method of corrective action depends on the particular problem and individual situation. Methods may include revision of policies or procedures, change of equipment, creation of a new information system, continuous monitoring, or on-site education.

Re-evaluate

After corrective action has been implemented, a re-evaluation is necessary to determine whether the applied corrective action resolves the problem. Frequently, re-evaluation is performed by repeating the first evaluation and comparing preaction data with postaction data.

Resolution

The final step in the process is resolution, which involves developing a plan to ensure the maintenance of the quality of care achieved with the corrective action. Periodic or continuous screening may be required.

Continuous Quality Improvement

The influence of Deming and others, who introduced the concept of total **quality improvement**—also called continuous quality improvement (CQI)—has had a great impact on quality in health care organizations. CQI provides a mechanism for examining the process, rather than the individual involved, and encourages participation across interdepartmental lines to improve the process itself. Quality improvement teams in an organization are appointed and study areas are identified. Process improvement is the direct result of the CQI program (see Box 2–4 for more information).

Measurement of Outcomes and Improvement

Interest in patient outcomes and their improvement continues to escalate. One reason for this is mounting evidence of wide and perplexing variations in outcomes of care, use of resources, and costs of care.

Outcome Improvement

Patient outcomes may include physiologic values (vital signs, chemical results), physical values (ability to self-administer IV therapy), mental or psychological terms (cog-

---

BOX 2–4 **Deming's 14-Point System for Managing Quality**

- Create consistency of purpose for continuous product improvement.
- Adopt the new philosophy across the organization.
- Cease dependence on inspection; improve the *process.*
- Avoid awarding business on price alone.
- Constantly seek to improve.
- Provide opportunities for training and staff development.
- Institute leadership; recognize the difference between management and leadership.
- Eliminate fear; fear inhibits innovation.
- Eliminate barriers among staff.
- Eliminate slogans; involve workers in the identification of new methods.
- Eliminate numerical quotas.
- Empower workers.
- Institute a broad-based education program to engage support.
- Be proactive in achieving transformation.

Adapted from Walton, M. (1991). *Deming management at work.* New York: Putnam.

---

nitive skill, affective interactions), social terms (ability to assume responsibility for self-care), and other health-related quality-of-life parameters (pain level, energy, sleep).

Process Improvement

The quality assurance technique operates on the assumption that the professional or institution is the sole cause of adverse outcomes and ignores the reality that sources of adverse outcomes are complex and include variations in policies, procedures, equipment, and techniques, as well as people (patients, professionals, support staff) and their interactions. In many cases, process improvement may be measured by developing a flow chart (**flow charting**) to identify patterns related to the basic process, the detailed process, errors and corrective measures, and redesigns (Batalden, Nelson, & Roberts, 1994).

The flow chart begins with the basic process at admission to the institution; the flow chart continues the detailed process by highlighting areas of possible duplication, complexity, and sources of error (Batalden et al., 1994). Using the flow chart as a basic tool, many institutions have developed ways to manage the improvement process by incorporating the model known as the Plan-Do-Check-Act (PDCA) improvement trial. Those who use this model proceed through the following sequence: state aim, identify measures of improvement, plan and do a pilot test, check and study results, act to improve, and reflect on learning (Batalden et al.):

- Aim—What are we trying to accomplish?
- Measure—How will we know that a change is an improvement?

- Possible changes—What changes can we make that we predict will lead to improvement?
- Plan—How shall we plan the pilot? Who does what? When? And with what tools and training? What baseline data need to be collected?
- Do—What are we learning as we do the pilot?
- Check—As we check and study what happened, what have we learned?
- Act—As we act to hold the gains or to abandon the pilot, what needs to be done? (Batalden et al., 1994)

A multidisciplinary quality council may be appointed within an organization to determine the best institution-wide approach to managing quality. A technique such as process management—consisting of merging comparative data analyses, operational and clinical analyses, **benchmarking** (comparing an institution with the best institutions nationwide), quality methods, and simulation methods—results in improvements in quality.

Some responsible and progressive hospitals and health networks have committed themselves to seeking significant improvements yearly. One goal, for example, is specific improvement in medication management by a certain year or other time frame. To achieve the overall outcome, the collaborative group may design an ideal plan for improved medication management. Some examples of the goals of the plan may be reducing medication errors within the respective facilities by 50% over a 3-year period; deploying an advanced adverse drug event detection technique in 100% of the collaborating systems; and introducing one breakthrough technology per year.

References and Selected Readings

Asterisks indicate references cited in text.

Alspach, G. (1998). Nurse-to-nurse recognition. *Critical Care Nurse, 18*(3), 6–9.

*American Association of Blood Banks. (1999). *Technical manual* (13th ed.). Bethesda, MD: Author.

*Batalden, P.B., Nelson, E.C., & Roberts, J.S. (1994). Linking outcomes measurement to continual improvement: The serial "V": Way of thinking about improving clinical care. *Journal on Quality Improvement, 20*(4), 168–169.

Bernzweig, E.P. (1981). *Nurse's liability for malpractice* (3rd ed., p. 68). New York: McGraw-Hill.

*Buerhaus, P.I. (1999). Lucian Leape on the causes and prevention of errors and adverse events in health care. *Image: Journal of Nursing Scholarship, 31*(3), 281–286.

*Centers for Disease Control and Prevention. (1998). Guidelines for prevention of intravascular infection. *Federal Register, 60* (187), 49978–50006.

*Conner, V.W. (1999). Patient confidentiality in the electronic age. *Journal of Intravenous Nursing, 22,* 199–201.

*Dorodny, V. (1998). The highwire act of medical records security. *Advice for Health Information Executives, 2,* 24–32.

Institute of Medicine of the National Academies. (1999). Report on preventing medical errors: To err is human: Building a safer health system. [On-line]. Available: http://www.ashp.org/public/news/breaking/IOM.num.

*Intravenous Nurses Society. (1998). Revised intravenous nursing standards of practice. *Journal of Intravenous Nursing, 21*(Suppl. 1), 517, 525.

*Joint Commission on Accreditation of Hospitals and Healthcare Organizations. (1999). *Accreditation manual for hospitals.* Chicago: Author.

Katz, J., & Green, E. (1997). *Managing quality: A guide to system-wide performance management in health care.* St. Louis: Mosby–Year Book.

Premier, Inc. (1999, December 21). San Diego, CA. Internal communications: Executive express (p. 1.)

Spielberg, A.R. (1998). Sociohistorical, legal and ethical implications of E-mail for the patient-physician relationship. *Journal of the American Medical Association, 280*(15), 1353–1357.

Terry, J., Baranowski, L., Lonsway, R.A., & Hedrick, C. (1995). *Intravenous therapy clinical principles and practice* (p. 68). Philadelphia: W.B. Saunders.

Weinstein, S. (1996). Legal implications/risk management. *Journal of Intravenous Nursing, 19*(3 Suppl), S16–S18.

Review Questions

Note: Questions below may have more than one right answer.

1. The statement, "every person is liable for his own tortious conduct" is known as the rule of:
   a. Negligent action
   b. Personal liability
   c. Tortious conduct
   d. Wrongdoing act

2. A nurse inserts an IV cannula against the wishes of a coherent adult patient. In this situation, the nurse could be charged with:
   a. Assault
   b. Battery
   c. Assault and battery
   d. Malpractice

3. Which of the following is *not* a component of the credentialing process?
   a. Accreditation
   b. Certification
   c. Diploma
   d. Licensure

4. Confidentiality of patient information involves all of the following issues except:
   a. Audits
   b. Confidentiality
   c. Privacy
   d. Security

5. Process improvement begins with which of the following patterns?
   a. Basic flow chart
   b. Identifying/reworking errors
   c. Redesigning flow chart
   d. Policy and procedure updates

6. Researchers who have affected the quality improvement process include:
   a. Conner
   b. Evanson
   c. Deming
   d. Dorodny

7. Benchmarking is the process of comparing:
   a. Institution to like institutions
   b. Institution to the best institutions
   c. Practitioner to practitioner
   d. Practitioner to the best practitioner

8. Quality improvement programs examine:
   a. Individuals
   b. Processes
   c. a only
   d. a and b

9. The Food and Drug Administration inspects devices on which of the following levels?
   a. Good manufacturing controls
   b. Application for a device existing before 1976 (still in common use)
   c. Implantable or hazardous device
   d. Nurse-inserted devices

10. Electronic patient records may include which of the following?
    a. E-mail
    b. Fax documents
    c. Computerized records
    d. Voice mail

Nursing Role and

Responsibilities

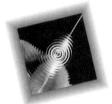

K E Y   T E R M S

Anesthesia   Resource Personnel
Blood Bank   Intravenous Nurse Specialist
Intravenous Nursing Teams   Staff Nurse
Pharmacist

■ COLLABORATIVE ROLE OF THE NURSE

Administration of safe, high-quality infusion therapy today depends on a collaborative practice environment in which many members of the health care team play a key role. The nurse, in particular, plays a primary role in collaborating with other health care providers to maintain an infusion and to protect the patient from the hazards and complications associated with routine intravenous (IV) therapy. Policies regarding the responsibilities of a **staff nurse** in relation to infusion therapy vary significantly among health care institutions and are often influenced by the presence or absence of a full-service IV team.

■ ROLE OF INTRAVENOUS NURSING TEAMS

Research findings show that an **IV nursing team** enhances the level of care that an organization provides. To ensure that the team approach provides safe IV care, the role of the team and the delineation of responsibilities must be part of the orientation program and ongoing education for all nurses. Specialized teams of IV nurses provide clinical expertise and cost-effective care. In the ideal setting, registered nurses with clinical and theoretic expertise should be responsible for administering IV therapy. This improves the quality of patient care because specialized nurses, freed from other responsibilities, can focus their attention on developing a high standard of performance. Such nurses, aware of the inherent risks of infusion therapy, are vigilant and meticulous in performing and maintaining IV therapy. Their advanced skills promote trauma-free venipunctures, conserve veins for future use, and reduce routine complications. The knowledge, skills, and abilities of these specialized nurses ensure patient safety. IV nursing teams succeed in those institutions in which their value is recognized and appreciated.

ROLE OF RESOURCE PERSONNEL

In lieu of a full-service IV team, the health care facility may use the services of one or more IV nurse specialists as resource personnel. In such situations, the IV specialist may serve as educator, clinician, or team leader to a number of integrated health care organizations or home care agencies. The role for the IV nursing specialist is continually evolving. Changes in clinical practice and in the practice setting direct this process (Lozins Miller, 1998).

LEADERSHIP RESPONSIBILITY

Traditionally, the responsibility for IV therapy is allocated to director of the **blood bank,** the **pharmacist,** or the **anesthesia** department. Obviously, the IV department nurses fulfill several important functions. Not only do they administer blood and blood components, but they are in close alliance with the pharmacy. IV department nurses administer infusions of which 50% to 80% contain additives. Moreover, they execute many of the functions performed by the anesthesiologist.

In some health care settings, IV departments may also function as self-contained cost centers within an institution's infrastructure. The IV team has become an integral part of the nursing department, engaging in increased interaction and collaboration with nursing colleagues.

Departmental Philosophy and Objectives

In organizing a department, the first consideration should be to establish a philosophy and the objectives necessary to support such a philosophy (Box 3–1).

BOX 3–1 **Example of Mission and Objectives of an IV Department**

Mission

To administer safe and successful IV therapy in the best interests of the patient, the hospital, and the nursing profession.

Objectives

The objectives of an IV department are:

1. To develop skills and impart knowledge that will provide a high level of safety in the practice of IV therapy
2. To encourage further education and knowledge in the field of IV therapy
3. To assist in keeping the nursing staff educated in the maintenance of IV therapy and other nursing needs relevant to IV therapy
4. To collaborate with other personnel in the development and implementation of continuing education in IV therapy
5. To develop nursing judgment and critical thinking in IV therapy
6. To keep abreast of the latest scientific and medical advances and their implications in the practice of IV therapy
7. To attain and maintain certification

Departmental Functions

In organizing an IV department, the functions to be performed must be delineated (Box 3–2).

Departmental Policies and Procedures

Policies and procedures play a vital role in the functioning of a department, serving as a guide to its operations, providing the nurse with adequate instruction, and ensuring the patient a high level of nursing care. They may also provide legal protection in determining whether a person involved in negligent conduct has had adequate instruction in performing the act.

Policies and procedures should comply with state and federal laws, and national guidelines should be followed. The Joint Commission on Accreditation of Hospitals and Healthcare Organizations publishes a manual for both hospital and home care accreditation. The American Association of Blood Banks provides a technical manual with standards for care and administration of blood and component therapy. The Centers for Disease Control and Prevention (CDC) and the Intravenous Nurses Society (INS) provide guidelines as well as Standards of Practice (CDC, 1998; INS, 1998, 2000) (see Chap. 2 for more information).

BOX 3–2 **Functions of an IV Department**

IV Administration

Parenteral fluids
Blood and blood components
Total parenteral nutrition
Antineoplastic therapy
Intra-arterial therapy
Pain management

IV Access and Monitoring

Peripheral lines
Pediatrics
Administration set and dressing changes
Therapeutic phlebotomy
Venous sampling
Peripherally inserted central catheters
Ommaya reservoirs
Other alternative access devices

Patient/Family Education

Self-care
Home infusion therapy

Preparation

Drugs in solution

Collaborative Practice

Safety committee
Quality improvement
Code team
Product evaluation
Development of policies and procedures

Policies describing the responsibilities of the IV nurse vary significantly among hospitals and should be outlined to prevent confusion or misunderstanding. Examples of such policies are found in Box 3–3.

Delineation of Qualifications

Because IV therapy involves specialized judgment and skills, the IV nurse must be qualified to meet the job requirements and scope of practice (CDC, 1998; INS, 1998, 2000).

BOX 3-3 **Examples of Policies Describing IV Nurse's Responsibilities**

Administration of Parenteral Fluids

- IV nurses will, on written order, initiate all infusions, with the exception of those not approved for administration by the nurse.
- No more than two attempts at venipuncture will be allowed.
- Venipunctures should be avoided in the lower extremities except when the patient's condition may necessitate this use and this location has specifically been ordered by the physician.

Preparation and Administration of Intravenous Drugs

- Nurses will, on written order, prepare and administer only those solutions, medications, and combinations of drugs approved in writing by the pharmacy and the therapeutics committee.
- Nurses must check the patient's clinical record and question the patient regarding sensitivity to drugs that may cause anaphylaxis. They must observe the patient after initial administration of such drugs.

Nursing Care Plan

- A nursing care plan should be established within 24 hours of date/time of admission.

Peripheral Catheter Selection

- The catheter selected should be of the smallest gauge and shortest length to accommodate the prescribed therapy.
- Only radiopaque catheters may be used.

Because of the highly specialized therapy and the responsibility involved, the success of the department depends on the selection of its personnel. Ideally, a credentialed **IV nurse specialist** meets this goal.

These nurses must be meticulous in their actions, conscientious, and dedicated to the specialty practice. There is no margin for error. Collaboration and teamwork are essential to the success of the department.

Mental and emotional stability are equally important to the nurse's success as an IV specialist. Manual dexterity, necessary in administering an IV infusion, is greatly affected by the mental and emotional attitude of the nurse. Moreover, the performance of few other procedures is so easily affected by stress as a difficult venipuncture.

Outstanding verbal and written communication skills are other assets necessary to the success of the nurse and the department.

Processing Requests for Service

A system for receiving calls must be developed, with special emphasis on emergency calls. Some systems work better than others under various conditions. The size of the hospital, number of patients, size and location of the department, and the functions to be performed must be considered when deciding which system would be most adaptable. Voice mail may be used for routine scheduling and nonemergencies. Pagers are effective, as are facsimile (fax) transmissions to ensure accuracy and save time.

Many IV teams make routine rounds focused on patients with complex conditions and therapies, all patients, or designated patient care units. This system contributes to enhanced communication between staff nurses and IV specialists.

Preparation of Equipment

To maximize safety and minimize response time, the facility may choose to set up an equipment cart or designated supply cabinet on each floor. The cart contains all necessary, single-use equipment for parenteral administration, including:

- IV fluids
- Alcohol wipes or povidone–iodine preparation pads
- Venous access devices
- Syringes
- IV securement devices
- Administration sets
- IV start kits
- IV filters
- Transparent dressings
- Tape
- Gloves

Before using the equipment, the professional IV nurse ascertains the accuracy of the physician's order and then assembles the needed supplies from the cart if it is maintained on each nursing unit, or from supply storage areas located elsewhere.

Regardless of the method of obtaining equipment for venipuncture, the IV nurse has a crucial role in determining the accuracy of the order, assembling the appropriate equipment consistent with the therapy that has been ordered, and using the equipment in a safe manner.

During their hospital stay, patients with infusions in progress may visit ancillary hospital departments, including medical imaging, nuclear medicine, and surgery. To ensure the success and viability of an IV therapy department or team, other departments in the institution must be oriented to the team's functions. If orders are written early in the day, it will be easier to meet all requests and ensure timely delivery of therapy to each patient under the team's care (Lozins Miller, 1998, INS 1998, 2000).

text continues on page 34

BOX 3–4 **Suggested Teaching Outline for IV Team Nurses**

I. Legal implications of IV therapy
A. State and institutional policy: review of state rulings and joint policies related to IV therapy
B. Health institution or agency policy
  1. Responsibilities of nurse in administering IV therapy
  2. List of fluids and drugs delineated for administration by the nurse
C. National guidelines and published standards
  1. Centers for Disease Control and Prevention
  2. Intravenous Nurses Society
D. Legal requirements
  1. Qualification by education and experience
  2. Adherence to institutional policy
  3. Knowledge base and skills sets
  4. Order by licensed physician for specific patient
  5. Skilled judgment
E. Review of policy and procedure books
  1. Policy statements do not provide immunity if the nurse is negligent.
  2. The nurse is legally responsible for own actions.

II. Equipment
A. Review all types of equipment, their characteristics, and usage.
B. Review procedures for the proper handling of equipment, changing of administration sets, safe use of products.
C. Adhere to established infection control procedures and safety guidelines.

III. Anatomy and physiology applied to IV therapy

IV. Safety
A. Choice of catheter (steel needle, catheter)
B. Hazards and complications (observing the patient, reporting reactions, and taking measures to prevent complications are the nurse's legal and professional responsibilities)
  1. Systemic complications, including infection (septicemia, fungemia)
  2. Local complications, including phlebitis (mechanical, chemical, and septic)
  3. Preventive measures:
    a. Do not use veins located over an area of joint flexion.
    b. Anchor catheters well to prevent motion and reduce the risk of introducing microorganisms into puncture wound.
    c. Adequately dilute medications.
    d. Use a catheter relatively smaller than the vein.
    e. Use aseptic and antiseptic technique.
    f. Remove catheter within 48 hours or consistent with institutional policy.
    g. Remove catheter for:
      (1) Erythema
      (2) Induration
      (3) Tenderness by palpation of venous cord
      (4) Nonfunctioning needle
      (5) Infiltration (recognize extravasation): check questionable extremity against normal extremity, then apply a tourniquet tightly enough to restrict venous flow proximal to the injection site. If infusion continues regardless of this venous obstruction, extravasation is evident.
C. Intra-arterial therapy
  1. Arterial puncture

continued

2. Constant arterial pressure monitoring
3. Arterial blood gases
4. Swan-Ganz catheter
   a. Basic knowledge
   b. Insertion
   c. Complications

V. Rationale of fluid and electrolyte therapy
A. Fundamentals of fluid and electrolyte metabolism
   1. Body fluid compartments
   2. Electrolyte composition
   3. Acid–base balance
B. Principles of fluid therapy
   1. Deficit
   2. Maintenance
   3. Replacement
C. IV fluids: Classification and effect

VI. Drug therapy
A. Hazards
   1. Incompatibilities
   2. Vascular trauma
   3. Speed shock
   4. Bacterial and fungal contamination
   5. Particulate contamination
   6. Medication errors
B. Knowledge of the drug
   1. Dose and effect
   2. Recommended rate of infusion
   3. Reactions
   4. Contraindications
C. Factors controlling stability and compatibility of admixtures
D. Preparation of admixture
   1. Procedure for transcribing orders on medication label
   2. Frequency with which medication order should be renewed
   3. Reconstitution of drug using aseptic and antiseptic technique
   4. Procedure for adding drug to fluid container
   5. Stability of the admixture
   6. Labeling
E. Administration of drugs
   1. Verify identity of patient and admixture.
   2. Check for sensitivities of patient to any drug that may cause anaphylaxis.
   3. Observe patient for untoward reactions when administering an initial dose of an antibiotic.
   4. Patients known to be sensitive to a drug require the presence of a physician.
   5. Inspect admixture each time before administration.
   6. Record drug, dosage, and amount of fluid on fluid intake chart and medication sheet.

VII. Transfusion therapy
A. Principles of immunohematology
B. Blood and blood components

Didactic Program: Education and Review

An adequate teaching program and criteria for evaluating the IV nurse must be established. The program curriculum and performance criteria depend on the role of the IV nurse as dictated by hospital policies. The nurse's competency must be evaluated and maintained, particularly when the IV nurse receives on-the-job training.

The length of time involved in teaching depends on the individual and may range from 6 to 8 weeks. Box 3–4 provides a suggested outline for teaching IV, drug, and transfusion therapy. The outline is consistent with that defined in the Core Curriculum for Intravenous Nursing (Corrigan, Pelletier, & Alexander, 2000).

■ IMPACT OF COST CONTAINMENT ON INFUSION TEAMS

In today's managed care environment, it is becoming increasingly difficult for established IV teams to justify their existence and for new teams to gain approval. The health care setting has changed dramatically; fiscal constraints are often overwhelming, forcing institutions to scrutinize methods of IV delivery for efficiency and cost effectiveness (see Chap. 23).

As a result, hospitals have downsized, restructured the workplace, and developed new patient care delivery models. Such models have had a significant impact on IV teams because ancillary services are not regarded as appropriate to the new, centralized, unit-based approach to patient care. In all practice settings, IV teams must be innovative and adaptable while maximizing capabilities and analyzing complementary practice roles and multidisciplinary care (Baranowski, 1995; CDC, 1998; Nursing Spectrum, 1996). The teams must work with their professional society to

T A B L E   3 – 1
REASSESSING THE ROLE OF THE IV TEAM

Reassessment Objective	Time Frame	Accountability
Reduce IV team full-time equivalents (FTEs)	60 days	Task force
Develop and implement training plan for staff nurse generalists	30 days	IV team leader, nurse educator, IV resource clinicians
Transfer 3.0 FTEs to staff nurse positions	30 days	Chair, co-chair, nurse recruiter
Develop clinical practice guidelines for infusion therapy based on Intravenous Nurses Society Standards of Practice	60 days	Task force
Establish advanced practice skills with 2.0 FTEs determined by caseload	60 days	IV team leader, nurse educator, medical director
Maintain level of quality	Ongoing	Task force

Adapted from Lozins Miller, P.K. (1998). Downsizing. *Journal of Intravenous Nursing*, 21(2), 107.

lead the way toward designing new directions for IV nursing practice (Baranowski, 1995).

The CDC document "Guidelines for Prevention of Intravascular Device-Related Infections: An Overview" and Part 2, "Recommendations for Prevention of Intravascular Device-Related Infections," published in *Infection Control and Hospital Epidemiology* and the *American Journal of Infection Control*, suggested that eliminating IV teams downgrades patient care by raising the risk of infection (CDC/Federal Register, 1998). Lozins Miller (1998) studied the use of IV clinicians to maintain high-quality venous access care in a health care system involved in downsizing its ranks. Reassigning the role of the IV team member to an IV nurse clinician added new skill sets and an expanded role (Table 3–1).

References and Selected Readings

Asterisks indicate references cited in text.

*Baranowski, L. (1995). Presidential address: Take ownership. *Journal of Intravenous Nursing, 18*(4), 163.

*Centers for Disease Control and Prevention. (1998). Guidelines for prevention of intravascular infection. *Federal Register, 60*(187), 49978–50006.

*Corrigan, A.M., Pelletier, G., & Alexander, M. (Eds.). (2000). *Intravenous Nurses Society core curriculum for intravenous nursing* (2nd ed.). Philadelphia: Lippincott Williams & Wilkins.

*Intravenous Nurses Society. (1998). Revised intravenous nursing standards of practice. *Journal of Intravenous Nursing, 21*(Suppl. 1), S8–11.

*Lozins Miller, P.K. (1998). Downsizing. *Journal of Intravenous Nursing, 21*(2), 105–112.

Review Questions

Note: Questions below may have more than one right answer.

1. IV specialists may provide clinical support in which of the following settings?

    A. Home care

    B. Acute care

    C. Infusion centers

    D. All of the above

2. The core curriculum may provide

    A. Didactic content

    B. Answers to procedural questions

    C. Policies

    D. Procedures

3. Policies and procedures should comply with which of the following?

    A. State and federal laws

    B. Local ordinances

    C. County rules and regulations

    D. Local law

4. The first step in developing an IV department is to:

    A. Establish philosophy

    B. Define objectives

    C. Order supplies

    D. Create requisitions

5. A catheter selected for peripheral infusion therapy should be:
   A. Largest gauge and longest length
   B. Smallest gauge and shortest length
   C. Largest gauge and shortest length
   D. Smallest gauge and longest length

6. Methods of reaching the IV specialist include which of the following?
   A. Pager
   B. Voice mail
   C. Computerized requisition
   D. All of the above

7. Equipment readily available for IV use includes which of the following?
   A. Administration sets and starter kits
   B. Reusable tourniquet tray
   C. Needle cutter

8. The IV specialist must have which of the following attributes?
   A. Mental and emotional stability
   B. Manual dexterity
   C. Verbal and written communication skills
   D. All of the above

9. A nursing care plan should be established within how many hours of admission?
   A. 6
   B. 12
   C. 18
   D. 24

10. The IV specialist may serve as:
   A. Resource nurse/clinician
   B. Educator
   C. a and b
   D. a only

Application of Intravenous Nurses Society Standards of Practice

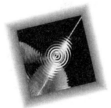

K E Y   T E R M S

Competencies
Educational Requirements
Practice Criteria
Scope of Practice
Standards of Practice

■ THE STANDARDS

The Intravenous Nurses Society (INS) has established the **scope of practice, competencies,** and **educational requirements** for the administration of infusion therapy and has set forth **Standards of Practice.** In 1998, the INS revised the Standards and published the revision as a supplement to the *Journal of Intravenous Nursing* (INS, 1998, 2000).

Because intravenous (IV) practice changes continually, practice Standards are updated to reflect those changes. The latest edition of the Standards, for example, eliminates the procedural aspects of IV practice; however, a Policy and Procedures Manual, also developed by INS, can be used as a companion to the Standards to complete the information base (INS, 2000).

■ POLICIES, PROCEDURES, AND INFUSION THERAPY

Each nurse in an organization must be cognizant of the policies and procedures relevant to infusion therapy and familiar with the nurse's responsibilities to provide a safe level of care for the patient. All nurses responsible for administering IV therapy should be familiar with established Standards of Practice.

The INS Standards of Practice establishes the educational, experiential, and technical criteria required to successfully perform at various levels in the specialty practice of infusion therapy. The Standards systematically direct practice and provide guidelines for assessing competency.

■ COMPETENCIES IN PRACTICE

The Standards allow for those inside and outside the profession to judge the competency of nurses practicing infusion therapy. The recently drafted edition of the Standards provides a framework for nurses to evaluate patient outcomes. Tools used for evaluation include nursing plans of care, assessment and monitoring processes, appropriate IV site selection and assessment, and various criteria for safe and effective clinical management of infusion therapy. Key standards and the practice criteria related to them are summarized in the following sections. (*Standards are printed in italics; practice criteria are not in italics.*) How well the nurse integrates the Standards and practice criteria is one way to evaluate competence in specialty IV nursing practice.

Care Planning and Practice Criteria

Care plans shall be established upon completion of the initial nursing assessment of the patient.

The methodology for content and construction of care plans should be defined in organizational policy and procedure and should reflect collaboration with the physician, pharmacist, dietitian, and appropriate others. The plan should set forth measurable goals and time frames as a means to evaluate the patient's progress and the effectiveness of nursing care (INS, 2000).

Assessment and Practice Criteria

Patient assessment by the registered nurse shall be an ongoing process to determine the appropriateness of infusion therapy and to ensure desired patient outcomes.

The use of infusion therapy assessment and monitoring tools should be established in policy and procedure. Initial assessment of the patient for whom IV therapy has been ordered includes the patient's primary medical diagnosis, nursing diagnosis, medical and surgical histories, allergies, vascular access history, patient preferences regarding vascular access device types and site locations, and long-range plans for infusion therapy when appropriate. It is essential that information obtained during the assessment and monitoring process be communicated to other health care professionals responsible for patient care (INS, 2000).

Clinical Management: Standards Applied

Site Selection and Practice Criteria

Site selection for vascular access includes assessment of the patient's condition, age and diagnosis; vascular condition, size and location; and type and duration of therapy. The vascular site should accommodate the gauge and length of the cannula required by the prescribed therapy.

Specific practice criteria address peripheral sites, midline sites, peripherally inserted central catheters (PICCs), and central and arterial lines. Procedures have been developed for peripheral-short, peripheral-midline, arterial, peripherally inserted central, and central catheterizations. The method and choice should be clearly delineated in organizational policy. The application of this standard is essential in producing positive patient outcomes. Considerations in the catheterization of a peripheral vein are featured in Boxes 4–1 and 4–2 (INS, 2000).

Catheter Selection and Practice Criteria

The catheter [or cannula] shall be the smallest gauge and shortest length to accommodate the prescribed therapy.

The tip of central vascular access catheters shall reside in the superior vena cava. Femorally-placed central vascular access catheters shall have the distal tip residing in the inferior vena cava. Midline catheters shall have the distal tip residing in or at the junction of the axillary vein. All catheters shall be radiopaque.

Defined practice criteria identify the properties of a peripheral, midline, PICC, central, and arterial line (INS, 2000).

BOX 4–1 Considerations in Site Selection for a Peripheral–Short Catheter

- Age
- Patient's condition
- Diagnosis
- Vein condition
- Size
- Location
- Type and duration of therapy
- Other therapies in progress

> BOX 4–2 **Considerations in Site Selection for Peripherally Inserted Central Catheters (PICC)**
>
> - Patient's condition
> - Age
> - Diagnosis
> - Vein condition
> - Size
> - Location
> - Type and duration of therapy
> - Anatomic measurements to ensure full advancement of the catheter and catheter tip placement in a central vein
>
> _____
>
> *Note:* Site selection of central catheters, other than for peripherally inserted central catheters, is a medical *responsibility.*

Hair Removal and Practice Criteria

Excess hair shall be removed by clipping with scissors or clippers.

Using a razor may potentially cause microabrasions of the skin that increase the risk of infection. Depilatories should not be used because of the potential of allergic reaction or irritation (INS, 2000).

Insertion Site Preparation and Practice Criteria

Prior to placement, the intended insertion site shall be cleaned with antimicrobial solution(s) using aseptic technique.

Maximum barrier precautions, including sterile gown and gloves, mask, surgical scrub, and large sterile drapes and towels, should be used for midline, PICC, arterial, and central line insertions. Talc-free sterile gloves should be used as well. Antimicrobial solutions include

- 2% tincture of iodine
- 70% isopropyl alcohol
- 10% povidone–iodine
- chlorhexidine (INS, 2000)

Catheter Placement and Practice Criteria

Placement of catheters shall reflect the state Nurse Practice Act. Catheters should be placed for definitive therapeutic and/or diagnostic purposes. Cannulas should be used one time only. The placement of central catheters other then PICCs shall be considered a medical act. [The Standard goes on to address the appropriate location of the PICC tip.]

Practice criteria address the need for a comprehensive understanding of human anatomy and physiology, vein assessment techniques, and insertion techniques specific to the device being used. The criteria further stress the need to consider manufacturer's recommendations for product use, including any modifications to be made to the catheter tip (INS, 2000).

Add-on Devices, Junction Securement, and Practice Criteria

The revised Standard emphasizes the need for aseptic technique and standard precautions in the use of all add-on devices.

A method of securing the catheter should be used at the juncture points of administration sets and add-on devices. All add-on devices should have a Luer-lock device. The criteria define add-on devices as stopcocks, extension sets, manifold sets, extension loops, solid catheter caps, infection/access ports, needle/needleless systems, and filters (INS, 2000).

Dressings and Practice Criteria

A sterile dressing, gauze or transparent semipermeable membrane (TSM), should be applied and maintained on all vascular access devices.

The use of dressings and frequency of dressing changes should be established in organizational policy and procedure (INS, 2000).

Biohazardous Waste Handling

Improper disposal and use of needles/stylets (sharps) increase potential risk to the practitioner, patient, and community (Pugliese & Salahuddin, 1999).

Needles and stylets should be disposed of in nonpermeable tamperproof containers. Needles and stylets (sharps) should not be broken, bent, or recapped with two hands. Safety products that are consistent with Occupational Safety and Health Administration (OSHA) guidelines should be utilized (see Chap. 11) (OSHA, 1999).

The practice criteria clearly suggest that all needles or other sharp devices have a safety device engineered to protect the nurse or other professional health care provider from injury. This is consistent with the recommendations for product selection found in Chapter 11 and Appendix.

Intravenous Administration Set Change and Practice Criteria

The Standards address primary and secondary continuous lines and the need to change the sets every 72 hours and immediately upon suspected contamination or when the integrity of the product has been compromised.

SAFE PRACTICE ALERT An organization may consider extending the maximum 72-hour interval for routine primary administration set change for peripheral catheters if a consistent monthly phlebitis rate of 5% or less is achieved for a minimum of 3 consecutive months.

Again, the criteria suggest defining rules for set changes in organizational policy and procedure, and identifying the need to maintain an ongoing phlebitis rate of less than 5% with administration set changes after 72 hours or reducing the time factor to 48 hours in the presence of redness, infiltration, or any ongoing phlebitis in excess of 5%.

Research Issues: WHAT IS THE PHLEBITIS RATE?

 A potential area of research is a study of the phlebitis rate in your organization and the impact that application of standards of Practice has on patient outcomes.

Infiltration is the inadvertent administration of a nonvesicant solution or medication into surrounding tissue (Tables 4–1 and 4–2).

T A B L E 4 – 1
INFILTRATION SCALE

Grade	Criteria (Indicators)
0	No symptoms
1	Skin blanched
	Edema <1 inch
	Affected area cool to touch
2	Skin blanched
	Edema 1–6 inches
	Affected area cool to touch
	Patient may or may not have pain
3	Skin blanched, translucent
	Gross edema >6
	Affected area cool to touch
	Patient may have mild to moderate pain
	Possible numbness
4	Skin blanched, translucent
	Skin tight, leaking
	Gross edema >6
	Deep-pitting tissue edema
	Circulatory impairment
	Patient may have moderate to severe pain

To calculate the infiltration grade of any amount of blood product, irritant, or vesicant, use the following formula:

$$\frac{\text{Number of infiltration indicators}}{\text{Total number of IV peripheral lines}} \times 100 + \% \text{ peripheral infiltration}$$

RECOGNIZING AND MANAGING INFILTRATION OR INFLAMMATION

	Infiltration	Inflammation
Characteristics	Damage to tissue (limits access to vessel in the future)	Presence of erythema, induration, tenderness
Intervention	Delay treatment	Obtain sterile equipment and select opposite extremity for replacement site.
Verification	Confirm by tourniquet, not backflow of blood*	Send a sample of catheter and infusate to the laboratory for culture.
		Record lot numbers catheter and infusate.

*An infusion has infiltrated if swelling occurs about the catheter site or a tourniquet applied above the catheter does not stop the flow of fluid. In small veins, the catheter may approach the side of the vein, occluding the lumen and obstructing blood flow; the solution flows undiluted so that no backflow of blood is obtained. The catheter may have punctured the vein, causing an infiltration, and at the same time be within the lumen of the vein, or the bevel may be only partially within the lumen of the vein, causing a swelling and still producing a backflow of blood on test.

The practice criteria clearly articulate the need to discontinue the infusion with an observed infiltration incident and to maintain statistical records including frequency, severity, and type of infusate for all such occurrences.

Change of Fluid Containers

Air embolism and blood embolism are significant hazards of infusion therapy and may be associated with delay in changing solution containers. Subsequent solutions should be added before the level of fluid falls in the drip chamber. Failure to do this results in some of the serious problems that follow.

PLUGGED CATHETER
Intravenous fluids flow into the vein by means of gravity. Once the fluid level has dropped in the tubing to approximately the level of the patient's chest, blood is forced back into the catheter, occluding its lumen.

An occluded catheter should be removed, not irrigated. Fibrinous material injected into the vein can propagate a thrombus, possibly resulting in an infarction. Irrigation may embolize small, infected catheter thrombi, which could result in septicemia. Aspiration efforts aimed at dislodging the fibrin may cause the vein to collapse around the catheter point, traumatizing the vessel wall.

TRAPPED AIR
If the bottle (in an air-venting system) is changed after the level of fluid drops in the tubing and before the catheter plugs, air becomes trapped in the tubing. The pressure of the fresh fluid then forces the trapped air into the patient, and fatal air embolism

KEY INTERVENTIONS: Managing a Stopped Infusion

Avoid potential complications of infusion therapy by knowing what to do when the infusion stops:

1. Check for infiltration.
2. Check the fluid level in the bottle.
3. Check for kinking of the tubing.
4. Open the clamp.
5. Check air vent.
6. Check the catheter for patency by kinking the tubing a few inches from the catheter while pinching and releasing the tubing between the catheter and the kinked tubing. Resistance, if encountered, should be treated with caution because a clot may have plugged the catheter. If the patient complains of pain, a sclerosed vein may be causing the cessation of flow. In either case, the catheter must be removed.
7. Consider whether the catheter is in line with the vein or up against the wall of the vein. A slight adjustment, by moving the catheter, may remedy the problem.
8. Consider the possibility of a venous spasm, which may result from cold IV fluid (eg, blood). Heat placed directly on the vein relieves the spasm and increases the flow of the infusion.
9. If the infusion is blood, check the filter; heavy sediment may be slowing the flow. Replace the filter if necessary.
10. Increase the height of the bottle to increase gravity.
11. If flow does not resume after following the preceding procedures, restart the infusion.

can result. Using plastic fluid bags, containers that contain no air, and administration sets that have no junctions through which air can leak has reduced the risk of introducing air into the patient's veins.

Air can be introduced at the beginning of an infusion, however, if the administration set is not completely cleared of air, or when containers are changed. Infusions administered through a central venous catheter carry an even greater risk of air embolism than do those administered through a peripheral vein. Air embolism can occur during tubing changes involving the central venous catheter.

It has been suggested, through animal experimentation, that a normal adult can tolerate air embolism of as much as 200 mL, but for people in poor health, smaller amounts may be fatal; fewer than 10 mL might be fatal in a gravely ill person (INS, 1998, 2000) (see Chap. 11).

Nonfunctioning (leaking or plugged) sets should be removed. In functioning sets, the old fluid should be replaced with fresh fluid before the flow ceases and the bottle empties. The following procedure should be used:

1. Vent a fresh bottle if venting is required.
2. Kink the tubing to prevent air from being introduced into the flowing fluid.
3. Change the fluid container, hanging the infusion bottle before unkinking the tubing.
4. Readjust flow rate if necessary.

Filters and Practice Criteria

Filters prevent the passage of undesirable substances into the vascular system.

Particulate matter filters should be used when preparing infusion medications for administration and blood filters should be used to filter blood or its components (see Chap. 17).

Air-eliminating filters, such as a 0.2-μm filter, protect the patient from air embolism, bacteria, and particulate matter. The INS advocates using 0.2-μm air-eliminating filters for routine administration of IV fluids as follows:

1. The filter should be placed at the terminal end of the administration set, that is, as close to the catheter as possible.
2. The filter should be changed at the time of administration set change.
3. Lipid emulsions, blood, and blood products should not be administered through the filter.
4. Follow the manufacturer's recommendations regarding administration, particularly when infusing certain drugs whose dosage may be affected by the filter.
5. The pounds per square inch (psi) of the filter must be compatible with the electronic infusion device in use (INS, 2000).

Monitoring and Practice Criteria

Ongoing monitoring provides information regarding a patient's response to the prescribed therapies.

Patients receiving IV therapies should be monitored at frequent, established intervals based on practice setting, prescribed therapy, condition, and age. Monitoring should

- Be established in policies and procedures
- Minimize risk of potential complications of routine IV therapy
- Include documentation of the catheter site, flow rate, clinical data, and patient response (INS, 1998, 2000; Perucca, 1995).

Documentation and Practice Criteria

Documentation of care provides a mechanism to record and retrieve information. Documentation of IV therapy should include the following:

- Catheter
- Site
- Patient's response to treatment
- Type of treatment
- Date and time
- Name of the professional providing care

Documentation should provide sufficient information to identify procedures, prescribed treatments, complications, and nursing interventions (INS, 2000).

Discontinuation of Therapy, Catheter Removal, and Practice Criteria

The patient's need for and/or response to therapy determine discontinuation of therapy.
To discontinue an infusion, the following procedure should be used:

1. Stop flow by clamping off tubing.
2. Remove all tape from catheter. Do not use scissors, which could accidentally cut the tubing.
3. With a dry, sterile sponge held over the injection site, remove the catheter. The catheter must be removed nearly flush with the skin. This prevents the point from damaging the posterior wall of the vein, thus encouraging the process of thrombosis.
4. Visually ascertain that the length of the catheter removed corresponds with the length inserted, and note this information in the record.
5. Apply pressure instantly and firmly. Do not rub. A hematoma may result from catheters carelessly removed, thereby rendering veins useless for future catheterization.

Small adhesive bandages, such as Band-Aids, should not be used unless specifically ordered. An adhesive strip does not stop bleeding, nor does it take the place of pressure. When used, it should be applied only after pressure has been applied and the bleeding stopped (INS, 2000).

References and Selected Readings

Asterisks indicate references cited in text.

*Intravenous Nurses Society. (1998). Revised intravenous nursing standards of practice. *Journal of Intravenous Nursing, 21*(Suppl. 1).

*Intravenous Nurses Society. (2000). Draft revised intravenous nursing standards of practice.

Mazzola, J.R., Schott-Baer, D., & Addy, L. (1999). Clinical factors associated with the development of phlebitis after insertion of a peripherally inserted central catheter. *Journal of Intravenous Nursing, 22,* 36.

Miller, J.M., Goetz, A.M., Squier, C., et al. (1996). Reduction in nosocomial intravenous device-related bacteremias after institution of an intravenous therapy team. *Journal of Intravenous Nursing, 19,* 103–106.

*Occupational Safety and Health Administration. (1999, November). *Revised compliance directive.* Washington, DC: Author.

*Perucca, R. (1995). Changing and discontinuing intravenous therapy. In J. Terry, L. Baranowski, R.A. Lonsway, & C. Hedrick (Eds.). *Intravenous therapy: Clinical principles and practice* (pp. 400–405). Philadelphia: W.B. Saunders.

*Pugliese, G., & Salahuddin, M. (1999). *Sharps injury prevention program: A step-by-step guide.* Chicago, IL: American Hospital Association.

Reed, T., & Phillips, S. (1996). Management of central venous catheter occlusion and repairs. *Journal of Intravenous Nursing, 19,* 289–292.

Smith, R.L., & Sheperd, M. (1995). Central venous catheter infection rates in an acute care hospital. *Journal of Intravenous Nursing, 18,* 255.

Zaragosa, M., Salles, M., Gomez, J., Bayas, J. M., & Trilla, A. (1999). Handwashing with soap or alcoholic solution? *American Journal of Infect Control, 27*(3)258–261.

Review Questions

Note: Questions below may have more than one right answer.

1. The INS Standards document was most recently revised in:
   A. 1995
   B. 1996
   C. 1998
   D. 2000

2. Which of the following statements is true of Standards?
   A. They provide a framework for evaluation of outcomes.
   B. They must be implemented institution-wide.
   C. They are applicable throughout a facility.
   D. They should regularly be compared with existing policies.

3. Which of the following is *not* true about care plans?
   A. They are an integral component of the nursing process.
   B. They reflect nursing diagnosis.
   C. They should be established before assessment.
   D. They include time frames for goal achievement.

4. Antimicrobial solutions suitable for skin preparation include which of the following?
   A. Tincture of iodine 1% to 2%
   B. Iodophors
   C. 70% Isopropyl alcohol
   D. Chlorhexidine

5. The 0.2-μm filter protects the patient from which of the following?
   A. Air
   B. Bacteria
   C. Particulate matter
   D. All of the above

6. Junction securement devices include:
   A. Luer-lock devices
   B. Tape
   C. Clasps
   D. Needleless systems

7. Which of the following is *not* a sign of infusion phlebitis?
   A. Swelling
   B. Redness
   C. Tenderness
   D. Raised wheal

8. An organization may consider extending the interval for routine primary administration set changes beyond 72 hours for peripheral catheters in the presence of a consistent monthly phlebitis rate of:
   A. Less than 1%
   B. 3% or less
   C. 5% or less
   D. Less than 7.5%

9. Hematoma is the result of:
   A. Careless removal of catheters
   B. Lack of patient compliance
   C. a only
   D. a and b

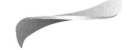

ASSESSMENT
AND
MONITORING

Anatomy and Physiology

Applied to

Intravascular Therapy

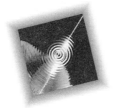

K E Y   T E R M S

Arterial Spasm
Arteriovenous Anastomosis
Integument
Radiopaque
Superficial Fascia

Tunica
Valves
Vascular System
Vasovagal Reaction

■ VASCULAR ANATOMY AND THERAPEUTIC GOALS

Because intravascular therapy involves the administration of fluids, blood, and drugs directly into the **vascular system,** that is, into arteries, bone marrow, and veins, the nurse and others responsible for administering therapy need to understand the anatomy and physiology of vascular structures and related systems.

Although the *veins*, because of their abundance and location, provide the most readily accessible route for intravascular therapies, the *arteries* and *bone marrow* are also used. Arteries provide the route for introducing **radiopaque** material for diagnostic purposes, such as arteriograms to detect cerebral disorders, blood pressure monitoring, determinations of arterial blood gas levels, and administration of chemotherapy. The dangers of **arterial spasm** and subsequent gangrene present problems that make this route of therapy hazardous for therapeutic use. The *bone marrow*, because of its venous plexus, is used for intravascular therapy by the intraosseous route.

The primary goal of intravenous (IV) therapy is to provide a positive outcome for the patient. Painless and effective therapy is desirable, promoting the patient's comfort, well-being, and often complete recovery from disease or trauma. An integral part of this goal is the recognition and prevention of complications. To achieve the goal and minimize the risk of complications, the IV nurse needs a solid knowledge of vascular anatomy and physiology.

Integration of Knowledge With Practice

By studying the superficial veins, for example, the nurse learns to discriminate the best veins to use for IV therapy. Factors to be considered in selecting a vein include size, location, and resilience. In addition, an understanding of the reaction of veins to the nervous stimulation of the vasoconstrictors and vasodilators enables the clinician to increase the size and visibility of a vein before attempting venipuncture and to relieve venous spasm and thus assist in infusion maintenance.

By studying the superficial veins of the lower extremities, the nurse becomes alert to the dangers resulting from their use. Avoiding venipunctures in veins susceptible to varicosities and sluggish circulation decreases the likelihood of complications, such as phlebitis and thrombosis, and reduces the secondary risk of pulmonary embolism.

Common Venous Complications

Phlebitis and thrombosis are by far the most common complications resulting from parenteral therapy (see Chap. 9). Although seemingly mild, phlebitis and thrombosis may have serious consequences. First they cause moderate to severe discomfort, often taking many days or weeks to subside. Second, they limit the veins available for future therapy. Injury to the endothelial lining of the vein contributes to these local complications.

Crucial to recognizing and preventing complications is a solid knowledge of the characteristics that differentiate veins from arteries and the positions of each. Understanding this helps the nurse avoid the complications of an inadvertent arterial puncture. The knowledge also helps to reduce the risk of necrosis and gangrene and to recognize the existence of an **arteriovenous anastomosis,** a congenital or traumatic abnormality in which blood flows directly from the artery into the vein.

Failure to recognize an arteriovenous anastomosis results in repeated and unsuccessful venipunctures performed in an attempt to initiate the infusion. Repeated punctures compound the trauma to the inner lining of the vein and increase the risk of the local complications already described, any one of which limits the number of available veins, interrupts the course of therapy, and causes unnecessary pain or, possibly, dire consequences for the patient.

■ SYSTEMS AND ORGANS INVOLVED IN INTRAVENOUS THERAPY

Among the organs and systems closely associated with intravascular therapy are the integumentary, neurologic, cardiovascular, and respiratory systems, as well as individual circulatory organs and structures.

Integumentary System and Connective Tissue

The **integument,** or skin, is the first organ affected in IV access. It protects the body from the environment and is a natural barrier to external forces. The skin is made up of two layers, the epidermis and the dermis.

Epidermis and Dermis

The epidermis is the uppermost layer, which forms a protective covering for the dermis. Its thickness varies in different parts of the body. It is thickest on the palms of the hands and the soles of the feet and thinnest on the inner surface of the limbs. Its thickness also varies with age. In an elderly patient, for example, the skin on the dorsum of the hand may be so thin that it does not adequately support the vein for venipuncture when parenteral infusions are required.

The dermis, or underlayer, is highly sensitive and vascular. It contains many capillaries and thousands of nerve fibers (Fig. 5–1).

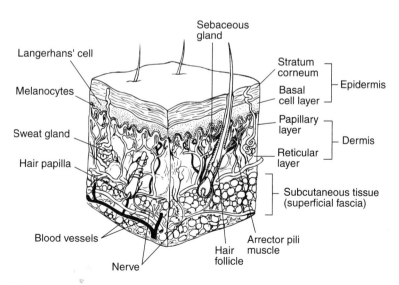

Figure 5–1. Layers of the skin. The epidermis protects the highly vascular dermis that lies above the superficial fascia (subcutaneous tissue)

Superficial Fascia

The **superficial fascia,** or subcutaneous areolar connective tissue, lies below the two layers of skin and is, in itself, another covering. The superficial veins are located in this fascia, which varies in thickness. When a catheter is inserted into this fascia, there is free movement of the skin above. Great care and meticulous aseptic technique must be observed because an infection in this loose tissue spreads easily. Such an infection is called *cellulitis* (Williams, Warwick, Dyson, & Bannister, 1995).

Neurologic System

The human nervous system responds to changes in the environment through sensory organs. The nervous system is responsible for:

- Sensory function, transmitting information from tactile, visual, and auditory receptors
- Motor functions, controlling skeletal and smooth muscle
- Autonomic function, controlling glands and smooth muscle

Nerve fibers under the skin include those that react to temperature, touch, pressure, and pain. The number of nerve fibers varies in different areas of the body. Some areas of the skin are highly sensitive; other areas are only mildly sensitive. The insertion of a needle in one area may cause a great deal of pain, yet another area may be virtually insensitive to pain. The inner aspect of the wrist is a highly sensitive area. Venipunctures are performed here only when other veins have been exhausted.

The anatomic divisions of the nervous system are the central nervous system (brain and spinal cord) and peripheral nervous system (12 cranial and 31 spinal nerves). The vagus nerve, which innervates the heart, is of prime importance. Stimulation of the vagus nerve produces a depressant effect on cardiac muscle, resulting in clinical signs such as bradycardia and hypotension. This condition is known as a **vasovagal reaction** or vasovagal syncope.

Cardiac System

The heart is encased in the pericardium, which has two layers. The outer, fibrous layer is composed of strong collagen fibers and covers the aorta, superior vena cava, right and left pulmonary arteries, and the four pulmonary veins. The inner, serous layer is further divided into the parietal and visceral layers. A thin film of fluid between these two layers enables the heart to move.

The superior vena cava returns blood from the upper part of the body and has no valve. The inferior vena cava returns blood from the lower part of the body and has a semilunar valve near the opening into the atrium. The atrium, in its role as reservoir, has sufficient capacity to move blood through the tricuspid valve into the right ventricle.

Cardiac output is regulated by changes in the volume of blood flowing into the heart and control of the heart by the autonomic nervous system.

Respiratory System

Parenteral fluid administration affects the trachea, bronchi, and lungs. Blood flows into the lungs from the pulmonary arteries, which carry deoxygenated blood. These arteries follow the path of the bronchi. Undissolved particles in infusates may enter the microcirculation of the lungs, which may lead to emboli (see Chap. 11).

Circulatory System

The blood volume and distribution, for which the circulatory system is responsible, result from complex interactions between cardiac output, excretion of fluids and electrolytes by the kidneys, and hormonal and nervous system factors. Total blood volume may be enhanced by pregnancy, large varicose veins, polycythemia, and inability of the heart to pump enough blood to perfuse the kidneys (see Chap. 17).

The circulatory system is divided into two main systems, the pulmonary and the systemic, each with its own set of vessels. The pulmonary system directs the blood flow from the right ventricle of the heart to the lungs, where it is oxygenated and returned to the left atrium.

The systemic circulatory system, the larger of the two, is the one that concerns the IV nurse. It consists of the aorta, arteries, arterioles, capillaries, venules, and veins through which the blood must flow.

The blood leaves the left ventricle, flows to all parts of the body, and returns to the right atrium of the heart through the vena cava. Systemic veins are categorized as superficial and deep.

Superficial Veins

The superficial or cutaneous veins are used in venipuncture. Located just beneath the skin in the superficial fascia, these veins and the deep veins sometimes unite, especially in the lower extremities. For example, the small saphenous vein, a superficial vein, drains the dorsum of the foot and the posterior section of the leg; it ascends the back of the leg and empties directly into the deep popliteal vein.

Before the small saphenous vein terminates in the deep popliteal, it sends out a branch that, after joining the great saphenous vein, also terminates in a deep vein, the femoral vein. Because of these deep connections, great concern arises when it becomes necessary to use the veins in the lower extremities. Thrombosis may occur, which could easily extend to the deep veins and cause pulmonary embolism. Understanding this, the nurse should refrain from using these veins.

Varicosities in the lower extremities, although readily available to venipuncture, are not a satisfactory route for parenteral administration. The relatively stagnant blood in such veins is likely to clot, resulting in a superficial phlebitis. Medication injected below a varicosity may result in another potential danger: a collection of the infused drug as a result of stagnated blood flow. This pocket of infused medication may delay the effect of the drug when immediate action is desired. Another concern is the danger of untoward reactions to the drug, which may occur when this accumulation finally reaches the general circulation.

Superficial Veins of the Upper Extremities

The superficial veins of the upper extremities are shown in Figures 5–2 and 5–3. They consist of the digital, metacarpal, cephalic, basilic, and median veins (Table 5–1).

Deep Veins

Deep veins are usually enclosed in the same sheath with the arteries. Occasionally an arteriovenous anastomosis may occur congenitally or as the result of past penetrating injury of the vein and adjacent artery. When such trauma occurs, the blood flows directly from the artery into the vein. As a result, the veins draining an arteriovenous fistula are overburdened with high-pressure arterial blood. These veins appear large and tortuous. In these unusual circumstances, the nurse's quick recognition of an arteriovenous fistula may prevent pain, complications, and loss of time resulting from repeated unsuccessful attempts to start the infusion.

Differences of Arteries and Veins

Possibly the most dramatic difference between arteries and veins is that arteries pulsate and veins do not. Less apparent differences involve location and structure. Although arteries and veins are similar in structure—both comprise three layers of tissue—a close examination of these layers reveals their differentiating characteristics.

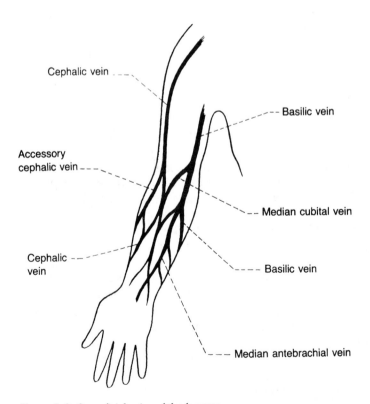

Figure 5–2. Superficial veins of the forearm.

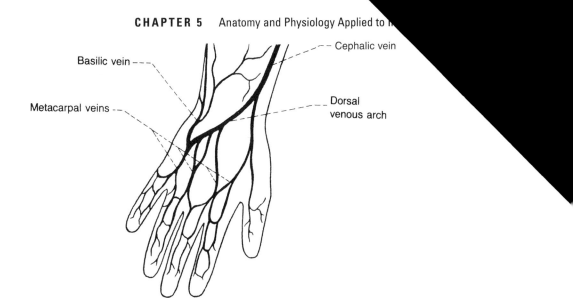

Figure 5–3. Superficial veins of the dorsal aspect of the hand.

TUNICA INTIMA: THE INNER LAYER

The first vascular layer is known as the **tunica** intima. It consists of an inner elastic endothelial lining, which also forms the valves in veins. Although these valves are absent in arteries, the endothelial lining is identical in the arteries and the veins, consisting of a smooth layer of flat cells.

This smooth surface allows the cells and platelets to flow through the blood vessels without interruption under normal conditions. Care must be taken to avoid roughening this surface when performing a venipuncture or removing a needle from a vein. Any trauma that roughens the endothelial lining encourages thrombin formation, a result of cells and platelets adhering or aggregating to the vessel wall.

Many veins contain **valves,** which are semilunar folds of the endothelium. Found in the larger veins of the extremities, these valves function to keep the blood flowing toward the heart. Where muscular pressure would cause a backup of the blood supply, these valves play an important role. They are located at points of branching and often cause a noticeable bulge in the veins. Applying a tourniquet to the extremity impedes the venous flow. When suction is applied, as occurs in the process of drawing blood, the valves compress and close the lumen of the vein, preventing the backward flow of blood. Thus, these valves interfere with the process of withdrawing blood. Recognizing the presence of a valve, the nurse may resolve the difficulty by slightly readjusting the needle.

These valves are absent in many of the small veins. However, if a thrombus obstructs an ascending vein, a small vein may be used instead. The catheter may be inserted below the thrombosis, directed toward the distal end of the extremity; this results in a rerouting of the fluid and avoidance of the thrombosed portion.

TUNICA MEDIA: THE MIDDLE LAYER

The second layer consists of muscular and elastic tissue. The nerve fibers, both vasoconstrictors and vasodilators, are located in this middle layer. These fibers, which constantly receive impulses from the vasoconstrictor center in the medulla, keep the

TABLE 5 – 1
THE APPROPRIATE PERIPHERAL VENIPUNCTURE SITE

...ation	Advantages	Disadvantages
...–distal ...gers	Ideal for short-term use	Fingers may require splinting and immobilization. Catheterization may create patient discomfort.
...of hand; ...e union of ...between the knuckles	Easily accessible; lies flat on the back of the hand	Wrist movement is decreased unless a short catheter is used. Insertion is painful because of increased nerve endings. Site may become phlebitic.
Accessory cephalic	Runs along radial bone	Large vein ideal for venipuncture; readily accepts large-bore needle; easily stabilized	May be difficult to align catheter hub flush with the patient's skin. Catheter may impair patient mobility if placed over a point of flexion.
Cephalic	Along radial side of forearm–upper arm	Excellent large vein; readily accessible; does not impair mobility	Proximity to elbow may compromise joint movement; site must be stabilized properly before venipuncture.
Medial antebrachial	Arises from palm and runs along ulnar side of forearm	Easily accommodates winged infusion needle access	Proximity to nerve endings; inherent danger of infiltration
Basilic	Runs along ulnar side of forearm–upper arm	Accommodates large-gauge needle; appropriate for large-gauge devices	May be difficult to position patient comfortably during insertion; penetration of dermal layer of skin and proximity of site to nerve endings may cause pain.
Antecubital	Located in the antecubital fossa: Median cephalic (radial side); median basilic (unlar side); median cubital (in front of elbow joint)	Large veins facilitate blood sampling; good for emergency use	Median cephalic crosses in front of brachial artery; scarred vessels due to frequent blood draws; difficult to stabilize properly

vessels in a state of tonus. They also stimulate both arteries and veins to contract or relax.

The middle layer is not as strong and stiff in the veins as it is in the arteries. Therefore, the veins tend to collapse or distend as the pressure within falls or rises. Arteries do not collapse.

Stimulation by a change in temperature or by mechanical or chemical irritation may produce spasms in the vein or artery. For example, interrupting a continuous infusion to administer a pint of cold blood may produce vasoconstriction; this results in spasm, impedes the flow of blood, and causes pain. Application of heat to the vein promotes vasodilation, which relieves the spasm, improves the flow of blood, and relieves the pain. The same results are obtained by heat when an irritating drug has caused vasoconstriction. In this situation, heat relieves the spasm, increases the blood flow, and protects the vessel wall from inflammation caused by the medication. With heat dilating the vein and increasing the flow of blood, the drug becomes more diluted and less irritating. The use of heat to achieve vasodilation is also helpful when the nurse must use a small or poorly filled vein.

Spasms produced by a chemical irritation in an artery may have dire consequences. A single artery supplies circulation to a particular area. If this artery is damaged, the related area experiences impaired circulation, with the possible development of necrosis and gangrene. If a chemical agent is introduced into the artery, the result may be a spasm—a contraction that could shut off the blood supply completely. This problem is not as serious when veins are used because many veins supply a particular area; if one is injured, others maintain the circulation.

TUNICA ADVENTITIA: THE OUTER LAYER

The third layer, which consists of areolar connective tissue, surrounds and supports the vessel. In arteries, this layer is thicker than in veins because it is subjected to greater pressure from the force of blood.

Arteries require more protection than veins and are placed where injury is less likely to occur. Whereas veins are superficially located, most arteries lie deep in the tissues and are protected by muscle. Occasionally an artery is located superficially in an unusual place; this artery is then called an aberrant artery. An aberrant artery must not be mistaken for a vein. If a chemical that causes spasm is introduced into an aberrant artery, permanent damage may result.

References and Selected Readings

Asterisks indicate references cited in text.

Terry, J. (1995). *Intravenous therapy: Clinical principles and practice.* Philadelphia: W.B. Saunders.

*Williams, P.L., Warwick, R., Dyson, M., & Bannister, L.H. (1995). *Gray's anatomy,* 39th ed. London: Churchill Livingstone.

Review Questions

Note: Questions below may have more than one right answer.

1. Blood volume and distribution result from which of the following interactions?
   A. Interaction between cardiac output and excretion of excessive amounts of fluids and electrolytes
   B. Excretion of excess fluids and electrolytes by the kidneys, and hormonal and nervous system
   C. a only
   D. a and b

2. Total fluid volume may be enhanced by:
   A. Pregnancy
   B. Large varicose veins
   C. Polycythemia
   D. Inability of the heart to pump enough blood to perfuse the kidneys

3. Which of the following statements is *not* true about valves?

   A. They may be found in many veins.

   B. They are semilunar folds of the endothelium.

   C. They are found in smaller veins of the extremities.

   D. They keep the blood flowing toward the heart.

4. Stimulation of which nerve produces a depressant effect on cardiac muscle?

   A. Vagus

   B. Brachial

   C. Ulnar

   D. Radial

5. All of the following statements is true about the epidermis except:

   A. It is the uppermost layer.

   B. It forms a protective covering.

   C. Its thickness varies.

   D. It is thinnest on the palms of the hands.

6. Which of the following veins is appropriate for peripheral access (short-term)?

   A. Digital

   B. Brachial

   C. Ulnar

   D. Femoral

7. Which vein is located on the surface of the hand?

   A. Ulnar

   B. Radial

   C. Metacarpal

   D. Brachial

8. Which of the following statements is true of an aberrant artery?

   A. It requires more protection than a vein.

   B. It lies deep in tissue.

   C. It is protected by muscle.

   D. It is located superficially in an unusual place.

9. A working knowledge of the anatomy and physiology of which systems enables the IV clinician to practice?

   A. Anatomy and physiology and peripheral vasculature

   B. Neurologic and cardiopulmonary systems

   C. a only

   D. a and b

10. Which of the following contributes to arterial spasm?

    A. Chemical irritation

    B. Impaired circulation

    C. Intra-arterial injection

    D. Necrosis

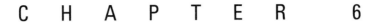

C H A P T E R 6

Laboratory Tests

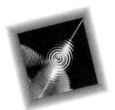

K E Y   T E R M S

Glycolysis
Hematoma
Hemoconcentration
Postprandial
Venous Blood Samples

■ COLLECTION OF VENOUS BLOOD

In the past, intravenous (IV) therapy departments included the collection of **venous blood samples** as one of their functions. Although collection of venous blood now is usually delegated to a team of laboratory phlebotomists or technologists, in many instances the IV nurse will be involved:

- When the patient is in a critical care unit
- When veins have become exhausted
- When the patient is to receive an IV infusion
- When the specimen is to be obtained from a central venous catheter that is to be removed, from a multilumen central venous catheter, from a Hickman-Broviac catheter, or from an implanted vascular access device

Role of Intravenous Nurse

Advantages are gained when the IV department is involved in collecting venous blood. First, the nurse, understanding the importance of preserving veins for infusion therapy, is cautious when choosing veins and in applying blood-drawing techniques. Second, the IV nurse is skilled at using a single venipuncture to permit both the withdrawal of blood and the initiation of an infusion, thereby preserving veins, reducing discomfort, and avoiding undue patient distress. Third, patient–blood identification is of paramount importance in preventing the error of infusing incompatible blood. Because the IV department assumes responsibility for patient–blood identification before transfusion and is aware of existing hazards, its personnel are well qualified and trained in the collection of samples for typing and crossmatching.

Significance of Blood Collection for Testing

The nurse in any clinical setting is often charged to collect blood in a specified amount and in a specified type of tube. This chapter is intended primarily to provide the nurse with information concerning the most commonly performed laboratory tests—their purpose and normal values—and the collection and proper handling of blood samples. Laboratory procedures are not explained.

Practice Standards in Testing

The nurse is responsible for maintaining the practice standard in diagnostic testing (Table 6-1). The collection of blood samples for certain tests must meet special requirements. Some tests call for whole blood, whereas others require components such as plasma, serum, or cells. The proper requirements must be met to prevent erroneous or misleading laboratory analysis. Practice standards cover a wide range of test procedures, techniques, and circumstances, such as those that follow.

Collecting Blood and Blood Components

Serum consists of plasma minus fibrinogen and is obtained by drawing blood in a dry tube and allowing the blood to coagulate. Serum is required for most of the laboratory tests in common use.

Plasma consists of the stable components of blood minus the cells and is obtained by using an anticoagulant to prevent the blood from clotting. Several anticoagulants are available in color-coded tubes. Choice of the anticoagulant depends on the test to be performed. Most of the anticoagulants, including sodium or potassium oxalate, citrate, and ethylenediamine tetra-acetic acid (EDTA), prevent coagulation by binding the serum calcium. Other anticoagulants, such as heparin, are valuable in specific tests but are not commonly used. Heparin prevents coagulation for only limited periods.

T A B L E 6 – 1
STANDARDS FOR DIAGNOSTIC TESTING*

Source and Standard	Applications to Testing
American Nurses Association (ANA) Council on Cultural Diversity and Nursing Practice prescribes culturally competent care.	The nurse serves as an advocate for the patient, communicates and collaborates with health care team from a cultural perspective. The nurse tailors instructions and care to patient's cultural needs.
Individual agency has a policy statement for specimen collection and procedure statement for monitoring patient after an invasive diagnostic procedure; policy for unusual witnessed consent situations.	The nurse observes universal precautions when handling any body fluid specimens. Labeled biohazard bags are used for transport of specimens. The nurse monitors and records vital signs for specific times before, during, and after completion of certain procedures. The nurse documents any deviations from basic consent policies and employs measures to obtain appropriate consents for the procedure.
U.S. Department of Transportation requires alcohol testing in emergency rooms in special situations.	The properly trained emergency room nurse performs blood and breath alcohol testing in unresponsive people and accident victims.
Occupational Safety and Health Administration (OSHA) standards apply to preventing transmission of hepatitis B and C and human immunodeficiency virus, safe work practices, vaccinations, and minimizing exposure to hazardous and toxic materials.	Nurses are exposed to bloodborne pathogens in the course of their work and are trained to observe universal precautions. Tasks and procedures in which occupational exposure may occur include: phlebotomy, injections, immunizations; handling contaminated materials, wastes, body fluids, and sharps; performing laboratory tests on body fluids; invasive procedures; vaginal exams and procedures; starting IVs; spinal taps; wound care; surgical procedures; cleaning.

*Nurses are accountable for safeguarding their patients within reasonable and prudent professional limits of practice.
(From Fischbach, F. [1998]. *Nurse's quick reference to common laboratory and diagnostic tests* [2nd ed.]. Philadelphia: Lippincott-Raven.)

Whole blood is required for many tests, including blood counts and bleeding time. Potassium oxalate is commonly used to preserve whole blood.

 SAFE PRACTICE ALERT *Hemoconcentration* through venous stasis should be avoided to avoid inaccurate results in some tests. Hemoconcentration, which occurs when a tourniquet is applied, increases proportionally with the length of time the tourniquet is in use. Once the venipuncture has been made, the tourniquet should be removed. This is a simple but important precaution, ignored by many.

Carbon dioxide and pH are examples of tests in which results are affected by hemoconcentration. If the tourniquet is required to withdraw the blood, it should be noted on the requisition that the blood was drawn with stasis.

Hemolysis causes serious errors in many tests in which lysis of the red blood cells (RBCs) permits the substance being measured to escape into the serum. When erythrocytes, which are rich in potassium, rupture, the serum potassium level rises, giving a false measurement. See Box 6–1 for a summary of special precautions for avoiding hemolysis.

Effect of Intravenous Fluids on Blood Sample

Intravenous fluids may contribute to misleading laboratory interpretations. Blood samples should never be drawn proximal to an infusion, but preferably from the contralateral extremity. If the fluid contains a substance that may affect the analysis, an indication of its presence should be made on the requisition–for example, "potassium determination during infusion of electrolyte solution."

Special Handling

Some samples require special handling when a delay is unavoidable. Some determinations, such as the pH, must be done within 10 minutes after the blood is drawn. When a delay is inevitable, the sample is placed in ice, which partially inhibits **glycolysis**—the production of lactic acid by the glycolytic enzymes of the blood cells—resulting in a rapid lowering of pH on standing.

Samples for blood gas analyses also require special handling and must be analyzed as soon as blood is collected. When the carbon dioxide content of serum is to be determined, the blood must completely fill the tube or carbon dioxide will escape. Several procedures are currently in use; in each, the escape of carbon dioxide must be prevented.

Fasting

Because absorption of food may alter blood composition, test results often depend on the patient fasting. Blood glucose and serum lipid levels are increased by ingestion of food. Serum inorganic phosphorus values are depressed after meals.

BOX 6–1 Avoiding Hemolysis When Drawing a Blood Sample

1. Use dry syringes and dry tubes.
2. Avoid excess pressure on the plunger of the syringe. Such pressure collapses the vein and may cause air bubbles to be sucked from around the hub of the needle into the blood.
3. Do not shake clotted blood specimens unnecessarily.
4. Avoid using force when transferring blood to a container or tube. Force of the blood against the tube results in rupture of the cells. In transferring blood to a vacuum tube, use no needle larger than 20-gauge.

Timely Examination

Immediate dispatch of blood samples to the laboratory is vital to accuracy of findings in some blood tests. Promptness in examining blood samples is necessary in the analysis of labile constituents of blood. In certain tests (eg, those involving potassium), the substance being measured diffuses out of the cells into the serum being examined. The result is a false measurement. To prevent this rise in serum concentration, the cells must be separated from the serum promptly.

Infected Samples

Special caution must be observed in the care of all blood samples because blood from all patients is considered infective. Blood samples should not be allowed to spill on the outside of the containers. Contaminated material should be placed in bags and treated according to institutional policies for disposal of infectious material. Catheters should not be recapped or broken but disposed of intact in catheter-proof containers. All personnel handling blood should wear gloves.

Emergency Tests

Blood for tests ordered on an emergency basis must be sent directly to the laboratory. Red cellophane tape or other special markings, according to the facility's preference, may be used to indicate a state of emergency. Tests most likely to be designated as emergency tests include amylase, blood urea nitrogen (BUN), carbon dioxide, potassium, prothrombin, sodium, glucose, and blood typing.

Effective Equipment: Vacuum System

The vacuum system, which has increased the efficiency of the blood sampling process, consists of a plastic holder into which screws a sterile, disposable, double-ended needle. A rubber-stoppered vacuum tube slips into the barrel. The barrel has a measured line denoting the distance the tube is inserted into the barrel; at this point, the needle becomes embedded in the stopper. The stopper is not punctured until the needle has been introduced into the vein. Advancing technology has made this process relatively bloodless and consistent with Occupational Safety and Health Administration and Centers for Disease Control and Prevention safety standards.

After entry into the vein, the rubber-stoppered tube is pushed the remaining distance into the barrel. As the needle is pushed into the vacuum tube, a rubber sheath covering the shaft is forced back, allowing the blood to flow. The tourniquet is released and several blood specimens may be obtained by simply removing the tube containing the sample and replacing it with another tube. As the tube is removed, the rubber sheath slips back over the needle, preventing blood from dripping into the holder.

If the vein is not located, removing the tube before the needle is withdrawn preserves the vacuum in the tube.

It sometimes is necessary to draw blood from small veins. If suction from the vacuum tube collapses the vein, drawing the blood becomes difficult. By pressing a finger against the vein beyond the point of the needle or by placing the bevel of the needle lightly against the wall of the vein, suction is reduced and the vein allowed to fill. In the latter process, the nurse should exercise particular caution to prevent injury to the endothelial lining of the vein. The pressure is intermittently applied and released, filling and emptying the vein. A small-gauge winged infusion needle with vacuum adapter may also be used; the smaller needle reduces the amount of suction and may prevent collapse of the vein. A syringe is often used to draw blood from small veins because the amount of suction can be more easily controlled.

Skillful Technique

Peripheral Venipunctures

When skillfully executed, a venipuncture causes the patient little discomfort. The numerous blood determinations necessary for diagnosis and treatment make good technique imperative.

The one-step entry technique should be avoided because too often it results in through-and-through punctures, contributing to hematoma formation. The needle should be inserted under the skin and then, after relocation of the vein, into the vessel.

The veins most commonly used are those in the antecubital fossa. The median antecubital vein, although not always visible, is usually large and palpable. Because it is well supported by subcutaneous tissue and least likely to roll, it is often the best choice for venipuncture. Second choice is the cephalic vein. The basilic vein, although often the most prominent, is likely to be the least desirable. This vein rolls easily, making the venipuncture difficult, and a hematoma may readily occur if the patient is allowed to flex the arm, which squeezes the blood from the engorged vein into the tissues.

Sufficient time should be spent in locating the vein before attempting venipuncture. Whenever the veins are difficult to see or palpate, the patient should lie down. If the patient is seated, the arm should be well supported on a pillow.

Central Access: Blood Withdrawal

Occasionally, venous samples must be drawn from a central line, especially because these catheters are commonly placed in patients with limited venous access. A dual-lumen catheter may facilitate this process. When multiple-lumen catheters are used for central venous blood sampling, the proximal lumen is the preferred site from which to draw the specimen. Aseptic technique is vital in preventing the introduction of bacteria into the catheter. A sterile IV catheter cap (Luer locking) reduces the risk of bacterial invasion. A recommended method is highlighted in Procedure 6-1.

**Procedure
6–1**

Steps for Obtaining Blood Samples From a Central Venous Catheter

Equipment

To collect a blood sample from a central venous catheter when the patient is not receiving medications, obtain the following:

Gloves

Alcohol wipes or other appropriate cleansing agent

Sterile 2″ × 2″ gauze sponge

Collection tubes

Vacutainer equipment or syringes as needed

Labels

Action	*Rationale*
Wash hands, put on gloves, and clamp the infusion line.	Ensures aseptic technique
Aseptically cleanse infusion port or injection cap.	Ensures closed system
Withdraw 4 mL blood and discard.	First sample contains flush solution, which may alter test results.
Withdraw required quantity of blood; then raise the patient's arm to shoulder level.	Reduces axillary pressure on catheter
Open clamp. Follow manufacturer's recommendations for preparing and using diluent. Then flush the line with the designated amount.	Maintains patency
Adjust flow at prescribed rate.	Ensures compliance with therapeutic regimen
Wash hands and dispose *properly* of all sharps and *any contaminated equipment*.	*Promotes safety and infection control*

Complications Resulting from Venipuncture

Complications related to venipuncture include hematomas, bloodborne diseases, syncope, and other problems.

Hematomas

Hematomas are the most common complication of routine venipuncture for withdrawing blood, and they contribute more to the limitation of available veins than any other complication. They may result from through-and-through puncture to the vein or from incomplete insertion of the needle into the lumen of the vein, which allows the blood to leak into the tissues through the bevel of the needle. In the latter case, advancing the needle into the vein corrects the situation. At the first sign of uncontrolled bleeding, the tourniquet should be released and the needle withdrawn.

Hematomas also result from the application of the tourniquet after an unsuccessful attempt to draw blood. The tourniquet should never be applied to the extremity immediately after a venipuncture.

Hematomas most frequently result from insufficient time spent in applying pressure and from the bad habit of flexing the arm to stop the bleeding. Once the venipuncture is completed, the patient should be instructed to elevate the arm; elevation causes a negative pressure in the vein, collapsing it and facilitating clotting. With patients who have cardiac disease, elevation of the arm should be avoided. Constant pressure is maintained until the bleeding stops. The pressure is applied with a dry, sterile sponge because a wet sponge encourages bleeding. Adhesive strips do not take the place of pressure and, if ordered, are not applied until bleeding stops. Ecchymoses on the arm indicate poor or haphazard technique.

Bloodborne Disease

Special caution must be exercised in caring for needles used to draw blood from patients suspected of harboring microorganisms. Contaminated needles should be placed immediately in a separate container for disposal and standard precautions should be followed. A vacuum tube with stopper provides adequate protection against accidental puncture from the contaminated needle until proper disposal can be made. Any needle puncture should be reported at once. See Chapter 11 for more information about equipment.

Other Complications

Other complications of venipuncture include syncope, continued bleeding, and thrombosis of the vein. Syncope is rarely encountered when the clinician is confident and skillful and when patient teaching has preceded the venipuncture process. Continued bleeding is a complication that may affect the patient receiving anticoagulants, the patient with a blood dyscrasia, or the oncology patient undergoing chemotherapy. To prevent bleeding and to preserve the vein, pressure to the site may be required for an extended period. The nurse should remain with the patient until the bleeding stops.

Thrombosis in routine venipuncture occurs from injury to the endothelial lining of the vein during the venipuncture. Antecubital veins may be used indefinitely if the clinician uses good technique.

■ COMMON LABORATORY TESTS

Laboratory tests are performed for several reasons:

- To indicate relatively common disorders
- To make a diagnosis
- To follow the course of a disease
- To regulate therapy

Standard laboratory values are listed in Table 6–2; examples of conversions of those values to Système International (SI) units are given in Table 6–3.

Blood Cultures

Blood cultures are performed to identify the causative microorganism when a bacteremia is suspected. Isolation of the organism facilitates appropriate treatment. Blood cultures are performed during febrile illnesses or when the patient is having chills with spiking fever. Intermittent bacteremia accompanies such infections as pyelonephritis, brucellosis, cholangitis, osteomyelitis, and others. In such cases, repeated blood cultures are usually ordered when the fever spikes.

In other infections, such as subacute bacterial endocarditis, the bacteremia is more constant during the 4 to 5 febrile days. Usually four or five cultures are obtained over a span of 1 to 2 days, and antimicrobial therapy is initiated once it is established that most cultures harbor the offending microorganism. If antimicrobial therapy is administered before the blood culture or before the patient's admittance to the hospital, the bacteremia may be suppressed, rendering isolation difficult.

Penicillinase may be ordered to be added to the blood culture medium to neutralize the existing penicillinemia and recover the organism. Antimicrobial therapy usually must be withheld to await report of culture to make a precise diagnosis. The penicillinase is added to the culture medium before or immediately after the blood sample is drawn.

Some bacteriology laboratories routinely culture blood under both aerobic and anaerobic conditions. If this is not done routinely and the clinician suspects bacteremia with strict anaerobes, the laboratory should be notified because a special culture broth is necessary.

Extreme care should be taken in ensuring a sterile field for venipuncture; the skin is a fertile field for bacterial growth. Colonization of organisms at the insertion site is associated with a high incidence of catheter-related infections. *Staphylococcus epidermidis*, diphtheroids, and yeast (common skin or environment contaminants) usually indicate contamination, whereas *Staphylococcus aureus* presents a greater problem, indicating either a contaminant or another serious pathogen.

Electrolyte Measurements

Electrolyte imbalances are serious complications in the critically ill patient, and must be recognized and corrected at once. Electrolyte determinations frequently are ordered on an emergency basis. Accurate measurement is essential and to a large degree depends on the proper collection and handling of blood specimens.

text continues on page 74

T A B L E 6 – 2
SELECTED LABORATORY VALUES

Parameter	Normal values
Blood chemistry/electrolytes	
Blood urea nitrogen (BUN)	10–20 mg/dL
Serum creatinine	0.7–1.5 mg/dL
Creatinine clearance	Male: 110–150 mL/min Female: 105–132 mL/min
BUN: creatinine ratio	10:1
Hematocrit	Male: 44%–52% Female: 39%–47%
Hemoglobin	Male: 13.5–18.0 g/dL Female: 12.0–16.0 g/dL
Red blood cells	Male: 4600–6000/mm³ Female: 4200–5400/mm³
Mean corpuscular volume	80–95 mm³
Mean corpuscular hemoglobin	26–34 pg
Mean corpuscular hemoglobin concentration	32%–36%
Complete blood count	
Total leukocytes	4500–11,000/mm³
Myelocytes	0
Band neutrophils	150–400/mm³ (3%–5%)
Segmented neutrophils	3000–5800/mm³ (54%–62%)
Lymphocytes	1500–3000/mm³ (25%–33%)
Monocytes	300–500/mm³ (3%–7%)
Eosinophils	50–250/mm³ (1%–3%)
Basophils	15–50/mm³ (0%–0.75%)
Platelets	150,000–300,000/mm³
Reticulocytes	0.5%–1.5%
Red cell volume	Male: 20–36 mL/kg Female: 19–31 mL/kg

Parameter	Normal values
Blood chemistry/electrolytes	
Magnesium	1.3–2.1 mEq/L or 1.8–3.0 mg/dL
Chloride	97–110 mEq/L
Carbon dioxide	24–30 mmol/L
Phosphate	Adults: 2.5–4.5 mg/dL (1.8–2.6 mEq/L) Children: 4.0–7.0 mg/dL (2.3–4.1 mEq/L)
Zinc	77–137 µg/dL (by atomic absorption)
Lithium	0.8 mEq/L (therapeutic level 8–12 h after administration)
Serum proteins	
Total	6.0–8.00 g/dL
Albumin	3.5–5.5 g/dL
Globulin	1.5–3.0 g/dL
Lactate (arterial blood)	4.5–14.4 mg/dL
Serum ketones	Often >50 mg/dL in diabetic ketoacidosis. Usually <20 mg/dL in salicylate intoxication
Serum salicylates	Therapeutic range: 20–25 mg/dL Toxic range: >30 mg/dL
Anion gap	12–15 mEq/L
Aspartate aminotransferase (AST)	5–40 U/L
Alanine aminotransferase (ALT)	10–60 U/L
Alkaline phosphatase (ALP)	Varies with testing method

Plasma volume	Male: 25–43 mL/kg Female: 28–45 mL/kg
Clotting time	8–18 min
Prothrombin time	11–15 s
Iron	60–90 μg/dL
Total iron-binding capacity (TIBC)	250–420 μg/dL
Serum transferrin	>200 mg/dL (measured directly)
Partial thromboplastin time	Standard: 68–82 s Activated: 32–46 s
Fibrinogen	160–415 mg/dL
Serum osmolality	280–295 mOsm/kg
Serum amylase	25–125 U/L
Serum glucose	70–110 mg/dL
Serum electrolytes	
Sodium	135–145 mEq/L
Potassium	3.5–5.0 mEq/L
Calcium	Total: 8.9–10.3 mg/dL or 4.6–5.1 mEq/L Ionized: 4.6–5.1 mg/dL
Serum bilirubin	
Total	0.3–1.1 mg/dL
Direct	0.1–0.4 mg/dL
Indirect	0.2–0.7 mg/dL (total minus direct)
Lactate dehydrogenase (LDH)	100–190 mμ/mL
Urine chemistry/electrolytes*	
Sodium	80–180 mEq/24 h (varies with Na^+ intake
Potassium	40–80 mEq/24 h (varies with dietary intake)
Chloride	100–250 mEq/24 h
Calcium	100–150 mg/24 h (if on average diet)
Osmolality	Varies with dietary intake Typical urine is 500–800 mOsm/L (extreme range is 50–1400 mOsm/L)
Specific gravity (SG)	Usually about $1\frac{1}{2}$–3 times greater than serum osmolality 1.002–1.030 (most random samples have an SG of 1.012–1.025)
pH	4.5–8.0
Arterial blood gases	
pH	7.35–7.45
Pa_{O_2}	80–100 mm Hg
Pa_{CO_2}	38–42 mm Hg
Bicarbonate	22–26 mEq/L
Base excess	−2 to +2

*Measurement of electrolytes may be of limited value because of recent administration of diuretics or lack of knowledge of dietary intake.

T A B L E   6 – 3
EXAMPLES OF CONVERSIONS TO SYSTEME INTERNATIONAL (SI) UNITS

Component	System	Present Reference Intervals	Present Unit	Conversion Factor	SI Reference Intervals	SI Unit
Alanine aminotransferase (ALT)	Serum	5–40	U/L	1.0	5–40	U/L
Albumin	Serum	3.9–5.0	mg/dL	10	39–50	g/L
Alkaline phosphatase	Serum	35–110	U/L	1.00	35–110	U/L
Aspartate aminotransferase (AST)	Serum	5–40	U/L	1.00	5–40	U/L
Bilirubin	Serum					
Direct		0–0.2	mg/dL	17.10	0–4	μmol/L
Total		0.1–1.2	mg/dL	17.10	2–20	μmol/L
Calcium	Serum	8.6–10.3	mg/dL	0.2495	2.15–2.57	mmol/L
Carbon dioxide, total	Serum	22–30	mEq/L	1.00	22–30	mmol/L
Chloride	Serum	98–108	mEq/L	1.00	98–108	mmol/L
Cholesterol	Serum					
Age <29 y		<200	mg/dL	0.02586	<5.15	mmol/L
30–39 y		<225	mg/dL	0.02586	<5.80	mmol/L
40–49 y		<245	mg/dL	0.02586	<6.35	mmol/L
>50 y		<265	mg/dL	0.02586	<6.85	mmol/L
Complete blood count	Blood					
Hematocrit						
Men		42–52	%	0.01	0.42–0.52	1
Women		37–47	%	0.01	0.37–0.47	1
Hemoglobin						
Men		14.0–18.0	g/dL	10.0	140–180	g/L
Women		12–16	g/dL	10.0	120–160	g/L
Red cell count						
Men		$4.6–6.2 \times 10^8$	/mm^3	10^6	$4.6–6.2 \times 10^{12}$/L	
Women		$4.2–5.4 \times 10^8$	/mm^3	10^6	$4.2–5.4 \times 10^{12}$/L	
White cell count		$4.5–11.0 \times 10^3$	/mm^3	10^6	$4.5–11.0 \times 10^9$/L	
Platelet count		$150–300 \times 10^3$	/mm^3	10^6	$150–300 \times 10^9$/L	
Cortisol	Serum					
8 AM		5–25	μg/dL	27.59	140–690	nmol/L
8 PM		3–13	μg/dL	27.59	80–360	nmol/L
Cortisol	Urine	20–90	μg/24 h	2.759	55–250	nmol/24 h
Creatine kinase (CK)	Serum					
High CK group (black men)		50–520	U/L	1.00	50–520	U/L
Intermediate CK group (nonblack men, black women)		35–345	U/L	1.00	35–345	U/L
Low CK group (nonblack women)		25–145	U/L	1.00	25–145	U/L
Creatinine kinase isoenzyme, MB fraction	Serum	>5	%	0.01	>0.05	1

(continued)

T A B L E   6 - 3
EXAMPLES OF CONVERSIONS TO SYSTEME INTERNATIONAL (SI) UNITS (*Continued*)

Component	System	Present Reference Intervals	Present Unit	Conversion Factor	SI Reference Intervals	SI Unit
Creatinine	Serum	0.4–1.3	mg/dL	88.40	35–115	μmol/L
Men		0.7–1.3	mg/dL	88.40		
Women		0.4–1.1	mg/dL	88.40		
Digoxin, therapeutic	Serum	0.5–2.0	ng/mL	1.281	0.6–2.6	nmol/L
Erythrocyte indices	Blood					
Mean corpuscular volume (MCV)		80–100	μm^3	1.00	80–100	fL
Mean corpuscular hemoglobin (MCH)		27–31	pg	1.00	27–31	pg
Mean corpuscular hemoglobin concentration (MCHC)		32–36	%	0.01	0.32–0.36	1
Ferritin	Serum					
Men		29–438	ng/mL	1.00	29–438	μg/L
Women		9–219	ng/mL	1.00	9–219	μg/L
Folate	Serum	2.5–20.0	ng/mL	2.266	6–46	nmol/L
Follicle-stimulating hormone (FSH)	Serum					
Children		12 or <	mIU/mL	1.00	12 or <	IU/L
Men		2.0–10.0	mIU/mL	1.00	2.0–10.0	IU/L
Women, follicular		3.2–9.0	mIU/mL	1.00	3.2–9.0	IU/L
Women, midcycle		3.2–9.0	mIU/mL	1.00	3.2–9.0	IU/L
Women, luteal		2.0–6.2	mIU/mL	1.00	2.0–6.2	IU/L
Gases, arterial	Blood					
Po_2		80–95	mm Hg	0.1333	10.7–12.7	kPa
Pco_2		37–43	mm Hg	0.1333	4.9–5.7	kPa
Glucose	Serum	62–110	mg/dL	0.05551	3.4–6.1	mmol/L
Iron	Serum	50–160	μg/dL	0.1791	9–29	μmol/L
Iron-binding capacity (IBC)	Serum					
Total IBC		230–410	μg/dL	0.1791	41–73	μmol/L
Saturation		15–55	%	0.01	0.15–0.55	1
Lactic dehydrogenase	Serum	120–300	U/L	1.00	120–300	U/L
Luteinizing hormone	Serum					
Men		4.9–15.0	mIU/mL	1.00	4.9–15.0	IU/L
Women, follicular		5.0–25	mIU/mL	1.00	5.0–25	IU/L
Women, midcycle		43–145	mIU/mL	1.00	43–145	IU/L
Women, luteal		3.1–31	mIU/mL	1.00	3.1–31	IU/L
Magnesium	Serum	1.2–1.9	mEq/L	0.4114	0.50–0.78	mmol/L
Osmolality	Serum	278–300	mOsm/kg	1.00	278–300	mmol/kg
Osmolality	Urine	None defined	mOsm/kg	1.00	None defined	mmd/kg
Phenobarbital, therapeutic	Serum	15–40	μg/mL	4.306	65–175	μmol/L
Phenytoin, therapeutic	Serum	10–20	μg/mL	3.964	40–80	μmol/L

(continued)

T A B L E 6 – 3

EXAMPLES OF CONVERSIONS TO SYSTEME INTERNATIONAL (SI) UNITS (*Continued*)

Component	System	Present Reference Intervals	Present Unit	Conversion Factor	SI Reference Intervals	SI Unit
Phosphate (phosphorus, inorganic)	Serum	2.3–4.1	mg/dL	0.3229	0.75–1.35	mmol/L
Potassium	Serum	3.7–5.1	mEq/L, g/mL	1.00	3.7–5.1	mmol/L
Protein, total	Serum	6.5–8.3	g/dL	10.0	65–83	g/L
Sodium	Serum	134–142	mEq/L	1.00	134–142	mmol/L
Theophylline, therapeutic	Serum	5–20	μg/mL	5.550	28–110	μmol/L
Thyroid-stimulating hormone (TSH)	Serum	0–5	μIU/mL	1.00	0–5	mIU/L
Thyroxine	Serum	4.5–13.2	μg/dL	12.87	58–170	nmol/L
T_3 uptake ratio	Serum	0.88–1.19		1.00	0.88–1.19	1
Triiodothyronine (T_3)	Serum	70–235	ng/mL	0.01536	1.1–3.6	nmol/L
Triglycerides	Serum	50–200	mg/dL	0.01129	0.55–2.25	mmol/L
Urate (uric acid)	Serum					
Men		2.9–8.5	mg/dL	59.48	170–510	μmol/L
Women		2.2–6.5	mg/dL	59.48	130–390	μmol/L
Urea nitrogen	Serum	6–25	mg/dL	0.3570	2.1–8.9	mmol/L
Vitamin B$_{12}$	Serum	250–1000	pg/mL	0.7378	180–740	pmol/L

(From Fischbach, F.T. [2000]. *A manual of laboratory and diagnostic tests* [6th ed., pp. 1138–1141]. Philadelphia: Lippincott Williams & Wilkins.)

Potassium Level

Potassium is an electrolyte essential to body function. Approximately 98% of all body potassium is found in the cells; only small amounts are contained in the serum.

The kidneys normally do not conserve potassium. When large quantities of body fluid are lost without potassium replacement, a severe deficiency occurs. Chronic kidney disease and the use of diuretics may cause a potassium deficit. Adrenal steroids play a major role in controlling the concentration of potassium: hyperadrenalism causes increased potassium loss, with deficiency resulting; steroid therapy promotes potassium excretion.

An elevated potassium level results from potassium retention in renal failure or adrenal cortical deficiency. Hypoventilation and cellular damage also result in an elevated potassium level.

Because intracellular ions are not accessible for measurement, determination must be made on the serum. Because the concentration of potassium in the cells is roughly 15 times greater than that in the serum, the blood for potassium determination must be carefully drawn to prevent hemolysis.

BLOOD COLLECTION

Blood (2 mL) is drawn in a dry tube and allowed to clot or, preferably, placed under oil, which minimizes friction and hemolysis of the RBCs. The blood should be sent to the laboratory immediately because potassium diffuses out of the cells and gives a falsely high reading.

TEST RESULT

Normal serum range is 3.5 to 5.0 mEq/L (Fischbach, 2000).

Sodium Level

The main role of sodium is the control of the distribution of water throughout the body and the maintenance of a normal fluid balance.

The excretion of sodium is regulated to a large degree by the adrenocortical hormone aldosterone. Water excretion is regulated by antidiuretic hormone, and as long as these two systems are in harmony, the sodium and water remain in isosmotic proportion. Any change in the normal sodium concentration indicates that the loss or gain of water and sodium is in other than isosmotic proportion. Increased sodium levels may be caused by excessive infusions of sodium, insufficient water intake, or excess loss of fluid without a sodium loss, as in tracheobronchitis. Decreased sodium levels may be caused by excessive sweating accompanied by intake of large amounts of water by mouth, adrenal insufficiency, excessive infusions of nonelectrolyte fluids, or gastrointestinal suction accompanied with water by mouth.

BLOOD COLLECTION

Blood (3 mL) is drawn carefully to prevent hemolysis and placed in a dry tube or a tube with oil.

TEST RESULT

Normal serum range is 135 to 145 mEq/L.

Chloride Level

Chlorides are usually measured along with other blood electrolytes. The measurement of chlorides is helpful in diagnosing disorders of acid–base balance and water balance of the body. Chloride reciprocally increases or decreases in concentration whenever changes in concentration of other anions occur. In metabolic acidosis, a reciprocal rise in chloride concentration occurs when the bicarbonate concentration drops.

Elevation in the blood chloride level occurs in such conditions as Cushing's syndrome, hyperventilation, and some kidney disorders. A decrease in blood chloride levels may occur in diabetic acidosis and heat exhaustion, and after vomiting and diarrhea.

BLOOD COLLECTION

Venous blood (5 mL) is withdrawn and placed in a dry tube to clot.

TEST RESULT

Normal serum range is 97 to 110 mEq/L.

Calcium Level

Calcium, an essential electrolyte of the body, is required for blood clotting, muscular contraction, and nerve transmission. Only ionized calcium is useful, but because it cannot be satisfactorily measured, the total amount of body calcium is determined; 50% of the total is believed to be ionized (Metheny, 2000). In acidosis, there is a higher level of ionized calcium; in alkalosis, a lower level.

Hypocalcemia (decrease in blood calcium) occurs whenever impairment of the gastrointestinal tract, such as sprue or celiac disease, prevents absorption. Deficiency, which also occurs in hypoparathyroidism and in some kidney diseases, is characterized by muscular twitching and tetanic convulsions.

Hypercalcemia (excess of calcium in the blood) occurs in hyperparathyroidism and in respiratory disturbances where the carbon dioxide blood content is increased, such as in respiratory acidosis.

BLOOD COLLECTION

Venous blood (5 mL) is placed in a dry tube and allowed to clot. Analysis is performed on the serum.

TEST RESULT

Normal serum range in adults is 8.9 to 10.3 mg/100 mL. The range is slightly higher in children.

Phosphorus Level

Phosphorus metabolism is related to calcium metabolism and the serum level varies inversely with calcium.

Phosphorus concentrations may be increased in conditions such as hypoparathyroidism, kidney disease, or excessive intake of vitamin D. Decreased concentrations may occur in hyperparathyroidism, rickets, and some kidney diseases.

BLOOD COLLECTION

Because RBCs are rich in phosphorus, hemolysis must be avoided. Analysis is performed on the serum; 4 mL blood is placed in a dry tube to clot.

TEST RESULT

Normal serum range is 2.5 to 4.5 mg/100 mL (Metheny, 2000). In infants in the first year, the upper limit of the range rises to 6.0 mg/100 mL.

Venous Blood Measurements of Acid–Base Balance

The body's major buffer system is the bicarbonate (HCO_3)-carbonic acid (H_2CO_3) buffer system. Normally, there are 20 parts of bicarbonate to one part of carbonic acid. When deviations occur in the normal ratio, the pH changes. The change is accompanied by a change in bicarbonate concentration.

Carbon Dioxide Content

Carbon dioxide content is the measurement of the free carbon dioxide and bicarbonate content of the serum, which provides a general measure of acidity or alkalinity. An increase in carbon dioxide content usually indicates alkalosis; a decrease indicates acidosis. This test, along with clinical findings, is helpful in determining the severity and nature of the disorder. Measurement of pH is necessary for accuracy—a change in carbon dioxide does not always signify a change in pH because pH depends on the buffer ratio, and not the carbon dioxide content. When the carbon dioxide and pH are known, the buffer ratio can be determined.

An elevated carbon dioxide content is present in metabolic alkalosis, hypoventilation, loss of acid secretions (such as occurs in persistent vomiting or drainage of the stomach), and excessive administration of corticotropin or cortisone. A low carbon dioxide content usually occurs in loss of alkaline secretions such as in severe diarrhea, certain kidney diseases, diabetic acidosis, and hyperventilation.

BLOOD COLLECTION

Several procedures are now used to collect blood: collection in a heparinized syringe with immediate placement on ice; collection in a heparinized vacuum tube; or collection in a dry tube without an anticoagulant. The procedure used depends on the laboratory. The containers must always be filled with blood to prevent carbon dioxide from escaping.

 SAFE PRACTICE ALERT In all methods, it is important that the patient avoid clenching his or her fist; excess muscular activity of the arm can increase the carbon dioxide level in the blood.

TEST RESULT
Normal serum range is 22 to 31 mEq/L.

Blood pH

The pH, a measure of acidity, indicates the serum concentration of hydrogen ions. The pH becomes lower in acid conditions, such as hypoventilation, diarrhea, and diabetic acidosis. The pH rises in alkaline conditions, such as hyperventilation and excessive vomiting.

BLOOD COLLECTION
The blood is collected without stasis in a heparinized 2-mL syringe; the syringe is then capped. The blood may be drawn with a small-vein needle, the needle discarded, and the tubing tied off. The specimen is left in the syringe and packed in ice.

Loss of carbon dioxide from contact with the air is thus avoided and excess production of lactic acid by enzymic reaction reduced. Blood (5 mL) may also be collected in a green-stoppered vacuum tube containing heparin.

TEST RESULT
Normal blood pH ranges between 7.35 and 7.45.

Enzyme Analyses

Amylase

Amylase determination is helpful in the diagnosis of acute pancreatitis or the acute recurrence of chronic pancreatitis. Amylase is secreted by the pancreas; a rise in the serum level occurs when outflow of pancreatic juice is restricted. This test is usually performed on patients with acute abdominal pain or on surgical patients in whom injury may have occurred to the pancreas. Amylase levels usually remain elevated for only a short time (3 to 6 days).

BLOOD COLLECTION
Venous blood (6 mL) is allowed to clot in a dry tube.

TEST RESULT
Normal serum range is 4 to 25 U/mL. The range may depend on the normal values established by clinical laboratories because the method may be modified.

Lipase

Lipase determination is used for detecting damage to the pancreas and is valuable when too much time has elapsed for the amylase level to remain elevated. When secretions of the pancreas are blocked, the serum lipase level rises.

BLOOD COLLECTION
The test is performed on serum from 6 mL of clotted blood.

TEST RESULT
Normal serum level is 2 U/mL or less.

Acid Phosphatase

Acid phosphatase levels are useful in determining metastasizing tumors of the prostate. The prostate gland and prostatic carcinoma are rich in phosphatase but do not normally release the enzyme into the serum. Once the carcinoma has spread, it starts to release acid phosphatase, increasing the serum concentration. In addition to carcinoma of the prostate, other conditions that produce increased serum acid phosphatase levels are Paget's disease, hyperparathyroidism, metastatic mammary carcinoma, renal insufficiency, multiple myeloma, some liver disease, arterial embolism, myocardial infarction, and sickle cell crisis.

BLOOD COLLECTION
Blood (5 mL) is allowed to clot in a dry tube. Hemolysis should be avoided. Analysis should be immediate, or the serum should be frozen.

TEST RESULT
Normal serum range: 0–3, 1 ng/mL

Alkaline Phosphatase

Alkaline phosphatase is a useful test in diagnosing bone diseases and obstructive jaundice. In bone diseases, the small amount of alkaline phosphatase usually present in the serum rises in proportion to the number of new bone cells. When excretion of alkaline phosphatase is impaired, as in some disorders of the liver and biliary tract, the serum level rises and may give some evidence of the degree of blockage in the biliary tract.

BLOOD COLLECTION
Blood (5 mL) is drawn and the test is performed on the serum. Sodium sulfobromophthalein dye should be avoided.

TEST RESULT
Normal serum range is 13 to 39 U/mL.

Aspartate Aminotransferase

The transaminases are enzymes found in large quantities in the heart, liver, muscle, kidney, and pancreas cells. Any disease that damages these cells results in an elevated serum transaminase level. Clinical signs and other tests are used in diagnosis.

The aspartate aminotransferase (AST; formerly known as serum glutamic-oxaloacetic transaminase) level is used to distinguish between myocardial infarction and acute coronary insufficiency without infarction. It is also useful as a liver function test to follow the progression of liver damage or ascertain when the liver has recovered.

BLOOD COLLECTION
The test is performed on serum from 5 mL clotted blood.

TEST RESULT
Normal serum range is 10 to 40 U/mL. In myocardial infarction, the level is increased 4 to 10 times, whereas in liver involvement a high of 10 to 100 times normal may occur. The serum level remains elevated for approximately 5 days.

Alanine Aminotransferase

The alanine aminotransferase (formerly known as serum glutamic-pyruvic transaminase level is more specific for hepatic malfunction than the AST value.

BLOOD COLLECTION
The test is performed on 5 mL of serum.

TEST RESULT
Normal serum range is 10–60 U/L.

Serum Lactate Dehydrogenase

The transaminase lactate dehydrogenase is present in all tissues and in large quantities in the kidney, heart, and skeletal muscles. Elevated serum levels usually parallel AST levels. Elevation occurs in myocardial infarction and may continue through the sixth day. Elevations have been found in lymphoma, disseminated carcinoma, and some cases of leukemia.

BLOOD COLLECTION
Blood (3 mL) is collected and allowed to coagulate. Care must be taken to avoid hemolysis because only a slight degree may give an incorrect reading.

TEST RESULT
Normal serum range is 60 to 120 U/mL.

Liver Function Tests

Liver function tests measure albumin, globulin, and total protein levels and the albumin/globulin ratio. These tests may be useful in diagnosing kidney and liver disease or in judging the effectiveness of treatment. The chief role of serum albumin is to maintain osmotic pressure of the blood; globulin assists. The globulin molecule, because it is larger than the albumin, is less efficient in maintaining osmotic pressure and does not leak out of the blood. With the loss of albumin through the capillary wall, the body compensates by producing more globulin. The osmotic pressure is reduced, which may result in edema. Certain conditions, such as chronic nephritis, lipoid nephrosis, liver disease, and malnutrition, result in a lowered albumin concentration.

BLOOD COLLECTION
The test is performed on serum from 6 mL clotted blood.

TEST RESULT
Normal serum ranges:

- Total protein: 6.0 to 8.0 g/100 mL
- Albumin: 3.2 to 5.6 g/100 mL
- Globulin: 1.3 to 3.5 g/100 mL

Bilirubin (Direct and Indirect)

The bilirubin test, which is becoming less common, differentiates between impairment of the liver by obstruction and hemolysis. Bilirubin arises from the hemoglobin liberated from broken-down RBCs. It is the chief pigment of the bile, excreted by the liver. Impairment by obstruction of the excretory function of the liver leads to an excess of free (non–protein-bound) circulatory bilirubin. Measurement of free bilirubin (direct) usually indicates obstruction.

When increased RBC destruction (hemolysis) occurs, the increased bilirubin is believed to be bound to protein (indirect).

A total bilirubin determination detects increased concentration of bilirubin before jaundice appears.

BLOOD COLLECTION
The test is performed on serum from 5 mL clotted blood.

TEST RESULT
Normal serum range is 0.1 to 1.0 mg/100 mL.

Cholesterol

Cholesterol, a normal constituent of the blood, is present in all body cells. In various disease states, the cholesterol concentration in the serum may rise or fall. Cholesterol is transported in the blood by the low-density lipoproteins (LDLs; 60% to 75%) and high-density lipoproteins (HDLs; 15% to 35%). Cholesterol measurements may be part of a total lipid profile or an absolute test value.

BLOOD COLLECTION
The test is performed on serum from 5 mL of clotted blood.

TEST RESULT
Normal serum range is 120 to 260 mg/100 mL.

Lipoproteins

A high level of HDL indicates a healthy metabolic system in a patient free of liver disease. Very–low-density lipoproteins (VLDLs) are major carriers of triglyceride. Degradation of VLDL is a major source of LDLs.

Prothrombin Time

The prothrombin time, considered one of the most important screening tests in coagulation studies, indirectly measures the ability of the blood to clot. During the clotting process, prothrombin is converted to thrombin. It is thought that when the prothrombin level falls below normal, the tendency for the blood to clot in the blood vessel decreases. The prothrombin time is an important guide to drug therapy and is commonly used when anticoagulants are prescribed. The prothrombin content is reduced in liver diseases.

BLOOD COLLECTION
Venous blood (4 mL) is collected, added to the coagulant, and quickly mixed. It is important to avoid clot formation and hemolysis. The blood should be examined as soon as possible.

TEST RESULT
The normal value is between 11 and 18 seconds, depending on the type of thromboplastin used.

Thymol Turbidity

Thymol turbidity detects damaged liver cells and differentiates between liver disease and biliary obstruction. Turbidity is usually increased when the serum of patients with liver damage is mixed with a saturated solution of thymol. Turbidity is usually normal in biliary obstruction without liver damage.

BLOOD COLLECTION
The test is performed on serum from 5 mL of clotted blood.

TEST RESULT
Normal serum range is 0 to 4 U.

Kidney Function Tests

Creatinine

The creatinine test measures kidney function. Creatinine, the result of the breakdown of muscle creatine phosphate, is produced daily in a constant amount in each person. A disorder of kidney function prevents excretion, and an elevated creatinine value gives a reliable indication of impaired kidney function. A normal serum creatinine value does not indicate unimpaired renal function, however.

BLOOD COLLECTION
The test is performed on serum from 6 mL of clotted blood.

TEST RESULT
Normal serum range is 0.6 to 1.3 mg/100 mL.

Blood Urea Nitrogen

The BUN is a measure of kidney function. Urea, the end product of protein metabolism, is excreted by the kidneys. Impairment in kidney function results in an elevated concentration of urea nitrogen in the blood. Rapid protein metabolism may also increase the BUN above normal limits. The nonprotein nitrogen is a similar test for measuring kidney function.

BLOOD COLLECTION
The test is performed on blood or serum. Blood (5 mL) is added to an oxalate tube and shaken, or placed in a dry tube to clot.

TEST RESULT
Normal range is 10 to 20 mg/100 mL.

Blood Glucose Tests

The tests for blood glucose detect a disorder of glucose metabolism, which may result from any one of several factors, including inability of pancreatic islet cells to produce insulin, inability of the intestines to absorb glucose, and inability of the liver to accumulate and break down glycogen.

An elevated blood glucose level may indicate diabetes, chronic liver disease, or overactivity of the endocrine glands. A decrease in blood glucose concentration may result from an overdose of insulin, tumors of the pancreas, or insufficiency of various endocrine glands.

Fasting Blood Glucose

A fasting blood glucose test requires that the patient fast for 8 hours.

BLOOD COLLECTION
Venous blood (3 to 5 mL) is collected in an oxalate tube and shaken to prevent microscopic clots.

TEST RESULT
Normal serum range is 70 to 100 mg/100 mL (true blood glucose method). The normal value depends on the method of determination. Values greater than 120 mg/100 mL on several occasions may indicate diabetes mellitus.

Postprandial Blood Glucose Determinations

The **postprandial** blood glucose test, which is performed approximately 2 hours after the patient has eaten, is helpful in diagnosing diabetes mellitus. If the blood glucose value is above the upper limits of normal for fasting, a glucose tolerance test is performed.

The glucose tolerance test is indicated for the following conditions:

• When the patient has glycosuria
• When the fasting or 2-hour blood glucose concentration is only slightly elevated

- When Cushing's syndrome or acromegaly is a suspected diagnosis
- When the cause of hypoglycemia needs to be determined

BLOOD COLLECTION

First, a sample of blood is drawn from the fasting patient. The patient then drinks 100 g of glucose in lemon-flavored water (some laboratories use 1.75 g glucose/kg of ideal body weight). Blood and urine samples are then collected at 30, 60, 90, 120, and 180 minutes after ingestion of glucose.

TEST RESULT

Normal (true blood glucose) values are:

- Fasting blood glucose below 100 mg/100 mL
- Peak below 160 mg/100 mL in 30 or 60 minutes

The values depend on the standards used.

Blood Group Identification

Blood typing, which is one of the most common tests performed on blood, is required for all donors and for all patients who may need blood. The ABO system denotes four main blood groups: O, A, B, and AB. The designations refer to the particular antigen present on the RBCs: group A contains RBCs with the A antigen, B with B antigen, AB with A and B antigens, and O erythrocytes contain neither A nor B antigens.

When erythrocytes containing antigens are placed with serum containing corresponding antibodies under favorable conditions, agglutination (clumping) occurs. Therefore, an antigen is known as an agglutinogen and an antibody as an agglutinin.

A person's serum contains antibodies that react with corresponding antigens not usually found on the person's own cells. For instance, serum of group O contains antibodies A and B, which react with the corresponding antigens A and B found on the RBCs of group AB.

Although agglutination occurs in antigen–antibody reactions in the laboratory, hemolysis occurs in vivo; antibody attacks RBCs, causing rupture with liberation of hemoglobin. Hemolysis results from infusion of incompatible blood and may lead to fatal consequences.

Rh Factor and Blood Collection

The antigens belonging to the Rh system are D, C, E, c, and e. They are found in conjunction with the ABO group. The strongest of these factors is the Rho(D) factor, found in approximately 85% of the white population. Therefore, the Rho(D) factor is often the only factor identified in Rh typing. When the Rho(D) factor is not present, further typing may be done to identify the less common Rh factors.

Venous blood is collected and allowed to clot. Usually one tube (10 mL) sets up 4 to 5 U blood. Positive patient identification must be made before the blood is drawn; the name and number on the identification bracelet must correspond with that on the requisition and label. The label is placed on the blood tube at the patient's bedside.

Blood Typing

Various methods are used in typing blood, but all involve the same general principle. The patient's cells are mixed in standard saline serum samples of anti-A and of anti-B. The type of serum, A or B, that agglutinates the patient's cells indicates the blood group. As a double check, the patient's serum is mixed with saline suspensions of A and of B erythrocytes. The ABO group is determined on the basis of agglutination or absence of agglutination of A and of B cells (see Chapter 17).

Coombs' Test

Not all antibodies cause agglutination in saline; some merely coat the RBCs by combining with the antigen, which is not a visible reaction. Coombs' test is performed to detect antibodies that cannot cause agglutination in saline; these are known as incomplete antibodies. Anti-human globulin serum is used. This serum is obtained by the immunization of various animals, usually rabbits, against human gamma globulin by the injection of human serum, plasma, or isolated globulin. This antiserum, when added to sensitized RBCs (erythrocytes coated with incomplete antibody), causes visible agglutination.

DIRECT METHOD

Coombs' test is performed in two ways. The direct Coombs' test is performed when the patient's RBCs have become coated in vivo. This test is a valuable procedure in diagnosing the following:

- Erythroblastosis fetalis. The erythrocytes of the infant are tested for sensitization.
- Acquired hemolytic anemia. The patient may have produced an antibody that coats his or her own cells.
- Investigating reactions. The patient may have received incompatible blood that sensitizes the RBCs.

INDIRECT METHOD

The indirect Coombs' test detects incomplete antibodies in the serum of patients sensitized to blood antigens. It tests the patient's serum, in contrast to the patient's RBCs in the direct Coombs' test. When pooled, normal erythrocytes containing the most important antigens are exposed in a test tube to the patient's serum and to Coombs' serum, the RBCs agglutinate, indicating the presence of incomplete antibody. This test is valuable in the following:

- Detecting incompatibilities not found by other methods
- Detecting weak or variant antigens
- Typing with certain antiserums, such as anti-Duffy or anti-Kidd, which require Coombs' serum to produce agglutination
- Detecting anti-agglutinins produced by exposure during pregnancy

---

References and Selected Readings

Asterisks indicate references cited in text.

*Fischbach, F. T. (2000). *A manual of laboratory and diagnostic tests* (6th ed.). Philadelphia: Lippincott Williams & Wilkins.

*Fischbach, F. (1998). *Nurses' quick reference to common laboratory and diagnostic tests* (2nd ed.). Philadelphia: Lippincott Williams & Wilkins.

*Metheny, N. M. (2000). *Fluid and electrolyte balance* (3rd ed.). Philadelphia: Lippincott-Raven.

National Institute for Occupational Safety and Health. (1997). *NIOSH Alert: Preventing allergic reactions to natural rubber latex in the workplace* (NIOSH Publication 97-135). Washington, DC: Author.

Tereskerz, P.M., Bentley, M., Coyner, B.J., & Jagger, J. (1996, July/August). Percutaneous injuries in health care workers. *Adverse Exposure Prevention, 2*(4), 1–3.

Review Questions

Note: Questions below may have more than one right answer.

1. A glucose tolerance test is indicated in which of the following clinical situations?

   A. When the patient shows glycosuria

   B. When fasting or 2-hour blood glucose concentration is only slightly elevated

   C. When Cushing's syndrome or acromegaly is a suspected diagnosis

   D. To establish the cause of hypoglycemia

2. Venous sampling through the central vein may be required in which of the following situations?

   A. When it is difficult to obtain an adequate vein

   B. When the practitioner wants to minimize patient stress

   C. When frequent sampling is required

   D. When the patient requests it

3. Which of the following statements is true of creatinine?

   A. Elevated creatinine level is a reliable indication of impaired kidney function

   B. Normal serum creatinine level does not indicate normal renal function

   C. Normal serum creatinine level indicates normal renal function

   D. Decreased creatinine level is a reliable indication of impaired kidney function

4. Measurement of chlorides is effective in diagnosing what type of disorders?

   A. Acid–base

   B. Water balance

   C. Anion concentration

   D. Hypoventilation

5. Which of the following is true of blood glucose and serum lipid levels?

    A. They are increased by ingestion of food

    B. They are depressed after meals

    C. a only

    D. b only

6. To prevent an elevated serum potassium concentration, which of the following is true?

    A. Samples must be processed in a timely manner

    B. False measurements must be avoided

    C. Potassium should be allowed to diffuse from the cells

    D. Cells must be separated

7. Complications of venipuncture (for venous sampling) include which of the following?

    A. Syncope

    B. Continued bleeding

    C. Thrombosis

    D. All of the above

8. Coombs' test is valuable in which of the following clinical situations?

    A. Detecting incompatibilities not found by other methods

    B. Detecting weak or variant antigens

    C. Detecting anti-agglutinins produced by exposure during pregnancy

    D. All of the above

9. All of the following statements about prothrombin are true *except*:

    A. Prothrombin indirectly measures the ability of the blood to clot.

    B. Prothrombin is converted to thrombin during the coagulation cascade.

    C. A low level of prothrombin increases the blood's tendency to clot.

    D. Prothrombin is reduced in liver disease.

10. Urea is an end product of which metabolism?

    A. Carbohydrate

    B. Fat

    C. Protein

    D. Mineral

C H A P T E R 7

Fluid and

Electrolyte Balance

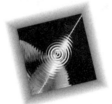

K E Y   T E R M S

Glycosuria
Homeostatic Mechanisms
Hyperkalemia
Hypernatremia
Hyponatremia
Hypovolemia

Metabolic Acidosis
Metabolic Alkalosis
Respiratory Acidosis
Respiratory Alkalosis
Stress Response

■ OVERVIEW OF PHYSIOLOGY

An imbalance of fluid or electrolyte levels is recognized as a threat to life. Never before has the nurse's responsibility for fluid and electrolyte administration and monitoring been more intense, regardless of the clinical setting in which care is provided. Patient outcomes depend in large part on specialty practice skills (see Chap. 10), which are based on a sound knowledge of physiology, in particular of fluid and electrolyte interplay.

The body loses water from the lungs, skin, gastrointestinal tract, and kidneys on a regular basis. There is a small, but significant, amount of water lost in the stool in normal conditions. The renal and stool loss of water is known traditionally as sensible water loss. Although the kidney can minimize the loss of fluid, it can never totally conserve water (Klotz, 1998).

The evaporative water loss that occurs through the lungs and skin is known as insensible water loss. Insensible water loss is independent of the body water and solute (electrolytes) and content. It does, however, depend on the patient's body surface area and environmental temperature (Adelman & Solhung, 1996).

At least 80% of all fluids administered today contain some electrolytes. Because electrolyte therapy is often a life-saving procedure, its safe and successful administration is essential. Knowledge of the fundamentals of fluid and electrolyte metabolism contributes to safe electrolyte therapy.

Abnormalities of body fluid and electrolyte metabolism present therapeutic problems. Treatment is complex when the mechanisms that normally regulate fluid volume, electrolyte composition, and osmolality are impaired. An understanding of these metabolic abnormalities enables the nurse to recognize the problems involved. Such clinical challenges arise in patients with renal insufficiency, adrenal insufficiency, adrenal hyperactivity, and other kinds of impaired organ function.

The two following examples illustrate how knowledge of fluid and electrolyte metabolism contributes to safe, successful therapy in the critically ill patient. Correction of a severe potassium deficit resulting from vomiting and diarrhea presents a problem in the dehydrated patient. Potassium replacement is imperative. However, potassium administered to patients with renal insufficiency results in potassium toxicity because the kidneys are unable to excrete electrolytes. The adverse effects of excess potassium on the heart muscle are arrhythmia and heart block. The nurse must recognize the importance of both hydrating the patient before potassium can be administered safely and watching for diminished diuresis that could necessitate a change in therapy. Once antidiuresis occurs, the potassium infusion must be interrupted and the physician notified.

Another example relates to therapeutic problems in patients with impaired liver function. When excessive loss of gastric fluid occurs, replacement fluid is necessary. Most deficits caused by gastric suction, unless severe, are treated with 0.9% sodium chloride in 5% dextrose in water or 0.33% sodium chloride in 5% dextrose in water. However, severe loss may call for gastric replacement fluids containing ammonium chloride, which can be potentially dangerous when administered to patients with impaired liver function. Ammonium chloride administered to a patient with severe liver damage may result in ammonia intoxication because of the liver's inability to convert ammonia to hydrogen ion and urea.

Fluid Content of the Body

The total body water content of a person varies with age, weight, and sex. The amount of water depends on the amount of body fat. Body fat is essentially water-free; the greater the fat content, the lower the water content.

In contrast to infants, who have a high body fluid content (approximately 70% to 80% of body weight), approximately 60% of a typical adult's weight consists of fluid (water and electrolytes; Fig. 7–1). After 40 years of age, mean values for total body fluid in percentage of body weight decrease for both men and women; a sex differentiation, however, remains. After 60 years of age, the percentage may decrease to 52% in men and 46% in women. With aging, lean body mass decreases in favor of fat (Metheny, 2000).

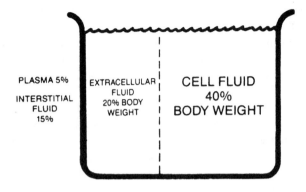

Figure 7–1. Total body fluid is 60% of body weight.

Fluid Compartments

The total body fluid is functionally allocated into two main compartments: the intracellular and the extracellular compartments (Fig. 7–2). The intracellular compartment consists of the fluid inside the cells and comprises approximately two thirds of the body fluid, or 40% of the body weight. The extracellular compartment consists of the fluid outside the body cells—the plasma, representing 5% of the body weight, and the interstitial fluid (fluid in tissues), representing 15% of the body weight (Metheny, 2000).

In newborn infants, the proportion is approximately three fifths intracellular and two fifths extracellular. This ratio changes and reaches the adult level by the time the infant is approximately 30 months of age.

There is one additional compartment, the transcellular compartment. The transcellular fluid is the product of cellular metabolism and consists of secretions such as gastrointestinal secretions and urine. An analysis of the secretions may assist the practitioner in tracing lost electrolytes and prescribing proper fluid and electrolyte replacement. Excessive fluid and electrolyte loss must be replaced to maintain fluid and electrolyte balance in the two main compartments. The amount of body water loss is easily computed by weighing the patient and noting loss of weight: 1 L body water is equivalent to 1 kg, or 2.2 lb, of body weight. Up to 5% weight loss in a child or adult may signify moderate fluid volume deficit—more than 5% may indicate severe fluid volume deficit. Weight changes are also valuable as indicators of body water gains—acute weight gain may indicate water excess.

Body Fluid Composition

Body fluid contains two types of solutes (dissolved substances): the electrolytes and the nonelectrolytes. The nonelectrolytes are molecules that do not break into particles in solution but remain intact. They consist of dextrose, urea, and creatinine.

Electrolytes are molecules that break into electrically charged particles called *ions*. The ion carrying a positive charge is called a *cation*, the ion with a negative charge, an *anion*. Potassium chloride is an electrolyte that, dissolved in water, yields

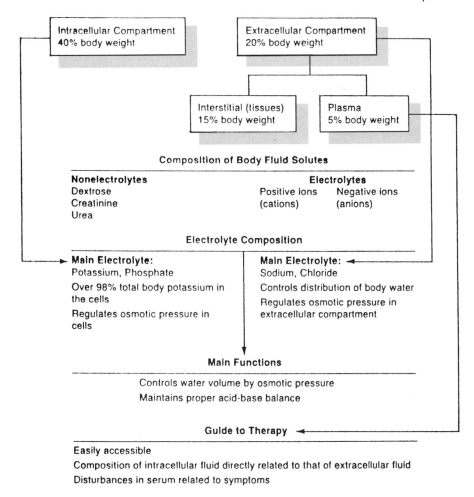

Figure 7–2. Total body water composition.

potassium cations and chloride anions. Chemical balance is always maintained; the total number of positive charges equals the total number of negative charges. The quantity of charges and their concentration is expressed as milliequivalents (mEq) per liter of fluid. Because the number of negative charges must equal the number of positive charges for chemical balance, the milliequivalents of cations must equal the milliequivalents of anions (Baxter Healthcare, 1999).

Electrolyte Composition

Each fluid compartment has its own electrolyte composition. The extracellular compartment (plasma and interstitial fluid) contains a high concentration of sodium, chloride, and bicarbonate and a low concentration of potassium. The composition of the intracellular fluid is quite different; the concentrations of potassium, magnesium, and phosphate are high, whereas the sodium and chloride concentrations are relatively low.

Electrolyte composition of the intracellular fluid is in part related to electrolyte composition of the plasma and interstitial fluids. Disturbances in the extracellular fluid are reflected in the patient's symptoms; this information, combined with an analysis of plasma, is thus a valuable guide to therapy.

Occasionally, however, the electrolyte determination of plasma may be misleading. For example, concentration of potassium in plasma may be high while there is a body deficit. This surplus is due to the shift of potassium from intracellular to extracellular fluid in the process of large potassium losses through the kidneys. Determination of plasma sodium may also present a false picture. In the case of an edematous cardiac patient, the plasma concentration may be low despite excess body sodium because total body sodium is equal to the sum of the products of volume times concentration in the various compartments.

Electrolytes serve two main purposes: to act in controlling body water volume by osmotic pressure and to maintain the proper acid–base balance of the body.

Characteristics of Fluids

Fluids are described in various ways. Significant characteristics of fluids include their concentration, or osmolality, as well as their acidity or alkalinity (pH).

Osmolality

Osmolality is the total solute concentration and reflects the relative water and total solute concentration because it is expressed per liter of serum. Osmotic pressure is determined by the amount of solutes in solution. If the extracellular fluid contains a relatively large number of dissolved particles and the intracellular fluid contains a small amount of dissolved particles, the osmotic pressure causes water to pass from the less concentrated fluid to the more concentrated. Therefore, fluid from the intracellular compartment passes into the extracellular compartment until the concentration becomes equal.

The unit of osmotic pressure is the osmole, and the values are expressed in milliosmoles (mOsm). Normal blood plasma has an osmolality of approximately 290 mOsm/kg water. The determination of serum osmolality is sometimes used to detect dehydration or overhydration. Measurement of sodium concentration also indicates the water needs of the body. At times, the osmolality reading may falsely indicate dehydration. Because the osmolality is the total solute concentration, nonelectrolytes are included in the reading. An elevated blood urea level can therefore increase the osmolality without exerting osmotic pressure. A determination of blood urea nitrogen (BUN) may supply a correction to the osmolality reading in cases of increased serum urea.

CONCENTRATION AS A METRIC VALUE
Concentrations of solutes may be expressed in several ways in addition to milliequivalents per liter, such as, milligrams per deciliter (mg/dL) or millimoles per

liter (mmol/L). Each of these units of measure may be used in a clinical setting. A milliequivalent of an ion is its atomic weight expressed in milligrams divided by the valence. This is the measure most often used for expressing small concentrations of electrolytes in body fluids because it emphasizes the principles that ions combine milliequivalent for milliequivalent.

CONCENTRATION AS A SYSTÈME INTERNATIONALE VALUE

Milligrams per 100 mL (deciliter) expresses the weight of the solute per unit volume. In those countries where the Système Internationale (SI) is used, electrolyte content in body fluids is expressed in millimoles. One mole (mol) of a substance is defined as the molecular (or atomic) weight of that substance in grams. For example, a mole of sodium is equivalent to 23 g (the atomic weight of sodium is 23). A millimole is one-thousandth of a mole, or the molecular or atomic weight expressed in milligrams. Therefore, a millimole of sodium equals 23 mg. Sometimes it is necessary to convert from millimoles per liter to milliequivalents per liter (Fig. 7–3). The following formula applies:

$$mEq/L = mmol/L \times valence$$

Acid–Base Balance

The acidity or alkalinity of a solution depends on the degree of hydrogen ion concentration. An increase in the hydrogen ions results in a more acid solution; a decrease results in a more alkaline solution. Acidity is expressed by the symbol pH, which refers to the amount of hydrogen ion concentration. A solution having a pH of 7 is regarded as neutral.

The extracellular fluid has a pH ranging from 7.35 to 7.45 and is slightly alkaline. When the pH of the blood is higher than 7.45, an alkaline condition exists; when lower than 7.35, an acid condition exists.

The biologic fluids, both extracellular and intracellular, contain a buffer system that maintains the proper acid–base balance. This buffer system consists of fluid with salts of a weak acid or weak base. A base or hydroxide neutralizes the effect of an acid. These weak acids and bases maintain pH values by soaking up surplus ions or releasing them; acids yield hydrogen ions, bases accept hydrogen ions.

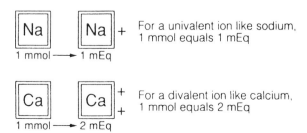

Figure 7–3. Millimoles versus milliequivalents for univalent and divalent ions.

The carbonic acid–sodium bicarbonate system is the most important buffer system in the extracellular compartment. The normal ratio is 1 part of carbonic acid to 20 parts of base bicarbonate, which represents 1.2 mEq carbonic acid to 24 mEq base bicarbonate.

Acid–Base Imbalance

Acid–base imbalances are normally the result of an excess or a deficit in either base bicarbonate or carbonic acid. Deviations of pH from 7.35 to 7.45 are combatted by the buffer system and by the respiratory and renal regulatory mechanisms. Two types of disturbance can affect the acid–base balance: respiratory and metabolic. A diagrammatic presentation of the following information is found in Figure 7–4.

RESPIRATORY DISTURBANCES

Respiratory disturbances affect the carbonic side of the balance by increasing or decreasing carbonic acid; when carbon dioxide unites with extracellular fluid, carbonic acid is produced.

Respiratory alkalosis results when excess carbon dioxide is exhaled during rapid or deep breathing. Carbonic acid is depleted because of the carbon dioxide loss. Respiratory alkalosis may occur as the result of emotional disturbances, such as anxiety and hysteria, and also from lack of oxygen or from fever (Metheny, 2000).

Symptoms are convulsions, tetany, and unconsciousness. Laboratory determination is a urinary pH above 7 and a plasma bicarbonate concentration less than 24 mEq/L. The body attempts to restore the ratio to normal by depressing the bicarbonate to compensate for the deficit in the carbonic acid.

Respiratory acidosis occurs when exhalation of carbon dioxide is depressed and the excess retention of carbon dioxide increases the carbonic acid. It may occur in conditions that interfere with normal breathing, such as emphysema, asthma, and pneumonia. Symptoms are weakness, disorientation, depressed breathing, and coma. Urinary pH is below 6, and plasma bicarbonate concentration is above 24 mEq/L. The bicarbonate increase is due to the body's attempt to restore the carbonic acid–bicarbonate ratio.

METABOLIC DISTURBANCES

Metabolic disturbances affect the bicarbonate side of the balance. Kidney function controls the bicarbonate concentration by regulating the amount of cations (hydrogen, ammonium, and potassium) in exchange for sodium ions to combine with the reabsorbed bicarbonate in the distal tubular lumen. As hydrogen ions are excreted, bicarbonate is generated, maintaining the proper acid–base balance of the blood. Ammonia excretion is increased in response to a high acidity; bicarbonate replaces the ammonia.

Metabolic alkalosis is a condition associated with excess bicarbonate; it occurs when chloride is lost. Chloride and bicarbonate are both anions, and the total number of anions must equal the total number of cations. When chloride anions are lost, the deficit must be made up by an equal number of anions to maintain electrolyte equilibrium; bicarbonate increases in compensation and alkalosis occurs.

Metabolic alkalosis is also associated with decreased levels of intracellular potassium. Potassium escapes from the cell into the extracellular fluid and is lost through the transcellular fluid. When body potassium is lost, the shift of sodium and hydrogen ions from the extracellular fluid causes alkalosis, whereas the increase of hydrogen ions in the intracellular fluid causes cellular acidosis.

Muscular hyperactivity, tetany, and depressed respiration are symptoms of metabolic alkalosis. Muscular hyperactivity and tetany are symptoms of the deficit in ionized calcium that exists in alkalosis. Laboratory determinations are urinary pH above 7, plasma pH above 7.45, and bicarbonate level above 24 mEq/L.

Treatment consists of the administration of fluids containing chloride to replace bicarbonate ions. An excess of bicarbonate ions is accompanied by potassium deficiency, so potassium must also be replaced.

Metabolic acidosis is a condition associated with a deficit in the bicarbonate concentration. This occurs when

- Excessive amounts of ketone acids accumulate, as in uncontrolled diabetes or starvation
- Inorganic acids, such as phosphate and sulfate, accumulate, as in renal disease
- Excessive losses of bicarbonate occur from gastrointestinal drainage or diarrhea

Acidosis may occur also from intravenous (IV) administration of excessive amounts of sodium chloride or ammonium chloride, causing chloride ions to flood the extracellular fluid.

Stupor, shortness of breath, weakness, and unconsciousness are the symptoms of metabolic acidosis, and laboratory determinations of metabolic acidosis are a urinary pH below 6, plasma pH below 7.35, and plasma bicarbonate concentration below 24 mEq/L.

Treatment and clinical management consist of increasing the bicarbonate level. Solutions of sodium lactate are often used, but because lactate ion must be oxidized to carbon dioxide before it can affect the acid–base balance, it is advisable to use sodium bicarbonate solutions, which are effective even when the patient is suffering from oxygen lack.

Homeostatic Mechanisms

The body uses regulating mechanisms called **homeostatic mechanisms** to maintain the constancy of body fluid volume, electrolyte composition, and osmolality. These mechanisms consist of the renocardiovascular, endocrine (adrenal, pituitary, and parathyroid), and respiratory systems. The kidneys, skin, and lungs are the main regulating agents (Metheny, 2000).

Kidney Function

The kidney plays a major role in fluid and electrolyte balance. To function adequately, the kidney depends on its own soundness as well as on the coordination of

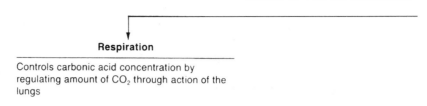

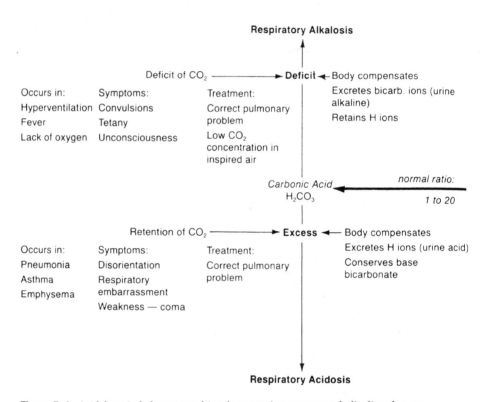

Figure 7–4. Acid–base imbalances resulting from respiratory or metabolic disturbances.

all the regulating organs. The distal renal tubules in the kidney are important in regulating body fluid. They selectively retain or reject electrolytes and other substances to maintain normal osmolality and blood volume. Sodium is retained and potassium is excreted (Baxter Healthcare, 1999).

The kidneys also play an important part in acid–base regulation. The distal tubule has the ability to form ammonia and exchange hydrogen ion (in the form of ammonia) for bicarbonate to maintain the carbonic acid–bicarbonate ratio.

Skin and Lung Function

The skin and lungs play an important role in fluid balance—the skin in loss of fluid through insensible perspiration and the lungs in loss of fluid by expiration. Normal

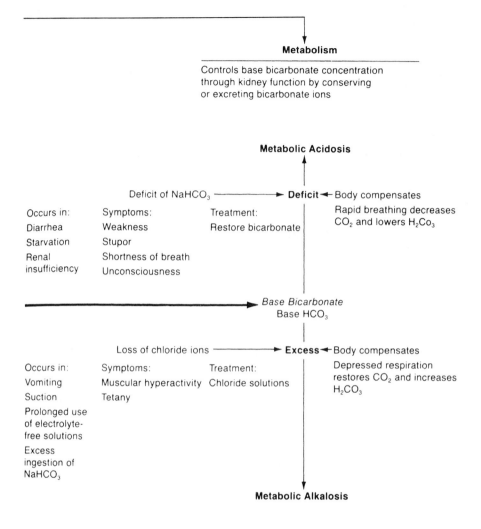

intake of 2500 mL from all sources delivers a loss of approximately 1000 mL in breath and perspiration, 1400 mL in urine, and 100 mL in feces.

Other Functions of Systems and Organs

The renocardiovascular system maintains fluid balance by regulating the amount and composition of urine. Plasma must reach the kidneys in sufficient volume to permit regulation of water and electrolyte balance. Renal disease, cardiac failure, shock, postoperative stress, and alarm impair this regulating mechanism.

The adrenal glands influence the retention or excretion of sodium, potassium, and water. These glands secrete aldosterone, a hormone that increases the reabsorption of sodium from the renal tubules in exchange for potassium, thus maintaining normal sodium concentration. Any stress, such as surgery, increases the secretion of aldosterone, thus increasing the reabsorption of sodium bicarbonate. Adrenal hyperactivity also increases the secretion of aldosterone and causes excess sodium retention. Excess loss of sodium occurs with adrenal insufficiency.

The pituitary gland is another important organ in the control of fluid and electrolyte balance. The posterior lobe of the pituitary releases antidiuretic hormone (ADH), which inhibits diuresis by increasing water reabsorption in the distal tubule. Increased concentration of sodium in the extracellular fluid stimulates the pituitary to release ADH. This hormone increases the reabsorption of water to dilute the sodium to the normal level of concentration. Increased body fluid osmolality, decreased body fluid volume, stress, and shock are conditions that increase ADH secretion. Increased body fluid volume, decreased osmolality, and alcohol inhibit ADH secretion.

The parathyroid glands, pea-sized glands embedded in the corners of the thyroid gland, regulate calcium and phosphate balance by means of parathyroid hormone (PTH). When the calcium level is low, PTH secretion is stimulated. This acts on bone to increase reabsorption of bone salts, releasing large amounts of sodium into ECF. When the extracellular calcium concentration is too high, PTH secretion is depressed so that almost no bone reabsorption occurs (Metheny, 2000).

The pulmonary system regulates acid–base balance by controlling the concentration of carbonic acid through exhalation or retention of carbon dioxide.

Electrolytes of Biologic Fluids

Electrolyte content of the intracellular fluid differs from that of extracellular fluid. Because specialized techniques are required to measure electrolyte concentration in the intracellular fluid, it is customary to measure the electrolytes in the extracellular fluid, chiefly plasma. Plasma electrolyte concentrations may be used to assess and manage patients with a diversity of electrolyte imbalances. Although some tests are performed on serum, the terms *serum electrolytes* and *plasma electrolytes* are used interchangeably. Table 7–1 identifies intracellular and extracellular concentrations and serum values. Table 7–2 lists plasma electrolyte values.

Potassium

Potassium is one of the most important electrolytes in the body. An excess or deficiency of potassium can cause serious impairment of body function and even result in death. Potassium is the main electrolyte in the intracellular compartment, which houses more than 98% of the body's total potassium. The healthy cell requires a high potassium concentration for cellular activity. When the cell dies, there is an exchange of potassium into the extracellular fluid with a transfer of sodium into the cell. This process also occurs to some degree when cellular metabolism is impaired, as in catabolism (breaking down) of cells from a crushing injury.

Serum concentration of potassium is 3.5 to 5.0 mEq/L. In the cell, the normal concentration is 115 to 150 mEq/L fluid. Variations from either of these levels can produce critical effects. When the potassium level is repeatedly above 5 to 6 mEq/L,

TABLE 7 – 1
INTRACELLULAR AND EXTRACELLULAR CONCENTRATIONS AND RELATED SERUM VALUES

Elements	Normal Concentrations and Values		
	Intracellular	Extracellular	Serum Laboratory Value
Na^+	10 mEq/L	142 mEq/L	135–145 mEq/L
K^+	140 mEq/L	4 mEq/L	3.5–5.2 mEq/L
Ca^{2+}	<1 mEq/L	5 mEq/L	8.5–10.5 mg/dL
Mg^{2+}	58 mEq/L	3 mEq/L	1.5–3.5 mEq/L
Cl^-	4 mEq/L	103 mEq/L	100–106 mEq/L
HCO_3^-	10 mEq/L	28 mEq/L	24–31 mEq/L
pH	7.0	7.4	7.35–7.45
Osmolality			280–294 mOsm/kg

a potassium excess is indicated; renal impairment usually is shown by renal function studies.

High serum concentrations have an adverse effect on the heart muscle and may cause cardiac arrhythmias. Serum potassium levels that are elevated two to three times normal may result in cardiac arrest. The electrocardiogram (ECG) may detect signs of potassium excess with peaked and elevated T waves; P waves later disap-

TABLE 7 – 2
PLASMA ELECTROLYTES

Electrolytes	mEq/L
Cations	
Sodium (Na^+)	142
Potassium (K^+)	5
Calcium (Ca^{2+})	5
Magnesium (Mg^{2+})	2
Total cations	154
Anions	
Chloride (Cl^-)	103
Bicarbonate (HCO_3^-)	26
Phosphate (HPO_4^{2-})	2
Sulfate (SO_4^{2-})	1
Organic acids	5
Proteinate	17
Total anions	154

(From Metheny, N. M. [2000]. Fluid and electrolyte balance [4th ed., p. 115]. Philadelphia: Lippincott Williams & Wilkins.)

pear, and, finally, decomposition and prolongation of the QRS complex (Metheny, 2000).

HYPOKALEMIA

Hypokalemia is the term that expresses a serum potassium level below normal, whereas **hyperkalemia** denotes a serum potassium level above normal. Hypokalemia, or a serum potassium level less than 4 mEq/L, may result when any one of the following conditions occurs:

- Total body potassium is below normal
- Concentration of potassium in cells is below normal

Hypokalemia and hyperkalemia are often caused by variations in the intake or output of potassium. A decreased intake of potassium from prolonged fluid therapy (lacking potassium replacement) may result in hypokalemia. Hypokalemia also may occur during a "starvation diet" because the kidneys do not normally conserve potassium. An increased loss of potassium usually results from polyuria, vomiting, gastric suction (prolonged), diarrhea, and steroid therapy.

Potassium deficiency may be unrelated to intake and output. It can be caused by a sudden shift of potassium from extracellular to intracellular fluid, such as that occurring from anabolism (building up of cells), healing processes, or the use of insulin and glucose in the treatment of diabetic acidosis. The shifts resulting from anabolism and healing processes are not usually of severe consequence unless accompanied by intervening factors. During treatment of diabetic acidosis, for example, the potassium shift may occur suddenly with grave consequences. When cells are anabolized, potassium shifts into the cells. When glucose is used in the treatment of diabetic acidosis, the glucose in the cells is quickly metabolized into glycogen for storage, causing a sudden shift of potassium from the extracellular to the intracellular fluid. This process results in hypokalemia.

The signs and symptoms of hypokalemia are malaise, skeletal and smooth muscle atony, apathy, muscular cramps, and postural hypotension. Treatment consists of administration of potassium orally or parenterally.

HYPERKALEMIA

Hyperkalemia may result from renal failure with potassium retention or from excessive or rapid administration of potassium in fluid therapy. It may also occur in conditions unrelated to retention or excessive intake. A sudden shift of potassium from intracellular to extracellular fluid results when catabolism of cells occurs, as in a crushing injury; potassium shifts from cells to plasma.

The signs and symptoms of hyperkalemia are similar to those of hypokalemia. In addition to the signs already listed, the patient may experience tingling or numbness in the extremities, and the heart rate may be slow. A serum potassium level greater than 5.5 mEq/L confirms the diagnosis.

Treatment consists of stopping the potassium intake. Dialysis may be necessary for a long-term renal problem. If the cause is a shift of potassium from cells to plasma, glucose and insulin therapy may be used.

Sodium

Sodium is the main electrolyte in the extracellular fluid; its normal concentration is 135 to 145 mEq/L plasma. The main role of sodium is to control the distribution of water throughout the body and maintain a normal fluid balance. Alterations in sodium concentration markedly influence the fluid volume: the loss of sodium is accompanied by water loss and dehydration; the gain of sodium, by fluid retention.

The body, by regulating urine output, normally maintains a constant fluid volume and isotonicity of the plasma. Urine output is controlled by ADH, secreted by the pituitary gland. If a hypotonic concentration results from a low sodium concentration, the fluid is drawn from plasma into the cells. The body attempts to correct this process; the pituitary inhibits ADH and diuresis results, with a loss of extracellular fluid. This loss of fluid increases sodium concentration to a normal level.

If a hypertonic concentration results from increased concentration of extracellular sodium, fluid is drawn from the cells. Again the body reacts, and the pituitary is stimulated to secrete ADH. This causes a retention of fluid that dilutes sodium to normal concentrations.

Therefore, increased sodium concentration stimulates the production of ADH, with retention of water, thus diluting sodium to the normal level; a decrease in sodium concentration inhibits the production of ADH, resulting in a loss of water, which raises the concentration of sodium to the normal level.

In the kidneys, sodium is reabsorbed in exchange for potassium. Therefore, with an increase in sodium there is loss of potassium; with a loss of sodium, there is an increase in potassium.

HYPONATREMIA

A sodium deficit (hyponatremia) may be present when the plasma sodium concentration falls below 135 mEq/L. It is caused by excessive sweating combined with a large intake of water by mouth (salt is lost and fluid increased, thus reducing the sodium concentration), excessive infusion of nonelectrolyte fluids, gastrointestinal suction plus water by mouth, and adrenal insufficiency, which causes large loss of electrolytes.

The symptoms of a sodium deficit are apprehension, abdominal cramps, diarrhea, and convulsions. Dehydration results from loss of sodium and leads to peripheral circulatory failure. When sodium and water are lost from the plasma, the body attempts to replace them by a transfer of sodium and water from the interstitial fluid. Eventually water is drawn from the cells and circulation fails; plasma volume cannot be sustained.

HYPERNATREMIA

Sodium excess (hypernatremia) may be present when the plasma sodium rises above 145 mEq/L. Its causes are excessive infusions of saline, diarrhea, insufficient water intake, diabetes mellitus, and tracheobronchitis (excess loss of water from lungs because of rapid breathing). The symptoms of sodium excess are dry, sticky mucous membranes, oliguria, excitement, and convulsions.

Calcium

Calcium is an electrolyte constituent of the plasma present in a concentration of approximately 4.6 to 5.1 mg/dL ionized calcium. The total calcium range is 8.5 to 10.5 mg/dL. Calcium serves several purposes. It plays an important role in formation and function of bones and teeth. As ionized calcium, it is involved in normal clotting of the blood and regulation of neuromuscular irritability.

The parathyroid glands control calcium metabolism. By acting on the kidneys and bones, PTH regulates the concentration of ionized calcium in the extracellular fluid. Impairment of this regulatory mechanism alters the calcium concentration. Hyperparathyroidism typically elevates the serum calcium level and decreases the serum phosphate level.

HYPOCALCEMIA

Calcium deficit may occur in patients who have diarrhea or problems in gastrointestinal absorption, extensive infections of the subcutaneous tissue, or burns. This deficiency can result in muscle tremors and cramps, excessive irritability, and even convulsions.

Calcium ionization is influenced by pH; it is decreased in alkalosis and increased in acidosis. With no loss of calcium, a patient in alkalosis may have symptoms of calcium deficit (eg, muscle cramps, tetany, and convulsions). This is due to the decreased ionization of calcium caused by the elevated pH.

A patient in acidosis may have a calcium deficit with no symptoms because the acid pH has caused an increased ionization of available calcium. Symptoms of calcium deficit may appear if acidosis is converted to alkalosis.

HYPERCALCEMIA

It is estimated that 98% of patients with hypercalcemia, or calcium excess, have cancer or hyperparathyroidism, or they use thiazide diuretics. Characteristics of hypercalcemia include muscular weakness, tiredness, lethargy, constipation, anorexia, polyuria, polydipsia, shortened QT interval on the ECG, and a serum calcium concentration greater than 10.5 mg/dL.

Other Electrolytes

The primary role of magnesium is in enzyme activity, where it contributes to the metabolism of both carbohydrates and proteins. Its serum concentration is 1.3 to 2.1 mEq/L. A magnesium deficit is a common imbalance in critically ill patients. Deficits may also occur in less acutely ill patients, such as those experiencing withdrawal from alcohol and those receiving parenteral or enteral nutrition after a period of starvation. Neuromuscular irritability, disorientation, and mood changes are indicative of hypomagnesemia. Hypermagnesemia is uncommon, but it may be seen in patients with advanced renal failure. Magnesium is excreted by the kidneys; therefore, diminished renal function results in abnormal renal magnesium retention.

Chloride, the chief anion of the extracellular fluid, has a plasma concentration of 97 to 110 mEq/L. A deficiency of chloride leads to a deficiency of potassium, and vice versa. There is also a loss of chloride with a loss of sodium, but because this loss can be compensated for by an increase in bicarbonate, the proportion differs.

Phosphate is the chief anion of the intracellular fluid; its normal level in plasma is 1.7 to 2.3 mEq/L.

■ OBJECTIVES OF FLUID AND ELECTROLYTE THERAPY

Parenteral therapy has three main objectives: to maintain daily body fluid requirements, to restore previous body fluid losses, and to replace present body fluid losses.

Maintenance

Maintenance therapy is aimed at providing all the nutrient needs of the patient: water, electrolytes, dextrose, vitamins, and protein. Of these needs, water is the most important. The body may survive for a prolonged period without vitamins, dextrose, and protein, but without water, dehydration and death occur.

Water

The body needs water to replace the insensible loss that occurs with evaporation from the skin and from expired air. An average adult loses from 500 to 1000 mL water per 24 hours through insensible loss. The skin loss varies with the temperature and humidity. Water balance is closely correlated to energy expenditure (Klotz, 1998).

Water is essential for kidney function. The amount needed depends on the amount of waste products to be excreted as well as the concentrating ability of the kidneys. Protein and salt increase the need for water.

A person's fluid requirements are based on age, height, weight, and amount of body fat. Because fat is water free, a large amount of body fat contains a relatively low amount of water; as body fat increases, water decreases in inverse proportion to body weight. The normal fluid and electrolyte requirements based on body surface area are more constant than when expressed in terms of body weight. Many of the essential physiologic processes such as heat loss, blood volume, organ size, and respiration have a direct relationship to the body surface area.

Fluid and electrolyte requirements are also proportionate to surface area, regardless of the patient's age. These requirements are based on square meters of body surface area and are calculated for a 24-hour period. Nomograms are available for determining surface area (see Chaps. 11 and 12). Table 7–3 highlights maintenance requirements based on body weight (assuming that renal function, gastrointestinal status, and temperature are normal).

Balanced electrolyte fluids are available for maintenance. The average requirements of fluid and electrolytes are estimated for a healthy person and applied to a patient. The balanced fluids contain electrolytes in proportion to the daily needs of the patient, but not in excess of the body's tolerance, as long as adequate kidney

T A B L E   7 – 3
FLUID AND ELECTROLYTE MAINTENANCE REQUIREMENTS*

Weight Range	Required Volume
Premature infant (<3 kg)	60 mL/kg
Younger patient	
0–10 kg	100 mL/kg/d
10–20 kg	1000 mL + 50 mL/kg/d
21 kg to average adult weight	1500 mL + 20 mL/kg/d
Adult (nonpregnant)	30–35 mL/kg/d

*Based on body weight.

function exists. When a patient's water needs are provided by these maintenance fluids, the daily needs of sodium and potassium are also met. For maintenance, 1500 mL/m^2 body surface area is administered over a 24-hour period.

Glucose

Because it is converted into glycogen by the liver, thereby improving hepatic function, glucose has an important role in maintenance. By supplying necessary calories for energy, it spares body protein and minimizes the development of ketosis caused by the oxidation of fat stores for essential energy in the absence of added glucose.

The basic daily caloric requirement of a 70-kg adult at rest is approximately 1600 calories. However, the administration of 100 g glucose a day is helpful in minimizing the ketosis of starvation; 100 g is contained in 2 L of 5% dextrose in water or 1 L 10% dextrose in water (Terry et al., 1995).

Protein

Protein is another nutrient important to maintenance therapy. Although a patient may be adequately maintained on glucose, water, vitamins, and electrolytes for a limited time, protein may be required to replace normal protein losses over an extended period. Protein is necessary for cellular repair, wound healing, and synthesis of vitamins and some enzymes. The usual daily protein requirement for a healthy adult is 1 g/kg body weight. Protein is available as amino acid. Taken orally, protein is broken down into amino acids before being absorbed into the blood.

Vitamins

Vitamins, although not nutrients in the true sense of the word, are necessary for the utilization of other nutrients. Vitamin C and the various B complex vitamins are the most frequently used in parenteral therapy. Because these vitamins are water soluble, they are not retained by the body but lost through urinary excretion.

Because of this loss, larger amounts are required parenterally to ensure adequate maintenance than may be required when administered orally. The B complex vitamins play an important role in the metabolism of carbohydrates and in maintaining gastrointestinal function. Vitamin C promotes wound healing and is frequently used for surgical patients. Vitamins A and D are fat-soluble vitamins, better retained by the body and not usually required by the patient on maintenance therapy.

Restoration of Previous Losses

Restoration of previous losses is essential when past maintenance has not been met—that is, when output exceeds intake. Severe dehydration may occur from failure to replace these losses. Therapy consists of replacing losses from previous deficits in addition to providing fluid and electrolytes for daily maintenance. Kidney status must be considered before electrolyte replacement and maintenance can be initiated; urinary suppression may result from decreased fluid volume or renal impairment. A hydrating fluid such as 5% dextrose in 0.2% (34.2 mEq) sodium chloride solution is administered. Urinary flow is restored if the retention is functional. The patient must be rehydrated rapidly to establish adequate urine output. Only after kidney function proves adequate can large electrolyte losses be replaced.

Replacement of Present Losses

Replacement of present losses of fluid and electrolytes is also an objective of therapy. Accurate measurement of all intake and output is a significant means of calculating fluid loss. Fluid loss may be estimated by determining loss of body weight; 1 L body water equals 1 kg, or 2.2 lb, body weight. An osmolality determination may indicate the water needs of the body. If necessary, a corrective BUN determination may be performed with the osmolality evaluation.

The type of replacement depends on the type of fluid being lost. A choice of appropriate replacement fluids is available. For example, excessive loss of gastric fluid may be replaced by fluids resembling the fluid lost, such as gastric replacement fluids. Excessive loss of intestinal fluid must be replaced by an intestinal replacement fluid. Examples of conditions that may result from current losses are alkalosis and acidosis (Table 7–4).

■ FLUID AND ELECTROLYTE DISTURBANCES IN SPECIFIC PATIENTS

Understanding how the endocrine system responds to stress helps the nurse better understand the imbalances and problems associated with stress. It also contributes to safe and successful parenteral therapy. The nurse anticipates what to expect, knows the possible dangers of imbalances, and recognizes early symptoms.

T A B L E   7 – 4
DIFFERENTIATING ACIDOSIS FROM ALKALOSIS

Cause	Physiology	Symptoms	Intervention
Alkalosis			
Loss of NaCl/KCl gastric fluid	Concentration of bicarbonate Gastric ions; anions must equal cations.	Slow shallow respiration, pallor	Administer appropriate replacement fluids.
	Ammonia is converted into urea and hydrogen ion. If liver fails to convert ammonia to urea, ammonia retention and toxicity result.	Sweating, tetany, coma	
Acidosis			
Excess fluid is alkaline.	Intestinal secretions contain excessive bicarbonate ions; with loss, chloride ion	Shortness of breath; rapid breathing	Administer base salts; ie, sodium lactate or sodium.

The Surgical Patient

The neuroendocrine response stimulated by many anesthetic agents is further heightened by surgical stress. Apprehension, pain, and duration and severity of trauma give rise to surgical stress and contribute to an increased endocrine response during the first 2 to 5 days after surgery.

The **stress response** is normal and is nature's way of protecting the body from hypotension resulting from trauma and shock. Correction is often unnecessary and may, in fact, be harmful.

The two major endocrine homeostatic controls affected by stress are pituitary gland and adrenal gland function (Fig. 7–5). The posterior pituitary controls quantitative secretions of ADH. The anterior pituitary controls secretions of corticotropin, which stimulates the adrenal gland to increase mineralocorticoid secretions (aldosterone) and glucocorticoid secretions (hydrocortisone). The adrenal medulla secretes vasopressors (epinephrine and norepinephrine) to help maintain the blood pressure.

A direct physiologic effect occurs when stress increases the secretions of these various hormones. When the posterior pituitary increases ADH secretions, antidiuresis is effected, thus helping maintain blood volume. When the anterior pituitary increases corticotropin secretions, the adrenal gland is stimulated to increase aldosterone.

Fluid Replacement Mechanisms

Adrenal hormones help maintain blood volume by causing the retention of sodium ions and chloride anions, thereby causing water retention and promoting the excretion of potassium (loss of cellular potassium ions causes loss of cellular water into extracellular space, where it is retained by ADH to maintain blood volume).

Hydrocortisone also promotes the catabolism of protein to provide necessary

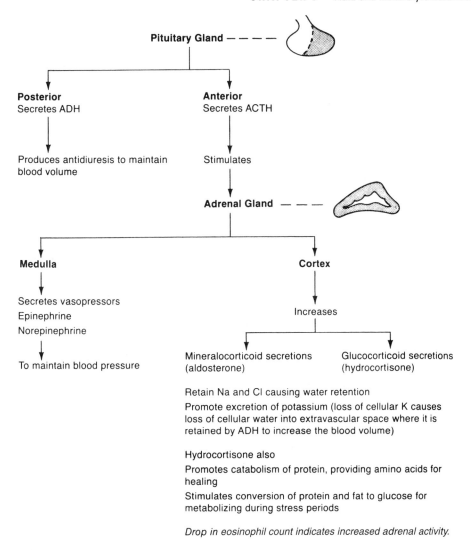

Figure 7–5. Endocrine response to stress.

amino acids for healing and stimulates the conversion of protein and fat to glucose for metabolism during the stress period. This metabolic activity may elevate the blood glucose level, a finding that may mistakenly suggest diabetes mellitus. A drop in the eosinophil count and an elevated level of serum 17-hydroxycorticosteroid hormones indicate increased adrenal activity.

Fluid Needs

Accurate records of intake and output are important for assessing fluid requirements and preventing serious fluid imbalances during the early postoperative period. The daily requirement of 1500 to 2000 mL varies with the patient's needs. Caution must be taken not to overhydrate the patient—the intake should be adequate but should not exceed the fluid losses.

The adrenocortical secretions, increased by trauma and stress of surgery, cause some water and sodium retention. This retention may be severe enough to present a false picture of oliguria. Excessive quantities of nonelectrolyte fluids (such as 5% dextrose in water) administered at a time when antidiuresis is occurring may cause hyponatremia, a serious electrolyte imbalance.

In hyponatremia, the serum sodium concentration is lower than normal. Water-yielding fluids, infused in excess of the body's tolerance, expand the extracellular compartment, lowering the electrolyte concentration. By osmosis, water invades the cells, with a resulting excess accumulation of intracellular fluid. Usually there is no edema because edema is the result of an excess accumulation of fluid in the extracellular compartment.

Symptoms of water excess include confusion, hallucinations, delirium, weight gain, hyperventilation, muscular weakness, twitching, and convulsions. If these occur during the early postoperative stages, the nurse should suspect water excess. This is of particular concern in young and elderly patients. Serious consequences, even death, can result.

Restricting the fluid intake may correct mild water excess, but for more severe cases, the administration of high concentrations of sodium chloride may be indicated. The electrolyte concentration of the plasma, increased by the concentrated saline, causes an increase in the osmotic pressure, drawing fluid from the cells for excretion by the kidneys.

Parenteral therapy during the stress period often consists of administering conservative amounts of 5% dextrose in water. Because some sodium retention results from the endocrine response to stress, care must be taken to avoid administering excessive quantities of saline at a time when there is an interference in the elimination of salt. During this early period, the physician frequently gives 5% dextrose in quarter- or half-strength saline to avoid sodium excess.

In hypernatremia, the serum sodium concentration is higher than normal. This excess may expand extracellular fluid volume or cause edema and possible disruption of cellular function (in potassium-depleted patients, the sodium may replace the intracellular potassium).

Symptoms of sodium excess include flushed skin, elevated temperature, dry and sticky mucous membranes, thirst, and a decreased or absent urine output. Treatment consists of reducing the salt and water intake and promoting diuresis to eliminate the excess salt and water from the plasma.

Nutrient Needs

Among the various nutrients needed by postsurgical patients are carbohydrates, proteins, fats, potassium, and vitamins.

CARBOHYDRATES

Carbohydrates provide an indispensable source of calories for the postoperative patient unable to receive food orally. When carbohydrate supplies are inadequate, the body uses its own fat to supply calories; the by-products are ketone bodies. These acid bodies neutralize bicarbonate and produce metabolic acidosis. The only by-products excreted in the metabolism of carbohydrates are water and carbon dioxide.

By providing calories for essential energy, carbohydrates also reduce catabolism of protein. During the **stress response,** the renal excretion of nitrogen (from the catabolism of protein) exceeds the intake. By reducing the protein breakdown, glucose helps prevent a negative nitrogen balance.

Carbohydrates do not provide adequate calories for the patient receiving prolonged therapy. Approximately 1 L of 5% dextrose in water provides 170 calories. Many liters, a volume too great for most patients to tolerate, would be required to provide a patient with 1600 calories. Greater concentrations of glucose, 20% and 50%, may be administered to provide calories for patients unable to tolerate large volumes of fluid (eg, patients with renal insufficiency). The concentrated fluids must be administered slowly for glucose utilization to occur. Rapid administration results in diuresis; the concentrated glucose acts as a diuretic, drawing interstitial fluid into the plasma for excretion by the kidneys.

ALCOHOL

Alcohol fluids may be administered to the postoperative patient for nutritional and physiologic benefits. Nutritionally, the alcohol supplements calories provided by the glucose, with 1 g ethyl alcohol yielding 6 to 8 calories. Because alcohol is quickly and completely metabolized, it provides calories for essential energy, sparing fat and protein. Metabolized in preference to glucose, alcohol allows the infused glucose to be stored as glycogen.

Physiologically, alcohol produces a sedative effect, reducing pain; 200 to 300 mL of a 5% solution per hour produces sedation without intoxication in the average adult. Alcohol also inhibits the secretion of ADH, promoting water excretion.

Fluids containing alcohol, particularly hypertonic fluids, can cause phlebitis. These fluids, if allowed to infiltrate, may cause tissue necrosis. The IV catheter should be carefully inserted within the lumen of the vessel and inspected frequently to detect any infiltration.

PROTEIN

Patients who receive parenteral fluid therapy for a prolonged time require protein for cellular repair, wound healing, and growth. Stress states accompanying surgical procedures and trauma frequently result in protein deficiency.

During the stress period, increased secretions of glucocorticoids from the adrenal cortex cause protein breakdown and the conversion of protein and fat to glucose for energy. More urinary nitrogen is lost than normal. When nitrogen loss exceeds intake, the patient is said to be in a negative balance. This response to stress is normal. However, protein losses must be counteracted; preservation of body cell mass is essential. A depleted body cell mass can be restored only by hyperalimentation. Approximately 1 g/kg body weight is required by a healthy adult to replace normal protein loss.

Because of their high ammonia level, extreme caution is required if proteins are administered to patients with hepatic insufficiency or emaciation. Organ-specific formulas have been developed for the patient with renal or hepatic disease.

SAFE PRACTICE ALERT   Supplemental medications added to the fluid may result in incompatibilities. Always check with the pharmacist before adding any medication to fluids.

Fluids, once opened, must be used immediately. Storing a partially used container of fluid in the refrigerator for future use provides a culture medium for the growth of bacteria. No fluids that are cloudy or contain precipitate should be used.

LIPID EMULSIONS

Lipid emulsions offer calories and essential fatty acids for metabolic processes. They are rich in calories, yielding 9 kcal/g, compared with 4 kcal/g from carbohydrates.

POTASSIUM

Once the stress period passes, adrenal activity decreases and diuresis begins. At this time, usually after the second to the fifth postoperative day, potassium is given daily to prevent a deficit. Potassium is not conserved by the body but is lost in the urine. Electrolyte maintenance fluids may be used or potassium may be added to parenteral fluids. When potassium is added to parenteral fluids, the container, bag, or bottle should be thoroughly shaken to mix and dilute the potassium. Potassium should never be added to a hanging container while the infusion is running. Such an action could result in a bolus injection of the drug. Rapid injection, which increases the drug concentration in the plasma, can result in trauma to the vessel wall and even in cardiac arrest. Potassium should never be given by IV push or bolus administration.

 SAFE PRACTICE ALERT   Potassium chloride must be used with considerable caution and is considered potentially dangerous if administered when renal function is impaired. A buildup of potassium, caused by the kidney's inability to excrete salts, can prove hazardous; arrhythmia and heart block can result from the effect of excess potassium on the heart muscle.

The status of the kidneys must be considered. If kidney function is inadequate, the patient must be **rehydrated.** During this infusion, the nurse must watch for diminished diuresis and notify the physician if antidiuresis occurs.

An amount of 40 mEq/L usually is sufficient to replace normal potassium loss. It is usually infused over an 8-hour period. Premixed potassium replacement fluids are available in a variety of strengths.

In extreme cases of hypokalemia, when the serum potassium concentration is lower than 2.0 mEq/L, the nurse may need to infuse potassium at a much faster rate—but not faster than 40 mEq/hour. When the serum potassium concentration reaches 2.5 mEq/L and ECG manifestations of hypokalemia diminish, the rate should be decreased to no more than 10 mEq/hour, using a fluid that contains no more than 30 mEq/L.

Continuous ECG monitoring is required when high doses of potassium are infused. The fluid containing potassium should be conspicuously labeled and must never be used when positive pressure is indicated—rapid infusion may result in cardiac arrest.

Potassium is irritating to the vein and may cause a great deal of discomfort, especially if infused into a vein where a previous venipuncture has been performed. Slowing the rate may decrease the pain.

VITAMINS

The B complex vitamins and vitamin C are usually added to parenteral fluids if, after 2 or 3 days, the patient cannot take fluids orally. Vitamin C is important in promoting healing in the surgical patient, and B complex vitamins aid carbohydrate metabolism.

Nursing Diagnoses

Nursing diagnoses for the postsurgical patient should address relevant fluid and electrolyte disturbances. Table 7–5 lists selected nursing diagnoses.

The Burn Patient

The patient with burns presents special clinical challenges (Table 7–6). The "rule of nines" (Table 7–7) is commonly used to estimate burned area. The body's surface area is divided into sections equal to 9% or multiples of 9% of total body area. The portion of the areas sustaining second- or third-degree burns is identified and the percentages are totaled to represent the full percentage of body surface area burned. This method may be inaccurate in children, and other charts are available for accurately determining percentage of body surface area burned.

Formulas for Fluid Replacement

Fluid requirements for the first 24 hours after burn injury range from 2 to 4 mL/kg body weight depending on percentage of body surface area burned. Several factors must be considered, including age of the patient, size and depth of the burn, type of fluid, and complication factors such as inhalation injury, electrical burns, or multiple trauma. Numerous formulas have been developed for this purpose, but an ideal rate of infusion is one that maintains perfusion, as reflected by a urinary output of 0.5 mL/kg body weight per hour in the adult patient.

Assessment

Ongoing assessment of the patient is needed to tailor fluid replacement to individual patient needs. Monitoring parameters include urine volume, sensorium, vital signs, and central venous pressure.

T A B L E   7 – 5

SELECTED NURSING DIAGNOSIS FOR POSTOPERATIVE PATIENT AFTER ABDOMINAL SURGERY

Nursing Diagnosis	Etiologic Factors	Defining Characteristics
Fluid volume deficit related to actual fluid loss and third-space fluid shift during surgical procedure	Vomiting after reaction to anesthesia GI suction Third-space fluid shift at surgical site	Postural tachycardia Postural hypotension initially; later, low blood pressure in all positions Decreased skin turgor Decreased capillary refill time Oliguria (<30 mL/h in adult) Weight change depends on cause (decreased if actual fluid loss, as in GI suction; usually increased if fluid loss is due to third-space shift, provided parenteral fluids are given in an attempt to correct hypovolemia)
Altered tissue perfusion (renal) related to hypotension during surgical procedure	Hypotensive effects of anesthesia Hypovolemia due to direct or indirect loss of fluid **Hypovolemia** due to inadequate parenteral fluid replacement	Oliguria or polyuria in presence of elevated serum creatinine
Alteration in sodium balance (hyponatremia) related to excessive ADH activity	Major surgery with its premedication, anesthesia, decreased blood volume, and postoperative pain results in increased ADH release (causing water retention with sodium dilution)	Serum sodium <135 mEq/L May be asymptomatic if Na >120 mEq/L Lethergy, confusion, nausea, vomiting, anorexia, abdominal cramps, muscular twitching
Alteration in acid–base balance (metabolic alkalosis) related to vomiting or gastric suction	Vomiting after reaction to anesthesia Gastric suction, particularly if patient is allowed to ingest ice chips freely	Tingling of fingers, toes, and circumoral region, due to decreased calcium ionization pH >7.45, bicarbonate above normal, chloride below normal
Altered nutrition (less than body requirements) related to negative nitrogen balance after surgical stress, and inadequate caloric intake	Catabolic response to stress of surgery Inability to tolerate oral feedings during first few postoperative days due to decreased GI motility, anorexia, nausea, and general discomfort Failure of health care providers to administer sufficient calories via the parenteral route	Weight loss of approximately $\frac{1}{4}$ to $\frac{1}{2}$ lb/d in adult (provided fluids are not abnormally retained) Perhaps a decrease in serum albumin, transferrin, and retinol binding protein levels (although delivery of a large volume of blood products or the long half-life of certin secretory proteins can interfere with correct interpretation)

ADH, antidiuretic hormone; GI, gastrointestinal.
(From Metheny, N. M. [2000]. *Fluid and electrolyte balance* [4th ed., p. 308]. Philadelphia: Lippincott Williams & Wilkins.)

T A B L E   7 – 6
THE BURN PATIENT RECEIVING PARENTERAL FLUID THERAPY

	Objectives of Parenteral Fluid Therapy	Intervention
First 48 Hours	Maintain fluid volume relative to loss and third spacing.	Ensure venous access; administer fluids consistent with clinical condition and physician's orders.
Intravascular to interstitial shift	Treat volume depletion.	Administer albumin as ordered to correct third-space shifts; maintain fluid status and IV access.
Shock	Re-establish inadequate tissue perfusion.	Replace water, electrolytes, and protein (from skin).
	Deliver oxygen to metabolically active cells.	In a patient with a 50% burn, edema, may exceed total plasma volume of patient.
Dehydration	Water and electrolyte loss is less than protein loss.	Determine replacement needs and administer fluids adequate to restore perfusion.
	Osmotic pressure draws fluid from undamaged tissues.	Administer colloids to draw fluid in from other compartments—thus increasing vascular volume.
Hypovolemia	Exudate from burned area, water (as vapor) and blood loss occurs.	Ensure adequate venous access to provide fluid volume.
Decreased urine output	Ensure that kidneys are working before administration of potassium replacement.	Replace blood volume and maintain kidney output.
	Antidiuretic hormone exceeds water reabsorption by kidneys.	Monitor intake and output to ensure elimination of wastes.
Potassium excess	Hyperkalemia; cells release potassium and decreased renal flow obstructs normal excretion of potassium.	Fluid replacement initiated with albumin, dextran, Hetastarch.
Sodium deficit	Due to loss of edema and exudate.	Administer nonelectrolyte solution to replace insensible losses.
Metabolic acidosis	Due to accumulation of fixed acids released from tissue.	Administer only enough fluid to maintain blood volume/urine output.
Second to third day	Shift from interstitial fluid to plasma.	Reduce parenteral fluids accordingly; excess urinary output is evidence of need to decrease fluid therapy.
	Avoid circulatory overload.	Maintain fluid volume and monitor patient for hypophosphatemia.

Urine output is the best indicator of adequate fluid resuscitation. Adult output should be 30 to 50 mL/hour. Lack of urine output or a substantial decrease in volume may be attributed to inadequate fluid replacement, gastric dilation, or renal failure. Daily weights are a helpful tool for monitoring the burned patient. A weight gain of 15% to 20% may indicate fluid retention. Adequacy of tissue perfusion is measured by assessing the patient's sensorium. Sensorium should remain normal with appropriate fluid replacement unless other factors, such as head injury, are present.

TABLE 7-7
RULE OF NINES FOR ESTIMATING
BURNED BODY AREA IN ADULTS

Body Parts	Percentage of Body
Head and neck	9
Anterior trunk	18
Each arm	9
Posterior trunk	18
Genitalia	1
Each leg	18

Vital signs should be monitored hourly in the burned patient. Blood pressure should remain at near normal values with consideration given to the patient's baseline pressure. Temperature may be elevated and tachycardia may be present. Rate and character of respirations should be evaluated. Peripheral pulses and capillary refill times should be monitored. Vasoconstriction of unburned skin is a compensatory response to help preserve normal blood flow in the hours immediately after a severe burn. Hence, unburned skin may be cool to the touch and appear pale at first.

Central venous and arterial pressure monitoring may be used to evaluate the effects of fluid replacement. Signs of inadequate fluid replacement are decreased urine output, thirst, restlessness and disorientation, hypotension, and increased pulse rate. Circulatory overload may be suspected with an elevated central venous pressure reading (15 to 20 cm H_2O), shortness of breath, and moist crackles.

The Diabetic Patient

Diabetic acidosis is an endocrine disorder causing complex fluid and electrolyte disturbances. It occurs when a lack of insulin prevents the metabolism of glucose, and essential calories are provided instead by the catabolism of the patient's own fat and protein. Acidosis results from the accumulation of acid by-products. Understanding the physiologic changes in diabetic acidosis aids the nurse in detecting early imbalances and the subsequent treatment.

Physiologic Changes in Diabetic Acidosis

Lack of insulin prevents cellular metabolism of glucose and its conversion into glycogen. Glucose accumulates in the bloodstream (hyperglycemia). When the blood glucose level rises above 180 mg/100 mL, glucose spills over into the urine (**glycosuria**). The kidneys require 10 to 20 mL water to excrete 1 g glucose; water excretion increases (polyuria).

The body's fat and protein are used to provide necessary calories for energy. Ketone bodies, metabolic by-products, reduce plasma bicarbonate, and acidosis occurs.

Fluid and Electrolyte Disturbances

Dehydration results from excessive fluid and electrolyte losses. Cellular fluid deficit occurs when water is drawn from the cells by the hyperosmolality of the blood. Extracellular fluid deficit occurs when

- Glycosuria increases the urinary output
- Ketone bodies raise the load on the kidneys and increase the water to excrete them
- Vomiting causes loss of fluid and electrolytes
- Oral intake falls because of the patient's condition
- Hyperventilation is induced by the acidotic state

DEHYDRATION

Dehydration lowers the blood volume, decreasing renal blood flow, and the kidneys produce less of the ammonia needed to maintain acid–base balance. Severe dehydration may lower the blood volume enough to cause circulatory shock and oliguria.

KETOSIS

Ketosis is the excessive production of ketone bodies in the bloodstream. Ketone bodies are the end products of oxidation of fatty acids. Ketosis occurs when a lack of insulin results in excessive fatty acids being converted by the liver to ketones and the decreased utilization of ketones by the peripheral tissues. Electrolytes and ketone bodies, retained in high serum concentration, increase the acidosis; the increase in the number of hydrogen ions, from the retention of ketone bodies, may drop the blood pH to 7.25 and lower. The bicarbonate anions decrease to compensate for the increase in ketone anions and may drop the bicarbonate level to 12 mEq/L or less.

HYPERGLYCEMIC HYPEROSMOLAR NONKETOTIC COMA

Hyperglycemic hyperosmolar nonketotic coma (HHNC) is a syndrome that may develop in the middle-aged or elderly type 2 diabetic patient. The condition is often associated with the stress of cardiovascular disease, infection, or pharmacologic treatment with steroids or diuretics. It is also precipitated by too-rapid infusion of parenteral nutrition fluid. Blood glucose levels may reach 4000 mg/dL but without the ketosis of diabetic ketoacidosis. Fluid volume deficit is profound and may lead to death. Underlying factors contributing to development of diabetic ketoacidosis or HHNC are found in Table 7–8. Signs and symptoms of diabetic acidosis are summarized in Box 7–1.

Parenteral Therapy

Insulin is given to metabolize the excess glucose and combat diabetic acidosis. Because absorption is quickest by the bloodstream, insulin is administered IV. When

T A B L E 7 – 8

FACTORS CONTRIBUTING TO DEVELOPMENT OF DKA OR HHNC IN SUSCEPTIBLE PERSONS

DKA	HHNC
Infections, illness	Chronic renal disease
Physiologic stresses (eg, trauma, surgery, myocardial infarction, dehydration, pregnancy)	Chronic cardiovascular disease
	Acute illness, infection
Psychological/emotional stress	Surgery burns, trauma
Omission/reduction of insulin	Hyperalimentation, tube feedings
Failure of insulin delivery system (pump)	Peritoneal dialysis
Excess alcohol intake	Mannitol therapy
	Pharmacologic agents
	Chlorpromazine
	Cimetidine
	Diazoxide
	Diuretics (thiazide, thiazide related, and loop diuretics)
	Glucocorticoids and immunosuppressive agents
	L-Asparaginase
	Phenytoin
	Propranolol

DKA, diabetic ketoacidosis; HHNC, hyperglycemic hyperosmolar nonketotic coma.
(From Metheny, N. M. [2000]. *Fluid and electrolyte balance* [4th ed., p. 335]. Philadelphia: Lippincott Williams & Wilkins.)

given subcutaneously or intramuscularly, the slower rate of absorption of insulin may be further decreased by peripheral vascular collapse in the presence of shock. The dose of insulin, when administered by continuous infusion, is usually 4 to 8 U/hour. Many types of infusion pumps are available to ensure accurate and continuous administration of medications.

Parenteral fluids are administered to increase the blood volume and restore kidney function. Early treatment of the hypotonic patient usually consists of the administration of 0.9% sodium chloride solution to replace sodium and chloride losses and to expand the blood volume. Later, hypotonic fluids with sodium chloride may be used. Bicarbonate replacement may be necessary in severe acidosis.

Potassium administration is contraindicated in the early treatment of diabetic acidosis. During the later stages (10 to 24 hours after treatment), the plasma potassium level falls; improved renal function increases potassium excretion and, in anabolic states, as the glucose is converted into glycogen, a sudden shift of potassium from extracellular fluid to intracellular fluid further lowers the plasma potassium level. If the patient is hydrated, potassium should be administered when the plasma potassium concentration falls.

A severe potassium deficit may occur if symptoms are not recognized and early treatment begun. Symptoms include weak grip, irregular pulse, weak picking at the bedclothes, shallow respiration, and abdominal distention.

BOX 7–1 **Signs and Symptoms of Diabetic Ketoacidosis**

Intravenous nurses need to become familiar with the signs and symptoms that characterize diabetic acidosis. By recognizing impending diabetic acidosis, early treatment may be initiated and complications prevented.

Hyperglycemia—When a lack of insulin prevents glucose metabolism, glucose accumulates in the bloodstream.

Glycosuria—When the accumulation of glucose exceeds the renal tolerance, glucose spills over into the urine.

Polyuria—Osmotic diuresis occurs when the heavy load of nonmetabolized glucose and the metabolic end products increase the osmolality of the blood. In turn, the increased renal solute load requires more fluid for excretion.

Thirst—Cellular dehydration, arising from the osmotic effect produced by hyperglycemia, prompts thirst.

Weakness and fatigue—The body's inability to use glucose and a potassium deficit lead to weakness and fatigue.

Flushed face—Flushing results from the acid condition.

Rapid, deep breathing—The body's defense against acidosis, expiration of large amounts of carbon dioxide reduces carbonic acid and increases the pH of the blood.

Acetone breath—Increased accumulation of acetone bodies results in acetone-scented breath.

Nausea and vomiting—Distention resulting from atony of gastric muscles causes nausea and vomiting.

Weight loss—An excess loss of fluid (1 L body water equals 2.2 lb, or 1 kg, body weight) and a lack of glucose metabolism contribute to weight loss.

Low blood pressure—Severe fluid deficit leads to low blood pressure.

Oliguria—Decreased renal blood flow that results from a severe deficit in fluid volume produces oliguria.

References and Selected Readings

Asterisks indicate references cited in text.

*Adelman, R.D., & Solhung, M.J. (1996). Pathophysiology of body fluids and fluid therapy. In: R.E. Behrman, R.M. Kliegman, & A.M. Arvin (Eds.). *Nelson textbook of pediatrics* (15th ed., pp. 185–222). Philadelphia: W.B. Saunders.

*Baxter Healthcare. (1999). *Clinical guide to infusion therapy: Water and electrolytes.* S. Weinstein (Ed.).

Foley, M. (1998). *Lippincott's need-to-know nursing reference facts* (pp. 107–148). Philadelphia: Lippincott-Raven.

*Klotz, R. (1998). The effects of intravenous solutions on fluid and electrolyte balance. *Journal of Intravenous Nursing, 21,* 20–24.

*Metheny, N.M. (2000). *Fluid and electrolyte balance* (4th ed.). Philadelphia: Lippincott Williams & Wilkins.

*Terry, J., et al. (1995). *Intravenous therapy: Clinical principles and practice* (pp. 111–115). Philadelphia: W.B. Saunders.

Review Questions

1. Which of the following contributes to respiratory alkalosis?
   A. Inhalation of excess carbon dioxide
   B. Shallow breathing
   C. Depletion of carbon monoxide
   D. Increased oxygenation

2. Symptoms associated with respiratory alkalosis include all of the following *except:*
   A. Tetany
   B. Unconsciousness
   C. Convulsions
   D. Lethargy

3. Respiratory acidosis is associated with all of the following *except:*
   A. Diabetes
   B. Emphysema
   C. Asthma
   D. Pneumonia

4. Kidney function controls which of the following?
   A. Bicarbonate concentration
   B. Sodium exchange
   C. Intracellular potassium
   D. Acidity

5. Symptoms associated with metabolic alkalosis include:
   A. Muscular hyperactivity
   B. Tetany
   C. Depressed respirations
   D. Increased respirations

6. Metabolic acidosis is associated with a deficit of:
   A. Bicarbonate ion
   B. Carbon dioxide
   C. Sodium
   D. Chloride

7. Symptoms of metabolic acidosis include which of the following?
   A. Stupor and shortness of breath
   B. Weakness and unconsciousness
   C. A plasma pH below 7.35
   D. Plasma bicarbonate concentration below 24 mEq/L

8. Regulating mechanisms that maintain the constancy of body fluid volume, electrolyte composition, and osmolality include which of the following?
   A. Renocardiovascular
   B. Endocrine
   C. Respiratory
   D. Kidneys

9. Normal intake of 2500 mL from all sources is estimated to deliver a loss of approximately how many milliliters in breath and perspiration?
   A. 1000 mL
   B. 1400 mL
   C. 1500 mL
   D. 1800 mL

10. The major electrolyte of the intracellular compartment is which of the following?
    A. Calcium
    B. Potassium
    C. Sodium
    D. Bicarbonate

C H A P T E R   8

Principles of Parenteral

Fluid Administration

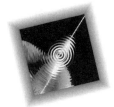

K E Y   T E R M S

Acidifying Infusions
Alkalizing Fluid
Dehydration
Hemolysis
Hexoses
Hydrating Fluids
Hyperinsulinism
Hypertonic

Hypodermoclysis
Hypotonic
Isotonic
Osmolality
Osmolarity
Turgor
Water Intoxication

■ PARENTERAL FLUIDS

To help enhance patient outcomes, a knowledge of parenteral fluids is essential when delivering infusion therapy. This is particularly important because rapid and critical changes in fluid and electrolyte balance may be caused by infusates.

Until the 1930s, intravenous (IV) fluids consisted of dextrose and saline solutions. Little was known about electrolyte therapy (see Chap. 1). Today, however, more than 200 types of commercially prepared fluids are available. The great increase in their use leads to a more common occurrence of fluid and electrolyte disturbances. Moreover, with the increased administration of fluids in alternative care settings, nurses must know the chemical composition and the physical effects of the infusions they administer.

▲ **Legal Issues:** FLUID INJECTIONS

Nurses have a legal and professional responsibility to know the:

• Normal amount of any IV infusion they administer
• Desired and untoward effects of any IV infusion
• Type of fluid, the amount, and the rate of flow, determined only after the physician has carefully assessed the patient's clinical condition

■ INTRAVENOUS INFUSION

Today, methods of infusion have changed dramatically, and small-volume parenteral *fluids* may be administered as a secondary infusate or in a volume-controlled reservoir for electronic drug delivery.

An infusion is usually regarded as an amount of fluid in excess of 100 mL designated to be infused parenterally because the volume must be administered over a long period. However, when medications are administered as a piggyback (secondary to and delivered with the initial infusion) small-volume (50 to 100 mL) parenteral infusion, a shorter period (usually 30 to 60 minutes) may be required. However, volumes of 150 to 200 mL may require more than 1 hour. Today, methodologies have changed to be consistent with the clinical needs of patients, and alternate delivery systems are readily available (see Chaps. 11 and 12).

Intravenous fluids are mistakenly referred to as *IV solutions*. The term *solution* is defined in the *United States Pharmacopeia* (USP) as a liquid preparation that contains one or more soluble chemical substances usually dissolved in water. Solutions are distinguished from injections, for example, because they are not intended for administration by infusion or injection (USP, 1999). Moreover, methods of preparation may vary widely. The USP refers to parenteral fluids as injections, and methods of preparation must follow standards for injection.

Official Requirements of Intravenous Fluids

Intravenous injections must meet the tests, standards, and all specifications of the USP applicable to injections. This includes quantitative and qualitative assays of infusions, including tests for pyrogens and sterility.

Particulate Matter

Each fluid container must be carefully examined to detect cracks. The fluid must be examined for cloudiness or particles. The final responsibility falls on the pharmacist and the nurse who administers the fluid. Tests to detect particulate matter, and standards for an acceptable limit of particles, have been established by the USP. A large-volume injection for single-dose infusion meets the requirements of the test if it contains not more than 50 particles per milliliter that are equal to or larger than 10.0 μm, and not more than 5 particles per milliliter that are equal to or larger than 25.0 m in effective linear dimension.

pH Value

The pH indicates hydrogen ion concentration or free acid activity in solution. All IV fluids must meet the pH requirements set forth by the USP. Most of these requirements call for a fluid that is slightly acid, usually ranging in pH from 3.5 to 6.2. Dextrose requires a slightly acid pH to yield a stable fluid. Heat sterilization, used for all commercial fluids, contributes to the acidity. It is important to know the pH of the commonly used IV fluids because it may affect the stability of an added drug and cause the drug to deteriorate. The acidity of dextrose fluids has been criticized for its corrosive effect on veins.

Tonicity

Parenteral fluids are classified according to the tonicity of the fluid in relation to the normal blood plasma. The **osmolality** of blood plasma is 290 mOsm/L. Fluid that approximates 290 mOsm/L is considered isotonic. IV fluids with an osmolality significantly higher than 290 mOsm (+50 mOsm) are considered **hypertonic,** whereas those with an osmolality significantly lower than 290 mOsm (−50 mOsm) are **hypotonic.**

Parenteral fluids usually range from approximately one-half isotonic (0.45% sodium chloride) to 5 to 10 times **isotonic** (25% to 50% dextrose). The tonicity of the fluid infused into the circulation affects fluid and electrolyte metabolism and may result in disastrous clinical disturbances (see Table 8–1 for more information on the effects of isotonic, hypertonic, and hypotonic fluids).

Knowing the osmolality of the infusion and the physical effect it produces alerts the nurse to potential fluid and electrolyte imbalances. The choice of veins used for an infusion is affected by the tonicity of the fluid; hyperosmolar fluids, for example, must be infused through veins that carry a large blood volume to dilute the fluid and prevent trauma to the vessel.

The tonicity of the fluid also affects the rate at which it can be infused. Hypertonic dextrose infused rapidly may result in diuresis and dehydration.

TABLE 8–1
RESULTS OF INFUSION OF FLUIDS WITH DIFFERENT TONICITIES

Tonicity	Effect
Hypertonic fluid	Increases osmotic pressure of plasma Draws fluid from the cells
Hypotonic fluid	Lowers the osmotic pressure of plasma Causes fluid to invade the cell
Isotonic fluid	Increases extracellular volume

Because of the direct and effective role osmolality plays in IV therapy, the nurse involved in administering IV fluids needs to be familiar with various terms and calculations. For instance, the *osmotic pressure* is proportional to the total number of particles in the fluid. The *milliosmole* (mOsm) is the unit that measures the particles or the osmotic pressure. By converting milliequivalents to milliosmoles, an approximate osmolality may be determined. A quick method for approximating the tonicity of IV injections follows.

FLUIDS CONTAINING UNIVALENT ELECTROLYTES

Each milliequivalent is approximately equal to a milliosmole because univalent electrolytes, when ionized, carry one charge per particle. An injection of normal saline (0.9% sodium chloride) contains 154 mEq sodium and 154 mEq chloride per liter of fluid, making a total of 308 mEq/L, or approximately 308 mOsm/L.

FLUIDS CONTAINING DIVALENT ELECTROLYTES

Because each particle carries two charges when ionized, the milliequivalents per liter of fluid or the number of electrical charges per liter when divided by the charge per ion (2) gives the approximate number of particles or milliosmoles per liter. As an example, when 20 mEq magnesium sulfate is introduced into a liter of fluid, each ionized particle carries two charges. By dividing 20 mEq or 20 charges by 2, an approximate 10 particles or 10 mOsm/L is reached for each component, or 20 mOsm/L total.

The osmolality of electrolytes in solution may be accurately computed but involves using the atomic weight and the concentration of the given electrolytes in milligrams per liter. The methods for accurately computing the osmolality of an electrolyte, such as potassium (K), in solution follow:

$$\frac{\text{milligrams of electrolyte/L}}{(\text{Atomic weight}) \, (\text{valance})} = \text{milliosmoles/L}$$

Example: 35 mg K/L

$$\frac{35}{35 \times 1} = 1 \text{ mOsm/L}$$

Example: 40 mg K/L

$$\frac{40}{40 \times 2} = 0.5 \text{ mOsm/L}$$

■ KINDS AND COMPOSITION OF FLUIDS

Various kinds of fluids are used for parenteral injections. These fluids are composed of dextrose in water, sodium chloride in water, sodium bicarbonate, ammonium chloride, and other substances.

Dextrose in Water

When glucose is part of parenteral injections, it is usually referred to as dextrose, a designation by the USP for glucose of requisite purity. Dextrose is available in concentrations of 2.5%, 5%, 10%, 20%, and 50% in water. To determine the osmolality or the caloric value of a dextrose fluid, the nurse needs to know the total number of grams or milligrams per liter. Because 1 mL water weighs 1 g, and 1 mL is 1% of 100 mL, milliliters, grams, and percentages can be used interchangeably when calculating solution strength. Thus, dextrose 5% in water equals 5 g dextrose in 100 mL, or 50 g dextrose in 1 L. The metabolic effects of dextrose are listed in Box 8–1.

Calories

Hexoses (glucose or dextrose and fructose) do not yield 4 calories per gram, as do dietary carbohydrates (eg, starches). Each gram of hydrous or anhydrous dextrose provides approximately 3.4 or 3.85 calories, respectively. One liter of 5% glucose infusion yields 170 calories; 1 liter of 10% glucose yields 340 calories (American Association of Healthcare Pharmacists [ASHP], 1998) (see Chap. 16 for more information).

Tonicity of Dextrose 5% in Water

Dextrose 5% in water is considered an isotonic fluid because its tonicity approximates that of normal blood plasma, or 290 mOsm/L. Because dextrose is a nonelectrolyte and the total number of particles in solution does not depend on ionization, the osmolality of dextrose fluids is determined differently from that of electrolyte fluids. One millimole (one formula weight in milligrams) of dextrose represents

---

BOX 8–1 **Metabolic Effects of Dextrose**

- Provides calories for essential energy
- Improves hepatic function because glucose is converted into glycogen by the liver
- Spares body protein (prevents unnecessary breakdown of protein tissue)
- Prevents ketosis or excretion of organic acid (which may occur when fat is burned by the body without an adequate supply of glucose)
- Stored intracellularly in the liver as glycogen, causes the shift of potassium from the extracelluar to the intracellular fluid compartment (*Note: This effect is desired as treatment for hyperkalemia. It is achieved by infusing dextrose and insulin.*)

1 mOsm (unit of osmotic pressure). One millimole of monohydrated glucose is 198 mg, and 1 liter of 5% dextrose in water contains 50,000 mg. Thus:

$$\frac{50,000 \text{ mg}}{198} = 252 \text{ mOsm/L}$$

pH Value

The USP requirement for the pH of dextrose fluids is 3.5 to 6.5. This broad range may at times contribute to an incompatibility in one bottle of dextrose and not in another when an additive is involved (see Chap. 16).

Indications for Use

Dextrose fluids are used for patients with dehydration, hyponatremia, and hyperkalemia. They are also vehicles for drug delivery and nutrition.

DEHYDRATION
In cases of **dehydration,** dextrose 2.5% in water and dextrose 5% in water provide immediate hydration for medical as well as surgical patients. Dextrose 5% in water is considered isotonic only in the bottle. Once infused into the vascular system, the dextrose is rapidly metabolized, leaving water. The water decreases the osmotic pressure of the blood plasma and invades the cells, providing immediately available water to dehydrated tissues.

HYPERNATREMIA
If the patient is not in circulatory difficulty with extracellular expansion, dextrose 5% in water may be administered to decrease the concentration of sodium.

MEDICATION ADMINISTRATION
Many of the drugs for IV therapy are added to infusions of dextrose 5% in water.

NUTRITION
Concentrations of dextrose 20% and 50% in conjunction with electrolytes provide long-term nutrition. Insulin is frequently added to prevent overtaxing the islet tissue of the pancreas.

 SAFE PRACTICE ALERT   Because the kidneys do not store potassium, prolonged fluid therapy with electrolyte-free fluids may result in **hypokalemia.** This happens when cells are anabolized by the metabolism of glucose, and potassium shifts from the extracellular to the intracellular fluid. Conversely, when renal function is impaired, IV potassium should be used cautiously. Remain alert for signs of **hyperkalemia.** If such signs develop, notify the physician and be prepared to replace fluid *components* with more appropriate electrolytes.

HYPERKALEMIA

Infusions of dextrose in high concentration with insulin cause anabolism (buildup of body cells), which results in a shift of potassium from the extracellular to the intracellular compartment, thereby lowering the serum potassium concentration.

Dangers of Use

Among abnormalities resulting from infusion of dextrose are dehydration, hypokalemia, hyperinsulinism, and water intoxication.

DEHYDRATION

Osmotic diuresis occurs when dextrose is infused at a rate faster than the patient's ability to metabolize it. A heavy load of nonmetabolized glucose increases the osmolality of the blood and acts as a diuretic; the increased solute load requires more fluid for excretion. A normal, healthy person with a urine specific gravity of 1.029 to 1.032 requires 15 mL water to excrete 1 g solute, whereas people with poor kidney function or low concentrating ability of the kidneys require much more water to excrete the same amount of solute (Metheny, 2000).

HYPERINSULINISM

A rapid infusion of hypertonic carbohydrate solutes may result in **hyperinsulinism**. In response to a rise in blood glucose level, extra insulin pours from the beta cells of the pancreatic islets in an attempt to metabolize the infused carbohydrate. Terminating the infusion may leave excess insulin in the body, resulting in symptoms such as nervousness, sweating, and weakness caused by the severe hypoglycemia that may be induced. Typically, after infusion of hypertonic dextrose, a small amount of isotonic dextrose is administered to cover the excess insulin (Metheny, 2000).

WATER INTOXICATION

An imbalance resulting from an increase in the volume of the extracellular fluid from water alone is known as **water intoxication**. Prolonged infusions of isotonic or hypotonic dextrose in water may cause this condition, which is compounded by stress and leads to inappropriate release of antidiuretic hormone (ADH) and fluid retention. The average adult can metabolize water at a rate of approximately 35 to 40 mL/kg/day, and the kidney can safely metabolize only approximately 2500 to 3000 mL/day in an average patient receiving IV therapy (Metheny, 2000). Under stress, the patient's ability to metabolize water decreases (Box 8–2).

BOX 8–2 **Potential Consequences of Infusing Specific Fluids**

- **Cellular dehydration** may result from excessive infusions of hypertonic fluids.
- **Water intoxication** results when hypotonic fluid is infused beyond the patient's tolerance for water.
- **Circulatory overload** can result from isotonic fluid administration.

Administration

Isotonic dextrose may be administered through a peripheral vein. Hyperosmolar fluids, such as dextrose 50% in water, should be infused into the superior vena cava through central venous access. Hypertonic dextrose administered through a peripheral vein with small blood volume may traumatize the vein and cause thrombophlebitis. Infiltration can result in tissue necrosis.

Sodium-free dextrose injections should not be administered by **hypodermoclysis** (direct administration into subcutaneous tissue to enhance hydration). Dextrose fluids, by attracting body electrolytes in the pooled area of infusions, may cause peripheral circulatory collapse and anuria in sodium-depleted patients.

Electrolyte-free dextrose injections should not be used in conjunction with blood infusions. Dextrose mixed with blood causes **hemolysis** of the red blood cells.

The amount of water required for hydration depends on the clinical condition and the needs of the patient. The average adult patient requires 1500 to 2500 mL water each day. For example, in patients with prolonged fever, the water requirement depends on the degree of temperature elevation. The 24-hour fluid requirement for a patient with body temperature between 101°F and 103°F increases by at least 500 mL; the requirement for a prolonged temperature above 103°F increases by at least 1000 mL.

The rate of administration depends on the patient's condition and the purpose of therapy. When the infusion is used to supply calories, the rate must be slow enough to allow complete metabolism of the glucose (0.5 g/kg/hour in normal adults). The maximum rate usually should not exceed 0.8 g/kg/hour (ASHP, 1998). When the infusion is used to produce diuresis, the rate must be fast enough to prevent complete metabolism of the dextrose, thereby increasing the osmolality of the extracellular fluid.

Isotonic Sodium Chloride Infusions

Sodium chloride injection (0.9%), USP (normal saline), contains 308 mOsm/L (sodium, 154 mEq/L; chloride, 154 mEq/L). It has a pH between 4.5 and 7.0 and is usually supplied in volumes of 1000, 500, 250, and 100 mL. The term *normal* (or *physiologic*) is misleading because the chloride in normal saline is 154 mEq/L, compared with the normal plasma chloride value of 103 mEq/L, whereas the sodium is 154 mEq/L, or approximately 9% higher than the normal plasma value of 140 mEq/L. Because normal saline lacks the other electrolytes present in plasma, the isotonicity of the fluid depends on the sodium and chloride ions, resulting in a higher concentration of these ions (ASHP, 1998).

Indications for Use

Normal sodium chloride injection is indicated for the following:

- Extracellular fluid replacement when chloride loss is relatively greater than or equal to sodium loss.

- Treatment of metabolic alkalosis in the presence of fluid loss; the increase in chloride ions provided by the infusion causes a compensatory decrease in the number of bicarbonate ions.
- Sodium depletion. When there is an extracellular fluid volume deficit accompanying the sodium deficit, an isotonic solution of sodium chloride is used to correct the deficit (Metheny, 2000).
- Initiation and termination of blood transfusions. When 0.9% sodium chloride is used to precede a blood transfusion, the hemolysis of red blood cells, which occurs with dextrose in water, is avoided.

 SAFE PRACTICE ALERT   Sodium chloride 0.9% solution (normal saline) provides more sodium and chloride than the patient needs. Marked electrolyte imbalances have resulted from the almost exclusive use of normal saline. Hypernatremia, acidosis, and circulatory overload may result when normal saline is administered in excess of the patient's tolerance.

Dangers of Use

An adult's dietary requirement for sodium is approximately 90 to 250 mEq/day, with a minimum requirement of 15 mEq and a maximum tolerance of 400 mEq (ASHP, 1998). When 3 L 0.9% sodium chloride or dextrose 5% in 0.9% sodium chloride is administered, the patient receives 462 mEq sodium (154 mEq/L), a level that exceeds normal tolerance.

HYPERNATREMIA
Infusion of saline during a period of sodium retention–for example, during stress—can result in hypernatremia. The danger of hypernatremia increases in the elderly, in patients with severe dehydration, and in patients with chronic glomerulonephritis; these patients require more water to excrete the salt than do patients with normal renal function. Isotonic saline does not provide water but requires most of its volume for the excretion of salt.

ACIDOSIS
One liter of 0.9% sodium chloride solution contains one-third more chloride than is present in the extracellular fluid. When infused in large quantities, the excess chloride ions cause a loss of bicarbonate ions and result in acidosis.

HYPOKALEMIA
Infusion of saline increases potassium excretion and at the same time expands the volume of extracellular fluid, further decreasing the concentration of the extracellular potassium ion.

CIRCULATORY OVERLOAD
Continuous infusions of isotonic fluids expand the extracellular compartment and lead to circulatory overload.

Requirements

In an average adult, the daily requirements of sodium chloride are met by infusing 1 L of 0.9% sodium chloride or 1 to 2 L of 4.5% sodium chloride, but the dosage depends on the patient's age, weight, clinical condition, and fluid, electrolyte, and acid–base status (ASHP, 1998).

Dextrose 5% in 0.9% Sodium Chloride

Dextrose 5% in 0.9% sodium chloride (normal or isotonic saline solution), which contains 252 mOsm dextrose (chloride, 154 mEq/L; sodium, 154 mEq/L), has a pH of 3.5 to 6.0 and is available in volumes of 1000, 500, 250, and 150 mL. When normal saline is infused, the addition of 100 g dextrose prevents both the formation of ketone bodies and the increased demand for water the ketone bodies impose for renal excretion. The dextrose prevents catabolism and, consequently, loss of potassium and intracellular water.

Indications for Use

Isotonic saline with dextrose injection is indicated for the following:

- Temporary treatment of circulatory insufficiency and shock caused by hypovolemia in the immediate absence of a plasma expander
- Early treatment along with plasma or albumin for replacement of loss caused by burns
- Early treatment of acute adrenocortical insufficiency

Dangers of Use

The hazards are the same as those for normal saline injection (see preceding section).

Dextrose 10% in 0.9% Sodium Chloride

Dextrose 10% in 0.9% sodium chloride contains 504 mOsm/L dextrose (sodium, 154 mEq/L; chloride, 154 mEq/L), has a pH of 3.5 to 6.0 and is usually supplied in volumes of 1000 and 500 mL.

Indications for Use

This fluid is used as a nutrient and an electrolyte (sodium and chloride) replenisher.

Administration

Dextrose 10% in 0.9% sodium chloride, because of its hypertonicity, must be administered IV, preferably through a wide vein to dilute the fluid and reduce the risk of trauma to the vessel. Close observation and precautions are necessary to prevent infiltration and damage to the tissues.

Hypertonic Sodium Chloride Infusions

These infusions include 3% sodium chloride (sodium, 513 mEq/L; chloride, 513 mEq/L) and 5% sodium chloride (sodium, 850 mEq/L; chloride, 850 mEq/L).

Indications for Use

Infusion of hypertonic sodium is indicated for

- Severe dilutional hyponatremia (water intoxication). Hypertonic sodium chloride, on infusion, increases the osmotic pressure of the extracellular fluid, drawing water from the cells for excretion by the kidneys.
- Severe sodium depletion. Infusions of hypertonic saline replenish sodium stores. An estimate of the sodium deficit can be made by taking the difference between the normal sodium concentration and the patient's current sodium concentration and multiplying it by 60% of the body weight in kilograms; sodium depletion is based on total body water, and not on extracellular fluid.

Administration

Hypertonic sodium chloride injection must be administered with great caution to prevent pulmonary edema. Cautions include frequent re-evaluation of the patient's clinical and electrolyte status during administration. A 3% or 5% solution of sodium chloride is used to correct the deficit, providing the fluid volume is normal or excessive; the amount of sodium administered depends on the sodium deficit in the plasma (Metheny, 2000).

Hypertonic saline solutions should be infused slowly (eg, 200 mL over a minimum of 4 hours), and the patient should be observed constantly. The fluid must be infused, with great care taken to prevent infiltration and trauma to the tissues. Box 8–3 summarizes the important nursing considerations in the administration of hypertonic saline infusion.

Hypotonic Sodium Chloride in Water

One-half hypotonic saline (0.45% saline containing sodium, 77 mEq/L, and chloride, 77 mEq/L) is used as an electrolyte replenisher. When there is a question regarding

---

BOX 8–3 **Nursing Considerations for Administering Hypertonic (3% and 5%) Saline Solution**

- Check the serum sodium level before administering the solution and frequently thereafter.
- These solutions are dangerous and should be used only in critical situations in which the serum sodium level is very low (ie, <110 mEq/L) and the patient exhibits neurologic signs.
- Administer the solution only in intensive care settings where the patient can be closely monitored. Watch for signs of pulmonary edema and worsening of neurologic signs. Use with great caution in patients with congestive heart failure or renal failure.
- Only small volumes are needed (eg, 5 or 6 mL/kg body weight of 5% sodium chloride) to elevate the serum sodium level by 10 mEq/L. For example, elevating the serum sodium level of a 70-kg patient from 110 to 120 mEq/L requires approximately 350 to 420 mL.
- The serum sodium should not rise more rapidly than 2 mEq/L/hour unless the clinical state of the patient indicates the need for more rapid treatment.
- The fluid can be administered with an electronic infusion device. The device should be monitored closely because no instrument is foolproof.
- Therapy aims to elevate the serum sodium level enough to alleviate neurologic signs—not to raise the serum sodium level to normal quickly. Recommendations include raising the serum concentration no higher than 125 mEq/L with hypertonic saline. The health care provider may prescribe furosemide to promote water loss and prevent pulmonary edema. Urine should be saved because renal sodium and potassium losses may need to be measured to allow for replacement.

---

the amount of saline fluid required, hypotonic saline is preferred over isotonic saline. In general, 0.45% sodium chloride is preferable to 0.9% sodium chloride.

Hydrating Fluids

Because fluids consisting of dextrose with hypotonic saline provide more water than is required for excretion of salt, they are useful as **hydrating fluids.** These fluids include dextrose 2.5% in 0.45% saline (dextrose, 126 mOsm/L, with sodium, 77 mEq/L, and chloride, 77 mEq/L), dextrose 5% in 0.45% saline (dextrose, 252 mOsm/L, with sodium, 77 mEq/L, and chloride, 77 mEq/L), and dextrose 5% in 0.2% saline (dextrose, 252 mOsm/L, with sodium, 34.2 mEq/L, and chloride, 34.2 mEq/L).

Indications for Use

Commonly called *initial hydrating fluids*, hypotonic saline dextrose infusions are indicated as follows:

- To assess the status of the kidneys before electrolyte replacement and maintenance is initiated
- To provide hydration for medical and surgical patients
- To promote diuresis in dehydrated patients

Administration

To assess the status of the kidneys, the fluid is administered at the rate of 8 mL/m^2 body surface area (BSA) per minute for 45 minutes. The restoration of urine flow shows that the kidneys have begun to function. The hydrating fluid then may be replaced by more specifically needed electrolytes. If after 45 minutes the urine flow is not restored, the rate of infusion is reduced to 2 mL/m^2 BSA per minute for another hour. If this does not produce diuresis, renal impairment is assumed (Metheny, 2000).

Initial hydrating fluids must be used cautiously in edematous patients with cardiac, renal, or hepatic disease. Once good renal function is obtained, appropriate electrolytes should be administered to prevent hypokalemia.

Hypotonic Multiple-Electrolyte Fluids

Hypotonic multiple-electrolyte fluids are patterned after the type devised by Butler and colleagues at the Massachusetts General Hospital, who were the first to emphasize that basic water and electrolyte requirements are proportionate to the BSA. Butler-type fluids are one third to one half as concentrated as plasma. They provide fluid to meet the patient's fluid volume requirement. In so doing, they provide cellular and extracellular electrolytes in quantities balanced between the minimal needs and the maximal tolerance of the patient. These fluids, because of their hypotonicity, provide water for urinary elimination and metabolic needs and take advantage of the body's homeostatic mechanisms to retain the electrolytes and reject those not needed, thereby maintaining water and electrolyte balance.

Hypotonic fluids should contain 5% dextrose for its protein-sparing and antiketogenic effect. The dextrose increases the tonicity of the fluid in the container, but once infused, the dextrose is metabolized, leaving the water and salt. Whether the patient has received too much or too little water depends on the tonicity of the electrolyte and not the osmotic effect of dextrose.

A balanced solution of hypotonic electrolytes is ideal for routine maintenance. Of the various modifications of the Butler-type fluids, those containing 75 mEq total cations per liter are used for older infants, children, and adults.

Administration

A useful formula for maintenance water requirements, based on studies by Crawford, Butler, and Talbot, is maintenance water equals 1600 mL/m^2 BSA per day. For obese or edematous patients, this should be calculated on ideal weight rather than actual weight. The water requirement must be patterned after the condition of the patient.

When infection, trauma involving the brain, or stress lead to inappropriate release of ADH, maintenance requirements are less. Excessive fluid losses through urine, stool, expired air, and so forth, require increased water. The rate of infusion is usually 3 mL/m^2 BSA per minute.

Dangers of Use: Water Intoxication

The patient's tolerance limits for water can be exceeded. Care should be exercised in maintaining the prescribed flow rate and in ensuring that the patient receives the prescribed volume of fluid. Water intoxication is more likely to occur when inappropriate release of ADH, in response to stress, causes water retention. These patients should be carefully watched to detect any early signs of an imbalance, so that a change in therapy can be initiated before the condition becomes precarious. Weighing the patient is the best way to monitor the status of water balance. Daily weights are extremely important in following the state of hydration in extremely ill patients.

Isotonic Multiple-Electrolyte Fluids

Many types of commercial replacement fluids are available. When severe vomiting, diarrhea, or diuresis results in a heavy loss of water and electrolytes, replacement therapy is necessary. Balanced fluids of isotonic electrolytes with an ionic composition similar to plasma are used.

Rapid initial replacement is seldom necessary. However, if a severely dehydrated patient shows signs of impaired circulation and renal function and it is necessary to restore the patient's blood pressure quickly, 30 mL/kg of an isotonic fluid may be provided in the first 1 or 2 hours.

Fluid overload must be prevented. Central venous pressure monitoring is especially helpful in elderly patients and in those with renal or cardiovascular disorders.

Extracellular replacement can usually be assumed to be complete after 48 hours of replacement therapy unless proved otherwise by clinical or laboratory evidence. To continue replacement fluids after deficits have been corrected may result in sodium excess, leading to pulmonary edema or heart failure. Patients receiving replacement therapy should be observed closely to detect any signs of circulatory overload.

Gastric replacement fluids provide the usual electrolytes lost by vomiting or gastric suction. They contain ammonium ions, which are metabolized in the liver to hydrogen ions and urea, replacing the hydrogen ion lost in gastric juices. They are useful in metabolic alkalosis caused by excessive ingestion of sodium bicarbonate. The usual adult dose is 500 to 2000 mL, and the rate should be consistent with the patient's clinical condition but not exceed 500 mL/hour.

Gastric replacement fluids are contraindicated in patients with hepatic insufficiency or renal failure. They require the same precautions as any fluid containing potassium and should be avoided in patients with renal damage or Addison's disease. Also, the low pH causes incompatibilities with many additives.

Lactated Ringer's injection is considered safe in certain conditions. Because the electrolyte concentration closely resembles that of the extracellular fluid, it may be used to replace fluid loss from burns and fluid lost as bile and diarrhea. Lactated Ringer's injection has been useful in mild acidosis, the lactate ion being metabolized in the liver to bicarbonate.

 SAFE PRACTICE ALERT Three liters of lactated Ringer's injection contain approximately 390 mEq sodium, which can quickly elevate the sodium level in a patient who is not sodium deficient. Lactated Ringer's injection is contraindicated in severe metabolic acidosis or alkalosis and in liver disease or anoxic states that influence lactate metabolism.

Alkalizing Fluids

When anesthesia or disorders, such as dehydration, shock, liver disease, starvation, and diabetes, cause a patient to retain chlorides, ketone bodies, or organic salts, or when a patient loses excessive bicarbonate, metabolic acidosis occurs. Treatment consists of infusing an appropriate **alkalizing fluid.** These fluids include one-sixth molar isotonic sodium lactate (1.9%, with sodium, 167 mEq/L, and lactate ions, 167 mEq/L, and a pH of 6.0 to 7.3), one-sixth molar sodium bicarbonate injection, USP (1.5%, with sodium, 178 mEq/L, and bicarbonate, 178 mEq/L, and a pH of 7.0 to 8.0), and hypertonic sodium bicarbonate injection (7.5% or 5%).

One-Sixth Molar Sodium Lactate

The lactate ion must be oxidized in the body to carbon dioxide before it can effect acid–base balance; the complete conversion of sodium lactate to bicarbonate requires approximately 1 to 2 hours.

Indications for Use

One-sixth molar sodium lactate is used when acidosis results from a sodium deficiency in such disorders as vomiting, starvation, uncontrolled diabetes mellitus, acute infection, and renal failure (ASHP, 1998).

Dangers of Use

Because oxidation is necessary to increase the bicarbonate concentration, sodium lactate is not used for patients experiencing oxygen lack, as in shock or congenital heart disease with persistent cyanosis. It is also contraindicated in liver disease because the lactate ions are improperly metabolized.

Administration

The usual dose is 1 L of a one-sixth molar solution, but the dosage depends on the patient's condition and the serum sodium level. One-sixth molar infusion may be administered by venoclysis or hypodermoclysis and usually at a rate not greater than 300 mL/hour (ASHP, 1998). The patient should be observed closely for any evidence of alkalosis.

Sodium Bicarbonate Injection

Sodium bicarbonate injection, USP (1.5%, with sodium, 178 mEq/L, and bicarbonate, 178 mEq/L) is an isotonic fluid that provides bicarbonate ions for conditions of excess depletion.

Indications for Use

Sodium bicarbonate injection is used for severe hyperpnea early in the treatment of severe acidosis until the signs of dyspnea and hyperpnea subside. The bicarbonate ion is released in the form of carbon dioxide through the lungs, leaving an excess of sodium cation behind to exert its electrolyte effect (Lonsway & Terry, 1995).

Recommendations and practice related to pharmacologic management of cardiopulmonary resuscitation suggest a cautious use of sodium bicarbonate to manage acidosis (Metheny, 2000).

Administration

The usual dose is 500 mL in a 1.5% solution. The dosage depends on the patient's weight, condition, and carbon dioxide content. If the isotonic infusion is not available, it may be made by adding two 50-mL ampules containing 3.75 g each of sodium bicarbonate to 400 mL hypotonic saline.

The fluid should be infused slowly IV. Rapid injection may induce cellular acidity and death.

The patient should be watched for signs of hypocalcemic tetany, and calcium supplement should be administered if required; calcium does not ionize well in an alkaline medium. Extravasation of hypertonic sodium bicarbonate injections must be avoided (ASHP, 1998). Bicarbonate therapy should cease when the pH reaches 7.2.

Acidifying Infusions

Normal saline (0.9% sodium chloride injection, USP) is not usually listed among the **acidifying infusions.** However, because metabolic alkalosis is a condition associated with excess bicarbonate and loss of chloride, isotonic saline provides conservative treatment. When the chloride ions are infused, the bicarbonate decreases in compensation and the alkalosis is relieved.

Ammonium chloride, the usual acidifying agent, is available as isotonic 0.9% ammonium chloride injection (ammonium, 167 mEq/L; chloride, 167 mEq/L) and hypertonic 2.14% ammonium chloride injection (ammonium, 400 mEq/L; chloride, 400 mEq/L). The pH range is 4.0 to 6.0. Both concentrations are supplied in 1-L bottles.

Indications for Use

Ammonium chloride is used as an acidifying infusion in severe metabolic alkalosis caused by loss of gastric secretions, pyloric stenosis, or other causes. The ammonium ion is converted by the liver to hydrogen ion and to ammonia, which is excreted as urea.

Administration

The 2.14% ammonium chloride is usually used in the treatment of the adult patient; 0.9% ammonium chloride is used for children.

The dosage depends on the condition of the patient and on an accurate chemical picture, including plasma carbon dioxide–combining power. Ammonium chloride must be infused at a very slow rate to enable the liver to metabolize the ammonium ion, not to exceed 5 mL/minute in adults. Rapid injection can result in toxic effects, causing irregular breathing, bradycardia, and twitching (ASHP, 1998). See Table 8–2 for more information on contents of fluids.

 SAFE PRACTICE ALERT   Because its acidifying effect depends on the liver for conversion, ammonium chloride must not be administered to patients with severe hepatic disease or renal failure. It is contraindicated in any condition in which the patient has a high ammonium level.

■ EVALUATION OF WATER AND ELECTROLYTE BALANCE

A rational approach is necessary if the patient is to receive safe and successful IV therapy. In the past, the nurse's technical responsibility in maintaining the infusion and patent venous access were emphasized. With the current increase in the use of IV therapy, however, clinical disturbances in fluid and electrolyte metabolism are more common.

Changes in the patient's status can occur quickly and in the absence of the physician. Today, the nurse's responsibility consists of monitoring the fluid and electrolyte status of the patient as well as the progress of the infusion. Greater emphasis must be placed on the causes and effects of fluid and electrolyte abnormalities so that these imbalances may be anticipated and recognized before they become disastrous.

Monitoring Parameters

The nurse should be familiar with the parameters used in evaluating fluid and electrolyte imbalances and in supplying fluid and electrolyte requirements.

TABLE 8 – 2
CONTENTS OF SELECTED WATER AND ELECTROLYTE SOLUTIONS

Solution	Cautions and Considerations
5% dextrose in water (D_5W): No electrolytes 50 g of dextrose	Supplies approximately 170 cal/L and free water to aid in renal excretion of solutes
	Should not be used in excessive volumes in patients with increased antidiuretic hormone activity or to replace fluids in hypovolemic patients
0.9% NaCl (isotonic saline): Na^+ 154 mEq/L Cl^- 154 mEq/L	Isotonic fluid commonly used to expand the extracellular fluid in presence of hypovolemia
	Because of relatively high chloride content, it can be used to treat mild metabolic alkalosis
0.45% NaCl ($\frac{1}{2}$-strength saline): Na^+ 77 mEq/L Cl^- 77 mEq/L	A hypotonic solution that provides Na^+, Cl^-, and free water; Na^+ and Cl^- provided in fluid allows kidneys to select and retain needed amounts
	Free water desirable as aid to kidneys in elimination of solutes
0.33% NaCl ($\frac{1}{3}$-strength saline): Na^+ 56 mEq/L Cl^- 56 mEq/L	A hypotonic solution that provides Na^+, Cl^-, and free water
	Often used to treat hypernatremia (because this solution contains a small amount of Na^+, it dilutes the plasma sodium while not allowing it to drop too rapidly)
3% NaCl: Na^+ 513 mEq/L Cl^- 513 mEq/L	Grossly hypertonic solutions used only to treat severe hyponatremia
	See Box 8–3 summary of important nursing considerations in administration
5% NaCl: Na^+ 855 mEq/L Cl^- 855 mEq/L	Dangerous solutions
Lactated Ringer's solution: Na^+ 130 mEq/L K^+ 4 mEq/L Ca^{2+} 3 mEq/L Cl^- 109 mEq/L	A roughly isotonic solution that contains multiple electrolytes in approximately the same concentrations as found in plasma (note that this solution is lacking in Mg and PO_4)
	Used in the treatment of hypovolemia, burns, and fluid lost as bile or diarrhea
Lactate (metabolized to bicarbonate) 28 mEq/L	Useful in treating mild metabolic acidosis
Sodium lactate solution, $\frac{1}{6}$ M: Na^+ 167 mEq/L Cl^- 167 mEq/L	A roughly isotonic solution used to correct severe metabolic acidosis (lactate is metabolized to bicarbonate in 1–2 h by the liver)
	Not used in patients with liver disease (lactate cannot be converted to bicarbonate in such patients); also, not used in patients with oxygen lack (unable adequately to convert lactate to bicarbonate)
Sodium bicarbonate, 5%: Na^+ 595 mEq/L Cl^- 595 mEq/L	A very hypertonic solution used to correct severe metabolic acidosis
	Should be cautiously administered at a slow rate, using EID
	Should be administered only with extreme caution to salt-retaining patients (eg, those with cardiac, renal, or liver damage)
Ammonium chloride, 2.14%:	Acidifying solution used to correct severe metabolic alkalosis
	Because of high ammonium content, must be administered cautiously with compromised hepatic function
Potassium chloride, 0.15%: K^+ 20 mEq/L Cl^- 20 mEq/L	Premixed potassium chloride solution
Potassium chloride, 0.30%: K^+ 40 mEq/L Cl^- 40 mEq/L	Premixed potassium chloride solution

Central Venous Pressure

Central venous pressure monitoring provides a simple, accurate, and valuable guide in detecting changes in blood volume and assessing fluid requirements. It is particularly valuable in assessing the ability of the heart to tolerate the infusion. Many erroneous conclusions are drawn from false values recorded when the infusion line is not properly responsive to right atrial pressures.

Normal venous pressure indicates an adequate circulatory blood volume; elevated venous pressure may mean an increase in circulatory volume and right heart pressure, with the possibility of circulatory overload. It may also indicate other problems such as a pulmonary embolus, myocardial infarction, or lack of digitalis. Determination of the hematocrit value supplements clinical information.

A low venous pressure, too low to measure, indicates that the patient has probably lost fluid or blood. The nurse must not overlook the fact that fluid loss can result from drug-induced vasodilation or improper administration of IV fluids. If rapid infusion of dextrose exceeds the patient's tolerance, massive diuresis with dehydration and diminished circulatory volume may occur. The decreased venous blood return into the right atrium is reflected by a decrease in the central venous pressure.

Pulse

The pulse quality and rate provide valuable clinical information for assessing fluid and electrolyte changes in the patient. A high pulse pressure, bounding and not easily obliterated by pressure, indicates a high cardiac output caused by circulatory overload. A regular pulse, easily obliterated by pressure, indicates low cardiac output resulting from a lowered blood volume.

A bounding, easily obliterated pressure signifies a drop in blood pressure with a wide pulse pressure, indicative of impending circulatory collapse. As the patient's condition deteriorates, the pulse becomes rapid, weak, thready, and easily obliterated, signifying circulatory collapse.

Hand Veins

Examination of the hand veins provides a means of evaluating the plasma volume. The hand veins usually empty in 3 to 5 seconds when the hand is elevated and fill in the same length of time when the hand is lowered to a dependent position. Peripheral vein filling takes longer than 3 to 5 seconds in patients with sodium depletion and extracellular dehydration.

Slow emptying of the hand veins indicates overhydration and excessive blood volume; slow filling indicates a low blood volume and often precedes hypotension. Hand veins that become engorged and clearly visible indicate an increase in plasma volume secondary to an interstitial-to-vascular fluid shift or an increase in extracellular fluid volume (Metheny, 2000). A rapid guide for fluid assessment is found in Table 8–3.

T A B L E   8 – 3
RAPID FLUID IMBALANCE ASSESSMENT GUIDE

Assessment Focus	Fluid Volume Excess	Fluid Volume Deficit
Cardiovascular system	Bounding pulse Elevated pulse rate Jugular distention Overdistended hand veins	Decreased blood pressure Decreased pulse rate Flat neck veins Narrow pulse pressure Slow hand vein filling
Integumentary system	Warm, moist skin Sternal fingerprinting	Decreased turgor over sternum/forehead Lowered skin temperature
Neurologic system		Altered orientation: confusion
Respiratory system	Moist crackles Respiratory rate >20/min Dyspnea Pulmonary edema	Clear lungs
Eyes	Periorbital edema	Dry conjunctiva Sunken eyes Decreased tearing
Lips	—	Dry and cracked
Mouth	—	Dry mucous membranes
Tongue	—	Dry, leathery texture Longitudinal furrows
Weight	Mild: 2% above normal Moderate: 5% above normal Severe: >8% above normal	Mild: <2% below normal Moderate: 5% below normal Severe: >8% below normal

Neck Veins

Changes in fluid volume are reflected by changes in neck vein filling, provided the patient is not in heart failure. In the supine position, the patient's external jugular veins fill to the anterior border of the sternocleidomastoid muscle. Flat neck veins in the supine position indicate a decreased plasma volume.

Weight

A sudden gain or loss in weight is a significant sign of a change in the fluid volume. A change in the volume of body fluid can be computed by weighing the patient daily at the same time of day, on the same scales, with the same amount of clothing. A loss or gain of 1 kg body weight reflects a loss or gain of 1 L body fluid. A rapid 2% loss of total body weight indicates mild fluid volume deficit, and a rapid loss of 8% or more represents severe fluid volume deficit. Conversely, weight gain occurs when total fluid intake exceeds total fluid output. A rapid 2% gain of total body weight indicates mild fluid volume excess; a 5% gain represents a moderate fluid volume excess; and 8% or greater indicates a severe fluid volume excess.

Thirst

Thirst is an important symptom denoting a deficit in body fluid or, more specifically, cellular dehydration. This type of dehydration occurs when the extracellular fluid becomes hypertonic, either as a result of water deprivation or the infusion of hypertonic saline. The increase in osmotic pressure causes fluid to be drawn from the cells, resulting in cellular dehydration, the stimulus to thirst. Normally, thirst governs the need for water but, in certain conditions, the lack of thirst may accompany dehydration. This is especially true in the aged, in whom thirst is not urgent. These patients may lose their thirst and as a result become severely dehydrated before the condition is recognized. In the severely burned patient, the great thirst experienced may lead to ingestion of excess water and to a serious sodium deficit.

Intake and Output

Water intake and output should be carefully measured and recorded. Hourly urine output measurements may be particularly important. A urine output of 200 mL/ hour indicates that too much water is being infused too rapidly. By regulating the urine output between 30 and 50 mL/hour, the patient receives at least enough fluid for the kidneys to work efficiently.

A decreased urinary output accompanies a decreased blood volume; changes in the arterial pressure and pressure in the glomeruli result in the oliguria or anuria of profound shock. The increase in urinary output accompanying an increase in blood volume is primarily caused by changes in arterial pressure and pressure in the glomeruli. Output should include urine, vomitus, diarrhea, drainage from fistulas, and drainage from suction apparatus.

Skin Turgor

Observing changes in skin **turgor** (elasticity) and texture is helpful in assessing the state of water balance. To test skin turgor, the skin is pinched over the sternum, inner aspect of the thigh, or forehead in the adult or the medial aspects of the thigh or abdomen in the child, and then released; in the normal person, the pinched skin returns to its original position. Skin that remains in a raised position for several seconds indicates a deficit in fluid volume.

Tongue Turgor

A dry, leathery tongue may indicate a fluid volume deficit or mouth breathing. To differentiate between the two, the mucous membrane may be checked for moisture by running the finger between the gums and the cheek; dryness indicates a fluid volume deficit.

Normally, the tongue has one longitudinal furrow. In the patient with fluid volume deficit, additional longitudinal furrows are present and the tongue is smaller because of the fluid loss. Not significantly affected by age, the tongue is a good parameter to measure in all age groups.

Edema

Edema reflects an increase in the extracellular fluid volume outside the circulating intravascular compartment. It depends on an imbalance or a disturbance in the exchange of water and electrolytes between the patient and the environment or the exchange of water and electrolytes between the compartments of the body. The fluid and electrolyte exchange between the body compartments may be affected by an alteration in the circulatory system, the lymphatic system, or the concentration of albumin in the serum; water and electrolytes escape from the circulation faster than they enter, and edema ensues.

Edema may be generalized, as in congestive failure; localized, as with ascites; or peripheral. By detecting edema early, a clinical imbalance may be corrected before the patient's condition deteriorates. Early peripheral edema may be detected by fingerprinting, a procedure in which the finger is rolled over the bony prominence of the sternum or tibia. As edema increases, pitting edema occurs and may be detected by pressure of the fingers on the subcutaneous tissue. Figure 8–1 shows the degrees of edema.

In generalized edema, such as that seen in cardiac failure, total extracellular water volume as well as interstitial edema increase. Symptoms such as venous engorgement, restlessness, dyspnea, cyanosis, and pulmonary rales indicate generalized edema.

Laboratory Values

Laboratory values, when used to supplement clinical observations, aid in forming diagnostic and therapeutic guidelines. Electrolyte studies (serum sodium, potassium, chloride, bicarbonate, and pH) performed daily are important in assessing the fluid and electrolyte status of the patient receiving IV fluids. In patients with massive electrolyte losses, such studies may be required two or three times a day. Blood cell

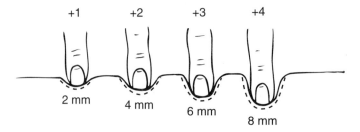

Figure 8–1. Edema scale. Severity of edema is ranked on a scale of +1 to +4, with +1 being barely perceptible and +4 being visible and remarkable.

count and hematocrit determinations are helpful in detecting hemoconcentration or hemodilution; hemoconcentration reflects a diminished plasma volume caused by dehydration, and hemodilution, an increased volume from overtreatment with water.

Measurement of serum protein with the albumin/globulin ratio helps in detecting a change in fluid volume; large quantities of parenteral fluid rapidly administered dilute and decrease the serum protein concentration. This determination is helpful when used to supplement clinical observation—otherwise, it may be misleading and interpreted as showing actual depletion. A decrease in serum protein reduces the osmotic pressure of the extracellular compartment, causing some edema and loss of plasma volume. Blood urea nitrogen should be measured frequently to evaluate kidney function, an important parameter in treating fluid and electrolyte imbalances.

■ CLINICAL DISTURBANCES OF WATER AND ELECTROLYTE METABOLISM

Most of the common clinical disturbances in water and electrolyte balance result from changes in the volume of total body water or in one or more of the fluid compartments of the body. Clinical disturbances in water and electrolyte metabolism have been classified into six types: isotonic, hypertonic, and hypotonic expansion and isotonic, hypertonic, and hypotonic contraction. These are discussed in the following sections.

Isotonic Expansion

Isotonic expansion (circulatory overload) occurs when fluids of the same tonicity as plasma are infused into the vascular circulation. Because fluids isotonic to plasma do not affect the osmolality, water does not flow from the extracellular to the intracellular compartment. The extracellular compartment expands in proportion to the fluid infused and is the only compartment affected. The increase in the volume of fluid dilutes the concentration of hemoglobin and lowers the hematocrit and total protein levels, but the serum sodium level remains the same.

Isotonic expansion is a critical complication of IV therapy. Patients who receive isotonic fluids around the clock are at particular risk and should be observed closely for early signs of circulatory overload. Sodium chloride (0.9%) or fluids containing balanced isotonic multiple electrolytes are used for pre-existing or continuing fluid and electrolyte losses and are not the ideal fluids for maintenance therapy. The electrolyte isotonicity of these fluids causes expansion of the extracellular compartment and does not provide the extra water that balanced hypotonic fluids provide for the kidney to retain or secrete as needed. The early postoperative or post-trauma patient is susceptible to this critical complication. The increased endocrine response to stress during the first 2 to 5 days after surgery results in retention of sodium chloride and water. When a patient under stress is receiving isotonic infusions, the nurse must anticipate and watch for signs of circulatory overload.

Elderly patients receiving isotonic fluids must be carefully monitored because they have a lower tolerance to fluids and electrolytes. Because they are also likely to have some degree of cardiac and renal impairment, the ability of the kidneys to eliminate fluid is likely to be diminished. The status of these patients can change quickly. In the patient who has had a craniotomy, large-volume isotonic infusions can increase the intracranial pressure and prove detrimental.

Patients who are potential candidates for isotonic expansion must be watched carefully and turned frequently to prevent fluid from settling in the lungs. Pulmonary edema can result from the cardiac and pulmonary side effects of IV therapy. The apices of the lungs, which are high, tend to be fairly dry, but the bases of the lungs, posteriorly and inferiorly, can be fairly wet (Metheny, 2000). As a result, hypostatic pneumonia secondary to gravity may develop.

Manifestations

The nurse who monitors IV infusions must be familiar with the early clinical manifestations that accompany isotonic expansion to recognize and prevent its development; mild pulmonary edema progressing to severe pulmonary edema is a late stage that must be prevented. Early clinical manifestations include (1) weight gain; (2) increased fluid intake over output; (3) high pulse pressure; (4) increase in central venous pressure; (5) peripheral hand vein emptying time; (6) peripheral edema; (7) hoarseness. If IV therapy is allowed to continue, isotonic expansion becomes more apparent and dangerous, with easily recognized signs: cyanosis, dyspnea, coughing, and neck vein engorgement. Laboratory characteristics include a drop in the hematocrit value and reduced concentrations of hemoglobin and total protein.

Treatment

Treatment for circulatory overload when detected early is relatively simple and consists of withholding all fluids until excess water and electrolytes have been eliminated by the body. After the condition is rectified, hypotonic maintenance fluids provide the patient with fluid and a minimum daily requirement of electrolytes. The hypotonicity of the fluid allows the kidneys to maintain the needed amount and selectively retain or excrete the excess.

Isotonic Contraction

Isotonic contraction occurs when there is loss of fluid and electrolytes isotonic to the extracellular fluid, such as whole blood or large volumes of fluid from diarrhea or vomiting. The extracellular compartment contracts. Because the fluid lost is isotonic, the osmolality of the extracellular compartment remains unchanged and no movement of water occurs between the compartments; only the extracellular volume is affected.

Manifestations

Because of the loss of fluid, the hematocrit level and the concentrations of hemoglobin and total protein are increased. The serum sodium concentration does not change. Clinical manifestations include:

- Weight loss
- Negative fluid balance (a decrease in urinary output but a greater output than total fluid intake)
- Regular pulse rate, easily obliterated by pressure, and, as the patient's condition deteriorates, becoming weak and thready
- Possible increase in peripheral hand vein filling time above the normal 3 to 5 seconds when the hand is moved from an elevated to a dependent position

Treatment

Treatment consists of replacing the fluid loss with isotonic fluids containing balanced electrolytes.

Hypertonic Expansion

Hypertonic expansion occurs when the volume of body water is increased by the IV infusion of hypertonic saline. Sodium chloride 3% or 5% is used to replace a massive sodium loss or remove excess accumulation of body fluids, but, if the infusion is administered rapidly, hypertonic expansion can result. The saline increases the osmotic pressure of the extracellular compartment, causing water to be drawn from the intracellular compartment until both compartments are isosmotic. The volume of the extracellular compartment increases and that of the intracellular compartment decreases. The osmolality of the extracellular fluid is higher than before the infusion but lower than the high level after the infusion because of the increased extracellular fluid volume (ASHP, 1998).

Caution must be used in the IV administration of hypertonic saline fluid. Circulatory overload with hypernatremia can occur. An understanding of the reason for the infusion, the condition of the patient, the proper rate of administration, and the signs and symptoms of hypertonic expansion provides a basis for sound IV practice.

Manifestations

Clinical manifestations include a gain in body weight dependent on the volume infused. A small volume (500 mL) does not contribute to a significant weight gain (Metheny, 2000).

An increased sodium load results in a decreased rate of water excretion; however, the abrupt increase in plasma volume may cause an increase in the rate of water excretion as the body attempts to excrete the excess salt and water. The degree of thirst depends on the hypertonicity of the plasma and consequently the amount of cellular dehydration.

Peripheral hand vein emptying time may be increased beyond the normal 5 seconds when the hand is elevated but depends on the degree of expansion of the extracellular compartment. A bounding pulse is significant in detecting hypertonic expansion. The serum sodium concentration is increased. The hematocrit level and the concentrations of hemoglobin and total serum protein are decreased as a result of the expanded fluid volume in the extracellular compartment.

Treatment

Treatment consists of stopping the infusion to allow the kidneys to eliminate the overload of salt and water. If no cardiovascular side effects are noted, dextrose 5% in water may be infused slowly to reduce the tonicity of the extracellular fluid and replace body water.

Hypertonic Contraction

Hypertonic contraction (hypertonic dehydration) occurs when water is lost without a corresponding loss of salt. This condition occurs in patients who are unable to take sufficient fluid for a prolonged period or in patients with excess insensible water loss through the lungs and skin.

In elderly patients, hypertonic dehydration is a common clinical disturbance; they frequently experience a decrease in the thirst stimuli in response to hypertonicity of body fluids, and adequate intake of fluid is not met. In the unconscious or incontinent patient, frequency and excess urination may go undetected or may be interpreted as a sign of good renal function. A loss of tubular ability to concentrate urine in the aged results in a large urinary volume when an increased solute load is presented to the patient (Metheny, 2000).

Elderly patients also have a diminished response to ADH. Large amounts of dilute urine may be lost, resulting in hypertonic dehydration (see Chap. 23). To prevent fluid imbalance, the nurse must recognize that individuals differ widely in the water they require; patients whose kidneys do not concentrate urine well require more water than those whose kidneys do concentrate urine well.

The daily fluid requirement must be met. In hypertonic contraction, the loss of water from the extracellular compartment results in an increase in the osmolality, causing water to flow from the cells to the extracellular compartment. Dehydration occurs as water leaves the cellular compartment to replace the plasma volume.

Both the intracellular and the extracellular compartments are affected by the water loss; there is a decrease in volume and an increase in osmolality in both compartments. In contrast, in isotonic contraction, only the extracellular compartment is affected and the contraction is more serious. Because signs of hypertonic contraction are not obvious in the early stages, the nurse must anticipate such an imbalance and be alert to any changes.

Manifestations

Clinically, thirst is an early and reliable sign of hypertonic contraction, but it may be absent in the elderly, complicating early recognition of this imbalance. Weight loss occurs. Negative fluid balance (output greater than intake) is present. Hourly output measurements show a decrease in the rate of excretion of water.

The pulse has a normal quality and is regular in the early stages of hypertonic contraction. The hand vein filling time may be within the normal limits; cellular fluid has partly replenished the plasma.

Irritability, restlessness, and possibly confusion may be present. Skin turgor diminishes and is a sign of dehydration in the later stages. A dry mouth with a furrowed tongue indicates dehydration. Laboratory studies show an increase in serum sodium concentration, hematocrit level, hemoglobin concentration, and total serum protein concentration.

Treatment

Treatment consists of hydrating the patient by administering a balanced hypotonic fluid such as the Butler-type fluids: 2400 mL/m^2 BSA per day for moderate pre-existing deficit and 3000 mL/m^2 BSA per day for severe pre-existing deficit. The usual rate for IV administration is 3 mL/m^2 BSA. A therapeutic test for functional renal depression may be necessary before infusing water and electrolytes for maintenance.

Hypotonic Expansion

Hypotonic expansion (water intoxication, dilutional hyponatremia) occurs when the increase in the volume of body fluids is caused by water alone. Water expands the extracellular compartment, causing a decrease in the concentration. Water then diffuses into the cells until both compartments are isosmotic. Both the extracellular and the intracellular compartments are affected; the volume is increased and the concentration is decreased.

The serum sodium concentration and the hematocrit, hemoglobin, and total serum protein levels are reduced. Hypotonic expansion occurs in patients who are receiving large quantities of electrolyte-free water to replace excessive fluid and electrolytes lost from gastric suction, vomiting, diarrhea, or diuresis, or insensibly through the skin.

Patients receiving continuous infusion of dextrose 5% in water are particularly susceptible to water intoxication. This fluid contains 252 mOsm dextrose per liter, making it an isotonic fluid in the container. Once introduced into the circulation, the dextrose is quickly metabolized, leaving the water free to dilute and expand the extracellular compartment. With the decreased osmolality of the extracellular fluid, water diffuses into the cells and hypotonic expansion occurs. The patient's tolerance to water can be exceeded by infusion of excess amounts of hypotonic fluids. The kidneys of the normal adult can metabolize water in amounts of 35 to 45 mL/kg/day, but the kidneys of the average patient can metabolize only 2500 to 3000 mL/day; above these volumes, abnormal accumulation of water occurs (Metheny, 2000).

Hypotonic expansion is more likely to occur during the early postoperative period, when retention of water is affected by the response to stress, particularly in the elderly patient, in whom the response to stress is compounded by impairment in renal function. Small amounts of adjusted hypotonic saline (sodium, 90 mEq/L; chloride, 60 mEq/L; and lactate, 30 mEq/L) may be used in the early postoperative management of the aged.

Manifestations

When acute onset of behavioral changes, such as confusion, apathy, and disorientation, occurs in the elderly postoperative patient, overhydration should be suspected.

Central nervous system disturbances such as weakness, muscle twitching, and convulsions are seen, as are headaches, nausea, and vomiting. Fluid intake is increased over fluid output. Weight gain is always present.

Blood pressure usually is normal but may be elevated. Peripheral hand veins are usually full, and hand emptying time is increased beyond the normal 5 seconds when the hand is elevated from a dependent position. The pulse may be regular and not easily obliterated when pressure is applied.

Treatment

Treatment consists of withholding all fluids until the excess water is excreted. In severe hyponatremia, it may be necessary to administer small quantities of hypertonic saline to increase the osmotic pressure and the flow of water from the cells to the extracellular compartment for excretion by the kidneys. Hypertonic saline must be used cautiously and must not be administered to patients with congestive heart failure.

Hypotonic Contraction

Hypotonic contraction (hypotonic dehydration) occurs when fluids containing relatively more salt than water are lost from the body. This loss results in a decrease in the effective osmolality of the extracellular compartment. Water is drawn into the cells until osmotic equilibrium is established. Because of the invasion of water, the intracellular compartment is expanded and the extracellular compartment is contracted. This imbalance may result from the loss of salt from any one of several sources: urine of patients receiving diuretics, fistula drainage, severe burns, vomitus, and sweat. The elderly are affected by the loss of small quantities of sodium.

Manifestations

Clinical manifestations include weight loss; negative fluid balance; pulse rate that is increased, weak or thready, and easily obliterated; increased hand filling time; and decreased skin turgor. Laboratory studies show a decrease in serum sodium concentration and an increase in hematocrit, hemoglobin, and total serum protein levels.

Treatment

Treatment of hypotonic contraction consists of replacing the fluids and electrolytes that have been lost. Because other electrolytes are usually lost along with the sodium loss, a balanced electrolyte fluid may be administered.

References and Selected Readings

Asterisks indicate references cited in text.

*American Society of Healthcare Pharmacists [ASHP]. (1998). Bethesda, MD: American Hospital Formulary Service, 1486, 1490, 1514–1517, 1527–1529.
Carpenito, L. J. (1995). *Nursing diagnosis applied to clinical practice* (6th ed., pp. 120–127). Philadelphia: J.B. Lippincott.
*Lonsway, R.A., & Terry, J. (1995). Fluids and electrolytes. In: J. Terry, L. Baranowski, & C. Hedrick (Eds.): *Intravenous therapy: clinical principles and practice* (p. 120). Philadelphia: W.B. Saunders.
*Metheny, N.M. (2000). *Fluid and electrolyte balance* (4th ed.). Philadelphia: Lippincott Williams & Wilkins.
*United States Pharmacopeia [USP]. (1999). (26th ed., pp. 803, 1027). Easton, PA: Mack Publishing.

Review Questions

Note: Questions below may have more than one right answer.

1. Which of the following IV dextrose fluids is considered isotonic?

   A. 2.5%

   B. 5%

   C. 0%

   D. 20%

2. A teaching plan for a patient diagnosed with hypermagnesemia should include:

   A. Preventing injury due to hypotension or weakness

   B. Availability of an antacid to prevent gastric acidity or reflux

   C. Preventing constipation by routine laxative administration

   D. Restricting fluid intake

3. Edema is the result of excess fluid in which of the following areas?

   A. Interstitial space

   B. Intracellular space

   C. Intrathecal space

   D. Intravascular space

4. One-sixth molar sodium lactate may be infused by which of the following methods?

   A. IV push

   B. Hypodermoclysis

   C. Venoclysis

   D. Syringe pump

5. The electrolyte concentration of lactated Ringer's injection closely resembles that of:

   A. Extracellular fluid

   B. Intracellular fluid

   C. Pericardium

   D. Intravascular compartment

Questions 6 and 7 are based on the following scenario:
A 55-year-old patient is admitted to the hospital with diabetic acidosis. A solution of dextrose 5% in 0.33% sodium chloride with insulin is ordered. After 2 hours of treatment, the patient is alert and states that she feels better, but 1 hour after that, the patient has a weak, irregular pulse and is restless.

6. The most likely cause of the patient's symptoms is:
   A. Hypokalemia
   B. Hyperkalemia
   C. Compensated metabolic acidosis
   D. Uncompensated metabolic acidosis

7. Given the clinical situation and likely cause, which of the following medications would be needed?
   A. Furosemide
   B. Potassium chloride
   C. Regular insulin
   D. Sodium bicarbonate

8. Slow filling of the hand veins indicates which of the following?
   A. Excessive blood volume
   B. Low blood volume
   C. Increased plasma volume
   D. Increased extracellular fluid volume

9. Gastric replacement fluids are contraindicated in patients with:
   A. Renal failure
   B. Hepatic insufficiency
   C. Increased pulse pressure
   D. Isotonic expansion

10. Which of the following is *not* appropriate for a patient with a diagnosis of bowel obstruction?
   A. Dextrose 5% in water
   B. Dextrose 5% in 0.45% sodium chloride with 20 mEq potassium chloride
   C. 0.9% Sodium chloride
   D. Lactated Ringer's injection

Potential Complications and

Ongoing Monitoring

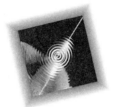

K E Y T E R M S

Air Embolism	Necrosis
Catheter Embolism	Phlebothrombosis
Cellular Toxicity	Speed Shock
Débridement	Thrombosis
Extravasation	Thrombophlebitis
Infiltration	Thrombogenicity
Ischemia	

■ UNDERSTANDING COMPLICATIONS

Complications are the major risks involved in administering intravenous (IV) therapy. The IV nurse needs to recognize complications and respond with appropriate nursing interventions to ensure quality of care. The various kinds of complications include those that are local and systemic. Local complications occur frequently but are rarely serious. Systemic complications, although rarer, are serious and frequently life-threatening. They require immediate recognition and medical attention.

■ LOCAL COMPLICATIONS

Occasionally, local complications are not recognized until considerable damage occurs, making early recognition of complications a key factor in infusion therapy. Early recognition may prevent the following:

- Extensive edema that deprives the patient of urgently needed fluid and medications
- **Necrosis** (localized death of tissue)
- Thrombophlebitis with the subsequent danger of embolism

Local complications usually occur as the result of trauma to the wall of the vein. Among the common local complications are thrombosis, thrombophlebitis, phlebothrombosis, and extravasation.

Thrombosis

Any injury that roughens the endothelial cells of the venous wall allows platelets to adhere and a thrombus to form. Because the point of the IV catheter traumatizes the wall of the vein where it touches, a thrombus or thrombi form on the vein and at the tip of the catheter. The result of local thrombi obstructing the circulation of blood is **thrombosis**. Thrombi not only obstruct circulation, they form an excellent trap for bacteria, whether the bacteria are carried by the bloodstream from an infection in a remote part of the body or enter the body through a subcutaneous orifice.

Thrombosis of the deep veins (axillary, subclavian, innominate, internal jugular, and superior vena cava) and subsequent risk of infection occurs when catheters are placed in the venous system (Fig. 9–1). The device that poses the greatest risk of iatrogenic bloodstream infection is the central venous catheter (CVC) in its numerous forms (Centers for Disease Control and Prevention [CDC], 1998). The reported inci-

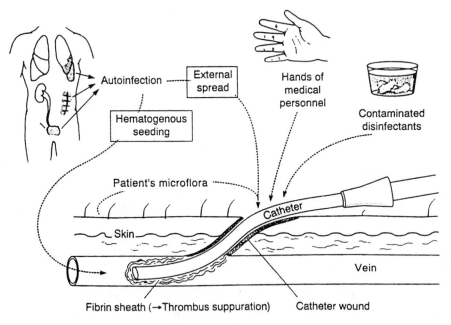

Figure 9–1. Sources of vascular catheter-related infection.

dence is difficult to determine, but studies indicate a variation from 0.02% to 13%. These studies included patients with peripherally inserted central catheters, implanted venous access ports, and CVCs (Bennett & Brachman, 1998) (Table 9–1).

Phlebothrombosis

Phlebothrombosis denotes thrombosis and usually indicates that the inflammation is relatively inconspicuous. It is thought to give rise to embolism because the thrombus is poorly attached to the wall of the vein. Both thrombophlebitis and phlebothrombosis have a degree of inflammation and are associated with potential embolism. Factors that promote thrombosis are summarized in Table 9–2.

Thrombophlebitis

Thrombophlebitis denotes a twofold injury–thrombosis plus inflammation. The development of thrombophlebitis is easily recognized. Classic symptoms of tenderness, erythema, and swelling are seen the longer a catheter remains in place. A painful in-

TABLE 9 – 1
APPROXIMATE RISKS OF BLOODSTREAM INFECTION ASSOCIATED WITH VARIOUS TYPES OF DEVICES FOR INTRAVASCULAR ACCESS*

Type of Device	Representative Rate	Representative Range
Short-term temporary access†		
Peripheral IV cannulas		
Winged steel needles	<0.2	0–1
Peripheral IV catheters		
Percutaneously inserted	0.2	0–1
Cutdown 6	0–1	
Midline catheters 0.7	0.7–0.8	
Arterial catheters 1	—	
Central venous catheters		
All-purpose, multilumen	3	1–7
Pulmonary artery 1	0–5	
Hemodialysis 10	3–18	
Long-term indefinite access‡		
Peripherally inserted, central venous catheters	0.20	—
Cuffed central catheters (eg, Hickman, Broviac)	0.20	0.10–0.53
Subcutaneous central venous ports (eg, Infusaport, Port-a-cath, Landmark) 0.04	0.00–0.10	

IV, intravenous.
*Based on data from recently published, prospective studies.
†Number of bloodstream infections per 100 devices.
‡Number of bloodstream infections per 100 device-days.
(Reproduced with permission from Bennett, J.V., & Brachman, P.S. [1998]. *Hospital infections* [4th ed., p. 696]. Philadelphia: Lippincott Williams & Wilkins.)

T A B L E   9 – 2
GENESIS OF THROMBOSIS

Type	Clinical Manifestation	Contributing Factors
Fibrin sheath thrombosis	Inability to aspirate blood; catheter occlusion	Thrombogenic catheter material
Vascular mural thrombosis	Vein obstruction; classic symptoms of thrombosis	Difficult insertions; multiple attempts at venipuncture; sustained contact of the catheter with the venous wall

flammation develops along the length of the vein. If the infusion is allowed to continue, the thrombosis progressively obstructs the circulation and the vein becomes hard, tortuous, tender, and painful. Early detection may prevent an obstructive thrombophlebitis that can slow and eventually stop the infusion. This condition, which is painful, may persist indefinitely, incapacitating the patient and limiting available veins for future therapy.

Contributing Factors

Any irritation involving the wall of the vein predisposes the patient to thrombophlebitis. *Duration of the infusion* is a significant factor in the development of thrombophlebitis. As the duration increases, so do the incidence and degree of inflammation.

The *composition of the solution* may play a role. Venous irritation and inflammation may result from the infusion of hypertonic glucose solutions, certain drug additives, or solutions with a pH significantly different from that of the plasma. Dextrose solutions are irritating to the vein. The *United States Pharmacopeia* (USP) specifications for pH of dextrose solutions range from 3.5 to 6.5; acidity is necessary to prevent "caramelization" of the dextrose during autoclaving and to preserve the stability of the solution during storage. Studies show a significant reduction in thrombophlebitis when buffered glucose solution have been infused. Neut, a sodium bicarbonate 1% solution, may be added to increase the pH of acid IV solutions. This additive, however, poses a problem of incompatibility when added to solutions containing drugs. The greatest number of incompatibilities may be produced by changes in pH (Bennett & Brachman, 1998). As an example, tetracycline hydrochloride, with a pH of 2.5 to 3.0, is unstable in an alkaline environment.

The *infusion site* can be a factor contributing to thrombophlebitis. The veins in areas over joint flexion undergo injury when motion of the catheter irritates the venous wall. The veins in the lower extremities are especially susceptible to trauma, which may be enhanced by stagnant blood in varicosities and stasis in peripheral venous circulation.

 SAFE PRACTICE ALERT   When used for infusing an irritating solution, small veins are subject to inflammation.

The *infusion catheter* may occlude the entire lumen of the vein, obstructing the flow of circulating blood; the solution then flows undiluted, irritating the wall of the vein.

Venipuncture technique can mean the difference between a successful infusion and the complication of thrombophlebitis. Only minimal trauma results from a skillfully executed venipuncture, whereas a carelessly performed venipuncture may seriously traumatize the venous wall. Phlebitis associated with sepsis may be related to the technique of the clinician. Infection is always a risk if sterile technique is not zealously observed. Thorough cleansing of the skin is important in preventing infections. Maintenance of asepsis is essential during long-term therapy, particularly in the use of the through-the-needle catheter (Bennett & Brachman, 1998).

Infusion methods for parenteral solutions may foster septic thrombophlebitis. This complication is most often associated with the through-the-needle catheter. The catheter threaded through the needle remains sterile and does not come in contact with the skin, but provides a large subcutaneous orifice facilitating entry of bacteria around the catheter and seepage of fluid.

The over-the-needle catheter is not without fault because it comes in direct contact with the skin before being introduced into the vein. However, the tight fit through the skin may bar further bacterial entry. Box 9–1 summarizes contributing factors.

Treatment

Most cases of superficial thrombophlebitis respond to prompt removal of the IV catheter and local application of heat, although the affected vein may remain firm for several months.

A sterile inflammation usually develops from a chemical or mechanical irritation. When the inflammation is the result of sepsis, however, the condition is much more serious and carries with it the potential danger of septicemia and acute bacterial endocarditis. Additional treatment measures are required, possibly including excision of the infected vein. The wound is then left to heal secondarily. Antibiotic therapy then begins and continues for 7 to 10 days.

An additional complication is embolism when thrombosis occurs. The more pro-

---

BOX 9–1 Factors Contributing to Venous Inflammation

Inflammation of the vein can occur from any foreign body and is mediated by the following:

- Duration of the infusion
- Composition of the solution
- Site of the infusion
- Venipuncture technique
- Method used

nounced the inflammation and the more intense the pain, the more organized the thrombus is likely to become. Embolism is less likely to occur from the well-attached clot of thrombophlebitis than from phlebothrombosis.

Preventive Measures

In performing venipunctures, the nurse exercises every caution to avoid injuring the wall of the vein needlessly. Multiple punctures, through-and-through punctures, and damage to the posterior wall of the vein with the point of the catheter can lead to thrombosis. The nurse can minimize the risk of phlebitis by implementing these measures:

- Refrain from using veins in the lower extremities.
- Select veins with ample blood volume when infusing irritating substances.
- Avoid veins in areas over joint flexion and use an arm board if the vein must be located in an area of flexion.
- Anchor the catheter securely to prevent motion, which may loosen the catheter.

To prevent septic phlebitis, thorough preparation of the skin, together with aseptic technique and maintenance of asepsis during infusion, is imperative. Periodic inspection of the injection site will detect developing complications before serious damage occurs.

Complaints of a painful infusion make it necessary to differentiate between early phlebitis and venospasm from an irritating solution. In the case of venospasm, slowing the infusion and applying heat to the vein dilates the vessel and increases the blood flow, thereby diluting the solution and relieving the pain. After a hypertonic solution infusion, infusion with an isotonic fluid flushes the vein of irritating substances.

If inflammation accompanies the pain, a change in the injection site should be considered. Continuing the infusion leads to progressive trauma and limits available veins. Adherence to time limits for removal of the catheter reduces the incidence of phlebitis (Intravenous Nurses Society [INS], 1998, 2000). Box 9–2 ranks the severity of phlebitis.

During removal of the infusion catheter, care must be taken to prevent injury to the wall of the vein; the catheter should be removed at an angle nearly flush with the skin. Pressure should be applied for a reasonable length of time to prevent extravasation of blood.

BOX 9–2 Phlebitis Scale

1+ = pain at site, erythema or edema, no streaking, no palpable cord
2+ = pain at site, erythema or edema, streak formation, no palpable cord
3+ = pain at site, erythema and/or edema, streak formation, palpable cord

Infiltration

Dislodgment of the catheter with consequent **infiltration** of fluid is common and frequently is considered of minor significance. With the increasing numbers of irritating solutions and the frequency with which potent drugs are infused in IV solutions, serious problems may occur when the fluid invades the surrounding tissues. Hypertonic, acid, and alkaline fluids are contraindicated for hypodermoclysis and are not intended for other than venous infusions. If they are allowed to infiltrate, necrosis may occur.

If necrosis is avoided, edema may nevertheless

- Deprive the patient of fluid and drug absorption at the rate essential for successful therapy
- Limit veins available for venipuncture, complicating therapy
- Predispose the patient to infection

 SAFE PRACTICE ALERT   To confirm an infiltration, apply a tourniquet proximal to the injection site tightly enough to restrict the venous flow. If the infusion continues regardless of this venous obstruction, extravasation is evident.

Extravasation

Extravasation can easily be recognized by increasing edema at the site of the infusion. Comparing the infusion area with the identical area in the opposite extremity can help the nurse identify swelling.

In many cases, the edema is allowed to increase to great proportions because of the misconception that backflow of blood into the adapter is significant proof that the infusion is entering the vein. This is not a reliable method for detecting possible infiltration because the point of the IV catheter may puncture the posterior wall of the vein, leaving the greater portion of the bevel in the lumen of the vein. Blood return is obtained on negative pressure, but if the infusion is allowed to continue, fluid seeps into the tissues at the point of the catheter, thereby increasing the edema (see Chaps. 8 and 9).

Occasionally, a blood return is not obtained on negative pressure. This may occur when the needle occludes the lumen of a small vein, obstructing the flow of blood. Evidence of backflow should not be the sole criterion for confirming extravasation.

Drugs that contribute to necrosis that results from extravasation are most often osmotically active or **ischemia** inducing, or they cause direct **cellular toxicity.** Mechanical compression in the infiltrated tissue can increase the extent of damage, as can infection of the resulting wound. If only superficial tissue loss occurs and the area remains free of infection, **débridement** yields a clean bed capable of granulation. If deep structures are involved, however, spontaneous wound healing may be averted, resulting in the need for wide excision, débridement, and grafting or amputation to restore tissue integrity.

■ SYSTEMIC COMPLICATIONS

Serious, even life-threatening systemic complications range from septicemia to embolism to shock and infection. These complications need to be prevented or identified as soon as possible and treatment interventions begun.

Septicemia

Septicemia is caused by invasion of the bloodstream by microorganisms or their byproducts, including bacteria, fungi, mycobacteria and, rarely, viruses. Clinical manifestations of septicemia include chills, fever, general malaise, and headache.

Contributing Factors

Certain predisposing factors put the infusion therapy patient at risk:

- Age younger than 1 year or older than 60 years
- Granulocytopenia
- Immunocompromised state
- Loss of skin integrity
- Distant infection that might contribute to hematogenous seeding.

Also contributing to the development of septicemia are catheter-related factors, such as the size of the catheter, number of lumens, function and use of the catheter, catheter material, bacterial adherence, and **thrombogenicity.**

Treatment

Supportive therapy for the patient with septicemia includes fluid replacement, blood pressure maintenance, oxygenation, cardiac output maintenance, nutritional support, and preservation of acid–base balance. Ancillary treatments involve administration of steroids, naloxone, and endotoxin vaccination.

Preventive Measures

Because intravascular systems should be considered potential portals for infection, prevention programs support the use of 0.2-μm air-eliminating, bacterial-retentive filters. In addition, good hand-washing techniques, line care protocols, and adherence to the INS Standards of Practice for monitoring, maintenance of infusion, tubing changes, and catheter care all contribute to an environment that does not readily support development of septicemia in patients receiving infusion therapies (see Chaps. 4, 9, and 10).

Pulmonary Embolism

Pulmonary embolism occurs when a substance, usually a blood clot, dislodges and floats freely, propelled by the venous circulation to the right side of the heart and into the pulmonary artery (Metheny, 2000). Emboli may obstruct the main pulmonary artery or the arteries to the lobes, occluding arterial apertures at major bifurcations (INS, 1998, 2000). Obstruction of the main artery, then, results in circulatory and cardiac disturbances. Recurrent small emboli may eventually result in pulmonary hypertension and right heart failure (Metheny, 2000).

Precautions for preventing this serious complication include the following:

- Filter infusions of blood or plasma through an adequate filter to remove any particulates that could promote small emboli formation.
- Do not perform venipuncture in the veins of the lower extremities. These veins are particularly susceptible to trauma that predisposes the patient to thrombophlebitis. Although superficial veins rarely seem to be the source of emboli (INS, 1998, 2000), a thrombus may extend into the deep veins, resulting in a potentially viable clot; superficial and deep veins unite freely in the lower extremities.
- Avoid applying positive pressure to relieve clot formation.

 SAFE PRACTICE ALERT Avoid irrigating a plugged catheter. Doing so may embolize small catheter thrombi, some of which are infected.

- Check for patency of the lumen of the catheter by kinking the infusion tubing approximately 8 inches from the catheter. Then kink and release the tubing between the catheter and the pinched tubing. If the tubing becomes hard and meets with resistance, obstruction is evident. The catheter should be removed and the infusion reinstated.
- Take special precautions with drug additives. Reconstituted drugs must be completely dissolved before being added to parenteral solutions because it is the inherent nature of red blood cells to adhere to particles, adding to the danger of clot formation.
- Examine fluids to detect particulate matter.

Air Embolism

Although **air embolism** is a significant possible complication with air-dependent containers, it is more frequently associated with central venous lines. There is a potential risk for air embolism to result from the insertion of a CVC, inadequate sealing of the tract before disconnecting a CVC, disconnection of central lines, and bypassing the pump housing of an electronic volumetric pump with an IV piggyback connection.

SAFE PRACTICE ALERT   Fatal embolism may occur when small bubbles accumulate dangerously and form tenacious bubbles that block the pulmonary capillaries. Recognition of the circumstances that contribute to this hazard and measures taken to prevent their occurrence are imperative for safe fluid therapy.

Symptoms associated with air embolism arising from sudden vascular collapse include cyanosis, drop in blood pressure, weak, rapid pulse, rise in venous pressure, and loss of consciousness.

 SAFE PRACTICE ALERT   If air embolism occurs, the source of air entry must be immediately rectified. The patient should be turned on the left side with his or her head down. This causes the air to rise in the right atrium, preventing it from entering the pulmonary artery. Oxygen is then administered and the physician notified.

Contributing Factors: Gravity Infusions

If a vented container is allowed to run dry, air enters the tubing and the fluid level drops to the proximity of the patient's chest. The pressure exerted by the blood on the walls of the veins controls the level to which the air drops in the tubing. A negative pressure in the vein may allow air to enter the bloodstream. Negative pressure occurs when the extremity receiving the infusion is elevated above the heart (Metheny, 2000).

Infusions flowing through a CVC carry an even greater risk of air embolism when the container empties than infusions flowing through a peripheral vein. Because the central venous pressure is lower than the peripheral venous pressure, there is more likely to be a negative pressure that could suck air into the circulation. The nurse therefore needs to take precautions while changing the administration set of a central venous infusion.

Running solutions simultaneously is a key factor. One empty vented container becomes the source of air for the flowing solution. This happens because the atmospheric pressure is greater in the open tubing to the empty container than below the partially restricted clamp on the infusion side. Recurrent small air bubbles are constantly aspirated into the flowing solution and on into the venous system. The introduction of air may be prevented by running one solution at a time. Vigilance is imperative if vented solutions are prescribed to run simultaneously. The tubing must be clamped off completely before the solution container is allowed to empty (Bennett & Brachman, 1998).

This same principle is involved in the piggyback setup for secondary infusions. The potential danger of air embolism exists whenever solutions from two vented sets run simultaneously through a common catheter. Advanced technologies have minimized the use of piggyback setups.

All connections of an infusion set must be tight. Any faulty opening or defective hole in the set allows air to be emitted into the flowing solution. If a stopcock is used, the outlets not in use must be completely shut off.

The regulating clamp on the infusion set should be located no higher than the pa-

KEY INTERVENTIONS:	Removing Air When Changing the IV Administration Set

If the fluid container on a continuous infusion should empty, fresh fluid will force trapped air into the circulation and air embolus may result. To help ensure that air does not enter the patient's system during an IV administration, take the following precautions:

1. Immediately before and during the time that the catheter will be open to the air, assist the patient to lie flat and supine in bed and perform the Valsalva maneuver (forced expiration with the mouth closed).
2. To remove the air from the administration set, first place a hemostat (clamp) close to the infusion catheter.
3. Hang the fresh solution container.
4. With an antiseptic agent, clean the section of the tubing proximal to the hemostat and below the air level in the tubing.
5. Insert a sterile needle to allow the air to escape.
6. *Unclamp the hemostat* and readjust flow.

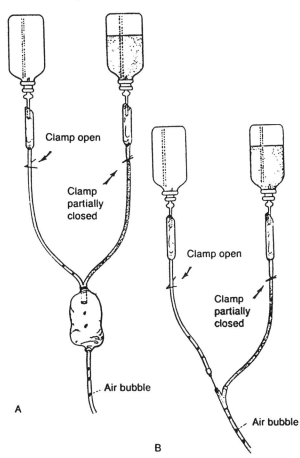

Clamp open

Clamp partially closed

Clamp open

Clamp partially closed

Air bubble

A

Air bubble

B

(A) When the infusate container runs dry during simultaneous infusion of fluids through a Y-type administration set, pressure below the partially constricted clamp is lower than the atmospheric pressure, allowing air from the empty container (atmospheric) to enter the infusion. (B) Without an automatic shut-off valve on a secondary infusion piggybacked through the injection site of a primary IV set, air from the empty infusate container will enter the patient's circulation.

The Y-type infusion set used with vented containers is a less obvious source of air embolism but one by which unknown quantities of air can be drawn into the bloodstream.

tient's chest. Because the pressure exerted by the blood on the venous wall normally raises a column of water from 4 to 11 cm above the heart, a restricting clamp placed above this point results in a negative pressure in the tubing. If great enough, the pressure can suck air into the flowing solution should a loose connection or a faulty opening exist between the clamp and the catheter (Bennett & Brachman, 1998). The lower the clamp, the greater the chance of defects occurring above the clamp, where positive pressure can force the solution to leak out (Bennett & Brachman, 1998).

An infusion set long enough to drop below the extremity gives added protection against air being drawn into the vein should the infusion bottle empty. Inlying pressure chambers on administration sets should be kept filled at all times. Manual compression of an empty chamber forces air into the bloodstream.

Catheter Embolism

Catheter embolism may occur during the insertion of a through-the-needle catheter if part of the catheter breaks off, which may happen if the proper procedure is not strictly followed. The catheter should never be pulled back through the needle. If it becomes necessary to remove the catheter, the entire unit should be removed and a new catheter inserted. Catheter embolism may also occur during the insertion of an over-the-needle catheter if the needle is either partially or totally withdrawn and then reinserted. If the catheter shears off into circulation, fluoroscopic cardiac catheterization may be necessary to visualize and remove the embolus.

Pulmonary Edema

Overloading the circulation is hazardous to any patient, but especially to elderly patients and to patients with impaired renal and cardiac function. Infusing fluids too rapidly increases the venous pressure, with the possibility of consequences such as cardiac dilation and pulmonary edema (see Chap. 22).

Signs and symptoms, such as venous dilation with engorged neck veins, increased blood pressure, and a rise in venous pressure, should alert the nurse to the danger of pulmonary edema. Rapid respiration and shortness of breath may occur.

Treatment

With signs of circulatory overload, the infusion should be slowed to a minimal rate and the physician notified. Raising the patient to a sitting position may facilitate breathing.

Preventive Measures

Several preventative measures may reduce the likelihood of pulmonary edema:

- Maintain infusions at the prescribed flow rate.
- Avoid applying positive pressure using the pressure-chamber administra-

tion sets to infuse solutions. If the patient requires fluids so rapidly that positive pressure is required, infusion then becomes the physician's responsibility.

- Use a controlled-volume infusion set for added protection. These sets control the volume from 10 to 150 mL and prevent large quantities of fluid from being accidentally infused.
- Discard solutions not infused within the 24-hour period prescribed. Do not infuse them with the following day's fluids. Fluids administered in excess of the quantity ordered can overtax the homeostatic controls, thereby increasing the danger of pulmonary edema.

Speed Shock

Speed shock is the systemic reaction that occurs when a substance foreign to the body is rapidly introduced into the circulation. Caution must be observed in administering IV push injections. Rapid injection permits medication to concentrate in the plasma and reach toxic proportions. The toxin may then flood the organs that are rich in blood, such as the heart and brain. As a result, syncope, shock, and cardiac arrest may occur (Metheny, 2000).

Some precautionary measures can minimize the potential danger of speed shock. Using a pediatric-type infusion set to reduce the size of the drops of infusate provides greater accuracy and thereby reduces the risks attendant on rapid administration. These sets are valuable when solutions containing potent drugs must be maintained at a minimal rate of flow. Electronic flow control devices may be used to control the rate of infusion, with the nurse who initiates the infusion making sure that the solution is flowing freely before adjusting the rate. The nurse also needs to keep in mind that movement of a catheter in which the aperture is partially obstructed by the wall of the vein can cause an increase in the flow, contributing to the danger of speed shock.

Intravascular Infection

Intravascular infection is related to many factors, such as the intravascular device (catheter/cannula), contaminated solution or other substances, and bloodborne pathogens, among others.

Intravascular device–related bloodstream infections are perhaps the least frequently recognized nosocomial infection (Bennett & Brachman, 1998). Catheter-related infections are those that originate from the catheter material itself or from migration of organisms through the open skin along the catheter (see Table 9–1). Solution-related infections are those that result from contamination of IV solutions, either in the manufacturing process or in use.

Sources of Infection

Bacteria responsible for IV-associated infection come from three main sources: air, skin, and blood. Microorganisms (flora and fauna) characteristic of a given location are referred to accordingly, hence the terms skin flora, intestinal flora, and so on. Table 9–3 identifies microbial pathogens associated with infusion-related septicemia (Bennett & Brachman, 1998).

AIR

The number of microbes per cubic foot of air varies depending on the particular area involved. Where infection is present, bacteria escape in bodily discharges, contaminating clothing, bedding, and dressings. Activity, such as making a bed, sends bacteria flying into the air on particles of lint, pus, and dried epithelium (Bennett & Brachman, 1998). Increased activity raises the number of airborne particles and pro-

T A B L E   9 – 3

MICROORGANISMS MOST FREQUENTLY ENCOUNTERED IN VARIOUS FORMS OF INTRAVASCULAR LINE–RELATED INFECTION

Source	Pathogens
Catheter related	
Peripheral IV catheter	Coagulase-negative staphylococci*
	Staphylococcus aureus
	Candida spp*
Central venous catheters	Coagulase-negative staphylococci
	S. aureus
	Candida spp
	Corynebacterium spp (especially JK-1)
	Klebsiella and *Enterobacter* spp
	Mycobacterium spp
	Trichophyton beiglii
	Fusarium spp
	*Malassezia furfur**
Contaminated IV infusate	Tribe Klebsielleae
	Enterobacter cloacae
	Enterobacter agglomerans
	Serratia marcescens
	Klebsiella spp
	Burkholderia cepacia
	Burkholderia acidivorans, Burkholderia pickettii
	Stenotrophomonas maltophilia
	Citrobacter freundii
	Flavobacterium, spp
	Candida tropicalis
Contaminated blood products	*E. cloacae*
	S. marcescens
	Ochrobactrum anthropi
	Flavobacterium spp
	Burkholderia spp
	Yersinia spp
	Salmonella spp

IV, intravenous.

*Also seen with peripheral IV catheters in association with the administration of lipid emulsion for parenteral nutritional support.

(Reproduced with permission from Bennett, J.V., & Brachman, P.S. (1998). *Hospital infections* [4th ed., p. 698]. Philadelphia: Lippincott Williams & Wilkins.)

vides an environment that interferes with aseptic technique and potentially contributes to contamination. Airborne microorganisms may be plentiful in patient areas and utility rooms. These contaminants find easy access to unprotected IV fluids.

SKIN

The skin is the source of bacteria mainly responsible for IV-associated infection. The bacteria found on the skin are referred to as resident or transient. Resident bacteria are those normally present, and they are relatively constant in a given individual. They adhere tightly to the skin and usually include *Staphylococcus albus* as well as diphtheroids and *Bacillus* species (Bennett & Brachman, 1998). Because not all bacteria are removed by scrubbing, meticulous care must be observed to avoid touching sterile equipment.

 SAFE PRACTICE ALERT Quaternary ammonium compounds such as aqueous benzalkonium chloride are inactivated by organic debris. Therefore, they are ineffective against gram-negative organisms and should not be used for skin disinfection.

The transient bacteria are responsible for infection carried from one person to another. Touch contamination is a potential hazard of infection because hospital personnel move about frequently, touching patients and objects. Frequent hand washing is imperative.

The patient's skin is fertile soil for bacterial growth. Some estimates indicate that a minimum of 10,000 organisms are present per square centimeter of normal skin (Parras et al., 1994). A square centimeter is equal to 0.155 square inches. Organisms such as gram-positive *Staphylococcus epidermidis, Staphylococcus aureus*, gram-negative bacilli (especially *Klebsiella, Enterobacter*, and *Serratia*), and enterococci are ubiquitous on the skin of hospitalized patients (Bennett & Brachman, 1998).

BLOOD

Like the skin, the blood may harbor potentially dangerous microorganisms. Therefore, care must be taken to prevent bacterial or other contamination from blood spills when drawing blood samples and performing venipunctures. Refer to Chapter 17 for a discussion of bloodborne pathogens; also see Box 9–3 for a summary of standard precautions for preventing infections, particularly bloodborne infections.

Survivability of Bacteria and Other Contaminants

Infection depends on the ability of bacteria to survive and proliferate. The factors that influence their survival are the specific organisms present, the number of such organisms, the resistance of the host, and the environmental conditions (Pearson, 1996).

SPECIFIC ORGANISMS

Bacteria are referred to as pathogenic or nonpathogenic. Pathogenic bacteria are capable of producing disease. All bacteria should be considered pathogenic because current data show that bacteria previously considered nonpathogenic may produce

---

BOX 9–3 **Standard Precautions**

Use Standard Precautions, or the equivalent, for the care of all patients, *Category IB**

A. Handwashing

(1) Wash hands after touching blood, body fluids, secretions, excretions, and contaminated items, whether or not gloves are worn. Wash hands immediately after gloves are removed, between patient contacts, and when otherwise indicated to avoid transfer of microorganisms to other patients or environments. It may be necessary to wash hands between tasks and procedures on the same patient to prevent cross-contamination of different body sites. *Category IB*

(2) Use a plain (nonantimicrobial) soap for routine hand-washing. *Category IB*

(3) Use an antimicrobial agent or a waterless antiseptic agent for specific circumstances (eg, control of outbreaks or hyperendemic infections), as defined by the infection control program. *Category IB* (see Contact Precautions for additional recommendations on using antimicrobial and antiseptic agents.)

B. Gloves

Wear gloves (clean, nonsterile gloves are adequate) when touching blood, body fluids, secretions, excretions, and contaminated items. Put on clean gloves just before touching mucous membranes and nonintact skin. Change gloves between tasks and procedures on the same patient after contact with material that may contain a high concentration of microorganisms. Remove gloves promptly after use, before touching non-contaminated items and environmental surfaces, and before going to another patient, and wash hands immediately to avoid transfer of microorganisms to other patients or environments. *Category IB*

C. Mask, Eye Protection, Face Shield

Wear a mask and eye protection or a face shield to protect mucous membranes of the eyes, nose, and mouth during procedures and patient-care activities that are likely to generate splashes or sprays of blood, body fluids, secretions, and excretions. *Category IB*

D. Gown

Wear a gown (a clean, nonsterile gown is adequate) to protect skin and to prevent soiling of clothing during procedures and patient-care activities that are likely to generate splashes or sprays of blood, body fluids, secretions, or excretions. Select a gown that is appropriate for the activity and amount of fluid likely to be encountered. Remove a soiled gown as promptly as possible, and wash hands to avoid transfer of microorganisms to other patients or environments. *Category IB*

E. Patient-Care Equipment

Handle used patient-care equipment soiled with blood, body fluids, secretions, and excretions in a manner that prevents skin and mucous membrane exposures, contamination of clothing, and transfer of microorganisms to other patients and environments. Ensure that reusable equipment is not used for the care of another patient until it has been cleaned and reprocessed appropriately. Ensure that single-use items are discarded properly. *Category IB*

F. Environmental Control

Ensure that the hospital has adequate procedures for the routine care, cleaning, and disinfection of environment surfaces, beds, bedrails, bedside equipment, and other frequently touched surfaces, and ensure that these procedures are being followed. *Category IB*

G. Linen

Handle, transport, and process used linen soiled with blood, body fluids, secretions, and excretions in a manner that prevents skin and mucous membrane exposures and contamination of clothing, and that avoids transfer of microorganisms to other patients and environments. *Category IB*

H. Occupational Health and Bloodborne Pathogens

(1) Take care to prevent injuries when using needles, scalpels and other sharp instruments or devices; when handling sharp instruments after procedures; when cleaning use instruments; and when disposing of used needles. Never recap used needles, or otherwise manipulate them using both hands, or use any other technique that involves directing the point of a needle toward any part of the body; rather, use either a one-handed "scoop" technique or mechanical device designed for holding the needle sheath. Do not remove used needles from disposable syringes by hand, and do not bend, break, or otherwise manipulate used needles by hand. Place used disposable syringes and needles, scalpel blades, and other sharp items in appropriate puncture-resistant containers, which are located as close as practical to the area in which the items were used and place reusable syringes and needles in a puncture-resistant container for transport to the processing area. *Category IB*

(2) Use mouthpieces, resuscitation bags, or other ventilatior devices as an alternative to mouth-to-mouth resuscitation methods in areas where the need for resuscitation is predictable. *Category IB*

I. Patient Placement

Place a patient who contaminates the environment or who does not (or cannot be expected to) assist in maintaining appropriate hygiene or environmental control in a private room. If a private room is not available, consult with infection control professionals regarding patient placement or other alternatives. *Category IB*

---

*Category IB. Strongly recommended for all hospitals and reviewed as effective by experts in the field and a consensus of HICPAC based on strong rationale and suggestive evidence, even though definitive scientific studies have not been done. (From Guideline for isolation precautions in hospitals developed by the Centers for Disease Control and Prevention and the Hospital Infection Control Practices Advisory Committee [HICPAC], January 1996.)

infection. In one study, *Serratia* species were implicated in 35% of cases of gram-negative septicemia resulting from IV therapy (Bennett & Brachman, 1998).

Bacteria are classified as gram positive and gram negative. In recent years, gram-negative bacteria have replaced gram-positive bacteria as the leading cause of death from septicemia (Pearson, 1996; INS, 1998, 2000). The single most important reason for the intensity of the problem is probably the increased use of antibiotics that are highly effective against gram-positive organisms but only selectively effective against gram-negative organisms. With the competitive inhibition of gram-positive bacteria eliminated, the more resistant gram-negative organisms have proliferated in the hospital environment (Metheny, 2000; Smith, 1998).

NUMBER OF ORGANISMS

The number of contaminants present influences the probability of an infection arising. The power of bacteria to proliferate must not be underestimated. It is simply not true that small amounts of bacteria from touch contamination are harmless. Contamination of IV fluids and bottles with even a few organisms is extremely dangerous because some fungi and many bacteria can proliferate at room temperature in a variety of IV solutions to more than 105 organisms/mL within 24 hours (Bennett & Brachman, 1998).

HOST RESISTANCE

The resistance of the host influences the development and course of infection, particularly septicemia. Underlying conditions such as diabetes mellitus, chronic uremia, cirrhosis, cancer, and leukemia may adversely affect the patient's capacity to resist infection. Treatment with immunosuppressive drugs, corticosteroids, anticancer agents, and extensive radiation therapy may depress immunologic response and permit the invasion of infection. Therapy may mask infection so that serious infection remains unrecognized until autopsy.

ENVIRONMENTAL CONDITIONS

Environmental conditions that affect the survival and propagation of bacteria in IV fluids are the pH, temperature, and the presence of essential nutrients in the infusion.

Some organisms grow rapidly in a neutral solution and are less likely to grow in an acid medium. Buffering of acidic dextrose solutions has been recommended for preventing phlebitis, although the neutral environment provided by the buffer may enhance the survival and proliferation of bacteria.

The temperature of the fluid may affect the ability of bacteria to multiply. At room temperature, strains of *Enterobacter cloacae, Enterobacter agglomerans,* and other members of the tribe Klebsielleae proliferate rapidly in commercial solutions of 5% dextrose in water.

Total parenteral nutrition fluids should be used as soon as possible after preparation. When they must be stored temporarily, they should be refrigerated at 4°C. At this temperature, growth of *Candida albicans* is suppressed (Bennett & Brachman, 1998).

Certain nutrients must be present to support bacterial growth. Blood and crystalloid solutions provide nutrients that broaden the spectrum of pathogens capable of proliferation. Maki and associates stated that the administration of blood or reflux of blood into the infusion system may provide sufficient nutrients to broaden this spectrum (Alhimyary, Fernandez, & Pizard, 1996). Accordingly, the American Association of Blood Banks requires blood to be stored at a constant controlled refrigeration of 1°C to 6°C (see Chap. 17).

Saline fluids are likely to contain enough biologically available carbon, nitrogen, sulfur, phosphate, and traces of other material to support, under favorable conditions, the survival and multiplication of any gram-negative bacillus introduced to as many as 1 million organisms per milliliter.

Contributors to Contamination and Infection

Extrinsic contamination and other factors that contribute to infection range from faulty handling of fluids to faulty devices and techniques.

FAULTY HANDLING AND FLAWED PROCEDURES

Containers of parenteral fluid are accepted as being sterile and nonpyrogenic on arrival from the manufacturer. The potential risk of contamination occurring in transit or in use is frequently overlooked by hospital personnel. However, through faulty handling or carelessness, glass containers may become cracked or damaged and plastic bags punctured. Bacteria and fungi may penetrate a hairline crack in an IV container, even though the crack is so fine that fluid does not leak from the container.

Besides providing carbon and energy, IV solutions of dextrose include the extra nutrients needed to support the growth of 10 million organisms per milliliter of fluid. If the fluid is not examined closely, its opalescence may be overlooked, and subsequent infusion of a few hundred milliliters of such contaminated fluid results in deep shock or possibly death.

The nurse has responsibility for examining containers of fluid before their use. They should be inspected against a light and dark background for cracks, defects, turbidity, and particulates. Plastic containers should be squeezed to detect any puncture hole. Accidental puncture may occur without being evident and provide a port for entry for microorganisms (Bennett & Brachman, 1998). Any container with a crack or defect must be regarded as potentially contaminated and unusable. Similarly, any glass container lacking a vacuum when opened should not be used.

UNSTERILE CONDITIONS

When a 1-L glass container is opened, approximately 100 mL of air rushes in to fill the vacuum. In areas with a high concentration of airborne particles, contamination of unprotected fluids is a potential risk. The sterile environment of a laminar flow hood prevents this problem.

OUTDATED SOLUTIONS

The longer the container is in use, the greater the proliferation of bacteria and the greater the risk of infection should contamination inadvertently occur. The risk of infusing outdated fluids can be avoided by adhering to special limits, supported by a strong monitoring policy. Every container should be labeled with the time it is opened. The guidelines of the CDC and INS Standards of Practice should be followed, in addition to adhering to the guidelines developed by the Hospital Infection Control Advisory Committee (Bennett & Brachman, 1998; CDC, 1998).

IMPROPERLY PREPARED ADMIXTURES

Allowing untrained hospital personnel to add drugs to IV containers contributes to the potential for contamination. This risk is reduced when admixtures are prepared under laminar flow hoods by skilled personnel adhering to strict aseptic technique in accord with a pharmacy additive program.

Nurses and physicians who have to prepare admixtures in an emergency, and other personnel involved in the preparation and administration of IV drugs, should receive special training in the preparation of admixtures and the handling of IV fluids and equipment. Adherence to strict aseptic methods is vital. It must be emphasized that touch contamination is the primary source of infection. Although laminar flow hoods prevent airborne contamination, they do not ensure sterility when a break in aseptic technique occurs (see Chap. 18).

MANIPULATION OF EQUIPMENT

Intravenous fluids can be inadvertently contaminated by faulty techniques in manipulating the equipment. In open systems, in which fluids are not protected by air filters, the simple procedure of hanging the container may be taken for granted and the risk of contamination overlooked.

When an administration set is inserted into the container and the container is inverted, the fluid tends to leak out the vent onto the unsterile surface of the container. Regurgitation of the contaminated fluid into the container occurs when the container vents. Instructions in the use of the equipment often go unread and unheeded. Squeezing the drip chamber of the administration set before inserting it into the container and releasing it when the container is inverted prevents regurgitation of fluid and minimizes the risk of contamination.

EXPOSURE OF INJECTION PORTS AND STOPCOCKS

Meticulous aseptic technique must be observed in using injection ports because they are a potential source of contamination when used to piggyback infusions. The injection port location, at the distal end of the tubing, exposes it to patient excreta and drainage, which enhance the growth of microorganisms.

The injection port must be scrubbed at least 1 minute with an accepted antiseptic, such as 70% isopropyl alcohol. Scrubbing the injection cap for 30 seconds with an antimicrobial (eg, povidone–iodine) fluid provides good protection.

Today's use of needleless systems has minimized the risk associated with connecting a needle to an injection port. However, when a needle must be used, it should be firmly engaged up to the hub in the injection site and securely taped to prevent any in-and-out motion of the needle from introducing bacteria into the infusion (see Chaps. 11 and 12).

Similarly, three-way stopcocks are potential mechanisms of bacterial transmission because their ports, unprotected by sterile coverings, are open to moisture and other contaminants. Connected to CVCs and arterial lines, they are still used for drawing blood samples. Accordingly, aseptic practices are vital in preventing bacteria from being introduced into the IV line. Attaching a sterile catheter plug when the stopcock is added and changing the devices after each use reduce the risk of contamination. Whenever fluid leakage is discovered at injection sites, connections, or vents, the IV set should be replaced.

CATHETER INSERTION

Within 24 to 48 hours after a plastic catheter is inserted into a vessel, a loosely constructed fibrin sheath develops around the intravascular portion of the device (see Fig. 9–1), forming a nidus within which microorganisms can multiply. The nidus shields them to an extent from host defenses and antibiotics. The thrombus or thrombi generated by the catheter material may play a role in systemic infection.

Infection Prevention

Catheter care and antibiotic lock technique are two interventions used to prevent catheter-related infection. Additional preventive measures involve careful adherence to policies and procedures based on INS standards with respect to rotating the infusion site and limiting the time that the catheter dwells in the vessel (in-dwell time). This may reduce the inherent problems of catheter-associated infection even though most device-related septicemias are actually caused by the patient's own skin flora or by microorganisms transmitted from the hands of the health care professional.

ANTIBIOTIC LOCK TECHNIQUE

The antibiotic lock technique has been used to reduce the potential for CVC-related infection in the immunocompromised patient (see Table 9–3). Vancomycin, amphotericin B, and fluconazole have all been successfully used as flush solutions. A small amount of concentrated antibiotic or antifungal agent is instilled in the catheter and the distal portion of the catheter is capped.

SKIN PREPARATION

Microbes on the hands of health care personnel contribute to hospital-associated infection. Too often, breaks in sterile technique occur from failure to wash the hands before changing containers or administration sets or preparing admixtures. Besides the usual skin flora, antibiotic-resistant gram-negative organisms frequently contaminate the hands of hospital personnel.

To maintain asepsis, the CDC recommends that the hands be thoroughly washed before insertion of CVCs. Further, guidelines support the use of sterile gloves.

In a study made of 118 patients receiving IV therapy through an indwelling polyvinyl catheter, 53 catheters were found to be contaminated with bacteria; in 28 of these, the organisms were comparable with those cultured from the skin of the patient before the skin was cleaned with iodine.

Frequently, the question arises of whether to shave the insertion site. The need to remove hair is not substantiated by scientific evidence. Antiseptics used to clean the skin also clean the hair. Moreover, shaving may produce microabrasions, which can enhance the proliferation of bacteria.

Alcohol 70% is typically used to prepare the skin site for venipuncture. Studies show that ethyl alcohol, 70% by weight, is an effective germicide for the skin when applied with friction for 1 minute, and INS standards support its use. It is as effective as 12 minutes of scrubbing and reduces the bacterial count by 75%. Because a minimum of 10,000 organisms/cm^2 is present on normal skin, the count is reduced to 2500. Too frequently, alcohol use consists of a quick wipe, which fails to reduce the bacterial count significantly (INS, 1998, 2000).

Iodine and iodine-containing disinfectants are still the most reliable agents for preparing the skin for venipuncture because they provide bactericidal, fungicidal, and sporicidal activity. Because of occasional patient allergy to iodine, the possibility of sensitivity should be investigated before its use. Tincture of iodine (2% iodine in 70% alcohol) is inexpensive and well tolerated. The solution should be liberally applied, allowed to dry for at least 30 seconds, and washed off with 70% alcohol. Both agents should be applied with friction, working from the center of the field to periphery. Iodophor preparations, when used for patients with sensitive skin, should not be washed off because the sustained release of free iodine may be necessary for germicidal action. Iodophor preparations require a 30-second contact time.

EQUIPMENT PREPARATION

The tourniquet itself may be a source of cross-infection and contamination owing to its potential for reuse from patient to patient. Using an IV start kit with a disposable tourniquet minimizes the problem. However, if reusable tourniquets are consistent with clinical practice, the tourniquet should be disinfected frequently.

Once the venipuncture is completed and the catheter is in the lumen of the vein, the catheter must be securely anchored. To-and-fro motion of the catheter in the puncture wound may irritate the intima of the vein and introduce cutaneous bacteria.

Thought should be given next to the possible contamination of the adhesive tape used to secure the catheter. Because rolls of tape last indefinitely, they may harbor contaminants; they are transported from room to room, placed on patients' beds and tables, and frequently roll to the floor. Furthermore, before venipuncture, strips of tape often are torn off the roll and placed in convenient locations on the bed, table, and uniform. These facts should be kept in mind. Adhesive tape should not be applied over the puncture wound. The puncture wound must be considered an open wound and asepsis must be maintained.

ACCESS DEVICE AND SITE CARE

The CDC recommends using a topical antibiotic or antiseptic ointment at the IV site after catheter insertion. The wound should be protected by a sterile, occlusive dressing. Dressing changes should be consistent with INS standards. The same applies to catheter site rotations. Frequent observations should be made for signs of malfunction of the catheter, infiltration, and phlebitis characterized by erythema, induration, or tenderness (Bennett & Brachman, 1998). Such signs require immediate removal of the catheter.

Research Issues: CENTRAL VENOUS CATHETERS

Krzywda, E. (1999). Predisposing factors, prevention, and management of central venous catheter occlusions. Journal of Intravenous Nursing, 22(6S), 14–16.
The author addressed current research on and clinical practices associated with central venous catheter occlusion. The summary demonstrated the effect of interruption of care on therapy, catheter replacement, limitations in vascular access, and other serious sequelae associated with thrombotic complications. The primary approach should be one of prevention.

Hadaway L.C. (1998). Major thrombotic and nonthrombotic complications: Loss of patency. Journal of Intravenous Nursing, 21(5S), 143–160.
In this study, the author demonstrated that maintaining catheter function depends on both catheter and vessel patency.

Besides monitoring for signs of catheter malfunction, the nurse needs to monitor the condition of the catheter. Contamination may result from a break in aseptic technique, from contaminated fluid or administration set, from bacterial invasion of the puncture wound, or from clinically undetected bacteremia arising from an infection in a remote area of the body, such as a tracheostomy, the urinary tract, or a surgical wound. The clot around or in the catheter serves as an excellent trap for circulatory microorganisms and as a source of nutrients for bacterial proliferation (Alhimyary, Fernandez, and Pizard 1996; Bennett & Brachman, 1998; Parras et al., 1994). See the accompanying CVC research display for more information.

Confirmation of Infection

Intravenous-associated sepsis is not always accompanied by phlebitis. Symptoms of infection consist of chills and fever, gastric complaints, headache, hyperventilation, and shock. Should infection develop from an unknown source in a patient receiving IV therapy, the IV system should be suspected and the entire system, including the catheter, removed. The catheter and the infusion fluid should then be cultured. See Procedure 9–1 for a step-by-step approach to culturing the catheter.

All containers of fluid previously administered to the patient should be suspected and, if possible, retained and cultured. All information and identification, in-

---

Procedure 9–1	**Step-by-Step Approach to Culturing the Catheter**

Equipment

Alcohol

Sterile scissors

Culture medium and labels

Action	*Rationale*
1. Cleanse the skin around the catheter site with alcohol and allow the alcohol to air dry.	1. Allowing the alcohol to air dry maintains a clean field.
2. Maintaining asepsis, remove the catheter.	2. Maintaining asepsis avoids contamination.
3. Snip 1 cm of the catheter tip into the culture medium.	3. Tip is immediately exposed to the medium.
4. Label and send the culture medium to the laboratory in accord with institutional policies and procedures.	4. Proper transit ensures accuracy of results.

cluding the lot number of the suspected fluid, should be recorded on the culture requisition and the patient's chart. The U.S. Food and Drug Administration, the CDC, and the local health authorities should be notified if contamination during manufacturing is suspected; fluids bearing implicated lot numbers should be stored for investigation. See the accompanying display, Culturing the Infusion Fluid, for more information.

CULTURES AND CULTURE PROFILES

Culture results identify microorganisms in suspected IV infections. Before removing a catheter for culture, the surrounding skin should be cleaned with 70% isopropyl alcohol and allowed to air dry. If purulent drainage is present, a specimen of the drainage should be obtained before the skin is cleaned.

When line sepsis is suspected, three blood culture specimens should be drawn, ideally from separate venipuncture sites. Deep candidal sepsis (systemic candidiasis) is often associated with negative culture results. It is common practice in a number of clinical settings, such as intensive care units, to develop a culture profile for the patient with suspected sepsis and routinely to culture the blood of patients receiving multiple infusion therapies. Quantitative blood cultures, using pour plates, are an excellent tool for diagnosing catheter-related infection.

SEMIQUANTITATIVE TECHNIQUE FOR CULTURING CATHETERS

In the presence of purulent drainage, before removing a catheter, the nurse cleans the skin around the insertion site with an alcohol-impregnated pad to reduce contaminating skin flora and to remove any residual antibiotic ointment. After the clean area dries, the nurse withdraws the catheter, taking care to avoid contact with the surrounding skin. If pus can be expressed from the catheter wound, it is prepared for Gram's staining and culture separately. For short indwelling catheters, the entire length of the catheter is cut from the skin–catheter junction (Fig. 9–2) using sterile scissors. With longer catheters, a 2-inch segment that includes the tip and the intracutaneous segment is cultured. Segments are cultured as soon as possible after removal and within 2 hours. In the laboratory, the segment is rolled back and forth across the surface of a 100-mm 5% blood agar plate four times. Plates are then incubated aerobically at 37°C for at least 72 hours. This technique has outstanding sensitivity and specificity in diagnosing catheter related infections. Box 9–4 lists criteria for defining a nosocomial bacteremia as catheter related.

KEY INTERVENTIONS: Culturing the Infusion Fluid

The following procedure should be used for culturing the infusion fluid:

1. Aseptically withdraw 20 mL of fluid from the IV line: Use 1 mL to prepare a pour plate; use the remaining fluid to inoculate two blood culture containers.
2. To the remaining IV fluid in the container, add an equal volume of brain–heart infusion broth enriched with 0.5% beef extract. Inoculate at 37°C. This is a more sensitive culture for detecting low-level contamination.

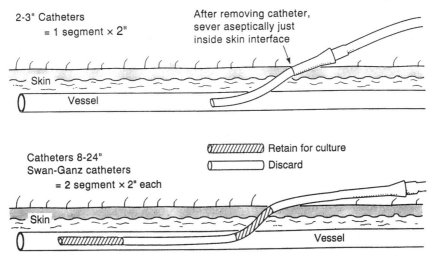

Figure 9–2. Segments of vascular catheters cultured semiquantitatively. (Reprinted with permission of D.G. Maki and Little, Brown & Co. © 1986.)

■ ADDITIONAL HAZARDS: PARTICULATES

Particulate matter comprises the mobile, undissolved substances unintentionally present in parenteral fluids. Such foreign matter may consist of rubber, glass, cotton fibers, drug particles, molds, metal, or paper fibers.

The pulmonary vascular bed acts as a filter for infused particles. Particles introduced into the vein travel to the right atrium of the heart, through the tricuspid valve, and into the right ventricle. From there they are pumped into the pulmonary artery and on through branches of arteries that decrease in size until the particles are trapped in the massive capillary bed of the lungs, where the capillaries measure 7 to 12 μm in diameter.

Five μm, the size of an erythrocyte suspended in fluid, has been suggested as the largest allowable size for a particle in the pulmonary capillary bed. Particles larger than 5 μm are recognized as potentially dangerous because they are likely to become lodged. Particles as large as 300 μm can pass through an 18-gauge catheter, and much larger particles may pass through an indwelling catheter with a larger lumen. Table 9–4 lists particle size comparisons.

If the occlusion of a small arteriole inhibits oxygenation or normal metabolic activities, cellular damage or tissue death may result. Where there is ample collateral circulation, the occlusion would have no appreciable biologic effect. However, a particle that is not biologically inert may incite an inflammatory reaction, a neoplastic response, or an antigenic, sensitizing response.

Particles may gain access to the systemic circulation, where occlusion of a small arteriole in the brain, kidney, or eye can be serious, for the following reasons:

- The pulmonary vascular bed cannot filter out all particles. Prinzmetal and associates demonstrated that glass beads up to 390 μm may pass through the

---

BOX 9–4 **Criteria for Defining a Nosocormial Bacteria Catheter-Related Infection**

- Isolation of the same species in significant numbers on semiquantitative culture of the catheter and from blood cultures obtained by separate venipunctures with negative culture of infusate
- Clinical and microbiologic data disclosing no other apparent source of septicemia
- Clinical features consistent with bloodstream infection

---

pulmonary capillary bed and reach the systemic circulation (Parras et al., 1994; Pearson, 1996).

- Large arteriovenous shunts exist in the human lung. Particles may bypass the pulmonary capillary bed and enter the systemic circulation, where a systemic occlusion could be serious.
- Particles larger than 5 μm may reach the systemic circulation by way of inter-arterial injection or infusion.

Sources of Particulates

The USP sets the acceptable limit of particles for single-dose infusion at not more than 50 particles/mL that are equal to or larger than 10.0 μm and not more than 5 particles/mL that are equal to or larger than 25.0 μm in effective linear dimension (see Chap. 11).

T A B L E   9 – 4
PARTICLE SIZE COMPARISONS

Micrometers		Inches
175	=	0.007
150	=	0.006
125	=	0.005
100	=	0.004
75	=	0.003
50	=	0.002
25	=	0.001

Note: One micrometer equals 40 millionths of an inch (approx.). A human hair is approximately 125 μm in thickness. Bacteria range in size from 0.3 to 0.5 μm. We cannot see a particle or hole smaller than 20 μm. A hole 25 μm in diameter in a HEPA filter is more than 75 times larger than the contaminants and bacteria passing through.

Over the years, manufacturers have made great efforts to produce high-quality products, but these efforts may be negated by manipulating the products before their infusion.

Medication Additives

Drugs constitute a major source of particulate matter. Improper technique in preparing drugs may result in the formation of insoluble particles. Use of an IV additive service precludes the need to mix drugs on the nursing unit (see Chap. 18).

Glass Ampules

Glass ampules may be responsible for the injection of thousands of glass particles into the circulation. Turco and Davis, in a classic study prompted by the frequency of high-dose administration of furosemide, showed that a dose of 400 mg, which at that time required the breaking of 20 ampules, could add 1085 glass particles larger than 5 μm to the injection. A dose of 600 mg, requiring 30 ampules, could result in 2387 particles larger than 5 μm.

Antibiotic Injectables

Particulate contamination of bulk-filled antibiotics may be 2 to 10 times greater than that of stable antibiotic solutions and lyophilized antibiotics. Filtration is impossible because packaging by the sterile bulk-fill method involves extracting and processing the antibiotic in sterile bulk powder form and then aseptically placing the bulk antibiotic into dry, presterilized vials.

In the lyophilized and the stable liquid packaging processes, the particulate matter can be terminally removed by filtration directly into presterilized vials. Most antibiotics are packed by the bulk-fill method, however.

Particulate matter in IV injections may be responsible for much of the phlebitis that so often occurs with the infusion of these drugs. Studies demonstrate the major pathologic conditions caused by particulate matter are direct blockage of vessels; platelet agglutination leading to formation of emboli; local inflammation caused by impaction of particles; and antigenic reactions with subsequent allergic consequence.

Reducing the Particulate Level

Because particulate matter infused through IV fluids may produce pathologic changes that can have an adverse effect on critically ill patients, every effort must be made to reduce the particulate count in IV injections. In general, nurses and physicians have been unaware of the potential dangers that exist and have unknowingly added to the contamination. To promote awareness, official agencies have developed standards for an acceptable particulate limit in IV fluids, and industry has provided the health care profession with filters to limit direct access of particulates, bacteria, fungi, and other contaminants to the bloodstream.

Filters

A filter aspiration needle specially designed to remove particulate matter from IV medications is available. With this device attached to a syringe, the medication is drawn from the vial or glass ampule and the particles are filtered out. The filter needle must then be discarded to prevent the particles trapped on the filter from being injected when the medication is added to the IV fluid.

Final Filters

The National Coordinating Committee on Large Volume Parenterals has recommended the inline filter that is both particulate and microbe retentive for patients receiving hyperalimentation and patients who are immunodeficient or immunocompromised. The particulate-retentive IV filter is usually recommended for patients receiving IV infusions when the fluid contains many additives or when drugs requiring constitution are known to be heavily particulated.

The INS policy advocates the routine use of 0.2-μm air-eliminating filters in delivering routine IV therapy because these filters remove particulates, bacteria, and air, and some remove endotoxins as well (INS, 1998, 2000).

Filters are manufactured in a variety of forms, sizes, and materials. Some block the passage of air under normal pressure when wet. Used with electronic infusion devices, they play an important role in preventing air from being pumped into the bloodstream should the fluid container empty.

A knowledge of filter characteristics, use, and proper handling is important for patient safety. Faulty handling can result in occlusion of the filter, with the patient not receiving prescribed fluids. In addition, the infusion may need to be discontinued and venipuncture repeated to insert a new line. Moreover, a ruptured filter may go undetected and introduce filter fragments, bacteria, and possibly air into the IV system. A thorough discussion of IV filtration and its benefits is provided in Chapter 11.

■ ONGOING MONITORING AND PRECAUTIONS

The practice setting in which care is delivered has no relevance to the level of diligence needed to provide high-quality infusion therapy. This theory is based on the fact that the patient is accustomed to the flora in his or her own environment. In any clinical environment, principles of asepsis must be adhered to in an effort to minimize the risk of IV catheter-related infection and to ensure a high level of IV patient care (see Chaps. 22 and 23).

Extensive guidelines for monitoring infusion therapy and preventing catheter-related infection have been published (CDC, 1998). Preventive measures described throughout this chapter should be adhered to. In addition, any device intended for vascular access must be thought of in fundamental terms as a direct conduit between the external world and the patient's bloodstream (CDC, 1998; INS, 1998, 2000).

Inappropriate catheter care and lack of monitoring and nursing interventions may contribute to catheter-related infections. The use of specialty IV teams to ensure a high level of aseptic technique during and after catheter insertion has been associated with substantially lower rates of catheter-related infection (Hadaway, 1998; Krzywda, 1999).

References and Selected Readings

Asterisks indicate references cited in text.

*Alhimyary, A., Fernandez, C., & Picard, M., et al. (1996). Safety and efficacy of total parenteral nutrition delivered via a peripherally inserted central venous catheter. *Nutrition in Clinical Practice, 11,* 199–203.

*Bennett, J.V., & Brachman, P.S. (1998). *Hospital infections* (4th ed., pp. 689–723). Philadelphia: Lippincott Williams & Wilkins.

*Centers for Disease Control and Prevention. (1998). *Guidelines for prevention of intravascular infection.* Atlanta, GA: Author.

**Hadaway, L.C. (1998). Major thrombotic and nonthrombotic complications: Loss of patency. *Journal of Intravenous Nursing, 21*(5S), 143–160.

*Intravenous Nurses Society. (1998, 2000). Revised intravenous nursing standards of practice. *Journal of Intravenous Nursing, 21*(Suppl. 1).

*Krzywda, E. (1999). Predisposing factors, prevention and management of central venous catheter occlusions. *Journal of Intravenous Nursing, 22* (6S), 14–16.

*Metheny, N.M. (2000). *Fluid and electrolyte balance* (4th ed.). Philadelphia: Lippincott Williams & Wilkins.

*Parras, F., Ena, J., Bouza, E., et al. (1994). Impact of an educational program for the prevention of colonization of intravascular catheters. *Hospital Epidemiology and Infection Control, 15,* 335–337.

*Pearson, M.L. (1996). The Hospital Infection Control Advisory Committee: Guideline for prevention of intravascular-device-related infections. *Hospital Epidemiology and Infection Control, 17,* 438–473.

*Smith, J.P. (1998). Thrombotic complications in intravenous access. *Journal of Intravenous Nursing, 21*(2), 96–98.

Review Questions

Questions below may have more than one right answer.

1. Gram-negative organisms include all of the following *except:*

   A. *Staphylococcus aureus*

   B. *Pseudomonas aeruginosa*

   C. *Klebsiella*

   D. *Escherichia coli*

2. Which of the following microorganisms is *not* associated with IV infusate contamination?

   A. *Coccidioides immitis*

   B. *Enterobacter cloacae*

   C. *Klebsiella pneumoniae*

   D. *Serratia marcescens*

3. The most accurate culture method to identify catheter sepsis is:

   A. Anaerobic

   B. Gram's stain

   C. Qualitative

   D. Semiquantitative

4. In the event of a suspected air embolism, the appropriate nursing intervention is to:

   A. Turn patient on left side, head down

   B. Turn patient on right side, head down

   C. Turn patient on left side, head raised

   D. Turn patient on right side, head raised

5. Which of the following is *not* a sign of impending pulmonary edema?

A. Venous dilation

B. Increased blood pressure

C. Engorged neck veins

D. Slow, shallow respirations

6. To minimize the danger of speed shock, it is necessary to:

A. Control volume

B. Avoid free flow

C. Catch up all solutions

D. Use positive pressure

7. Classic symptoms of air embolism include all of the following *except*:

A. Cyanosis

B. Dyspnea

C. Churning over precordium

D. Increase in pulse pressure

8. The recommended method of culture for purulent drainage is:

A. Agar

B. Broth culture

C. Semiqualitative

D. Semiquantitative

9. Factors influencing the survival of bacteria include all of the following except:

A. Number and type of organisms present

B. Environmental conditions

C. Resistance of the host

D. Use of filtration

10. Clinical manifestations of septicemia include which of the following?

A. Chills and fever

B. Chills and fever, headache, and general malaise

C. General malaise only

D. Fever and headache only

Defining and Documenting

Evidence-Based Practice

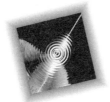

K E Y   T E R M S

Clinical Decision Making
Documentation
Evidence-Based Practice
Informatics

Outcomes
Performance Criteria
Research
Variable

■ EVIDENCE-BASED NURSING

Current trends in nursing reflect a continuing emphasis on evidence-based practice. **Evidence-based practice** is nursing activity that incorporates the findings of pertinent, valid, and reliable research studies into nursing care and process. Evidence-based practice calls for a nurse to select and review appropriate **research** studies from the health-related literature and apply relevant findings to patient care. Appropriate selections include studies that warrant immediate attention by nurses who are attempting to keep pace with important advances in the profession. Some specific purposes of evidence-based nursing are found in Box 10–1. Intravenous (IV) nurses, in particular, are consistently challenged to keep up with the rapidly growing and changing information base in their area of practice. In addition to knowing where to obtain the information (Box 10–2), nurses must evaluate the quality of the material.

Evidence-Based Practice and Outcomes

Evidence-based nursing integrates the best evidence from research findings with clinical expertise, patient preferences, and existing resources to form decision-

---

BOX 10–1 **Purposes of Evidence-Based Nursing**

- To identify, using predefined criteria, the best quantitative and qualitative original and review *studies on quality assurance; continuing professional development;* and, especially, the meaning, cause, course, diagnosis, prevention, treatment, or economics of health problems managed by nurses
- To summarize these *studies* in "structured abstracts" that describe their objectives, methods, results, and evidence-based conclusions in a reproducible and accurate fashion
- To provide brief, highly expert commentary on the context of each *study,* its methods, and clinical applications that its findings warrant
- To disseminate the summaries in a timely manner to nurses

Based on Banks, N. (1999). Positive outcome after looped peripherally inserted central catheter malposition. *Journal of Intravenous Nursing, 22*(1), 14–17.

---

making tools about the health care of individual patients (DiCenso, Cullum, & Ciliska, 1998a, b). The quality of information that nurses demand and how effectively they evaluate and use it for **clinical decision making** influences patient **outcomes** and, ultimately, the role of nurses in the health care delivery system.

Nurses comprise the greatest number of health care professionals in the largest area of practice in the most settings. In the past few decades, clinical research has proliferated in nursing-related health services and in **informatics** (the use of computer-based searches). The application of these research findings to practice is great. However, it requires an investment of attention, methods, and resources to achieve the best outcomes for a specific patient population.

BOX 10–2 **Sources of Information**

- Textbooks
- Journals
- Bibliographic databases
- Sources of distilled and consolidated information (some of the critical appraisal work has already been done for the reader and only a distillation of the best studies is presented), such as the journal *Evidence-Based Nursing*
- Internet sites
  - www.hopkins-aids.edu/default.htm (clinical experts respond to patient queries)
  - www.shef.ac.uk/uni/academic/R-Z/scharr/netting.html (references and sources related to evidence-based practice)

Applicable Research Evidence

An example of an IV therapy-related research study with findings that are applicable to nursing practice may be found in the article, "Fewer Patients Dislodged Peripheral Intravenous Catheters With Transparent Dressings Than With Gauze Dressings." This original work by Tripepi-Bova and colleagues appeared in the *American Journal of Critical Care* in 1997. Diane Palmer, lecturer at the School of Nursing, the University of Hull (United Kingdom), commented on the original manuscript, noting that the study evaluates the effectiveness of two frequently used dressings in a randomized, controlled trial. The authors measured adhesive properties, reduction in peripheral vein thrombophlebitis, dislodgment by patients, and infiltration. To ensure standardization of insertion and dressing techniques, nurses attended mandatory training sessions, received written instructions, and had access to diagrams. Patients were monitored until the IV catheter for that specific insertion site was discontinued (Tripepi-Bova, Woods, and Loach, 1997).

When recommending changes in procedure or policy, or both, based on others' studies, the nurse must also consider the local practice and published standards, such as the Intravenous Nurses Society (INS) *Standards of Practice*. A serious-minded review of published studies such as that of Tripepi-Bova and colleagues could be beneficial to clinicians evaluating the feasibility of specific dressing materials (INS, 1998, 2000).

Nurses know that patients benefit from the care that nurses provide. But how can that effectiveness be verified? Alvin Tarlov and colleagues in 1989 took into account the specific outcomes that gauge the effectiveness of nursing care (Kelly, 1994; Tarlov, 1989), including the patient's health status, quality of life, knowledge, and ability to function and manage symptoms. A more recent study documented significant relationships between nursing and patient outcomes, including mortality and patient satisfaction (Scott, Sochalski, Aiken, 1999).

By measuring patient outcomes, nurses can respond to two pivotal questions: Do our patients benefit from our care? And if so, how? A focus on outcomes may help nurses survive an unstable job market, evaluate the efficacy of IV teams, and ensure that the nursing perspective regarding outcome management is represented.

Outcomes are the consequences of a treatment or intervention. Indicators are valid and reliable measures related to performance. *Outcome indicators*, or measures, gauge how patients are affected by their nursing care; for example, is the rate of nosocomial infections down? Is the incidence of IV-related infections lower? *Process indicators*, such as pressure ulcers, evaluate the nature and amount of care that nurses provide. *Structure indicators* assess the organization and delivery of nursing care from a standpoint of staffing. Indicators are commonly reviewed to evaluate patient status in relation to outcomes—for example, the ability to bear weight is an indicator used to evaluate ambulation. (Other terms associated with outcomes, research, and evidence-based practice are given in Box 10–3.)

Evidence-Based Practice and Quality Assurance

Across the health care arena, organizations are developing national quality initiatives (Table 10–1). One such organization is ECRI (Plymouth Meeting, PA), a firm that tests medical devices and develops guidelines and test programs. Formerly known as Emergency Care and Research Institute, ECRI has developed

---

BOX 10–3 **Terms Used in Evidence-Based Practice**

Case control — (Dawson-Saunders, 1994): An observational study beginning with patients who have had the health problem and with control subjects who do not have the health problem; looks backward to identify possible causal factors

Cohort — A group of people with a common characteristic or set of characteristics

Constant comparison — (Crombie, 1996): A procedure in qualitative research wherein newly collected data are compared in an ongoing fashion with data obtained earlier to refine theoretically relevant categories

Data saturation — (Crombie, 1966): Process of collecting data in a qualitative research study without generating new themes

Double-blind study — A research design in which neither subject nor researcher knows to which group or study methods the various subjects are assigned

Effectiveness — Extent to which an intervention does more good than harm for participants who receive the intervention under usual conditions; answers the question *does it work?*

Random effects model — (Polit & Hungler, 1995): Provides a summary estimate of the magnitude of effect in meta-analysis; takes into account both within-study and between-study variance and gives a wider confidence interval to the estimate than a fixed-effects model if there is significant between-study variation

Relative risk: — Risk of adverse effects resulting from treatment as opposed to risks attendant to nontreatment

---

T A B L E   1 0 – 1
NATIONAL QUALITY INDICATORS

Organization	Initiative	Description
Joint Commission on the Accreditation of Hospitals and Healthcare Organizations (JCAHO)	ORYX	Integrates use of outcomes and performance measures
National Committee for Quality Assurance (NCQA)	Health Plan Employer Data and Information Set (HEDIS)	HEDIS targets effectiveness of care, access and availability, patient satisfaction, costs
American Nurses Association (ANA)	Nursing Report Card	Indicators and measurement tools for evaluating quality of nursing care in acute care settings
Health Care Financing Administration (HCFA)	OASIS (Outcome and Assessment Information Set)	Assessment questions used to collect clinical, financial and administrative data in home health care
Foundation for Accountability	Foundation for Accountability	Improves information available to consumers when they are choosing health plan, provider, hospital, treatment

a comprehensive guide to quality practice using the principles of evidence-based disease management. Disease management is an approach to patient care that coordinates medical resources for patients across the entire health care delivery system.

In 1997, the Agency for Health Care Policy and Research (AHCPR) restructured its popular clinical practice guideline and technology assessment programs. AHCPR's Evidence-Based Practice Program now sponsors the development of technology assessments and evidence reports by 12 designated evidence-based practice centers. The new initiative includes the development of a National Guideline Clearinghouse (NGC) that will be a comprehensive database. ECRI has been chosen to create the database, abstract existing guidelines, compare guidelines on similar topics, and establish the NGC web site. For each guideline, ECRI will produce:

- A standardized summary about the guideline and its development
- A comparison of guidelines covering similar topic areas, listing the major interventions addressed and the areas of agreement and disagreement
- The full text of guidelines or links to the full text

Measurements: Performance Criteria and Research Studies

Measurement in nursing may be traced to Florence Nightingale, who used mortality statistics as a quality-of-care measure for British soldiers during the Crimean War. The ORYX initiative of the Joint Commission on the Accreditation of Healthcare Organizations (JCAHO) integrates patient outcomes and other performance measures into the accreditation process. ORYX is defined as a "gazelle." The long-range goal of this program is to establish a data-driven continuous survey and accreditation process to complement the standards-based assessment. Although accreditation is still based on standards, trends in data and in an organization's response to its data are being used as part of JCAHO's overall assessment as the performance measures database expands (JCAHO, 1999).

The INS *Standards of Practice* were developed as a framework for establishing infusion policies and procedures in all practice settings and for defining **performance criteria** for nurses responsible for administering infusion therapy. The 1998 edition of the *Standards* define the criteria relative to nursing accountability in the delivery of infusion therapies. They provide a framework for nurses to evaluate patient outcomes. They also provide a tool for evaluating the quality of patient care and the *competency* of the nurse delivering infusion therapy (INS, 1998, 2000).

Whereas performance may be measured by established standards, health and other focuses can be measured in many different ways. The various measurable aspects of health are known as **variables.** In a treatment study, such as one by Banks (1999), in which the author demonstrated positive outcomes after looped, peripherally inserted central catheter (PICC) malposition, the intervention (independent variable) was the noninvasive approach. The outcome (dependent variable) was central tip placement of the catheter and prevention of additional costs and potential discomfort for the patient. Banks summarized documented PICC malpositions and resolutions (Table 10–2).

T A B L E 1 0 – 2
SUMMARY OF DOCUMENTED PICC MALPOSITIONS AND METHODS OF RESOLUTION

Source	Location of Malposition	Incidence of Malposition	Technique Use for Resolution	Successful Outcomes	Unsuccessful Outcomes
Frey	Curled in subclavian vein	2 of 269 insertions	Infusions with an infusion pump		
	"figure 8" in basilic vein	1 of 269 insertions	None cited	Used for 6 weeks	
	Looped in basilic vein	1 of 269 insertions	None cited	Used for 3 weeks	
	"several other" PICCS looped back on themselves in the upper arm during insertion	unknown	Removed		Classified as "unsuccessful inserts"
James et al.	R. basilic insertions: subclavian, axillary, jugular or right atrium	42 malpositions (34%) on first insertion	CXRs obtained with guidewire in place		
	R. cephalic insertions: subclavian, axillary, right atrium, or peripheral vein (1)		Removing guidewire and allowing tip to "fall" into SVC or partially withdrawing wire and readvancing catheter	11 of 42 lines (26%) successfully repositioned	11 of 42 in subclavian or axillary position (26%) could not be repositioned using any of these techniques
	L. basilic insertions: other locations (not specified)				
	R. cephalic insertions: other locations (not specified)		Rapid saline flush with patient in semi-Fowler's position	2 of 42 lines (4%) successfully repositioned	Unsuccessful in 3 of 42 lines (7%)
LaRue	May–Dec. 1992: unable to thread catheter past subclavian-jugular-innominate junction	14 of 100 attempts (14%)	Turning patient's head more severely in chin-to-shoulder position (toward insertion side), vigorous flush technique or changing arm position	1 out of 14 attempts at repositioning was successful (1%) using one or more of these techniques	13 of 14 attempts at repositioning were unsuccessful (99%) using one or more of these techniques

	Description	Incidence	Intervention	Outcome
	Dec–Oct 1993: change in insertion technique (7 cm withdrawal of guidewire after 1/2 of line inserted) jugular placement	99 of 100 lines (99%) successfully placed		Successful SVC placement
		1 of 100 lines (1%)	Withdrawn and reinserted with new technique	
LaFortune	Malpositioned tip in 26% of patients: looped or coiled in branches or tributaries off the axillary vein	6 of 11 malpositions	Readvancing catheter after withdrawing catheter 2–6 cm and performing one or more of the following actions: Withdrawal of catheter 2–6 cm; Hyperextension of arm; Rotation of arm; Traction applied to wrist; Having patient open and close fist; Relaxation and distraction	7 of 11 lines repositioned after one or two attempts
		5 of 11 malpositions		One patient needed repositioning under fluroscopy
				One line in an 8-year-old child was removed after one attempt at repositioning was unsuccessful
Lum and Soski	Internal jugular vein	20 of 62 (32.2%)	Patient positioning	80% (8 of 10 cases)
	Axillary vein	22 of 62 (35.5%)	Guidewire exchange	69% (9 of 13 cases)
	Opposite innominate vein	7 of 62 (11.3%)	Rapid flushing	55% (22 of 40 cases)
	Subclavian vein	4 of 62 (6.5%)	Partial withdrawal	94% (17 of 18 cases)
	Right atrium	6 of 62 (9.7%)	Removal	100% (22 of 22 cases)
	Innominate vein	1 of 62 (1.6%)		
	Basilic vein	1 of 62 (1.6%)		
	Unknown vein	1 of 62 (1.6%)		
Abi-Nader	Primary malposition (tip site not specified)	5 of 92 insertions (5%)	Line removed and reinserted	100% effective
	Tip located in heart	14 of 92 insertions (15%)	Pulled back to correr position using CXR	Effective
	Curled in axillary vein	1 of 92 insertions (1%)	Line left in place, second PICC line inserted in a different vein	Second PICC line found to have straightened out the first line on second CXR

(continued)

TABLE 10-2
SUMMARY OF DOCUMENTED PICC MALPOSITIONS AND METHODS OF RESOLUTION (*Continued*)

Source	Location of Malposition	Incidence of Malposition	Technique Used for Resolution	Successful Outcomes	Unsuccessful Outcomes
Alhimyary et al.	Coiling or malposition (site of tip not specified)	7 of 135 insertions (5%)	3 PICC lines removed and reinserted		
			3 PICC lines removed and replaced with subclavian catheters		
			1 PICC line successfully repositioned, technique not specified		
Ng et al.	Cephalad to internal jugular vein	27 of 963 insertions (2.8%)	Resolution techniques not discussed		
	Right atrium or right ventricle	13 of 963 insertions (1.3%)			
	Looped in subclavian or axillary vein	16 of 963 insertions (1.6%)			
		56 of 963 insertions (3.7%)			

CXR, chest x-ray; PICC, peripherally inserted central catheter; SVC, superior vena cava.

Evaluation of the Evidence

In reviewing the literature, the professional nurse is urged to determine whether the study and its methods and measures are reliable and valid. Reliability refers to the degree to which a measure gives the same result two or more times under similar circumstances. Validity is the ability of a measurement tool accurately to measure what it is intended to measure. Criterion-related validity requires comparing a given measure with a gold standard, such as the INS *Standards of Practice* (see Chap. 4).

Thus, readers of research reports should consider the types of measures used, the reliability and validity of the measures, and methods used in measuring the outcomes. Examples of published findings specific to infusion therapy may be found in the accompanying research display, Noteworthy Research Relevant to Infusion Therapy.

Research Issues: NOTEWORTHY RESEARCH RELEVANT TO
INFUSION THERAPY

Treatment
The influence of epidural analgesia on cesarean delivery rates: A randomized, prospective clinical trial. Clark, A., Carr, D., & Loyd, G. (1998). *American Journal of Obstetrics and Gynecology, 179,* 1527–1533.

Total parenteral nutrition in the critically ill patient: A meta-analysis. Heyland, D.K., MacDonald, S., & Keefe, L. (1998). *Journal of the American Medical Association, 280,* 2013–2019.

Applying current research to influence clinical practice: Use of midline catheters. Kupensky, D.T. (1998). *Journal of Intravenous Nursing, 21,* 271–279.

Prognosis
Central venous catheter related-thrombosis in children: Analysis of the Canadian Registry of Venous Thromboembolic Complications. Massicotte, M.P., Dix, D., & Monagle, P., on behalf of the Canadian Childhood Thrombophilia Program. (1998). *Journal of Pediatrics, 133,* 770–776.

Clinical factors associated with the development of phlebitis after insertion of a peripherally inserted central catheter. Mazzola, J.R., Schott-Baer, D., & Addy, L. (1999) *Journal of Intravenous Nursing, 22,* 36–41.

Outcome
The peripherally inserted central catheter: A retrospective look at three years of insertions. Goodwin, M.L., & Carlton, I. (1993). *Journal of Intravenous Nursing, 16,* 92–103.

Catheter-related colonization associated with percutaneous inserted central catheters. Pauley, S.Y., Vallande, N.C., & Riley, E.N. (1993). *Journal of Intravenous Nursing, 16,* 50–54.

■ COMPETENCY-BASED PROGRAMS AND DOCUMENTATION

The IV nurse specialist, through study, supervised practice, and validation of competency, acquires knowledge and develops skills necessary for the practice of IV nursing. Such a nurse is competent to practice.

Competency-based orientation programs are designed to orient the IV nurse who is new to an institution to that institution's or agency's practices, policies, and procedures. Such a program benefits the institution or agency as well as the patient (Weinstein, 2000). And such a program must be standardized but individualized, quality based but cost effective (Weinstein, 2000).

Orientation or institutional competencies are derived from standards of accrediting organizations, such as JCAHO, and the standards of practice of specialty nursing organizations. JCAHO, for example, requires **documentation** of competence not only at orientation but on an ongoing basis. State health departments also require documentation of clinical competence. Competency programs incorporate self-assessment tools, orientation curriculum, skills checklists, and in-house education, which includes simulated practice, written and didactic examination, and program evaluation. Adult learning principles, as described by Knowles, are an integral component of the program (Case, 1996).

Documentation is essential as a legal record of care provided, a communication tool for other health care professionals, and a determinant of eligibility for reimbursement. Detailed, accurate, adequate documentation prevents reinvention of the wheel (or duplication of effort and services) by saving time, ensures that the patient masters skill sets, and protects the health care provider or the institution. Tools used to document care include nursing care plans (see Chap. 4), flow sheets, progress notes, periodic updates developed by home care providers, and discharge summaries (Rankin & Stallings, 1996).

Documentation should include the intervention performed, the patient's response to the intervention, and the subsequent outcomes. Sentinel or adverse events should also be documented consistent with institutional policy. By providing an accurate record of the care delivered and by structuring that care on evidence-based nursing practice and published standards, the nurse who is responsible for providing IV care ensures safe practice.

References and Selected Readings

Asterisks indicate references cited in text.

*Alhimyary, A., Fernandez, C., & Pizard, M. (1996). Safty and efficacy of total parenteral nutrition. *Nutrition in Clinical Practice*, 11, 199–203.

*Banks, N. (1999). Positive outcome after looped peripherally inserted central catheter malposition. *Journal of Intravenous Nursing*, 22, 14–17.

*Case, B. (1996). Breathing air into adult learning. *Journal of Continuing Education in Nursing*, 27(4), 148–158.

Connor, V.W. (1999). Patient confidentiality in the electronic age. *Journal of Intravenous Nursing*, 22, 199–200.

*Crombie, I.K. (1996). *The pocket guide to critical appraisal: A handbook for healthcare professionals* (p. 47). London: BMJ Publishing Group.

*Dawson-Saunders, B., & Trapp, R.G. (1997). Basic and Clinical Biostatistics. Norwalk: Appleton, and Lange.

*DiCenso, A., Cullum, N., & Ciliska, D. (1998a). *Evidence-based nursing* (p. 66). Kent, United Kingdom: RCN Publishing.

*DiCenso, A., Cullum, N., & Ciliska, D. (1998b, April 1). Implementing evidence-based nursing: Some misconceptions. *Evidence-Based Nursing*, 38–40.

*Frey, A.M. (1995). Pediatric peripherally inserted catheter program report. *Journal of Intravenous Nursing*, 18, 280–291.

Hagland, M. (1998). The gap: HIPAA and secure information technology. *Health Management Technology*, 19, 24–30.

*Intravenous Nurses Society. (1998). Revised intravenous nursing standards of practice. *Journal of Intravenous Nursing, 21,* 516, 19 , 25.

*James, L., Bledsoe, L, Hadaway, L.C. (1993). A retrospective look at tip location and complications of peripherally inserted catheter liines. *Journal of Intravenous Nursing, 16,* 104–109.

*Joint Commission on Accreditation of Healthcare Organizations (JCAHO). (1999). ORYX: The next evolution in accreditation. [On-line]. Available: http://www.jacho.org/perfmeas/oryx_qa.html.0

*Kelly, K.C. (1994). The Medical Outcomes Study: A nursing perspective. *Journal of Professional Nursing, 10,* 209–216.

*LaRue, G.D. (1995). Improving central placement rates of peripherally inserted catheters. *Journal of Intravenous Nursing, 18,* 24–27.

Ouriel, K., Veith, F.J., & Sasahara, A.A. (1998). A comparison of recombinant urokinase with vascular surgery as initial treatment for acute arterial occlusion of the legs. *New England Journal of Medicine, 338,* 1105–1111.

*Polit, D.E., & Hungler, B.P. (1995). *Nursing research: Principles and methods* (p. 22). Philadelphia: Lippincott-Raven.

*Rankin, S.H., & Stallings, K.D. (1996). *Patient education issues, principle, practices.* (3rd ed., pp. 122, 162–164, 183–187). Philadelphia: Lippincott-Raven.

*Scott, J.G., Sochalski, J., & Aikenn, L. (1999). Review of magnet hospitals research. *Journal of Nursing Adminstration, 29* (1) 9–18.

*Tarlov, (1989). The medical outcomes study: Application of methods for monitoring. *Journal of the American Medical Association, 262,* 925–930

*Tripepi-Bova, K.A., Woods, K.D., & Loach, M.C. (1997, Sept. 6). A comparison of transparent polyurethane and dry gauze dressings for peripheral IV catheter sites: Rates of phlebitis, infiltration, and dislodgment by patients. *American Journal of Critical Care,* 377–381.

*Weinstein, S.M. (2000). Certification and credentialing to ensure competency-based practice. *Journal of Intravenous Nursing, 23,* 1, 21-28.

Review Questions

Note: Questions below may have more than one right answer.

1. Outcomes can best be described as which of the following?

   A. Use of protocols to render health care

   B. Ability to provide consistent care in all regions of the country

   C. End results of treatment or intervention

   D. Use of less invasive and less costly procedures

2. Measurable aspects of health are known as:

   A. Regional practices

   B. Variables

   C. Standards

   D. AHA requirements

3. Quality of care was originally measured by which of the following?

   A. Mortality rate

   B. Length of stay

   C. Functional ability

   D. Cost of service

4. Which of the following is *not* an example of a useful outcome indicator to measure quality of nursing care?

   A. Functional status

   B. Patient satisfaction

   C. Patient discomfort

   D. Health insurance plan

5. Measurement issues reviewed when perusing the literature include which of the following?

   A. Reliability

   B. Validity

   C. Length

   D. Bias

6. Patient outcomes are influenced by which of the following?

   A. Quality of information

   B. How information is used in clinical decision making

   C. a only

   D. a and b

7. Tools used to document care include which of the following?

   A. Nursing care plans

   B. Flow sheets

   C. Progress notes

   D. Discharge summaries

8. Reliability refers to:

   A. Validity of the measurements

   B. Degree to which the same results are achieved two or more times

   C. Degree to which results are achieved under same circumstances

   D. Determining what is important to measure

9. Data saturation refers to:

   A. Process of collecting data in qualitative research study

   B. Extent to which intervention does more harm than good

   C. Observational study of patients with similar health problems

   D. Comparison of new data with earlier data

10. Treatment-related research in the area of evidence-based nursing includes that by which of the following authors?

    A. Goodwin

    B. Heyland

    C. Mazzola

    D. Pauley

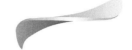

PRINCIPLES OF EQUIPMENT SELECTION AND CLINICAL APPLICATIONS

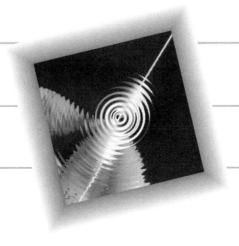

Principles and Use of

Intravenous Equipment

for Infusion Therapy

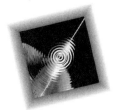

K E Y   T E R M S

Absorption
Bubble point
Calibrated
Controller
Differential Pressure
Elastomeric
Electronic Infusion Devices
Free Flow
Gravity
Hemorepellant
Hydrophobic
Hydrophilic
Hydrostatic

Hypovolemia
Linear
Needleless
Osmolality
Over-the-Needle
Point-of-Care
Psi
Pressure Pump
Ramping
Resealable Injection Site
Through-the-Needle
Wetted

■ PHYSICAL PRINCIPLES OF EQUIPMENT USE

As technology continues to keep pace with advances in medical science, the delivery of patient care has improved and more sophisticated devices and innovative equipment are available for administering infusion therapy. However, no matter how sophisticated and reliable or easy to use infusion devices and accessories are, the intravenous (IV) nurse first needs a solid understanding of the physical principles that govern flow and other facets of infusion therapy.

Flow Dynamics

Pressure, a principle of physics underlying infusion therapy, is the force that overcomes the natural resistance to flow created by infusion equipment, such as the IV administration set, in-line filters, narrow-gauge needles, and venous or arterial back pressure. Fortunately, the human body readily adapts to changes in pressure, which enables clinicians to deliver IV therapy safely.

Pressure

Pressure in the arterial system ranges from 80 mm Hg in the aorta to a low of 5 to 10 mm Hg in the venous return system. Intravenous pressure is created by the weight of a column of fluid in the catheter tubing—the weight is due to gravity—and we refer to it as **hydrostatic** pressure. Fluid always flows from an area of higher pressure to one of lower pressure. For a fluid to infuse by gravity, it is necessary to create a pressure only slightly more than normal, or 40 mm Hg in a peripheral line.

A number of resistance factors may interfere with or inhibit fluid flow. These factors include the patient's own vascular pressure, internal diameter of the tubing, in-line filters, viscosity of fluid, narrow-gauge needles, and the length of the tubing. Resistance to flow is determined by the smallest component in the IV system; this is usually the catheter. An example of equipment that incorporates principles of pressure for delivery of precise amounts of drugs and fluids is the electronic infusion device (EID), which is discussed later in the chapter (see section on Electronic Infusion Devices).

Gravity

Gravity is the physical force that propels the flow of the infusate, although this flow also depends on head pressure. Roller clamps and screw clamps used to adjust and maintain rates of flow on gravity infusions vary considerably in their efficiency and accuracy. Rate minders or flow-control mechanisms may also be used to regulate and adjust flow. When a rate minder is added to an IV administration set, the desired flow rate may be preset. Levels of accuracy vary with the type of device used. Factors such as venous spasm, venous pressure changes, patient movement, manipulations of the clamp, and bent or kinked tubing may cause variations in the flow rate.

To monitor consistency of the flow rate, preprinted or self-made time tapes may be attached to the IV container. The time tape should be attached to the container and hourly increments marked on the tape or strip, beginning with the time the infusion began (Fig. 11–1).

Flow

To determine the flow rate intelligently, the nurse must have a knowledge of parenteral solutions, their effect, and the rate of administration. The nurse must also understand other factors that influence the speed of the infusion. These factors include the patient's body surface area (BSA), condition, age, and tolerance to the infusion. The composition of the fluid is also a factor in the rate of administration.

BODY SURFACE AREA
The BSA is proportionate to many essential physiologic processes (organ size, blood volume, respiration, and heat loss) and, therefore, to total metabolic activity. Knowing the BSA helps the nurse determine fluid and electrolyte amounts and compute infusion rates. The larger the person, the more fluid and nutrients are required and the faster they can be used. The usual infusion rate is 3 mL/m^2 BSA/minute (see nomograms in Fig. 11–2). This rate applies to maintenance and replacement fluids. However, the speed must be adjusted carefully to each individual.

PATIENT'S CLINICAL CONDITION AND AGE
Because the heart and kidneys play a vital role in using infused solutions, the cardiac and renal status of the patient affects the desired rate of administration. Blood volume may expand when fluids, rapidly infused, overtax an impaired heart, and renal damage causes retention of fluid. Patients with **hypovolemia** must receive plasma and blood rapidly, but the desired rate of the infusion should be specified by the physician. Vital signs must be carefully observed and the speed of the infusion decreased as the blood pressure rises. For specific parameters regarding the influence that age has on the rate of administration, refer to Chapters 21 and 22.

COMPOSITION OF SOLUTION
The composition of the fluid may affect the rate of flow. When the solution is used as a vehicle for administering drugs, the speed of the infusion depends on the drug and the desired clinical effect. Because of its deleterious effect on the heart when infused at a rapid rate, potassium should be administered with caution. Approximately 20 to 40 mEq potassium in a liter of fluid infused over an 8-hour period is an average rate for administering potassium parenterally.

Concentration of solutions must be considered because the flow rate may alter the desired effect. When dextrose is administered for caloric benefits, it is infused at a rate that ensures complete utilization. Dextrose has been administered at a maximum rate of 0.5 g/kg body weight/hour without producing glycosuria in a normal person. At this rate, it would take approximately 1.5 hours to administer 1 L of 5% dextrose to a person weighing 70 kg, or twice as long for 1 L of 10% dextrose. This maximum rate is faster than usual and is not customarily used except in an emergency.

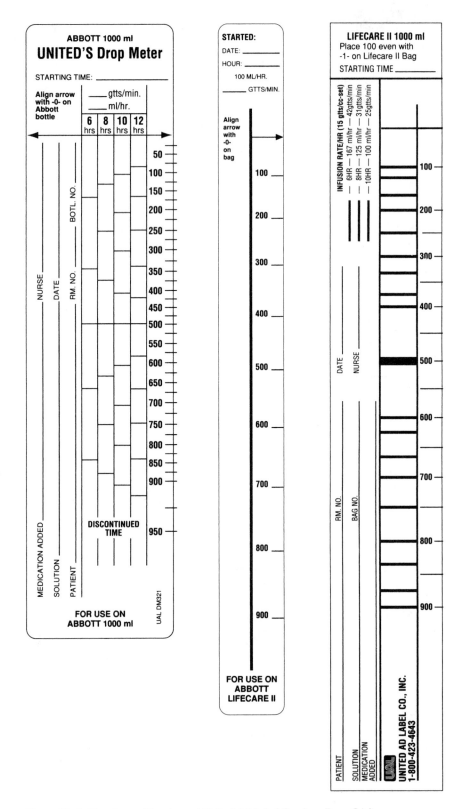

Figure 11-1. Time tapes. (Courtesy of United Ad Label Co., Inc., Brea, CA.)

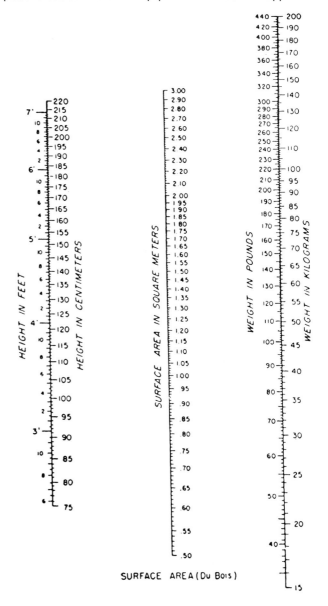

SURFACE AREA (Du Bois)

Figure 11–2. A nomogram.

When a diuretic effect is desired, a more rapid infusion is necessary. If the fluid is too rapidly infused for complete metabolism, the glucose accumulates in the bloodstream, increases the **osmolality,** and acts as a diuretic.

When oliguria or anuria occurs, the status of the kidneys must be determined before fluids containing potassium can be administered. Urinary suppression may be caused by a blood volume deficit or kidney damage. An initial hydrating fluid, to test kidney function, is usually administered at a rate of 8 mL/m^2 BSA/minute for 45 minutes. If urine does not flow, the rate is slowed to approximately 2 mL/m^2 BSA/minute for another hour. If urine output does not occur after this period, kidney damage is likely to be present (Metheny, 2000). For more information, refer to Chapters 7 and 8.

PATIENT'S TOLERANCE

Tolerance to fluids varies among individuals and influences the rate of infusion. A 5% infusion of alcohol has been administered at the rate of 200 to 300 mL/hour to sedate without intoxicating an average adult. However, when such a fluid is to be administered, the rate must be titrated to the individual and prescribed by the physician. The infusion should be checked frequently to maintain the required rate of flow. Because of certain factors, the rate is subject to change.

HEIGHT OF THE INFUSION CONTAINER

Intravenous fluids are propelled by gravity. Any change in gravity induced by raising or lowering the infusion container, relative to the patient's position, alters the rate of flow. When patients receiving infusions are ambulatory or transported to ancillary departments, the containers should be retained at the same height, or the speed of the infusion should be readjusted to maintain the prescribed rate of flow.

CLOT IN THE CATHETER

Any temporary stoppage of the infusion, such as a delay in hanging subsequent fluids, may cause a clot to form in the lumen of the catheter, partially or completely obstructing it. Clot formation may also occur when an increase in venous pressure in the extremity receiving the infusion forces blood back into the catheter. This results from restriction of the venous circulation. In arm infusion sites, this is most commonly caused by the blood pressure cuff on the infusion arm; restraints placed on or above the infusion catheter; and the patient lying on the arm receiving the infusion.

CHANGE IN CATHETER POSITION

A change in the catheter's position may push the bevel of the catheter against or away from the wall of the vein. Special precautions should be taken to prevent speed shock or vascular overload by making sure that the fluid flows freely before adjusting the rate.

OTHER CHANGES

Stimulation of vasoconstrictors from any infusion of cold blood or irritating fluid may cause venous spasm, impeding the rate of flow. A warm pack placed on the vein proximal to the infusion catheter offsets spasms. Any injury, such as phlebitis or thrombosis, that reduces the lumen of the vein decreases the flow of the fluid. In addition, a clogged air vent in the administration set used with air-dependent containers causes the infusion to stop.

If the nurse has any question as to the rate of administration, the physician should be consulted. This applies particularly to IV administration of drugs in fluid.

The rates should also be established for patients receiving two or more infusions simultaneously. Any change in the rate from that normally used should be prescribed by the attending physician.

Computation of Administration Rate

When determining drops per minute, the nurse rounds the drop rate to a whole number. The milliliters per hour also are rounded to a whole number when gravity infusion sets are being used. Flow rate calculations require the following base of information: amount of fluid to be infused, duration of the administration, and drop factor of the set to be used.

Calculating the appropriate infusion rate is easy. The nurse must first know the drop factor of the set that being used; then, he or she can set up a fraction showing the volume of infusate over the number of minutes in which the volume should be infused. For example, if the patient is to receive 100 mL of fluid within 1 hour, the fraction would be

$$\frac{100 \text{ mL}}{60 \text{ minutes}}$$

The fraction is multiplied by the drop factor to determine the number of drops per minute to be infused, using this simple equation:

$$\text{Drops per minute} = \frac{\text{total mL}}{\text{total minutes}} \times \text{drop factor}$$

If 1000 mL of fluid is ordered over an 8-hour period, the equation is modified as follows:

$$\text{Flow rate} = \frac{1000 \text{ mL}}{8 \text{ hours}} = 125 \text{ mL/hour}$$

For microdrip or pediatric systems, the equation is:

$$\text{mL/hour} = \text{drop factor}$$

■ SAFETY PRINCIPLES AND SELECTION OF EQUIPMENT

General IV equipment includes IV catheters and accessories, air-venting, microbe-retentive filters, administration sets, and EIDs. A working knowledge of the selection and use of these devices is vital for the nurse who must provide IV therapy and ensure the patient's safety and comfort. Although purchasing decisions are increasingly being made with a group purchasing contract in mind, nurses should be involved in selecting IV equipment as members of a product evaluation committee, equipment task force, or safety committee. The concept of safety will always have a profound impact on practice. Worker safety, in particular, is a top priority for health care institutions today (Pugliese, 1999). Protecting health care workers from injury is essential, especially in infusion therapy, where injuries resulting from sharp objects and devices—referred to as *sharps injuries*—are more prevalent than in other areas of nursing practice. Sharps injuries are related not only to needles but to any sharp objects and devices that have the potential to cause harm by exposing the nurse or others to the blood and body fluid of patients. Box 11–1 lists examples of these objects.

Safety Devices and Programs

Many IV nurses find that gathering information concerning the availability and use of safety devices in an institution or agency is helpful in implementing safety programs. Data on injuries may be gathered from local sources and from the more than 70 health care facilities participating in Exposure Prevention Information Network (EPINet) and the International Health Care Worker Safety Center (Ippolito, Puro, & Petrosillo, 1997; Tereskerz, Bentley, Coyner, & Jagger, 1996; Tokars et al., 1993). See the appendices for information on EPINet and needlestick tracking information.

Safety Assessment

Safety assessment should include the number of sharps-related injuries and the type of devices involved. Data from studies on human immunodeficiency virus (HIV) se-

---

BOX 11–1 Sharps Used in IV Practice

Disposable syringes with needles
Medication cartridge syringes
Needles (injection, vascular access, anesthetic, IV)
Suture needles
Intravascular catheters
Lancets
Scalpels
Razors
Surgical instruments
Glass vacuum blood tubes
Glass capillary tubes or pipettes
Glass medication vials or ampules
Glass IV bottles

roconversion after needlestick injuries show that injuries caused by large-gauge, hollow-bore needles directly inserted into a vein or artery are associated with a high risk of inadvertent intramuscular or subcutaneous injection (Cardo, Culver, & Ciesielski, 1997). Because they are hollow, blood-filled needles, IV introducer needles, and phlebotomy devices pose a significant risk for transmitting bloodborne infection (Tereskerz et al., 1996) (see Chap. 17).

Needleless Systems

In a study by the Centers for Disease Control and Prevention (CDC), 89% of occupational exposures to HIV were caused by percutaneous injuries; most were needlesticks (CDC, 1998). In today's practice arena, the **needleless** system has nearly revolutionized infusion therapy. In general, the product consists of a blunt-tipped plastic insertion device and an injection port that opens to reduce the incidence of accidental needlestick injuries and to promote safety in infusion practice. Again, diverse systems are available to meet clinical needs in many settings.

Peripheral Vascular Access Devices

Innovations in catheter technology have produced catheters to meet the patient's every need, from routine peripheral infusion to the most sophisticated therapy. Catheters vary in gauge, length, design, and composition. Their composition may be polyvinylchloride (PVC), polyurethane, or silicone. Thin-walled catheters promote increased flow rates, which allow smaller catheters to be used. Most catheters are radiopaque or contain a stripe of radiopaque material to enable radiographic visualization. Peripheral access catheters are available in two types: **over-the-needle** (ONC) and **through-the-needle** (or inside-the-needle).

Some products have wings, which confer all the advantages of a small-vein needle for insertion and taping. In these devices, the adapter of the IV set connection is located a few inches from the catheter, which provides ease and smoother technique when changing sets, thereby reducing the potential for mechanical phlebitis and contamination. Such catheters are available with injection sites as an integral part of the catheter; the mixing of drugs or blood components with primary parenteral fluid is reduced to a minimum (0.4 mL), minimizing the potential for incompatibilities.

Product Selection and Evaluation Criteria

A multidisciplinary health care team that includes front-line health care workers should be involved in selecting safety products. Other potential team members include infection control, safety, quality improvement, occupational health, materials management, medical staff, emergency/trauma, surgical, anesthesia, diagnostic radiology, home care, critical care, and laboratory staff. The IV specialist must be included in the team that assesses products used in infusion therapy.

BOX 11–2 U.S. Food and Drug Administration Suggested Criteria for Selecting a Safety Device

- Device provides a barrier between the hands and the needle following use.
- Device allows or requires worker's hands to remain behind the needle at all times.
- Safety constitutes an integral part of the device, is not an accessory.
- Safety features are effective before disassembly and remain in effect after disposal.
- Device should be simple and easy to use, requiring little or no training.

Adapted from U.S. Food and Drug Administration. (1995). Supplementary guidance on the content of premarket notification (510K) submission for medical devices with sharps injury prevention features (draft). Rockville, MD: General Hospital Device Branch, Pilot Device Evaluation Division, Office of Device Evaluation.

In determining the criteria for selecting IV safety devices, design and performance should be considered. Consideration should be given also to latex-free components of a device that may have prolonged contact with a patient, such as an IV catheter (U.S. Food and Drug Administration [FDA], 1996). The suggested FDA criteria are given in Box 11–2.

An evaluation survey instrument may also be developed to measure accurately staff opinion during product evaluation. Examples of forms used by the Training for the Development of Innovative Control Technology Project convened by Dr. June Fisher of the University of California at San Francisco are given in Figure 11–3 (Pugliese, 1999).

Intravenous Catheters

Most IV catheters consist of a flexible, nonthrombogenic tubing that remains within the lumen of the vessel, negating many of the formerly routine complications associated with IV therapy (see Chap. 9). Standard catheters include:

- ONCs: Once the venipuncture is made, the catheter is slipped off the needle into the vein and the steel needle removed. The use of obturators, which are inserted into the catheter to maintain patency for intermittent infusion, is infrequent today.
- Through-the-needle (or inside-the-needle) catheters: The venipuncture is performed and the catheter is then pushed through the needle until the desired length is within the lumen of the vein; the cutting edge is then protected by a shield to prevent the catheter from being severed (Intravenous Nurses Society [INS], 1998, 2000).

Date: _____ Department: _____ Occupation: _____

Product Evaluated: _____ Number of times used: _____

Please circle the most appropriate answer for each question. A rating of one (1) indicates the highest level of agreement with the statement, five (5) the lowest. Not applicable (N/A) may be used if the question does not apply to this product.

agree. . . . . .disagree

1. The safety feature can be activated using a one-handed technique.	1	2	3	4	5	N/A
2. The safety feature does not interfere with normal use of this product.	1	2	3	4	5	N/A
3. Use of this product requires you to use the safety feature.	1	2	3	4	5	N/A
4. This device does not require more time to use than a nonsafety device.	1	2	3	4	5	N/A
5. The safety feature works well with a wide variety of hand sizes.	1	2	3	4	5	N/A
6. The device allows for rapid visualization of flashback in the catheter or chamber.	1	2	3	4	5	N/A
7. Use of this product does not increase the number of sticks to the patient.	1	2	3	4	5	N/A
8. The product stops the flow of blood after the needle is removed from the catheter (or after the butterfly is inserted) and just prior to line connections or hep-lock capping.	1	2	3	4	5	N/A
9. A clear and unmistakable change (either audible or visible) occurs when the safety feature is activated.	1	2	3	4	5	N/A
10. The safety feature operates reliably.	1	2	3	4	5	N/A
11. The exposed sharp is blunted or covered after use and prior to disposal.	1	2	3	4	5	N/A
12. The product does not need extensive training to be operated correctly.	1	2	3	4	5	N/A

Figure 11–3. An intravenous-access devices' safety feature evaluation form. (From the American Hospital Association.)

The choice of catheter depends on the purpose of the infusion and the condition and availability of the veins. The ONCs are used routinely today to ensure a ready route for administering blood and fluid. Through-the-needle catheters are used when a longer catheter is desired. They afford less risk of infiltration than a steel needle, and they are often used for administering drugs or hypertonic fluids that may cause necrosis if extravasation occurs (see Chap. 9).

Variations on these products include a plethora of vascular access devices, from midline catheters to percutaneous ports, and from peripherally inserted central catheters to long-term central lines.

Catheters are made of diverse materials; for many years, PVC was used almost exclusively. Ideally, to reduce the risk of thrombus formation on the catheter, the catheter should be made of a **hemorepellant** material, such as silicone. Catheters should be radiopaque for detection by imaging equipment in the event the catheter is severed and lost in the circulation (INS, 1998, 2000).

Steel Needles

Steel needles are of two types: the steel needle (not recommended for infusion purposes) and the winged infusion device or small-vein needle. The gauge of the needle refers to both the inside and the outside diameters of the lumen—the smaller the gauge, the larger the lumen. Steel needles are typically thin walled. Because the wall of the needle is thinner than that of the standard needle, a larger lumen is obtained for the same external diameter, offering the advantage of enhanced flow rates. Today, the steel needle is most commonly used for sampling venous blood.

Factors to be considered in selecting a steel needle are length of bevel, gauge, and length of the needle. A short bevel reduces the risk of trauma to the endothelial wall, infiltration from a puncture to the posterior wall, and hematoma or extravasation occurring when the steel needle enters the vein. When a steel needle with a long bevel is inserted into the vessel, blood may leak into the tissues before the entire bevel is in the lumen of the vein.

Whenever possible, the gauge of the needle should be appreciably smaller than the lumen of the vein to be entered; when the gauge of the needle approaches the size of the vein, trauma may occur. When a large needle occludes the flow of blood, irritating fluids flowing through the vein with no dilution of blood may cause chemical phlebitis. Mechanical phlebitis may result from motion and pressure exerted by the needle on the endothelial wall of the vein.

When large amounts of fluid are required, a needle of adequate size must be used; a small lumen interferes with the flow of fluid. The flow of blood varies inversely as the fourth power of the radius of the lumen of the needle. Thus, a needle with an internal radius of 1 mm that delivers 1 mL of blood with a fixed pressure on the plunger or in the infusion bottle delivers only $\frac{1}{16}$ of a milliliter when the radius is reduced to 0.5 mm. A large needle is also required with fluids of high viscosity. The rate of flow of the fluid decreases in proportion to the viscosity of the fluid.

The flow of the fluid varies inversely with the length of the needle shaft. If the length of the needle is increased, other conditions being equal, the volume flowing is reduced. Use of a short needle for infusions reduces the risk of infiltration. Because a short needle affords more play than a long needle, more motion is needed to puncture the vessel wall.

Making a wise choice of a catheter for an infusion is a relatively straightforward process. Although the number and types of lines have increased dramatically, several factors remain considerations in all choices (Table 11–1). In addition, a number of safety devices are available to facilitate delivery of peripheral infusion therapy (Table 11–2 and Fig. 11–4).

TABLE 11-1
PERIPHERAL VENOUS ACCESS DEVICES AND THEIR USE

Device	Description	Advantages	Disadvantages
Catheter	ONC catheter Variety of sizes and lengths Radiopaque TNC(INC)	Easily inserted	Short-term use; site should be rotated consistent with institutional policy Infrequently used; essentially replaced by midline and PICC lines
Midline catheter	A mid-catheter device usually placed in either the basilic or cephalic vein; may be ONC or TNC	ONC: Aquavene elastomeric polymer expands 2 gauge sizes and up to 1 inch in length when hydrated; TNC design may have a breakaway needle or peel-away sheath Longer indwell time	Inherent risk of puncturing and shearing the catheter during insertion
PICC catheter	20 to 24 inches long and used for long-term access in patients with poor central access and those at risk for complications from central insertion	Reduced incidence of complications; may be placed by physician or nurse;* diversity of size ranges and manufacturers; may be inserted using guidewire, stylet, or introducer	Care must be taken when threading the catheter through the introducer needle not to withdraw or pull the catheter back through the needle (avoid shearing) May occlude smaller peripheral vessels
Winged infusion needle	Steel needle or flexible catheter with fixed extension set	Easily inserted and secured with wings; extension set ensures access	

ONC, over-the-needle catheter; TNC, through-the-needle catheter; INC, inside-the-needle catheter; PICC, peripherally inserted central catheter.
*Consistent with state Nurse Practice Act.

WINGED INFUSION NEEDLES

The winged infusion device or small-vein needle is similar to the steel cannula, with the hub replaced with two flexible wings. Originally designed for pediatric and geriatric use, it has been used in prolonged therapy for all ages. Two types of small-vein needles are available, one with a short length of plastic tubing and a permanently attached **resealable injection site,** the other with a variable length of plastic tubing permanently attached to a female Luer adapter that accommodates an administration set. The small-vein needle with the resealable injection site allows the intermittent administration of medications or fluids. Variations of the winged infusion needle are available for short-term infusion use. A dilute solution of heparinized saline or saline solution maintains patency of the needle when it is not in use. Winged infusion needles also enhance safety and protection (Figs. 11–5 and 11–6).

text continues on page 210

T A B L E   1 1 – 2

SAFETY EQUIPMENT: MANUFACTURERS AND PRODUCTS

Manufacturer	Injection Equipment (Needle Guards, Needleless Systems)	IV Medication Delivery Systems	IV Insertion Devices	Blood Collection Equipment
B-D	Safety Glide Safety-Lok Jetinjector	Interlink (Baxter/BD) POSIFLOW valve	Insyte Auto Guard™ Saf-T-Intima™	Eclipse VACUTAINER System Pronto VACUTAINER System Vacutainer Brand Safety-Gard phlebotomy system Vacutainer Safety-Lok Blood collection tubes
Johnson & Johnson			Protectiv Protective Plus Biovue PICC midline catheter with Protectiv Safety Introducer	
InjectiMed, Inc.	Protector Syringe and Safety Cap System			
Kendall Healthcare	Monoject Safety Syringe			
Sterimatic	Safety Needle Safety Tip			
Safety Medical Supply International				Angel Wing Safety Needle System

SIMS Portex	Needle-Pro	Needle-Pro™ venous/arterial needle protection
Bioject	Biojector 2000
Abbott Laboratories	Life Shield
Baxter Healthcare	Needle Lock Device Interlink (Baxter/BD)
New Medical Technology	NMT Safety Syringe
Wyeth-Ayerst	Tubex Blunt Point cartridge unit
Safety 1st Medical	Safety 1st Safety Syringe
Sanofi Wintrop/BD/Baxter	Carpuject with InterLink blunt cannula or Luer Lok
ICU Medical	Clave connector
	Click Lock/Piggy Lock
Tri-State Medical	Centurion Uni-Guard Piggy Back Connector
3M Health Care	AVI Checkvalve
Beech Medical	Versa-Lok and Pro-Lok
North American Medical Products	Safe Point Vac and Safe Point M-D
Sage Products Winfield Medical	Shamrock safety winged set Saf-T-Clik

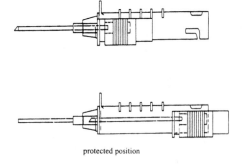

protected position

ProtectivᵀᴹI.V. Catheter
Safety System
Johnson & Johnson
Medical, Inc.
Arlington, TX
*A protective sleeve encases
the sharp stylet as it is
retracted from the catheter.*

Insyte® AutoGuardᵀᴹ
Shielded I.V. Catheter
Becton Dickinson
Vascular Access
Sandy, UT
*Stylet is instantly encased
inside a tamper-resistant
safety barrel by pressing the
activation button.*

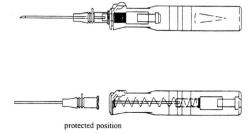

protected position

Figure 11–4. Safety devices for IV catheters.

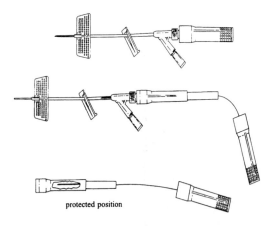

protected position

Saf-T-Intimaᵀᴹ I.V.
Catheter Safety
System
Becton Dickinson
Vascular Access
Sandy, UT
*Following catheter
insertion, the stylet is
withdrawn and
automatically covered
in a telescoping safety
chamber.*

Figure 11–5. IV catheter winged safety device.

Punctur-Guard™
Winged Set
Bio-Plexus
Tolland, CT
After placement, third wing is rotated to flat position which blunts needle point before it is removed from the patient.

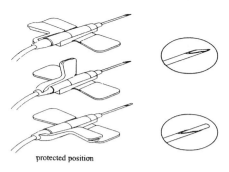

protected position

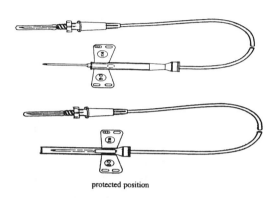

protected position

Vacutainer® Brand
Safety-Lok™
Winged Needle
Becton Dickinson
Vacutainer Systems
Franklin Lakes, NJ
After removal from patient, safety shield is advanced forward and locks in place beyond needle tip.

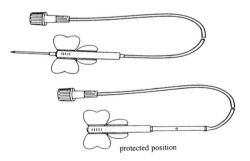

protected position

Shamrock™ Safety
Winged Needle
Winfield Medical
San Diego, CA
After removal from patient, needle is retracted backward and locks in covered position between wings.

Angel Wing™
Safety Needle
Sherwood Medical
St. Louis, MO
Stainless steel barrier tip is advanced forward to end of needle, locking over point as needle is withdrawn from the patient; one-handed activation.

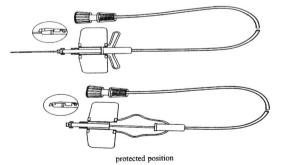

protected position

Figure 11–6. Winged safety devices.

Needle Shields

Manufacturers have incorporated safety needle shields into their respective designs. Shields or sheath covers help to prevent inadvertent needlesticks. Needle-Pro (Smith Industries Medical Systems) and SafetyTip are examples of these products (Fig. 11–7). The SafetyTip is a needlestick prevention device with distinct advantages. Composed of a standardized hypodermic needle with an integral safety shield that moves into place to protect the health care worker from accidental needlestick injury, it can be used by left- or right-handed people, permits one-handed activation, ensures that the user's hand is behind the needle at all times during shielding, and requires no assembly or disassembly. Most needle sheaths physically engage the needle to remain shut. Safety Tip avoids this flaw by using a simple catch mechanism to secure the safety sheath.

Midline Catheters

The introduction of the midline catheter brought an alternative to central line catheter placement for prolonged IV access. The materials that midline catheters are made of are significant safety features. For instance, polytetrafluoroethylene (Teflon) is less thrombogenic and less inflammatory than polyurethane or PVC. Vialon, a new material, is nonhemolytic and free of plasticizers. It is slick after immersion in fluid and softens after insertion, minimizing vein trauma and clot induction. Another catheter material, Aquavene, is an elastomeric hydrogel that softens and expands when hydrated (in contact with aqueous fluids, such as blood). Advantages of using the product include reduction of peripheral IV restarts, elimination of the need for central IV lines with their associated complications, and ease of midline insertion (see Chap. 12).

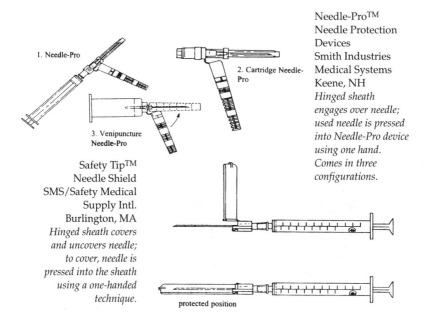

1. Needle-Pro

2. Cartridge Needle-Pro

3. Venipuncture Needle-Pro

Needle-Pro™
Needle Protection
Devices
Smith Industries
Medical Systems
Keene, NH
Hinged sheath engages over needle; used needle is pressed into Needle-Pro device using one hand. Comes in three configurations.

Safety Tip™
Needle Shield
SMS/Safety Medical
Supply Intl.
Burlington, MA
Hinged sheath covers and uncovers needle; to cover, needle is pressed into the sheath using a one-handed technique.

protected position

Figure 11–7. Safety shields for needles.

The complete softening and expansion process takes approximately 90 minutes. Aquavene catheters expand precisely two gauge sizes—they do not continue to expand beyond this. Catheter cannulas consist of an Aquavene outer layer and thin polyurethane inner lining. The polyurethane lining is impermeable and prevents hydration from the inner lumen. The outer, Aquavene layer hydrates by absorbing water and electrolytes from the blood and plasma. This product permits long-term placement when venous access is limited or when therapy is prescribed for a specific time. The product is considered a peripheral venous catheter according to INS standards. Professionals are encouraged to develop policies and procedures relevant to indwell time and consistent with INS standards and institutional guidelines (INS, 1998, 2000).

Fluid Containers

Sterile glass containers first became available in 1929. Although currently used much less frequently, glass remains the container of choice for those fluids that, because of their characteristics, may not be administered in plastic containers. For example, nitroglycerin can be absorbed into plastic containers and tubing, and lipid emulsions can absorb certain plastics from the container into the fluid.

GLASS CONTAINERS

At manufacture, glass IV containers are sealed under vacuum and therefore must be vented when delivered to the patient. The air vent on the administration set (typically as part of the piercing pin) should have an air filter to prevent the ingress of microbes as the fluid is vented. If a nonvented administration set is used with a glass container, the fluid will not flow. Air must displace the fluid in the container for flow to occur.

Medications should be added to glass containers through the rubber stopper. Glass is also an absolute barrier to gases such as carbon dioxide and oxygen. Some drugs such as lipids and bicarbonate are not stable in current plastic containers because of gas diffusion.

PLASTIC CONTAINERS

Baxter Healthcare (Deerfield, IL) was the first manufacturer to develop plastic containers for parenteral fluids. Plastic containers are easily transported, minimize the risk of damage to the container, and are easily disposed of. Air venting is not required because the container collapses as the fluid is delivered. This in turn reduces the risk of air embolism and airborne contamination. Because plastic containers do not have stoppers or bushings, the risk of coring and particulate matter is eliminated. Plastic IV containers range in size from 25 to 1000 mL for IV infusion.

SYRINGES AND SAFETY SYRINGES

A syringe may be a fluid container, especially when used with an infusion device that accommodates syringe delivery. Delivery of fluid or medication from a syringe is well suited to patient care areas in which small volumes of medication or fluid are required. The limiting feature of the syringe is its volume capacity (see Chap. 21). One manufacturer, I-Flow Corporation, Lake Forest, CA, provides a syringe system to deliver either intermittent or IV push medications in all clinical settings. Using standard syringes, delivery times vary from 15 to 60 minutes with an accuracy rate of ±15%.

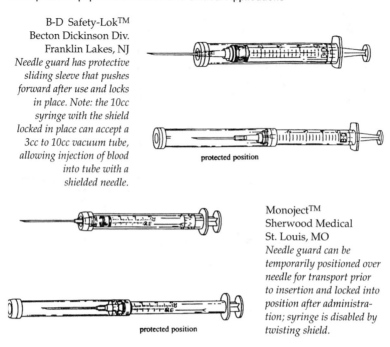

B-D Safety-Lok™
Becton Dickinson Div.
Franklin Lakes, NJ
*Needle guard has protective
sliding sleeve that pushes
forward after use and locks
in place. Note: the 10cc
syringe with the shield
locked in place can accept a
3cc to 10cc vacuum tube,
allowing injection of blood
into tube with a
shielded needle.*

protected position

Monoject™
Sherwood Medical
St. Louis, MO
*Needle guard can be
temporarily positioned over
needle for transport prior
to insertion and locked into
position after administration; syringe is disabled by
twisting shield.*

protected position

Figure 11–8. Safety syringes.

The development of safety syringes has contributed greatly to practice. Several manufacturers provide safety syringes with needle guards to protect the health care worker and patient (Fig. 11–8).

Drug Delivery Systems

Three of six IV drug delivery systems received superior ratings at a national panel of clinicians (Consensus Development Conference, September 27 and 28, 1999). The systems were manufacturer-prepared IV delivery systems, point-of-care–activated IV delivery systems, and pharmacy-based IV admixture programs. IV push, volume control chambers, and syringe pumps were ranked lower by the panel of experts. The use of these systems varies within a given institution and in specific clinical circumstances; for example, in a medical emergency, IV push may be preferred (Tereskerz et al., 1996; Occupational Safety and Health Administration, 1998, CDC, 1998).

MANUFACTURER PREPARED

Manufacturer-prepared fluids have revolutionized practice because increasing numbers of medications are marketed in this way. Premixed fluids are prepared under sterile conditions in the designated diluent and container with specific instructions for use. Easily transported and stable, manufacturer-prepared fluids have changed the way in which home care is delivered (see Chap. 23).

POINT-OF-CARE

A use-activated (**point-of-care**) container is compartmentalized, with premeasured drug in one compartment and the required fluid in another compartment. To activate the container for infusion, the nurse must remove or dislodge a diaphragm or seal between the compartments. This simplifies drug delivery by allowing the drug and the fluid to mix. It also eliminates the need for separate drug and diluent vials and yields an appropriate admixture for delivery.

PHARMACY-BASED INTRAVENOUS ADMIXTURE

Although many medications come in a prefilled container for IV piggyback administration, some medications must be added to fluid before administration. Methods for adding medications to fluid containers vary with each system, and new safety parameters have been added to currently available devices. The plastic bag contains a resealable medication port through which the medication is injected, although some products permit needleless access to the container.

When medications are added to the plastic containers during an infusion, care must be taken to ensure that the clamp on the administration set is closed and the flow interrupted before the medication is added. This prevents inadvertent administration of an undiluted and potentially toxic dose of medication that has not been fully diluted in the IV container. Medications and fluids should always be mixed thoroughly before administration, regardless of the system used. Most drug delivery systems use universal piercing pins. Use of such products eliminates the need to remove an existing air vent from the piercing pin.

Intravenous Administration Sets

An important factor in the administration set is the rate of flow the given set is gauged to produce. Commercial sets vary, delivering anywhere from 10 to 15 drops/mL, depending on the nature of the fluid. The nurse must be aware of the drop factor to set the rate of flow correctly. Increased fluid viscosity may slow the rate of infusion, but does not affect the drop factor.

Most conventional sets use the roller clamp or slide clamp for controlling the flow rate. Fluid temperature, room temperature, height of the fluid container, and the patient's catheter size all affect flow rate. The nurse should recheck the infusion rate regularly to ensure the prescribed flow rate is maintained.

Alternatives to the roller clamp are available from a number of manufacturers; they can save nurses valuable time and are helpful in maintaining the rate of infusion. One device has a flow-metering system that essentially eliminates changes in flow rate. The metering device consists of "an adjustable dam." The dam is usually added to a standard administration set and can be removed if desired. The rate can be set and is maintained as long as the head height of the fluid container remains constant. This minimizes the risk of runaway infusions and free flow, which can occur if the roller clamp fully opens accidentally.

SPECIALTY-USE SETS

Non-PVC IV administration sets are available for gravity and volumetric EIDs. Nitroglycerin and other drugs can be administered without altering the dosage of the drug through **absorption** into the walls of PVC tubing. Fat emulsion leaches plasticizers from the PVC tubing; these specialty sets may have non-PVC layers in fluid contact, or use plasticizers that do not leach as easily.

In many cases, the flow must be maintained at a minimal rate. One method is to reduce the drop size by using a microdrip set. These sets deliver 60 drops/mL. At the rate of 60 drops/minute, it would take 1 hour to infuse 60 mL. A variety of commercial sets are available for alternate or simultaneous infusion of two fluids. Some sets contain a filter (Fig. 11–9).

Positive-pressure sets are designed to increase the rate of infusion and are an asset when rapid replacement of fluid becomes necessary. When used with the collapsible plastic fluid container, the danger of air embolism is minimal because as the bag collapses, the risk of air in the system is reduced. In contrast to the collapsible plastic container, glass containers must be vented to allow the fluid to flow, and air is thus present in the system. As the last portion of fluid from the glass container is delivered to the patient, the air under pressure may rapidly enter the vein before the clamp can be applied, resulting in an embolus. The nurse should never apply positive pressure to infuse fluids.

CHECK-VALVE SETS

Check-valve sets were traditionally used to administer secondary medications as a piggyback into the injection site located below the valve. The valve automatically shut off the main-line infusion while the admixture was running and automatically allowed the main infusion to start when the medication had run in. Variations of this set are available for use with electronic flow control devices (EIDs), which enable the user to back-prime the small-volume container (piggyback) with primary fluid (see section on Electronic Infusion Devices).

VOLUME-CONTROLLED SETS

Accuracy in controlling the volume of IV fluids is facilitated by using a volume-controlled set. Several available devices permit accurate administration of measured volumes of fluids (Fig. 11–10). Sets contain vented, **calibrated** burette chambers that control the volume from 100 to 150 mL. The burette chamber of some sets contains a rubber float that prevents air from entering the tubing once the infusion is completed.

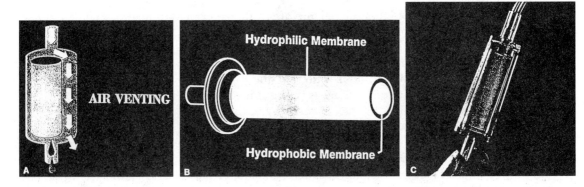

Figure 11–9. (A) Air-eliminating properties of an IV filter. (B) Hydrophilic/hydrophobic membrane properties of an IV filter. (C) Optimal IV filter for add-on or in-line use. (Courtesy of Abbott Laboratories, Abbott Park, IL)

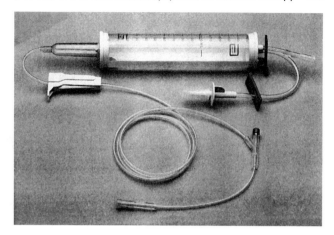

Figure 11–10. Volume-controlled infusion set. (Courtesy of Abbott Laboratories Abbott Park, IL)

Some calibrated burette chambers contain a microporous filter to block the passage of air when the chamber empties. Refilling these chambers requires a specific procedure. The word *oscar* is a memory helper to recall the procedure:

O—open clamp
S—squeeze drip chamber and hold
C—close clamp close to drip chamber
A—and
R—release drip chamber

The Rely-A-Flow rate-controlled set uses flow control tubing to administer an infusion at a preset rate with 6% to 10% accuracy.

ELECTRONIC INFUSION DEVICE–SPECIFIC SETS

Some administration sets are made specifically for use with EIDs. These sets also come in a number of configurations. Such sets and their respective electronic delivery systems ensure safe delivery of infusion therapy to patients of all ages in a variety of clinical settings. By extracting fluid from the IV container and ejecting it at predetermined intervals through the administration set, the EID delivers the appropriate preset amount of diluent.

Final Intravenous Filters

Filters prevent passage of undesirable substances into the vascular system (Fig. 11–11).

Particulate filters of 1 or 5 μm are recommended when IV medications are being prepared. A bacteria-retentive filter, in the range of 0.2 μm, is recommended for the routine delivery of IV therapies. The time of change should ideally coincide with the changing of the administration set (see Chap. 4).

Filters come in diverse configurations, including add-on and integral units. Add-on filters should be securely connected to the administration set and treated as

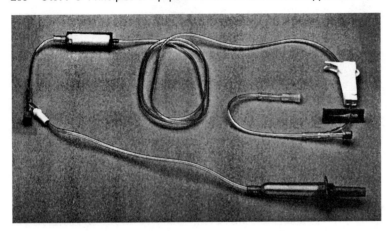

Figure 11–11. Primary venoset with IVEX-2 integral filter.

a part of that set. Integral filters are attached by the manufacturer to the administration set. To achieve final filtration, the filter should be located as close to the catheter site as possible. A 0.2-μm filter is considered an absolute, bacteria-retentive, air-eliminating filter and decreases the complications of infection and the potential for air embolism.

The industry standard is a membrane filter. Membrane filters are screen-type filters with uniformly sized pores that provide an absolute rating. A 0.2-μm screen-type filter retains on the flat surface membrane all particles larger than 0.2 μm.

The *United States Pharmacopeia* (1999) has established an acceptable limit of particles for single-dose infusion as not more than 50 particles/mL that are equal to or larger than 10.0 μm and not more than 5 particles/mL that are equal to or larger than 25.0 μm in effective linear dimension.

EFFECT OF PRESSURE AND AIR ON FILTERS

At a certain pressure, all filters allow air to pass from one side of the **wetted** hydrophilic membrane to the other. This pressure value is called the **bubble point** of that particular membrane. Distinguishing features that affect the bubble point are the different filter materials (eg, hydrophobic, hydrophilic, depth, screen), different wetting or nonwetting characteristics, and the test liquid. Water or saline solution, for example, is the test liquid of choice when testing hydrophilic membranes for IV filters because fluids that are administered IV are primarily water. Water is inexpensive, can be filtered easily for control of particulates and microorganisms, and is readily available. There are other advantages to using water as a bubble point test fluid. Water tests the wetting characteristics of hydrophilic membrane filters. To define this point further, an explanation of bubble point tests in relation to membranes is required.

BUBBLE POINT TESTS

Bubble point testing is particularly important in IV therapy because it is crucial that the filter in the IV line prevent air from passing through it at low pressures, such as those used in IV therapy.

Testing involves encapsulation of the membrane in an integral housing. Two different types of bubble point tests may be performed, open bubble and closed bubble point, depending on downstream flow and the ability to see the membrane (Fig. 11–12). An open bubble point test can be performed only if the direction of normal flow is such that the bubbles produced can be seen as they form. This means that the housing of the filter must be transparent and the "downstream" side of the membrane can be observed. This test is performed by first flowing the test liquid through the device at low pressures until it is wetted out. Usually, this pressure is the same as that used in administering fluid by gravity feed pressures (36 to 39 inches of water). Then, after the membrane is wetted out, air pressure is applied as before. The bubble point has been reached when a steady stream of bubbles is seen on the downstream side of the membrane.

A closed bubble point test must be performed when the downstream side of the membrane cannot be visualized. Closed bubble points result in slightly higher values than open bubble points because the air pressure during the test is steadily increasing, and it takes more time for the air bubbles to escape through the distal port. If the pressure is increased slowly, the test is more accurate.

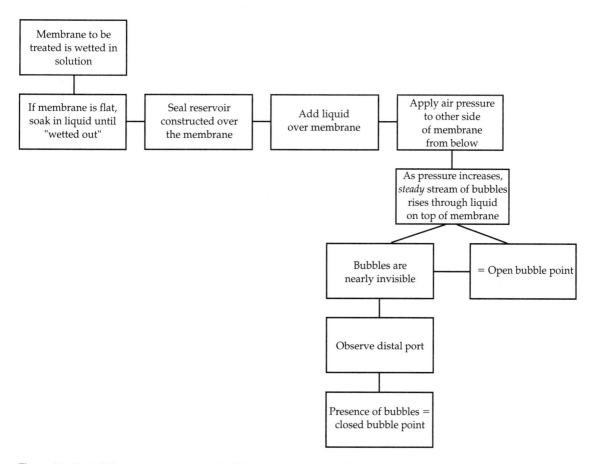

Figure 11–12. Bubble point tests. An open bubble point test can be performed only if the direction of normal flow permits bubbles to form.

Testing of IV membranes and filter devices with water is significant. Most hydrophilic membranes incorporate either external (applied after they are made) or internal (in the base formula) wetting agents to render them more wettable with water. It is particularly important in IV therapy because it is critical that the membrane should wet properly so that air does not pass the membrane at low pressures.

The 0.2-μm air-venting filters automatically vent air through a nonwettable (**hydrophobic**) membrane and permit uniform high gravity flow rates through large, wettable (**hydrophilic**) membranes. They prevent an air block, which could ultimately result in a plugged catheter.

Filters are also rated according to the pounds per square inch (**psi**) of pressure they withstand, an important consideration in selecting the proper filter. The filter should withstand the pressure exerted by the infusion pump or rupture may occur. If the psi rating of the housing is less than that of the membrane, excess force will break the housing, leaving the filter intact.

Optimal filters should (1) automatically vent air; (2) retain bacteria, fungi, and endotoxins; (3) not bind drugs; (4) allow high gravity flow rates; and (5) be able to withstand the pressure exerted by the infusion pump. The pressure rating of the housing, when less than that of the filter membrane, may provide added protection.

Intravenous Accessories

A plethora of accessories, such as injection caps, latex ports, and needleless systems, is available today (Fig. 11–13). Most include safety features. The injection port or catheter cap may be used to adapt any indwelling device to an intermittent infusion device. Available either as an individual unit or incorporated into the design of an

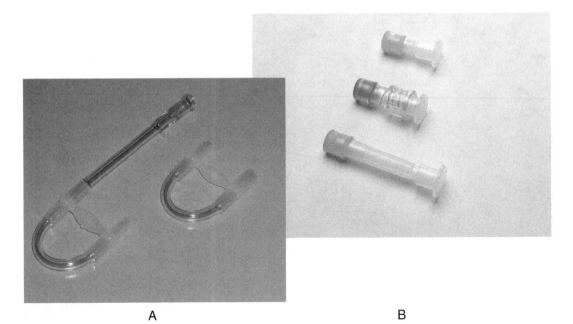

A   B

Figure 11–13. Among the many accessory items for IV therapy are (A) loops and (B) injection ports.

ONC or winged infusion set, injection ports have simplified the administration of intermittent therapies using needleless systems.

Intermittent infusion devices may also be called *heparin locks*, *INTS*, or *PRN adapters* because heparin or saline is routinely instilled into the cap and its housing to maintain patency. Most health care organizations routinely instill saline rather than dilute heparin in such devices.

The Click-Lock is a product of ICU Medical (San Clemente, CA) and was the first positive-locking IV catheter–connecting device (Fig. 11–14). It uses a removable stainless steel needle in a clear plastic housing that snap-locks onto the injection port. Abbott Laboratories (Abbott Park, IL) provides a number of needleless components, including LifeShield prepierced ports and blunt cannulas, Clave connectors, Aluer vials, and needleless male adapters. Figure 11–15 compares a needle catheter flush and the CLC 2000 positive displacement flush (Abbott, 1999).

Latex Devices and Sensitivity

At the turn of the century, **latex** sensitivity remains a challenge for health care workers and patients alike, with powdered latex gloves being the most common latex equipment to exacerbate allergies. In addition, many of the clinical supplies used to deliver IV fluids and fluids are made of latex.

The various types of latex reactions include irritant or contact dermatitis, allergic contact type IV hypersensitivity, and type I hypersensitivity. Allergic reactions are potentially avoidable for both the patient and clinicians. The nurse delivering IV therapy should be cognizant of the prevalence, symptoms, risk factors, diagnosis, and treatment of latex allergy (Warshaw, 1998; Beezhold et al., 1996; Gritter, 1999; National Institute for Occupational Safety and Health [NIOSH], 1997).

Standard precautions mandate that health care providers wear gloves for prolonged periods of patient care. Latex is a natural rubber product derived from the sap

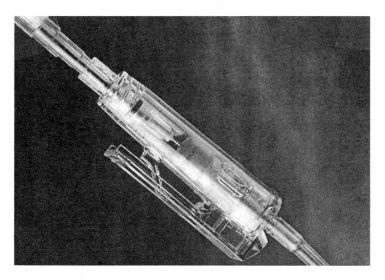

Figure 11–14. Click-Lock locking (junction securement) device. (Courtesy of ICU Medical, San Clemente, CA).

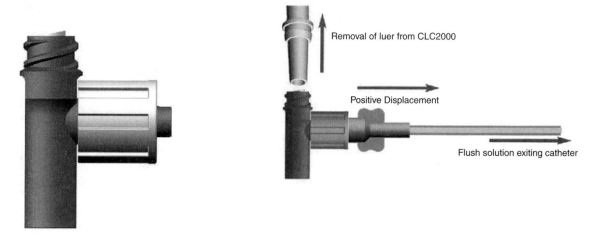

Figure 11–15. Comparison between needle catheter flush and CLC 2000 flush. (Courtesy of Abbott Needleless Systems CLC 2000, Abbott Park, IL.)

of the commercial rubber tree *Hevea brasiliensis*. The latex fluid is composed of carbohydrates, lipids, phospholipids, and *cis*-1,4 polyisoprene. Latex is a complex protein by-product of the rubber tree containing more than 28 antigenic peptide proteins and contributing to allergic reactions in people with hypersensitivity latex allergy (Table 11–3).

Exposure can occur through cutaneous, mucosal, parenteral, or aerosol routes. Parenteral exposure includes medications injected through latex IV injection sites or drawn through rubber stoppers of vials. Powder released into the air during the removal of a powdered latex glove may precipitate respiratory distress. Latex proteins may remain airborne for as long as 5 to 12 hours (Warshaw, 1998; Beezhold et al., 1996). Diagnosis is confirmed by detailed history, including risk factors and suspected reactions. Physical examination may reveal a lack of symptoms. A skin prick test is a reliable indicator of an antigen allergy. Radioallergosorbent testing (RAST) is

T A B L E   1 1 – 3
TYPE I REACTIONS TO LATEX

System Affected	Clinical Manifestation
Cardiovascular	Hypotension, sinus tachycardia, arrhythmias, cardiac arrest
Gastrointestinal	Nausea, vomiting, diarrhea, abdominal cramping
Respiratory	Bronchospasm, shortness of breath, cyanosis, laryngeal edema, wheezing, respiratory arrest
Cutaneous	Flushing, urticaria, pruritus, rash
Systemic	Faintness, generalized edema

an in vitro test for IgE antibodies to a specific antigen. The results of RAST may be inconclusive, however. Use, challenge, or patch tests may be performed, along with intradermal testing, basophil histamine release, and inhalation tests. Prevention is achieved by providing a latex-free environment. NIOSH recommends that if latex gloves are worn, they should be the low-antigen type and powderless (Warshaw, 1998). For more information, see Box 11–3.

Electronic Infusion Devices

The INS Standards of Practice address regulation of flow (see Chap. 4). **Electronic infusion devices** should be used when warranted by the patient's age and condition, setting, and prescribed therapy. The nursing professional is responsible and accountable for the use of EIDs. Use of EIDs, their deployment, selection criteria, and classifications should be outlined in institutional policy and procedure manuals. The nurse's knowledge base concerning EIDs should include, at the minimum, indications for use, mechanical operation, safe use and troubleshooting techniques, and the psi rating.

The psi rating is important because **differential pressure** is often a component of such devices. With a range of two or three levels, such equipment may sense a change in pressure, usually 5 psi over baseline, and some devices monitor and read out (display) line pressure. Operating or line pressure is the pressure generated by a pump that causes fluid to flow at a predetermined rate. Maximum occlusion pressure is the limit to operating pressure at which an occlusion alarm is triggered. Needle pressure is the same as venous pressure. During an infusion, pressure at the tip of the catheter is only slightly greater than the pressure in the vein or artery, regardless of the output pressure of the pump. The pressure at the needle tip needs to be slightly higher than vascular pressure for fluid to flow. An understanding of pressure and the psi rating is essential to safe use of EIDs, filters, and other components of the IV system.

Electronic infusion devices are invaluable in neonatal, pediatric, and adult intensive care units, where critical infusions of small volumes of fluid or doses of high-potency drugs are required. These devices have increased the level of safety in parenteral therapy. Today, the risk of air embolism is reduced by alarm systems and by

---

BOX 11–3 Web Site Sources of Information: Latex Sensitivity

- *Education for Latex Allergy/Support Team and Information Coalition (ELASTIC)*
  www.netcom.com/~ecdbmd/elastic.html
- *Latex Allergy Links*
  www.netcom.com/~naml/latex_allergy.html
- *National Institute for Occupational Safety and Health (NIOSH)*
  www.cdc.gov/niosh/latexalt.html

the automatic interruption of the infusion when a container empties. A controlled rate of flow reduces the risk of circulatory overload.

The devices have saved valuable nursing time; uniform control of fluid eliminates the need to count drops and continually adjust flow rates. Plugging of the catheter, which occurs when blood backs into the catheter because of an increase in venous pressure from coughing, crying, or straining, is eliminated. The pressure generated by the EID pump may exceed the maximum venous pressure.

AMBULATORY INFUSION DEVICES

Self-care is an important component of current health care delivery systems. The development of compact, battery-driven EIDs has simplified care in diverse ambulatory clinical settings, including home care. The AIM Plus (Abbott Laboratories) is an example of an ambulatory infusion device (Fig. 11–16).

EXTERNAL INFUSION PUMPS

The size, weight, and portability of the unit are important considerations in choosing a system. An active patient must be comfortable wearing the lightest pump possible; a sedentary patient may prefer the advantages of a larger device. Accessories and loading procedures vary with the manufacturer and the product selected. Infu-

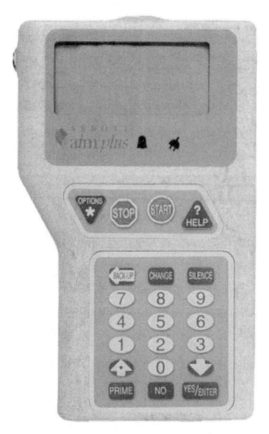

Figure 11–16. Aim Plus ambulatory pump. (Courtesy of Abbott Laboratories, Abbott Park, IL.)

sion capacity may dictate the choice of the system. Pump-specific sets may be required, such as with the patient receiving nutritional support or pain medication. Integral safety features include

- Occlusion alarm
- Low volume safety alarm
- Low battery alarm

Competition in this exciting area of growth has stimulated many new companies to enter the electronic infusion market, resulting in greater availability of more sophisticated products for the professional IV nurse.

ELASTOMERIC BALLOON DEVICES

An **elastomeric** device is made of a soft, rubberized material capable of inflating to a predetermined volume. The balloon deflates at a rate determined by the diameter of the restricting outlet located in the preattached tubing or in the neck of the container. The size of the tunnel controls the passage of fluid. The balloon, safely encapsulated inside a rigid, transparent container, becomes the reservoir for fluid. The shape of this device is manufacturer specific, and it may be round, disk shaped, or cylindrical. A tamper-proof port for injecting medication into the balloon is attached. Typically, the capacity is 50 to 100 mL and the devices are for one-time use only.

Baxter's Intermate (Fig. 11–17) provides fixed rates to ensure accurate dosages and pharmacokinetic consistency. No IV pole or electric cord is needed. The design, in various configurations, is small and lightweight. As a single-use disposable item, it simplifies single-dose infusion therapies.

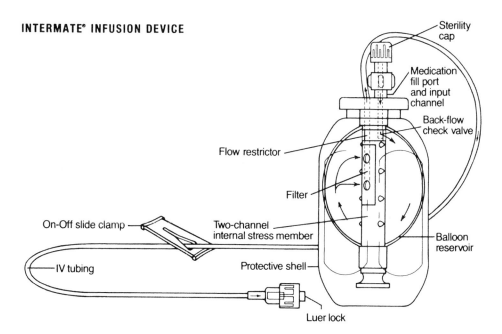

INTERMATE® INFUSION DEVICE

Sterility cap

Medication fill port and input channel

Back-flow check valve

Flow restrictor

Filter

On-Off slide clamp

Two-channel internal stress member

IV tubing

Protective shell

Balloon reservoir

Luer lock

Figure 11–17. Baxter Intermate. (Courtesy of Baxter Healthcare, Deerfield, IL.)

SPRING-COIL PISTON SYRINGES

The volume of a spring-coil piston syringe ranges from 30 to 60 mL, and a spring powers the plunger in the absence of manual pressure. Like the elastomeric balloon, this device has limited applications and is for one-time use only. The syringe is filled by withdrawing the piston and overextending the spring. As the spring regains its shape, it forces the piston down, expelling its contents.

SPRING-COIL CONTAINER

This container combines the principles of the spring-coil piston syringe in a multiuse and small volume container. An overextended spring in an enclosed space between two disks seeks to collapse, pulling the top and bottom together and forcing the fluid contents out of the restricting orifice. Handy and convenient for the ambulatory patient, the spring-coil container is ideal for home use.

THERAPY-SPECIFIC DEVICES

Electronic infusion devices are finding increasing use in keep-open arterial lines and infusion of drugs, blood, and viscous fluids such as hyperalimentation fluids. Advances in technology have provided us with more sophisticated devices. Many types and models are available. In general, pumps are devices that generate flow under positive pressure. Such devices may be peristaltic, syringe, or pulsatile. **Controllers** are devices that generate flow by gravity and are capable of either drop counting or volumetric delivery.

CONTROLLERS

Controllers do not exert positive pressure greater than the head height of the infusion container, which is usually 2 psi. The controller is used to monitor the infusion for accuracy, to sound an alarm if flow is interrupted, and to provide even, consistent delivery of fluid. A controller uses drop-sensor technology. Manufacturers have developed variations on this theme, specific to patient populations and clinical needs.

PUMPS

A diversity of pump products is available, including syringe, positive-pressure, and volumetric devices.

Syringe Pumps. Many manufacturers have met the demand for syringe infusion systems. Syringe pumps are calibrated in milliliters per hour, are used with standard disposable syringes, and provide smooth and precise delivery of low volumes of fluid to specific patient populations. A variety of new products on the market may be configured to suit special clinical situations, with options such as auto bolus reduction to minimize the possibility of administering an accidental bolus of drug, preset upper bolus rates, maintenance notification, and downloading capability between instruments. Alaris Medical's (San Diego, CA and Hampshire, United Kingdom) IVAC P3000 and IVAC P7000 syringe pump have multiple features (Fig. 11–18). Multi-instrument docking stations allow the user to administer sequential infusions (Fig. 11–19).

Positive-Pressure Infusion Pumps. A positive-pressure device overcomes vascular resistance, tubing compromises such as excessive length, and the normal physical limitations that cause an IV to function improperly.

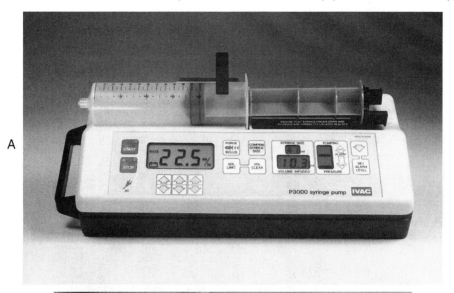

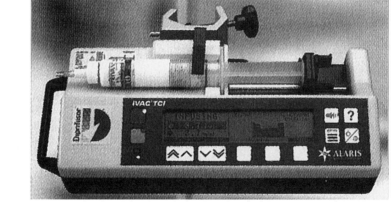

Figure 11–18. Syringe pumps. (Courtesy Alaris Medical, San Diego, CA and Hampshire, UK.)
(A) The IVAC P3000 uses standard disposable syringes and operates at low-level pumping pressure.
(B) The IVAC P7000 can deliver fluid over a preset time and in preset doses, using syringes ranging
from 5 to 100 mL.

Pressure exerted by the unit is expressed in pounds per square inch (psi) or millimeters of mercury. One pound per square inch and 50 mm Hg exert the same amount
of pressure. The psi rating of an EID is important because it may affect the type of filter
being used or the ability of the unit to infuse fluids through arterial lines. The pressure
exerted should not exceed the pressure the filter can withstand or a rupture may occur;
when the pump is used for arterial infusion, the pressure must be high enough to overcome arterial pressure. Positive **pressure pumps** are used in most clinical settings.

Volumetric Infusion Pumps. With the volumetric pump, the unit calculates the volume delivered by measuring the volume displaced in a reservoir that is a component

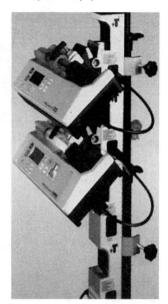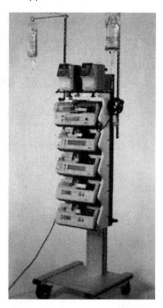

Figure 11–19. Alaris medical docking systems. (Courtesy of Alaris Medical Systems, San Diego and Hampshire, UK.)

of the disposable administration set. The mechanism of action may be piston generated or **linear.**

Volumetric pumps such as Abbott's Plum family offer cassette-based technology and the ability to deliver two simultaneous or intermittent infusions through one patient line. The cassette also allows the clinician to back-prime to eliminate air before it leaves the cassette. The Plum provides free-flow protection, is available in single-channel or dual-channel capacity, or as the XL3, which provides three pumping mechanisms in one device. The Omni-Flow pump is a four-channel device that allows programmable continuous or intermittent infusions on four lines with only one patient line, thus reducing the need for multiple IV sites (Fig. 11–20).

Computer-Generated Technology

The computer has become the focal point of the IV drug delivery system. Electronic flow is now the norm rather than the exception. EIDs today are available in diverse sizes and technologies for a broad range of purposes. Accompanying these computerized systems is a whole new lexicon of terms with which the nurse must become familiar to use the equipment safely and properly. For example, commonly heard terms include *tapering* or **ramping,** which describe the progressive increase or decrease of infusion rate. Another common term is **free flow.** Free-flow alarms may be life saving if the administration set has no intrinsic valves or reservoirs that require

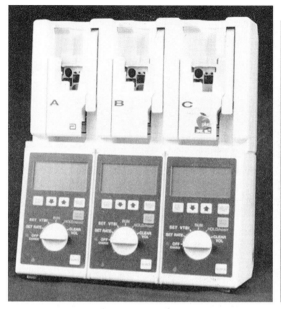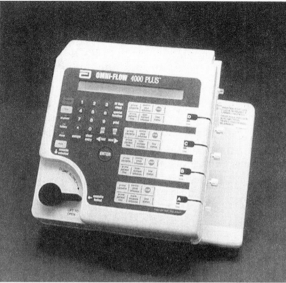

Figure 11–20. Infusion pumps. The pump on *left* has three channels; the pump on *right* has four. (Courtesy of Abbott Laboratories, Abbott Park, IL.)

motion of the pumping mechanism to propel the fluid. Many pumps incorporate free-flow alarms that are capable of detecting open flow of fluid to the patient. Others have internal clamps or devices that lock into place when tubing is removed from the pump, preventing free flow of fluid to the patient. Other safety features are available on a number of products.

■ EQUIPMENT SAFETY AND USE

ECRI (Plymouth Meeting, PA), an independent, nonprofit agency that tests equipment for safety and effectiveness and continually designs new criteria for evaluation of equipment, is dedicated to improving the safety, efficacy, and cost effectiveness of health care technology, facilities, and procedures. Among the products assessed are EIDs from various manufacturers. The organization develops strict evaluation criteria aimed at helping care providers in the clinical setting perform with a high degree of safety and accuracy.

In relation to EIDs and infusion therapy, evaluation criteria are wide ranging to meet the needs of nursing staff in today's complex health care setting. The impact of downsizing and the integration of health care organizations has affected staffing patterns nationwide; therefore, nurses must be familiar with the literature and with the device to be used. They must take all precautions to ensure safe, efficient operation. One thing, however, remains a constant. The EID should never be used as a substitute for high-quality care and patient monitoring (see Chaps. 2 through 4).

Product Selection and Evaluation

Selection of equipment is a complex task. Hospitalized patients now receive a multitude of therapies through their vascular systems. The type of device used to initiate flow depends on the complexity of care, the range of flow needed, pressure, the insertion site, and the delivery rate.

Product selection should be a serious consideration and should be based on needs assessed in the clinical setting. The ability to deliver a specified dose in μg/kg/minute, μg/kg/hour, mg/kg/minute, or mg/kg/hour by entering the appropriate concentration, patient weight, bolus amount, and mass units is a feature often required in the critical care setting. Demands for features such as bolus capabilities, syringe size sensing, and delivery in body weight, mass, continuous, or volume-over-time modes have challenged today's manufacturers to produce ever more advanced products.

Decision-Making Process

The product evaluation committee is usually involved in the selection of EIDs in the clinical setting. This focus should carry into the alternative care setting as well, so that the EIDs chosen clearly meet the patients' clinical and therapeutic needs while fulfilling a real function as accessories to high-quality IV nursing care. When selection is made by a group purchasing contract, nursing input is vital to the selection process.

Patient Selection and Education

Patients should be carefully evaluated for their ability to comprehend and perform self-care procedures, especially when EIDs are to be used. The patient should be taught how to wear the pump, how to operate and care for the equipment (pump and line as well), and what troubleshooting steps to take in case of technical problems (see Chap. 22).

References and Selected Readings

Asterisks indicate references cited in text.

Abbott, Laboratories (1999). CLC 2000 product literature.

*Beezhold, D.H., Sussman, G.L., Liss, G.M., et al. (1996). Latex allergy can induce clinical reactions to specific foods. *Clinical and Experimental Allergy, 26,* 416–422.

Blum, D.Y. (1995). Untoward events associated with use of midterm IV devices. *Journal of Intravenous Nursing, 18,* 116–119.

*Cardo, D.M., Culver, D.H., & Ciesielski, C.A. (1997). A case-control study of HIV seroconversion in health care workers after percutaneous exposures. *New England Journal Medicine, 177,* 1485–1490.

Centers for Disease Control and Prevention (1998). Guidelines for prevention of intravascular infection. Atlanta, GA: Author.

Chiarello, L.A. (1995). Selection of needlestick prevention devices: A conceptual framework for approaching product evaluation. *American Journal of Infection Control, 23,* 386–395.

ECRI (1999). Needlestick prevention devices. *Health Devices, 28* (10): 381-407.

Goetz, A.N., Miller, J., Wagener, M.M., & Muder, R.R. (1998). Complications related to intravenous midline catheter usage. *Journal of Intravenous Nursing, 21,* 76–79.

*Gritter, M. (1999). Latex allergy: Prevention is the key. *Journal of Intravenous Nursing, 22,* 281–285.

Hanchett, M., & Kung, L. (1999). Do needleless intravenous systems increase the risk of infection? *Journal of Intravenous Nursing, 22,* 117–119.

International Health Care Worker Safety Center (1997). Uniform needlestick and sharp-object injury report. *Adv Exposure Prev.,* 3 (2): 15-16.

*Intravenous Nurses Society. (1998). Revised intravenous nursing standards of practice. *Journal of Intravenous Nursing,* 21 (Suppl. 1) 41-45, 46, 50.

Intravenous Nurses Society. (2000). Draft document. Revised Standards of Practice.

*Ippolito, G., Puro, V., & Petrosillo, N. (1997). *Prevention, management and chemoprophylaxis of occupational exposure to HIV* (p. 12). Charlottesville, VA: International Health Care Worker Safety Center, University of Virginia.

Luebke, M.A., Arduino, M.J., & Duda, T.E. (1998). Comparison of microbial properties of a needleless and a conventional needle-based intravenous access system. *American Journal of Infection Control, 26,* 431–436.

*Metheny, N.M. (2000). *Fluid and electrolyte balance* (4th ed.). Philadelphia: Lippincott Williams & Wilkins.

*National Institute for Occupational Safety and Health. (1997). *NIOSH alert: Preventing allergic reactions to natural rubber latex in the workplace* (Publication 97-135). Washington, DC: Author.

National Symposium on Patient Safety (1999). Consensus Development Conference. Washington, DC.

*Occupational Safety and Health Administration. (1998). Occupational Safety and Health Administration docket no. H370A: Occupational exposure to bloodborne pathogens; request for information. *Federal Register, 63* (174), 48250–48252.

*Pugliese, G. (1999). *What is a sharps injury?* Chicago: American Hospital Publishing.

*Tereskerz, P.M., Bentley, M., Coyner, B.J., & Jagger, J. (1996). Percutaneous injuries in health care workers. *Advances in Exposure Prevention,* 2(5), 1–3.

*United States Pharmacopeia [USP]. (1999). (26th ed., pp. 803, 1027). Easton, PA: Mack Publishing.

*U.S. Food and Drug Administration. (1996). Latex-containing devices; user labeling; proposed rules. *Federal Register, 61,* 32618–32621.

U.S. Public Health Service. (1998). Guidelines for the management of healthcare worker exposures to HIV and recommendations for post-exposure prophylaxis. *Morbidity and Mortality Weekly Report Reports and Recommendations,* 47 (RR-7).

* Warshaw, E.M. (1998). Latex allergy. *Journal of the American Academy of Dermatology, 38,* 1–24.

Review Questions

Note: Questions below may have more than one right answer.

1. Which of the following factors should be considered in selecting IV equipment?

   A. Latex-free components

   B. Safety design

   C. Performance

   D. All of the above

2. The porosity rating of an inline IV filter is what size in micrometers (μm)?

   A. 0.2

   B. 0.5

   C. 1.0

   D. 1.2

3. Which of the following statements is true concerning syringe delivery of medication?

   A. Limiting feature in adult patient is volume

   B. It is a fluid container when used with a syringe-loaded EID

   C. a only

   D. a and b

4. Preferred IV drug delivery systems include which of the following?

   A. Manufacturer-prepared

   B. Point-of-care activated

   C. Pharmacy-based admixture

   D. Volume-control chambers

5. Which of the following statements is true concerning hypovolemic patients?

   A. Plasma and blood must be delivered rapidly

   B. Plasma and blood must be delivered slowly

   C. Rate of infusion decreases with increased blood pressure

   D. Rate of infusion increases with changes in blood pressure

6. An initial hydrating fluid to test kidney function is administered at 8 mL/m^2/minute over how many minutes?

   A. 10

   B. 30

C. 45

D. 60

7. Latex fluid is composed of which of the following?

A. Carbohydrates

B. Lipids and phospholipids

C. a only

D. a and b

8. Which of the following systems may reduce the incidence of needlestick injuries?

A. Needleless

B. Filters

C. Luer locks

D. Universal connectors

9. Examples of sharps involved in IV practice include which of the following?

A. Lancets

B. Needles

C. IV catheters

D. b and c

10. Type I latex reactions manifested by the respiratory system include which of the following?

A. Angioedema, respiratory arrest

B. Shortness of breath

C. Cyanosis and wheezing

D. Laryngeal edema, wheezing

Techniques of Peripheral

Intravenous Therapy

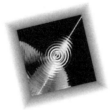

K E Y   T E R M S

Arteriospasm
Arteriovenous Fistula
Axillary Dissection
Fear Cascade

Sympathetic Reaction
Syncope
Vasovagal Reaction

■ APPROACH TO PREPARATION

How the nurse approaches the patient about to receive IV therapy may have a direct bearing on that patient's response to treatment. Because an undesirable response can affect the patient's ability to accept treatment, the nurse's manner and attitude are significant factors.

Although routine for the nurse, IV therapy may be a new and frightening experience for any patient unfamiliar with the procedure. Various factors enter into the patient's perception of IV therapy, including accounts in the mass media, rumors related to errors or fatalities, or simple miscommunications. The nurse who provides a careful explanation of the procedure does much to alleviate fear and ensure patient compliance. Considerations in preparing the patient for the procedure may be found in Box 12–1.

Clinical Conditions

The critically ill patient is particularly susceptible to fears, which can at times become exaggerated, triggering an undesirable autonomic nervous system response known

---

BOX 12–1 Considerations in Preparing the Patient for IV Therapy

---

Patient's clinical condition
Type of therapy ordered
Duration of treatment
Patient's experience level and IV history
Other treatment modalities
Vascular assessment

---

as the **vasovagal reaction,** which may manifest itself as **syncope.** In many cases, the nurse can prevent the vasovagal response and consequent syncope by appearing confident and reassuring the patient.

It is desirable to prevent syncope to avoid the **sympathetic reaction** that may follow and result in vasoconstriction. The peripheral collapse attendant to vaso-constriction then limits the supply of available veins, which complicates venipuncture. Repeated attempts at venipuncture can result in an experience so traumatic as to affect the further course of IV therapy. Only a skilled clinician should perform a venipuncture on an anxious patient who has limited access and difficult veins. (See Chaps. 21 and 22 for special considerations for special popu-lations.)

Exaggerated reactions to fear may trigger the **fear cascade** (Fig. 12–1), which not only makes therapy difficult, but may constitute a real threat to the patient, particu-larly one with severe cardiac disease.

Type of Therapy Prescribed

The type of therapy ordered often dictates the plan of care. The ambulatory surgical patient has decidedly different educational needs than the critically ill patient with multiple IV accesses. If the patient will be involved in self-care and self-administra-tion of IV medications and solutions, the approach must encourage and support the patient's independence and confidence. Plans for promoting self-care and indepen-dence should begin at the time of admission to the hospital or with the patient's first encounter with the IV service.

Duration of Therapy

A prolonged course of therapy requires multiple solutions, which makes preserva-tion of the veins essential. Performing the venipuncture distally with each subse-quent puncture proximal to the previous one and alternating arms contributes to ve-nous preservation.

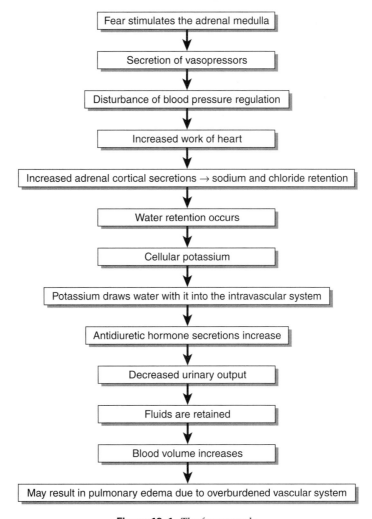

Figure 12–1. The fear cascade.

The patient's comfort also needs to be considered when solutions are required over an extended period. For instance, performing venipunctures on veins located on the dorsal surface of the extremities provides more freedom and comfort for the patient.

Patient's Experience and IV History

Prior experience with IV therapy, good or bad, affects the patient's acceptance of treatment. If venipuncture by an experienced clinician has been a positive experience for the patient, he or she may feel more comfortable and relaxed. If the patient's history includes complications associated with IV therapy, venipuncture may be difficult.

Other Treatment Modalities

Use of multiple clinical modalities (ie, nutritional support, antibiotics, and transfusions) has a significant effect on preparations for IV therapy. In such cases, the clinician may consider using a multilumen catheter so that administration of subsequent medications can be timed to avoid interference with the line providing nutrition or the line providing transfusional therapy. Other concerns include non-IV therapies. For example, if the patient is also undergoing physical or occupational therapy, the nurse may find it difficult to use the hand veins for an IV line because such placement makes maintaining secure, dry connections and a tightly sealed dressing difficult.

Vascular Assessment

Initially, the nurse makes a vascular assessment. If findings confirm that limited vascular access precludes successful venipuncture and long-term treatment, consideration should be given to the proposed course of therapy and use of alternative access devices, such as a midline or peripherally inserted central catheter (PICC). Then, after ensuring the patient's privacy and comfort, the nurse implements various procedures, including hand washing, making sure to avoid an **arteriovenous fistula** or graft inserted for dialysis (because catheterization of a graft or fistula is determined by institutional policy), and avoiding the dependent extremity of a patient who has had a mastectomy or cerebral vascular accident.

■ CONSIDERATIONS FOR VEIN SELECTION

The selection of the vein may be a deciding factor in the success of the infusion and the preservation of veins for subsequent treatment (Table 12–1). The most prominent vein is not necessarily the most suitable for venipuncture. Prominence may result from a sclerosed condition, which occludes the lumen and interferes with the flow of solution, or the prominent vein may be located in an area impractical for infusion purposes. Scrutiny of the veins in both arms is desirable before a choice is made. The prime factors to be considered in selecting a vein are

- Suitable location
- Condition of the vein
- Purpose of the infusion
- Duration of therapy

TABLE 12-1
SITE SELECTION: SUPERFICIAL VEINS OF THE ARM

Vein	Location	Device	Considerations
Cephalic	Radial aspect of lower arm along radial bone of forearm	18- to 22-gauge cannula; usually ONC	Large vein, easily accessed Start distal and work upward Good for infusing blood or chemically irritating drugs
Basilic	Ulnar aspect of lower arm along the ulnar bone	18- to 22-gauge ONC	Difficult to access Large vein, easily palpated Stabilize during venipuncture
Accessory cephalic	Branches off of cephalic vein along radial bone	18- to 22-gauge ONC	Medium–large vein, easily stabilized Valves at cephalic junction may inhibit catheterization Short length may require short (1-inch) catheter
Upper cephalic	Radial aspect of upper arm above elbow	16- to 20-gauge ONC	Difficult to visualize Good site for confused patients
Median antebrachial	Extends up front of forearm from median antecubital	18- to 22-gauge ONC	Nerve endings preclude cannulation Infiltration may occur
Median basilic	Ulnar aspect of forearm	18- to 22-gauge ONC	Appropriate site
Median cubital	Radial aspect of forearm	18- to 22-gauge ONC	Appropriate site
Antecubital fossa	Bend of elbow	Any size; may be used for midline or peripherally inserted central catheter insertion	Best for emergency interventions

ONC, over-the-needle catheter.

Location

Most superficial veins are accessible for venipuncture (Fig. 12–2), but some of these veins, because of their location, are not practical. Located over an area of joint flexion where any motion could dislodge the IV catheter and cause infiltration or result in mechanical phlebitis, the antecubital veins exemplify a poor choice for routine therapy. If these large veins are impaired or damaged, phlebothrombosis may occur, which can limit access to the many available hand veins. The antecubital veins offer excellent sources for withdrawing blood and may be used numerous times without damage to the vein, provided good technique and sharp needles are used. However, one infusion of long duration may traumatize the vein, limiting the availability of vessels that most readily provide ample quantities of blood when needed.

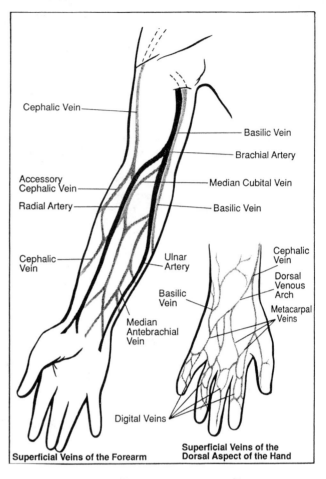

Figure 12–2. IV placement chart. (Courtesy of Becton Dickinson Vascular Access, Sandy, UT.)

Because of the proximity of the arteries to the veins in the antecubital fossa, special care must be taken to prevent intraarterial injection when medications are introduced.

Aberrant arteries in the antecubital area are present in 1 of 10 people. When a patient complains of severe pain in the hand or arm on infusion, an **arteriospasm** caused by an intra-arterial injection is to be suspected, and the infusion must be stopped immediately.

Surgery often dictates which extremity can be used. Veins should be avoided in the arm on the same side as an **axillary dissection,** as in radical mastectomy, because the circulation may be impaired, affecting the flow of the infusion and increasing edema. When the patient is turned sideways during the operation, the upper arm is used for the IV infusion; increased venous pressure in the lower arm may interfere with free flow of the solution.

Use of the veins in the lower extremities usually depends on a physician order because of the danger of pulmonary embolism caused by a thrombus extending into the deep veins. Complications may also arise from the stagnant blood in varicosities, which makes them susceptible to trauma. In addition, pooling of infused medications in stagnant blood can cause untoward reactions when drug concentrations reach toxic levels in circulating blood.

Guidelines from the Centers for Disease Control and Prevention (CDC) strongly recommend using upper extremity veins in adult patients, or if necessary, subclavian and jugular sites (CDC, 1998). Guidelines of the Intravenous Nurses Society (INS) support that premise (INS, 1998, 2000).

Condition of the Vein

Frequently, the dorsal metacarpal veins provide points of entry that should be used first to preserve the proximal veins for further therapy. The use of these veins depends on their condition. In some elderly patients, the dorsal metacarpal veins may be a poor choice; blood extravasation occurs more readily in small, thin veins, and it may be difficult adequately to secure the catheter because of thin skin and lack of supportive tissue. At times, these veins do not dilate sufficiently to allow for successful venipuncture; when hypovolemia occurs, the peripheral veins collapse more quickly than do larger, more proximal ones.

Palpation of the vein is an important step in determining the condition of the vein and in differentiating it from a pulsating artery. A thrombosed vein may be detected by its lack of resilience; its hard, cord-like feeling; and by the ease with which it rolls. Use of such traumatized veins results only in repeated attempts at venipuncture, pain, and undue stress.

Occasionally, when thrombosis from multiple infusions interferes with the flow of solution and limits available veins, the venipuncture may be performed with the catheter inserted in the direction of the distal end. Lack of valves in these small peripheral veins permits rerouting of the solution and bypassing of the involved vein.

Often, large veins may be detected by palpation and offer advantages over the smaller but more readily discernible veins. Because of the small blood volume, the more superficial veins may not be easily palpated and may not make a satisfactory choice for venipuncture.

Continual use by the nurse of the same fingers for palpation increases their sensitivity. The thumb should never be used because it is not as sensitive as the fingers; also, a pulse may be detected in the nurse's thumb, and this may be confused with an aberrant artery.

Although not apparent, edema may conceal an available vein; application of finger pressure for a few seconds may help to disperse the fluid and define the vein.

Purpose of the Infusion

The purpose of the infusion dictates the rate of flow and the solution to be infused—two factors that inherently affect the selection of the vein. When large quantities of fluid are to be rapidly infused, or when positive pressure is indicated, a large vein must be used. When fluids with a high viscosity, such as packed red blood cells, are required, a vein with an adequate volume of flow is necessary to ensure flow of the solution.

Large veins are used when hypertonic solutions or solutions containing irritating drugs are to be infused. Such solutions traumatize small veins; the supply of blood in these veins is not sufficient to dilute the infused fluid. Large vessels provide better hemodilution of the drug or solution, thereby minimizing the potential for developing phlebitis.

Selection of the Device

Many diverse infusion devices are available; particular consideration should be given to the use of safety equipment. See Chapter 11 for a discussion of safety devices for IV access.

Secure and Optimal Environment

The importance of proper lighting should not be overlooked. A few extra seconds spent in obtaining adequate light may actually save time and free the patient from unnecessary venipunctures. The ideal light is either ample daylight or a spotlight that does not shine directly on the vein but leaves enough shadow for clearly defining the vessel.

Venous Distention

Special care must be taken to distend the vein adequately. To achieve this, a soft, preferably latex-free, tourniquet is applied with enough pressure to impede venous flow while maintaining arterial flow. If the radial pulse cannot be felt, the tourniquet is too tight.

To fill the veins to capacity, pressure is applied until radial pulsation ceases and then released until pulsation begins. A blood pressure cuff may be used; inflate the cuff and then release it until the pressure drops to just below the diastolic pressure.

The tourniquet is applied to the mid-forearm if the selected vein is in the dorsum of the hand. If the selected vein is in the forearm, the tourniquet is applied to the upper arm.

Very little pressure is applied when performing venipuncture on patients with sclerosed veins. If the pressure is too great or the tourniquet is left on for an extended time, the vein becomes hard and tortuous, causing added difficulty when the catheter is introduced. For some sclerosed veins, a tourniquet is unnecessary and only makes the phlebotomy more difficult (see considerations for the geriatric patient in Chap. 22).

If pressure exerted by the tourniquet does not fill the veins sufficiently, the patient may be asked to open and close his or her fist. This action of the muscles forces the blood into the veins, causing them to distend considerably more. A light tapping usually fills the vein. It may be helpful, before applying the tourniquet, to lower the extremity below the heart level to increase the blood supply to the veins. On occasions when these methods are inadequate to fill the vein sufficiently, application of heat helps. To be effective, the heat must be applied to the entire extremity for 10 to 20 minutes and must be retained until the venipuncture is performed (see Table 12–1).

■ CONSIDERATIONS BEFORE BEGINNING THE INFUSION

Checking Solution and Container

Careful inspection must be made to ensure that the fluid is clear and free of particulates and the container intact—with no cracks in the glass bottle or holes in the plastic bag. The label must be checked to verify that the correct solution is being used and that the container is not outdated. The nurse also needs to check the time and the date of the container's opening. After 24 hours, the fluid is outdated and should not be used (see Chap. 4). Hang time is determined in institutional policy.

Attaching Administration Set to Fluid Container

The nurse attaches the IV administration set to the solution container by closing the roller clamp to equalize pressure, squeezing the drip chamber, and inserting the set into the container with a thrust, not a twisting motion. The drip chamber is released, causing the air vent to function immediately and the drip chamber to fill on suspension of the container. This prevents the fluid from leaking through the air vent and clears the infusion set of air, thereby preventing bubbles from entering the tubing. In systems that do not require air venting—plastic and semi-rigid containers—squeezing the drip chamber before insertion avoids the subsequent introduction of air into the container.

Establishing Height of the Fluid Container

The nurse suspends the fluid container approximately 3 feet above the injection site. The pressure from this height is adequate to ensure a maximum flow rate. The greater the height of the container, the greater the force with which the fluid flows into the vein should the flow-control clamp release, and the greater the risk of speed shock.

Ensuring Privacy and Comfort

The nurse may ask visitors to leave the room during the procedure and close bedside curtains if the patient has a roommate. The patient should be in a comfortable position with the arm on a flat surface. If necessary, a strip of tape can be used to secure the arm to an arm board to prevent an uncooperative or disoriented patient from jerking the arm during catheter insertion.

If the area selected for venipuncture is hairy, clipping the hair permits better cleansing of the skin and makes removal of the catheter less painful when the infusion is terminated. Shaving is not recommended, consistent with INS standards (INS, 1998, 2000). Products such as Skin-Prep decrease bacterial flora and may be considered for use before venipuncture.

Applying Anesthetic Products

Eutectic mixture of local anesthetics (EMLA; Astra Pharmaceuticals, Westborough, MA) is a cream mixture of two local anesthetics (lidocaine 2.5% and prilocaine 2.5%). If appropriate, EMLA may be applied to the skin under an occlusive dressing. The release of lidocaine and prilocaine into the epidermal and dermal layers of the skin provides anesthesia. The two agents stabilize neuronal membranes by inhibiting the conduction of impulses (Astra Pharmaceuticals, 1997). Use of the product is contraindicated in patients with a known history of sensitivity to local amide anesthetics (Procedure 12–1).

Between 1 and 2 mg of topical nitroglycerin (Nitro-Bid; Hoechst Marion Roussel, Kansas City, MO) may also be applied. Studies indicate that this product distends the veins without the need for tapping, pumping the hand, or clenching the fist. Alternatively, some professionals advocate administering intradermal lidocaine before venipuncture. This is done with 0.1 to 0.2 mL of 1% lidocaine and a tuberculin syringe. Lidocaine may, however, expose the patient to allergic reaction, anaphylaxis, inadvertent injection of the drug into the vascular system, and obliteration of the vein.

Procedure 12–1	**Applying EMLA Crème**

Equipment

    Antiseptic skin cleanser

    Sterile wipes or sponges

    EMLA cream

    Occlusive dressing

Action	*Rationale*
1. Cleanse skin with antiseptic	1. Prevents risk of infection
2. Apply 2.5 g EMLA cream thickly at intended site	2. Ensures covering entire dermal at surface
3. Place an occlusive dressing over the EMLA cream and smooth edges of the dressing. Keep dressing in place until it is time for venipuncture.	3. Ensures occlusivity
4. Record application time.	4. Ensures appropriate absorption time and documentation of procedure

■ CONSIDERATIONS FOR VENIPUNCTURE PROCEDURE

Variations in direct and indirect methods are described in Table 12–2.

The injection site should be scrubbed with an antiseptic that remains in contact with the skin for at least 30 seconds before venipuncture. Typical antiseptic preparations include tincture of iodine 1% to 2%, iodophor, or chlorhexidine. Isopropyl alcohol 70% is recommended if the patient is sensitive to iodine. If the vein has sustained a through puncture (evidenced by a developing hematoma) and the venipuncture is unsuccessful, the catheter should be immediately removed and pressure applied to the site.

 SAFE PRACTICE ALERT   Never reapply a tourniquet to the extremity immediately after a venipuncture; a hematoma will occur, limiting veins and providing an excellent culture medium for bacteria.

T A B L E   1 2 – 2
COMPARING APPROACHES TO VENIPUNCTURE

Direct (One-Step)	Indirect (Two Complete Motions)
Nurse thrusts catheter through skin and into vein with quick motion.	Nurse inserts catheter through skin below the point where vein is visible but above the vein.
Catheter enters directly over the vein.	This approach depresses the vein, obscuring its position.
Direct technique is not suitable for small veins because of potential for hematoma formation.	The catheter is adjacent to the vein but has not penetrated the vessel wall. Gently locate the vein, decrease catheter angle, and enter the vessel.

KEY INTERVENTIONS: A Step-by-Step Approach to Basic Venipuncture

1. To ensure sterility of field, wash hands and put on gloves before applying tourniquet.
2. Select appropriate site that will best enhance venous distention.
3. Prepare skin according to recommendations consistent with INS Standards of Practice.
4. Establish minimum rate of flow. To do this, adjust clamp. Then kink infusion tubing between third and fourth fingers of the dominant hand. (When the kinked tubing is released, the minimum rate of flow prevents the rapid fluid or drug infusion that has the potential to induce speed shock. (*Note: the tubing may also be kinked by placing it through the slots on the roller clamp.*)
5. Hold patient's hand or arm with other hand using your thumb to keep skin taut. This helps to anchor the vein and prevent rolling.

6. Align steel introducer needle with the vein, approximately one-half inch from entry site. Keeping the needle in bevel-up position facilitates easier venipuncture and is atraumatic. (*Note: In some cases, the bevel-down approach may be used in small veins to avoid extravasation. Then readjustment may be made before releasing the tourniquet to prevent puncturing the vein and producing a hematoma.*)
7. To ensure simultaneous entry through skin and tissue, insert the needle at a 45° angle.
8. Relocate vein and decrease angle slightly to minimize trauma.
9. Then, slowly (with a downward motion) pick up the vein. Doing this levels the introducer needle and catheter almost flush with the skin.
10. Watch for a flashback of blood, which may indicate successful entry. Also anticipate both a sense of increased resistance when the catheter meets the wall of the vein and a "snap" felt at the loss of resistance as the catheter enters the vein.
11. Release tourniquet, remove introducer needle, and activate the needleless cover (see Chap. 11 for information concerning safety devices). The catheter may then be advanced manually or with *infusing* fluid.
12. Release pressure exerted by little finger (Step 4).
13. Connect administration set to hub and release kinked tubing to initiate flow.
14. Check injection site for swelling.

Anchoring the Device

Once the catheter is in place, the nurse needs to make sure it stays securely in place and safe from dislodgment. This involves a special taping technique.

Taping

Using half-inch–wide tape over the hub of the catheter, the nurse anchors the device flush with the skin. No elevation of the hub is necessary because this would only increase the risk of puncturing through the vein (known as a through puncture) with the point of the introducer needle.

After placing a half-inch strip of tape—adhesive up—under the hub of the catheter, the nurse folds one end of the strip tightly and diagonally over the catheter and repeats the motion with the other end crossing the first end. This secures the catheter firmly and prevents any sideways movement. Tape should not be placed directly over the actual injection site.

Looping the Tubing

After the device is secured by tape, the IV tubing is looped to relieve tension and secured with tape independent of the catheter tape. This prevents dislodging the catheter by an accidental pull on the tubing.

Dressing and Documenting

An occlusive dressing is applied over the catheter entrance site to allow for routine, standardized inspection. The type, gauge, insertion date, and nurse's initials are written on tape near the dressing and documented in the clinical record. Variations in taping are shown in Figure 12–3.

Other Securement Devices

Other securement devices may also be used. Dyna-Lok consists of a specially designed, latex-free, foam anchor pad with 3M (Minneapolis, MN) adhesive. The anchor pad, along with two additional anchor strips made of the same material, neatly secures the IV tubing and catheter in place. Dyna-Lok is a securement and dressing product. ConMed's (Utica, NY) Veni-Gard is a stabilization dressing available in various configurations for use with peripheral lines, multilumen catheters, and long-term vascular access devices (Figs. 12–4 and 12–5).

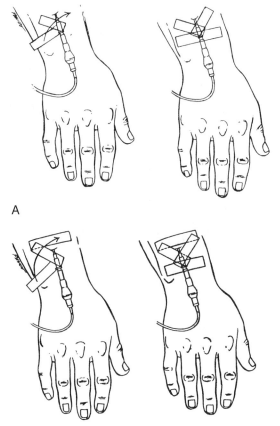

A

B

Figure 12–3. Variations in taping. (A) Chevron taping technique. (B) Taping variations for over-the-needle catheters.

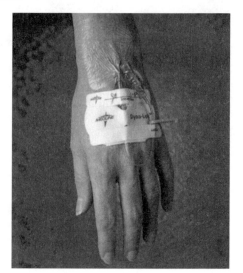

Figure 12–4. The Dyna-Lok IV securement device is a latex-free foam anchor pad that keeps the IV tubing and catheter safely in place. (Courtesy of Medline Industries, Inc., Mundelein, IL)

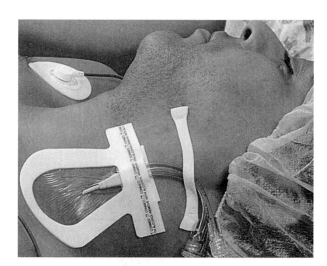

Figure 12–5. The Veni-Gard IV stabilization dressing (ConMed, Utica, NY) reduces complications related to movement and other problems and maximizes patient freedom.

Arm Boards

An arm board may be helpful for immobilizing the extremity when undue motion can result in infiltration or phlebitis. It is a valuable aid in restraining the arm when infusions are initiated on uncooperative, disoriented, or elderly patients or children, or when the catheter is inserted on the dorsum of the hand or in an area of joint flexion.

When the metacarpal veins are used, the fingers should be immobilized to prevent any movement of the catheter that could result in phlebitis. This complication results from failure to recognize that the hand has both transverse and longitudinal arches and that if the knuckle joints (metacarpophalangeal) are immobilized in a straight position, they develop motion-preventing contracture. Patients who are receiving long-term therapy and who have edema or muscular weakness are particularly vulnerable. Intensive physical therapy, splinting, and even surgery may be required to restore mobility.

To preserve maximal function, the hand should be immobilized in a functional position on the arm board. If a plastic arm board is used, the nurse can cover it with absorbent paper or a bandage to prevent the arm from perspiring and sticking to the board. Any tape placed on the catheter must be independent of the board so that a motion of the arm on the board does not cause a pull on the catheter. If the arm must be restrained, the restraint is secured to the board, not to the patient's arm above the puncture area. Such restraint might act as a tourniquet, causing a backflow of blood into the catheter and resulting in clotting and obstruction of the flow. Arm board design has changed dramatically, and many man-ufacturers now provide sophisticated devices aimed at ensuring patient comfort.

 SAFE PRACTICE ALERT The function of the hand may be endangered and even permanently impaired by the widespread practice of flattening the hand on an arm board during infusion therapy.

Dressings

Consistent with INS Standards of Practice, an occlusive dressing should be applied over the infusion site. The occlusive dressing may be gauze or tape, or a transparent, semipermeable membrane dressing.

The following procedure is applicable to the Tegaderm pouch dressings manufactured by 3M Healthcare (Fig. 12–6). The professional is encouraged to follow the manufacturer's recommendations for the use of a specific product.

Infusion sites should be labeled with type of catheter (Fig. 12–7), length and size, date, time, and initials of the person who initiated the infusion. Many labels are available to facilitate this practice (Fig. 12–8).

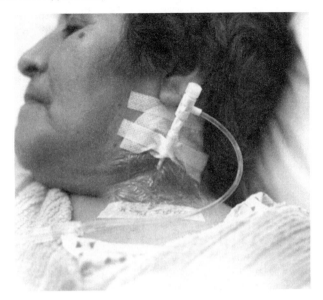

Figure 12–6. Using a dressing such as the Tegaderm IV transparent dressing allows the IV nurse to see the injection site without removing the dressing. (Courtesy of 3M Minneapolis, MN.)

■ OTHER INSERTION TECHNIQUES

Whether performing a basic IV insertion procedure or varying the procedure in accord with the patient's condition or equipment available, the IV nurse's competence in performing peripheral IV therapy should be assessed periodically. Of course, the competent IV nursing professional should be able successfully to perform the procedure using aseptic technique. Other competence criteria are summarized in Figure 12–9.

Variations in insertion techniques are common, and although they may depend on devices available (catheter products are covered completely in Chap. 11), this section addresses some products with regard to actual insertion technique.

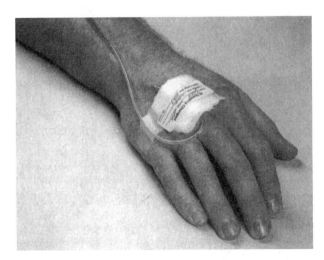

Figure 12–7. Labeling of the venipuncture site consistent with INS standards. (Courtesy of United Ad Label Co., Inc., Brea, CA.)

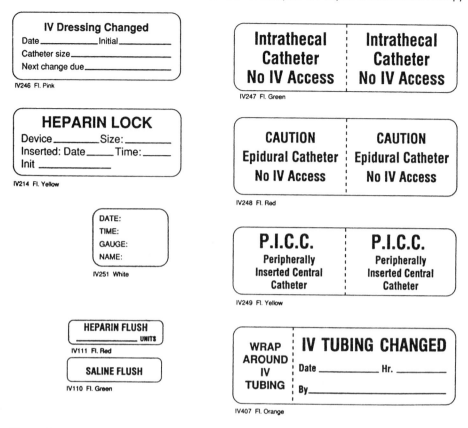

Figure 12–8.   Variety of labels used to identify catheter sites, types, dressings, and other products and procedures.

Insertion of the Through-the-Needle/Inside-the-Needle Catheter

The through-the-needle or inside-the-needle catheter (TNC/INC) is seldom used today because of the inherent danger of infection from bacteria invading the vein through the cutaneous opening or along the plastic catheter. Trauma caused by insertion of a large catheter increases when the procedure is performed by an inexperienced clinician.

Another drawback to the TNC/INC is the potential for severance by the cutting edge of the needle. This can result in a serious complication when the catheter is lost in the bloodstream. Moreover, a TNC/INC introduced into a vein over a joint flexion area increases the risk of complication if the extremity is not immobilized.

A TNC/INC facilitates prolonged therapy but increases the risk of thrombophlebitis. Limiting the time the catheter is used reduces the incidence of phlebitis, although a time limit may be difficult to enforce because veins may be exhausted in a critically ill patient whose life depends on infusion therapy. A new generation of TNC/INC uses a peel-away design (see the discussion on PICC placement, later).

Describe relevant anatomy/physiology	Meets expectations	Needs education
Skin	☐	☐
Layers of vein	☐	☐
Venous and arterial system	☐	☐
Determine appropriate placement of device		
Length and duration of therapy	☐	☐
Age and clinical condition	☐	☐
Verbalizes factors influencing selection	☐	☐
Verifies physician order		
Type, rate, volume to be delivered	☐	☐
Isotonic, hypertonic, hypotonic	☐	☐
Rate and volume	☐	☐
Inspects integrity of equipment		
Fluid container	☐	☐
Administration set	☐	☐
Infusion device, accessories	☐	☐
Performs successful venipuncture (initial attempt)		
One attempt per device (success rate >85%)	☐	☐
Implements Standards of Practice		
Occlusive dressing application	☐	☐
Ongoing monitoring	☐	☐
Site rotation	☐	☐
Set changes	☐	☐

Figure 12–9. Performance checklist for IV therapy.

Insertion of the Over-the-Needle Catheter

To insert the over-the-needle catheter, the nurse puts on gloves, applies a tourniquet above the injection site, selects the vein, and prepares the injection site according to authorized recommendations. If palpation of the vein is necessary, the nurse prepares the fingertip in the same manner. Without touching the proposed insertion site, the nurse performs the venipuncture in the usual manner and proceeds as follows:

1. Once the needle has punctured the venous wall, introduce the needle one-half inch farther to ensure entry of the catheter into the lumen of the vein.
2. Hold the needle in place and slowly slide the catheter hub until the desired length is in the vein. If the venipuncture is unsuccessful, do not reinsert the needle into the catheter. To do so can sever the catheter.
3. Remove the needle by holding the catheter hub in place. To minimize leakage of blood while removing the needle and connecting the infusion set, apply pressure on the vein beyond the catheter with the little finger.
4. Attach the IV administration set, which has been previously cleared of air, and regulate the flow rate.
5. Consider applying a topical antiseptic iodophor ointment, or a broad-spectrum antiseptic ointment for patients sensitive to iodine.
6. Tape the catheter securely to prevent motion that could contribute to phlebitis. However, avoid taping over injection site. Then cover the site with a sterile gauze sponge or transparent, semipermeable dressing.
7. Loop the tubing and tape independent of the catheter to prevent an accidental pull from withdrawing the catheter.

8. Initial the tape close to the dressing and indicate the length, gauge, and type of catheter and the date of insertion. Document the procedure in the clinical record.
9. Remove gloves and wash hands.

Insertion of the Midline Catheter

The midline catheter is designed for peripheral infusion of general IV solutions and medications and for venous sampling. Indications for midline IV therapy include administration of antibiotics, hydration, pain medication, peripheral nutrition solutions of 12.5% or less final glucose concentration, and selected antineoplastic agents (excluding vesicants, which the Oncology Nursing Society recommends be infused through a central line).

The procedure should be performed only by experienced nurses with excellent IV insertion skills, and then only after careful consideration of the possible risks, including thrombosis, phlebitis, air embolism, infection, vascular perforation, bleeding, and catheter transection (see Chap. 11).

As with any venipuncture, adequate assessment of the patient and the venous status is essential to ensure success. The basilic vein is the vein of choice for longer-line IV insertions because of its larger size, straighter course, and adequate hemodilution capability.

Before insertion, the clinician should carefully select the vessel site and aseptically prepare it consistent with institutional policy and recommended INS Standards of Practice, then establish a sterile field and apply gloves. Again, the technique is specific to the manufacturer's recommendations for the use of its product. A general procedure for insertion may be found in the accompanying Key Intervention display.

KEY INTERVENTIONS: Inserting a Midline Catheter

1. Gather equipment, ensure the patient's comfort, and explain the procedure to put the patient at ease.
2. Extend the patient's arm and support it with a rolled towel so that the arm is abducted at a 45-degree angle.
3. Prepare the work area and position a protective covering under the patient's arm to protect the patient's environment from blood or leakage.
4. Apply tourniquet to mid to upper arm for final assessment to ensure appropriate site selection; then remove tourniquet.
5. Wash hands and put on sterile gloves. Prepare skin and remove hair from the insertion site in accord with INS Standards of Practice. Then discard gloves.
6. Apply tourniquet and put on a second pair of gloves.
7. Use fenestrated drape to create a sterile field.
8. Complete venipuncture, inserting catheter in accord with the manufacturer's instructions.
9. Slowly advance the catheter to the desired length. If resistance is met, stop and reposition the arm, rotate the wrist, or ask the patient to open and close the fist. If resistance continues, discontinue catheter insertion.
10. Aspirate for blood return to confirm patency.
11. Remove guidewire slowly, gently retracting while stabilizing the device at the insertion site.

Note: Some manufacturers suggest immobilizing the arm for 30 minutes to allow catheter material to soften and minimize venous irritation.

Peripherally Inserted Central Catheter Placement

The INS has developed an extensive PICC Education Module for use by nurse instructors. The module contains a narrative outline and 179 slides to ensure consistency in the content of PICC presentations. The information in the module is based on INS Standards of Practice. Sample pre- and post-tests with answer sheets, a PICC insertion data collection form, competency/skills checklist, and a student syllabus are included.

The PICC should be placed by nurses with advanced IV therapy skills; the exception is in those states in which the Nurse Practice Act prohibits nurses from placing PICC lines. Insertion depends on the type of product used (see Chap. 11). Placement may be made through a breakaway needle or catheter with or without a guidewire. With this configuration, the catheter is advanced through a splittable needle. After placement is achieved, the needle is split and peeled from around the catheter. The catheter design uses an over-the-needle catheter as the introducer. The needle is removed, leaving the catheter in place, and the catheter is threaded through the plastic introducer.

A guidewire may be included to add firmness to the silicone catheter, requiring venous access to be established with a needle. Commonly known as the Seldinger technique, the guidewire is threaded through the needle, the needle is removed, and the catheter is threaded over the guidewire.

Placement of the PICC is specific to the type of product used and the manufacturer's instructions for use. A general procedural outline is given in Procedure 12–2.

Procedure 12–2	**Insertion of Nontunneled, Noncuffed Catheters: PICC**

Equipment

Mask and gown	Sterile towels
Several pairs of nonpowdered, sterile gloves	Sterile fenestrated drapes
Tourniquet	PICC insertion set
Sterile tape	Scissors for clipping body hair
Sutures	0.9% Sterile sodium chloride solution
Sterile gauze pads	Sterile heparinized saline solution
Sterile cleaning solution	Prepared IV catheter (administration set)

Action	*Rationale/Outcome*
1. Place patient in dorsal recumbent position; complete assessment.	1. Ensures comfort and safety
2. Wash hands and don mask, prepare work area.	2. Ensures integrity of area and/or procedure

Action	*Rationale/Outcome*
3. Apply tourniquet to mid to upper arm	3. Facilitates final venous assessment
4. Measure arm with sterile tape. Measure antecubital insertion site up arm to and across shoulder; continue to sternal notch and down to third intercostal space.	4. Ensures accurate length for superior vena cava placement
5. Select vein and release tourniquet; then clip hair per institutional procedure.	5. Promotes venous distention and selection and helps to prevent infection and discomfort when catheter is withdrawn
6. To avoid airborne contamination, apply nonpowdered sterile gloves; prepare skin in usual manner, then remove and discard gloves.	6. Ensures integrity and safety of the procedure
7. Apply tourniquet and don second pair of gloves.	7. Same as above
8. Drape arm with sterile towels.	8. Maintains sterile field
9. Perform venipuncture using shallow, 15- to 30-degree angle while applying reverse traction with other hand.	9. Stabilizes vein
10. After venipuncture is achieved, lower introducer angle, pull back stylet, and slowly advance introducer.	10. Secures placement within lumen of vein
11. Remove stylet and slowly advance catheter.	11. Prevents damage to the vein
12. Release tourniquet and, using smooth pick-up, continue to advance catheter over 5 to 10 inches through the introducer.	12. Promotes advancement of the catheter
13. When halfway done, ask patient to turn head toward insertion site with chin downward on the clavicle. Remove introducer and slowly advance remaining catheter to predetermined length.	13. Ensures catheter entry
14. Gently remove guidewire from	14. Prevents damage to catheter catheter.

Action	Rationale/Outcome
15. Attach prepared infusion line.	15. Facilitates infusion
16. Aspirate line using 0.9% sodium chloride solution to check for blood return; assess type of flow, color, consistency, pulsation.	16. Verifies placement of line and integrity of blood return
17. Flush line vigorously with remaining sodium chloride solution followed by heparinized saline solution.	17. Ensures patency of the line by preventing clotting
18. Tape or suture line in place. Apply occlusive dressing and document the procedure.	18. Secures catheter and ensures securement
19. Before initiating therapy, radiographically confirm that catheter tip is located within the vena cava.	19. Ensures appropriate placement

Hypodermoclysis

Although it is rarely used, the IV nursing professional should be familiar with the term *hypodermoclysis* and its clinical applications. When performing a hypodermoclysis, the subcutaneous route is used as a vehicle for absorption of IV isotonic hydration fluids, usually lactated Ringer's solution. One-half ampule of Wydase is added to each 500 mL of IV solution to enhance absorption of the solution within the subcutaneous tissue.

A clysis needle, resembling the standard winged infusion needle, is entered into the lateral aspect of the patient's thigh and the infusion is initiated. Standard skin preparation consistent with INS Standards of Practice should be followed before the procedure and for removal of the needles at the completion of the clysis. Some manufacturers provide therapy-specific clysis administration sets. In lieu of such a set, a standardized 78-inch administration set may be used.

Phlebotomy

The professional IV nurse performs phlebotomy in many institutions. The phlebotomy, a bleeding of between 400 and 500 mL blood, is performed for transfusion purposes, as well as therapeutically for acute pulmonary congestion, polycythemia vera, hemochromatosis, and porphyria cutanea tarda.

Phlebotomy for Transfusion Purposes

Routine Donation

When phlebotomy is performed for routine bank blood, donor selection is based on the medical history and the physical examination (weight, temperature, pulse, blood pressure, and hemoglobin). The procedure is performed according to the standards of the American Association of Blood Banks (AABB) (AABB, 1999).

Autotransfusion

Autotransfusion is used to return the patient's own blood to the circulation. The phlebotomy may be performed either by blood bank procedure or non–blood bank procedure.

When the phlebotomy is performed in the blood bank, the usual blood bank procedure is followed. The blood can be stored at 4°C or the red blood cells can be frozen.

When the bleeding is performed outside the blood bank, the same technique (according to the standards of the AABB) is used. However, the donor criteria can be modified. For example, people with a history of cancer cannot make a routine donation but may donate for themselves. Blood, which is suitable only for the donor, must be labeled with the donor's name and hospital number or Social Security number. The donated blood is then segregated from other donor bloods. The ABO type is confirmed just before transfusion.

An important fact to bear in mind is the possibility of sepsis; clinically undetected bacteremia may exist in the patient with a catheter, a tracheostomy, or a disease process.

Phlebotomy for Therapeutic Purposes

The therapeutic phlebotomy is performed to remove blood from and promote the health of the donor. The practice requires a written order by the physician specifying the date, the amount of blood to be drawn, the frequency for performing the procedure, and the hemoglobin or hematocrit value at which the patient's blood should be drawn. If the patient's physician approves and if the label conspicuously indicates the patient's diagnosis and that the blood was drawn therapeutically, the blood may be used for transfusion (see Chap. 17).

Relief of Acute Pulmonary Congestion

An inpatient phlebotomy may be performed to reduce venous pressure and relieve the workload on the heart of a patient with acute pulmonary edema resulting from cardiac failure or overtransfusion. Overtransfusion is much less likely to occur today because central venous pressure monitoring provides a valuable guide for fluid administration. Also, effective drugs are available to increase cardiac output and lower the central venous pressure.

Polycythemia Vera

Although it can be an inpatient or outpatient procedure, a therapeutic phlebotomy for polycythemia vera is most frequently performed on a hospitalized patient in an effort to obtain a remission of the disease, which is characterized by a striking increase in the number of circulating red blood cells. Either alone or in combination with radioactive phosphorus (^{32}P), phlebotomy reduces the red blood cell mass, lowers the blood volume, reduces blood viscosity, and improves circulatory efficiency. The number of and interval between phlebotomies should be specified by the physician and the hematocrit value determined after the blood donation.

SAFE PRACTICE ALERT   Because the patient with acute pulmonary congestion is critically ill, the phlebotomy should probably be done by or in the presence of the patient's physician.

Hemochromatosis

Excessive body stores of iron characterize hemochromatosis. The phlebotomy is usually an outpatient procedure performed to reduce the total body iron concentration. Because patients with hemochromatosis usually have a hematocrit value in the normal range, periodic checks on the hematocrit value are desirable.

Porphyria Cutanea Tarda

How outpatient phlebotomy acts to relieve the skin lesions of porphyria cutanea tarda is not clear. These patients may have a normal hematocrit reading; thus, they are likely to undergo phlebotomy too often.

Donor Phlebotomy Procedure

To allay apprehension and avoid a vasovagal reaction, the nurse should explain the procedure and reassure the patient before proceeding as follows.

Patient Preparation

1. Identify the patient. Match the donor with the record and the order for the phlebotomy.
2. Make sure that identically numbered labels are applied to the donor record, the blood collection container, and the test tubes for donor blood samples. In addition, make sure that the processing tubes are correctly numbered and kept with the container during the blood collection. Consult institutional policy for prep solutions.
3. Prepare the donor's arm to provide an aseptic site for venipuncture. This protects both the blood donor and the blood recipient. In preparing the area, always start at the venipuncture site and move outward in concentric spirals for at least $1\frac{1}{2}$ inches. Use only sterile materials and instruments.
4. Put on gloves. Then, using a 15% aqueous (not alcoholic) soap or detergent solution, scrub the donor's arm vigorously for at least 30 seconds with gauze or 60 seconds with cotton balls.
5. Apply 10% acetone in 70% isopropyl alcohol to remove the soap. Let the site dry.
6. Apply tincture of iodine (3% in 70% ethyl alcohol) to the site and allow it to dry.
7. Use 10% acetone in 70% isopropyl alcohol to remove the iodine; again allow the site to dry.
8. Place dry sterile gauze over the site until ready to perform the venipuncture.

 SAFE PRACTICE ALERT   Verifying the patient's identity is a safety imperative.

An alternative procedure is as follows:

1. Put on gloves
2. Use 0.7% aqueous scrub solution of iodophor compound (povidone–iodine or poloxamer–iodine complex). Scrub the area for 30 seconds. Remove the foam; it is not necessary to dry the arm.
3. Prepare the site with iodophor complex solution (eg, 10% povidone–iodine); allow to stand 30 seconds. The solution need not be removed.
4. Place a dry, sterile gauze sponge over the site until ready to perform the venipuncture. Do not repalpate vein.

Collection of Blood

The following procedure for collecting blood using a plastic bag is reproduced from the AABB's *Technical Manual* (AABB, 1999). This procedure may be modified when the blood is to be discarded.

1. Inspect bag for any defects. Apply pressure to check for leaks. The anticoagulant solution must be clear.
2. Position bag carefully, making sure it is below the level of the donor's arm.
   - If a balance system is used, ensure counterbalance is level and adjusted for the amount of blood to be drawn. Unless metal clips and a hand sealer are used, make a very loose overhand knot in tubing. Hang the bag and route tubing through the pinch clamp.
   - If balance system is not used, be sure there is some way to monitor the volume of blood drawn.
   - If vacuum-assist device is used, follow the manufacturer's instructions.
3. Reapply tourniquet or blood pressure cuff. Have donor open and close hand until previously selected vein is again prominent.
4. Uncover sterile needle and do venipuncture immediately. A clean, skillful venipuncture is essential for collection of a full, clot-free unit. Tape the tubing to hold needle in place and cover site with sterile gauze.
5. Open the temporary closure between the interior of bag and tubing, if present.
6. Have donor open and close hand, squeezing a rubber ball or other resilient object slowly every 10 to 12 seconds during collection. Keep donor under observation throughout phlebotomy. The donor should never be left unattended during or immediately after donation.
7. Mix blood and anticoagulant gently and periodically (approximately every 30 seconds) during collection. Mixing may be done by hand, by placing bag on a mechanical agitator, or by using a rocking vacuum-assist device.
8. Ensure blood flow remains fairly brisk, so that coagulation activity is not triggered. Rigid time limits are not warranted if there is continuous agitation, although units requiring more than 8 minutes to draw may not be suitable for preparation of platelet concentrates, fresh frozen plasma, or cryoprecipitate.
9. Monitor volume of blood being drawn. If a balance or vacuum-assist device is used, blood flow stops after the proper amount has been collected. One milliliter of blood weighs 1.053 g, the minimum allowable specific gravity for female donors. A convenient figure to use is 1.06 g; a unit containing 405 to 495 mL should weigh 425 to 520 g plus the weight of the container with its anticoagulant.

10. Clamp tubing temporarily using a hemostat. Collect blood-processing sample by a method that precludes contamination of the donor unit. This may be accomplished in several ways:
    - If the blood collection bag contains an in-line needle, make an additional seal with hemostat, metal clip, hand sealer, or tight knot made from a previously prepared loose knot just distal to the in-line needle. Open the connector by separating needles. Insert proximal needle into processing test tube, remove hemostat, allow tube to fill, and reclamp tubing. Carefully reattach slide connector. Donor needle is now ready for removal.
    - If the blood collection bag contains an in-line processing tube, ensure that the processing tube, or pouch, is full when the collection is complete and the original clamp is placed near the donor needle. The entire assembly may now be removed from donor.
    - If a straight-tubing assembly set is used, there are two alternative procedures. In the first method, remove the needle from donor's arm as soon as tubing is clamped. Take bag and assembly to the sealer area or collect the processing tube at the donor chair by placing a hemostat close to where donor tubing enters the bag, leaving the tubing full of blood. Remove clamp next to donor needle, empty contents of donor tubing into processing test tube, reapply clamp or permanently seal next to donor needle, remove hemostat next to donor bag, and allow donor tubing to refill with blood, well mixed, from donor bag.

        In the second method, place two hemostats or temporary seals on tubing. Cut tubing between the seals, put the cut end of tubing into the processing test tube, remove proximal hemostat, allow tube to fill, and reclamp tubing.
11. Deflate and remove tourniquet. Remove needle from arm. Apply pressure over gauze and have donor raise arm (elbow straight) and hold gauze firmly over phlebotomy site with the other hand.
12. Discard needle assembly into rigid container designed to prevent accidental injury to and contamination of personnel.
13. Strip donor tubing as completely as possible into the bag, starting at seal. Work quickly to avoid allowing the blood to clot in the tubing. Invert bag several times to mix thoroughly, then allow tubing to refill with anticoagulated blood from the bag. Repeat this procedure once.
14. Seal the tubing left attached to the bags into segments on which the segment number is clearly and completely readable. Knots, metal clips, or a dielectric sealer may be used to make segments suitable for cross-matching. It must be possible to separate segments from the container without breaking sterility of the container.
15. Reinspect container for defects.
16. Recheck numbers on container, processing tubes, and donation record. Be sure the expiration date of the unit is on the container label.
17. Place blood at appropriate temperature. Unless platelets are to be removed, whole blood should be placed at 1°C to 6°C immediately after collection. If platelets are to be harvested, blood should not be chilled but should be maintained at room temperature (approximately 20°C to 24°C) until platelets are separated. Platelets should be separated within 6 hours after collection of the unit of whole blood.

Treatment of Adverse Donor Reactions

Stop the phlebotomy at the first sign of reaction and call the physician. If the donor faints:

- Elevate the donor's feet above head level.
- Loosen tight clothing.
- Ascertain that the donor has an adequate airway.
- Apply cold compresses to forehead and back of neck.
- Check and record blood pressure, pulse, and respiration periodically.

If the donor experiences nausea and vomiting, instruct the donor to breathe slowly. If the patient exhibits muscular twitching or tetanic spasms of hands or face, assist him or her to rebreathe into a paper bag. Do not give oxygen.

If the donor has convulsions (rare), call for assistance. Then, prevent injury by turning the donor on the left side. For more serious reactions or if the donor does not respond, call for medical assistance.

Record the nature and treatment of all reactions on the donor's record; include opinion as to the future use of the donor for blood donations.

KEY INTERVENTIONS: Suggested Therapeutic Phlebotomy Procedure

---

In therapeutic phlebotomies, collected blood must be discarded. The procedure itself is not adequate for recipient protection. Equipment needed includes a phlebotomy pack, a counterbalance stand or small spring scale, blood pressure cuff or tourniquet, tincture of iodine (3% in 70% ethyl alcohol) or iodophor complex solution (10% povidone–iodine), 10% acetone in 70% isopropyl alcohol for use with tincture of iodine, and sterile sponges. The nurse then proceeds as follows:

1. Put on gloves.
2. Select the most suitable vein. Apply a tourniquet or a blood pressure cuff inflated to 50 to 60 mm Hg. Have the patient open and close his or her fist to make the vein more prominent, if necessary. Remove the tourniquet.
3. Prepare the venipuncture site with cleansing solution applied to sterile gauze sponges. Always start at the puncture site and move out in concentric spirals for 1}12} inches.
4. Apply tincture of iodine; allow to dry. Question patient before applying; some patients may be allergic to iodine.
5. Apply 10% acetone in 70% isopropyl alcohol to remove iodine. Allow to dry. Iodophor complex (10% povidone–iodine) may be substituted for iodine. It does not cause skin reactions even in iodine-sensitive people. Do not wash off iodophor complex. Cover the site with dry, sterile gauze to prevent contamination until the phlebotomy is begun.
6. Begin blood collection by suspending bag from donor scale as far below donor's arm as possible.
7. If counterbalance scales are used, adjust the balance for amount of blood to be drawn.
8. Make loose overhand knot in donor tube near needle.
9. Apply tourniquet (do not impair arterial circulation).
10. Do not touch or repalpate vein.
11. Perform phlebotomy.
12. Tape needle in place and cover with sterile sponge.
13. Pinch bead into bag from junction of donor tube and bag to open lumen and allow blood to flow.
14. Instruct patient to open and close fist slowly.
15. Collect blood until bag falls on scale. If spring scales are used, collect until prescribed amount has been withdrawn.

16. Pull knot tight.
17. Release tourniquet, withdraw needle, and apply pressure with gauze pad until bleeding has stopped. Do not flex arm. The arm may be elevated while applying pressure.
18. Dispose of blood and equipment as directed by hospital procedure.
19. Record procedure in clinical record.

Techniques associated with intravenous therapy remain consistent throughout the clinical settings in which care is delivered. Adherence to institutional guidelines and Standards of Practice ensures good-quality outcomes.

Research Issues: ADVANTAGES OF SECUREMENT DEVICES

 Sheppard, K., LeDesma, M., Morris, N., O'Connor, K. (1999). A prospective study of two intravenous catheter securement techniques in a skilled nursing facility. *Journal of Intravenous Nursing, 22*(3), 151–153. In this prospective, controlled study in a skilled nursing facility, the authors determined IV dwell times and outcomes associated with a securement device. The device resulted in significantly longer average catheter dwell times (3.95 days vs 2.45 days), and significantly fewer local complications (65 vs 155). The securement device also reduced clinical time in managing vascular access by 13.5 minutes.

References and Selected Readings

Asterisks indicate references cited in text.

*American Association of Blood Banks. (1999). *Technical manual* (13th ed., pp. 378, 456–458). Arlington, VA: Author.

*Astra Pharmaceuticals. (1997). Product literature. Westborough, MA: Author.

Banks, N. (1999). Positive outcome after looped peripherally inserted central catheter malposition. *Journal of Intravenous Nursing, 22*(1), 14–18.

*Centers for Disease Control and Prevention. (1998). *Guidelines for prevention of intravascular infection.* Atlanta, GA: Author.

ConMed. (1999). Product literature. Utica, NY: Author.

*Intravenous Nurses Society. (1998). Revised intravenous nursing standards of practice. *Journal of Intravenous Nursing, 21*(Suppl. 1), S53–58

Intravenous Nurses Society. (2000). Draft revised Standards of Practice.

Mazzola, J.R., Schott-Baer, D., & Addy, L. (1999). Clinical factors associated with the development of phlebitis after insertion of a peripherally inserted central catheter. *Journal of Intravenous Nursing, 22*(1), 36–39.

Medline Industries, Inc. (1999). Product literature. Mundelein, IL: Author.

Metheny, N.M. (2000). *Fluid and electrolyte balance* (4th ed.). Philadelphia: Lippincott Williams & Wilkins.

Sheppard K., Ledesma, M., Morris, N., & O'Connor, K. (1999). A prospective study of two intravenous catheter securement techniques in a skilled nursing facility. *Journal of Intravenous Nursing, 22*(3), 151–153.

3M Corporation. (1999). Product literature. Minneapolis, MN.

Review Questions

Note: Questions below may have more than one right answer.

1. The term *vasovagal reaction* refers to an autonomic nervous system response to:

   A. Stress

   B. Fluid resuscitation

   C. Sudden hydration

   D. Circulatory overload

2. Appropriate actions for the nurse to take if a patient's veins do not become prominent after application of a tourniquet include all of the following *except:*

   A. Asking the patient to pump his or her hand

   B. Placing the extremity in a dependent position

C. Tapping the vein gently

D. Tightening the tourniquet to restrict arterial flow

3. Which of the following catheter materials is associated with the greatest incidence of thrombosis?

A. Elastomeric hydrogel

B. Polyvinyl chloride

C. Silastic

D. Teflon

4. Which of the following veins should be assessed first to preserve veins for future use?

A. Dorsal metacarpal

B. Cephalic

C. Basilic

D. Digital

5. The dorsal metacarpal veins may be a poor choice in which of the following patients?

A. Elderly

B. Home care

C. Diabetic

D. Renal patient

6. A thrombosed vein may be detected by which of the following factors:

A. Resilience

B. Soft, pliable feel

C. Cord-like feel

D. Lack of resilience

7. Application of digital pressure applied to disperse fluid denotes presence of which of the following?

A. Circulatory collapse

B. Edema

C. Hypertension

D. All of the above

8. EMLA cream is a mixture of which of the following anesthetic agents?

A. Lidocaine, Novocain, and prilocaine

B. Novocain and lidocaine

C. Prilocaine and Novocain

D. Lidocaine and prilocaine

9. Before venipuncture, the injection site should be scrubbed with an antiseptic that is allowed to remain in contact with the skin for:

A. 15 seconds

B. 30 seconds

C. 45 seconds

D. 60 seconds

10. Dislodging of the catheter by an accidental pull may be accomplished by which of the following procedures?

A. Looping the tubing

B. Taping catheter flush with the skin

C. Placing tape over the injection site

D. All of the above

Central Venous

Catheterization

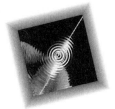

K E Y T E R M S

Axillary Vein
Basilic Vein
Cephalic Vein
Central Line
Central Venous Catheter
Central Venous Pressure
External Jugular Vein
Innominate Vein

Internal Jugular Vein
Ipsilateral
Subclavian Vein
Superior Vena Cava
Tip Placement
Valsalva Maneuver
Vascular Access Device

■ VASCULAR STRUCTURES USED IN CENTRAL VENOUS CATHETERIZATION

A **central venous catheter** is commonly referred to as a **central line,** the line being the device threaded into the central vasculature (Jensen, 1995). Advantages of central venous catheterization include placement, usually by percutaneous puncture, lower risk of infection, and catheter **tip placement** in the superior vena cava (Box 13–1). Catheter tip placement in the superior vena cava allows for rapid dilution of the infusate, thereby reducing the risk of phlebitis and venous sclerosis. It also facilitates **central venous pressure** (CVP) monitoring.

A review of both the vascular system and assessment criteria is essential for providing care to the patient with a central venous catheter. Vessels involved include the cephalic, basilic, axillary, jugular, subclavian, and innominate veins as well as the superior vena cava (Figs. 13–1 and 13–2 and Box 13–2).

> **BOX 13–1 Indications for Central Venous Placement**
>
> - Surgery, when there is a risk of overloading an anesthetized, traumatized patient who is continuously losing blood
> - Shock, when origin is unknown
> - Massive fluid replacement in open heart surgery and in critical cases, such as severely burned patients, in whom circulatory overload is a hazard
> - Anuria or oliguria, when questionable cause is dehydration

Cephalic Vein

The **cephalic vein** ascends along the outer border of the biceps muscle to the upper third of the arm. It passes in the space between the pectoralis major and deltoid muscles. It terminates in the axillary vein, with a descending curve, just below the clavicle. The cephalic vein is occasionally connected with the external jugular or subclavian vein by a branch that passes from it upward in front of the clavicle.

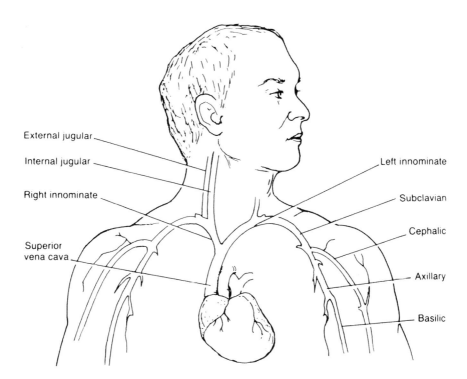

Figure 13–1. Central venous catheters are inserted through the subclavian and internal or external jugular veins.

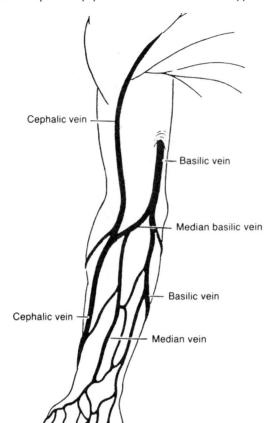

Figure 13–2. The cephalic and basilic veins are used for peripheral insertion of central venous catheters.

Basilic Vein

The **basilic vein** is larger than the cephalic. It passes upward in a smooth path along the inner side of the biceps muscle and terminates in the axillary vein.

Axillary Vein

The **axillary vein** starts upward as a continuation of the basilic vein, increasing in size as it ascends. It receives the cephalic vein and terminates immediately beneath the clavicle, at the outer border of the first rib, at which point it becomes the subclavian vein.

External Jugular Vein

The **external jugular vein** is easily recognized on the side of the neck. It follows a descending inward path to join the subclavian vein above the middle of the clavicle.

BOX 13–2 **Assessment Criteria for Selection of a Vascular Access Device**

Physician's order for IV therapy
   Therapy
   Duration and interval
Diagnosis
   Potential need for multiple therapies
   Potential for blood products/sampling
   Other therapies
Physical assessment
   Venous assessment
   Head-to-toe
Need for venous access (real or potential)
   Extended (2–7 days)
   Intermediate (7–30 days)
   Long term (>30 days)
Infusate properties (current or potential)
   Osmolarity
   pH
   Chemical properties
Clinical patient management
   Inpatient
   Extended care
   Home care
   Infusion center or other alternate site

Internal Jugular Vein

The **internal jugular vein** descends first behind and then to the outer side of the internal and common carotid arteries. The carotid plexus is situated on the outer side of the internal carotid artery. The internal jugular vein joins the subclavian vein at the root of the neck. At the angle of junction, the left subclavian receives the thoracic duct, whereas the right subclavian receives the right lymphatic duct.

Subclavian Vein

The **subclavian vein**, a continuation of the axillary vein, extends from the outer edge of the first rib to the inner end of the clavicle, where it unites with the internal jugular to form the innominate vein. Valves are present in the venous system until approximately 1 inch before the formation of the innominate vein.

Right and Left Innominate Veins

The **right innominate vein** is approximately 1 inch long. It passes almost vertically downward and joins the **left innominate vein** just below the cartilage of the first rib.

The left innominate vein is approximately 2.5 inches long and larger than the right. It passes from left to right across the upper front chest, in a downward slant. It joins the right innominate to form the superior vena cava.

Superior Vena Cava

The **superior vena cava** receives all blood from the upper half of the body. It is composed of a short trunk 2.5 to 3 inches long. It begins below the first rib close to the sternum on the right side, descends vertically slightly to the right, and empties into the right atrium of the heart.

■ EARLY USES OF CENTRAL VENOUS CATHETERS

Peripherally inserted central venous catheters were first used for monitoring central venous pressure (CVP), which denotes the pressure in the right atrium or vena cava of the venous blood as it returns from all parts of the body. The pressure varies among individuals, usually ranging between 4 and 11 cm H_2O in the vena cava, whereas the pressure in the right atrium is usually 0 to 4 cm H_2O (Metheny, 2000). In CVP monitoring, the normal pressure range has little significance because the true value lies in the change or lack of change in pressure after attempting to alter the blood volume or improve cardiac action.

Because CVP relates to a fully sufficient circulation, pressure measurement facilitates assessment of both the blood volume and the ability of the heart to tolerate an increased volume, thereby providing a valuable guide for fluid administration. Monitoring CVP requires no laboratory personnel and no expensive equipment; it is implemented by a simple technique that, once set up, allows the nurse to evaluate pressure changes quickly and as often as required (Metheny, 2000).

Central venous pressure also relates to an adequate circulatory blood supply. Pressure depends on the following:

- Blood volume
- Cardiac contractility (myocardial status)
- Vascular tone

Circulatory failure may result from deficiency in any one or a combination of these essential factors. Parameters used to evaluate a patient in shock appear in Box 13–3.

Blood Volume

Changes in blood volume alter the tone of the blood vessels and the ability of the heart to circulate the blood. Reduced blood volume results in less pressure at the

---

BOX 13–3 **Parameters for Assessing Shock**

The parameters used in evaluating a patient in shock consist of:

- Blood pressure
- Rate and quality of pulse
- Skin temperature and color
- Urinary output
- Peripheral venous filling
- Blood pH

---

right atrium, indicated by a drop in CVP; an increased blood volume produces more pressure at the atrium, with a rise in CVP (Metheny, 2000).

In managing inadequate circulation, the clinician must first establish a normal blood volume. If the inadequate circulation results from deficient blood volume, pressure may be manipulated by administering blood volume expanders. In instances of increased volume, phlebotomy may be used to reduce volume. If circulation is still insufficient, the clinician needs to evaluate the remaining two essential components: cardiac contractility (myocardial status) and vascular tone (Box 13–4).

Cardiac Contractility

Cardiac contractility may be affected by disease, drugs, fluids, or anesthetics. Because the CVP is a measure of the capacity of the myocardium as well as the blood volume, it is invaluable in monitoring the effects of anesthesia and surgery on elderly patients with arteriosclerosis or patients with myocardial insufficiency. The CVP rises if the heart muscle is impaired—the pressure of the volume of blood at the heart increases because the heart muscle can no longer pump an adequate flow of blood

---

BOX 13–4 **The Role of Blood Volume in Circulation**

Prolonged hypovolemia may cause poor tissue perfusion with the inherent risk of renal and myocardial complication; uncorrected hypovolemia can eventually lead to shock and death. Blood volume is not necessarily reflected by the blood pressure. In cardiogenic shock, for example, the blood volume is increased and the blood pressure is low. In septic shock, hypotension accompanies normal blood volume.

out of the right atrium (Metheny, 2000). A high CVP may suggest cardiac failure, which is one of the most common causes of elevated CVP in shock.

Drugs or chemicals are administered to improve myocardial response, thus increasing cardiac output and lowering the CVP.

Vascular Tone

The third essential component, vascular tone, depends on the arterial pressure and on external and internal pressures on the veins. The arterial pressure arises from the contractile force of the left ventricle and is transmitted through the capillaries to the veins.

The external pressures on the veins result from muscular and fascial pumping action in the extremities, the intra-abdominal pressure from straining and distention, and the intrathoracic pressure from contraction of the diaphragm and chest wall. CVP of patients on positive-pressure respirators is usually increased by 4 cm H_2O; patients on negative pressure show a decreased CVP (INS, 1998, 2000).

The blood volume, myocardial response, and sympathomimetic amines (epinephrine, norepinephrine) produce internal pressure on the veins. By stimulating contraction of the venous wall, vasopressors decrease the capacity of the venous system and improve vascular tone. Various methods are used to detect change in a patient's blood volume, including hematocrit, changes in patient weight, and blood volume computations. CVP is a parameter used to assess blood volume.

■ EXPANDED USES OF CENTRAL VENOUS CATHETERS

Besides monitoring pressure changes to detect potential problems or evaluate patient improvement, central venous catheters have many more uses.

Central lines inserted in the subclavian vein were first used for administering total parenteral nutrition (Fischer, 1991). This subject is thoroughly discussed in Chapter 16. Then, with the advent of catheter tunneling techniques, antithrombogenic catheter materials, new designs, and lowered infection rates, central venous catheters increased in popularity for patients with cancer. They may be used for administering antineoplastic agents over the long term, blood or blood components, and antibiotics, as well as for obtaining specimens of venous blood (see Chap. 19.)

In a hospitalized patient who requires venous access and whose peripheral veins cannot be catheterized, a long-term central catheter may be used. The same is true for many home care patients, including those who have learned to self-administer continuous or intermittent medications through a central device (see Chap. 23).

Measuring and Interpreting Central Venous Pressure

Central venous pressure is a measure of right heart function or the pressure of blood in the right atrium or vena cava (Miller, 1995). The CVP waveform reflects the contraction of the atria and the concurrent effect of the ventricles and surrounding major vessels. Normal parameters vary with the patient's clinical condition and the measurement methodology; values are affected by circulating volume, cardiac contractility, and vascular tone.

Central venous pressure monitoring may be accomplished by using a water manometer, which records pressure in units of centimeters of water (between 4 and 12 cm H_2O), or by transducer and monitor, which records pressure in units of millimeters of mercury (between 0 and 8 mm Hg). CVP readings indicate changes in preload (filling pressure in the right ventricle). Abnormal readings may indicate inadequate or increased preload, decreased contractility, or increased afterload (pressure against which the left ventricle contracts). Abnormal pressures may appear in many patients (Box 13–5).

Use of Water Manometer to Measure Central Venous Pressure

A common way to measure CVP is by attaching an IV administration set to a three-way stopcock and to an extension tube with a radiopaque catheter of approximately 24 inches. A vertical length of infusion tubing serves as the manometer. This tubing is connected to the stopcock and attached to the IV stand against a tape measure device marked in centimeters. Most facilities use CVP sets that are available with disposable water manometers and graduated unit measures (Fig. 13–3). In general, the nurse adjusts the zero mark on the tape so that it is level with the patient's right atrium. The pressure is measured at either the superior vena cava by introducing the catheter through the antecubital, jugular, or subclavian vein, or at the inferior vena cava through the femoral vein.

The superior vena cava is the most commonly used insertion site because more complications have been associated with catheters placed in the inferior vena cava. Use of the femoral vein and the length of time the catheter is in the vein increase the risk of thrombotic complications. A second disadvantage is the accompanying abdominal distention that interferes with accurate right atrial pressure readings.

BOX 13–5 Abnormal Central Venous Pressure Readings

Patients in whom abnormal readings may be found include those with

- Tricuspid stenosis
- Mitral value regurgitation
- Cardiac tamponade
- Constrictive pericarditis
- Pulmonary hypertension
- Chronic left ventricular failure
- Volume overload
- Volume depletion

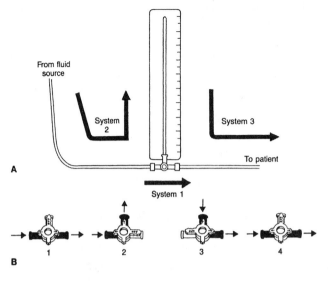

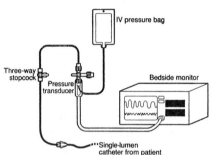

Figure 13–3. Instruments used to monitor central venous pressures. At *top* (A) is the water manometer system. Fluid is administered through system 1; fluid fills the manometer through system 2 and system 3 takes the fluid from the manometer to the patient and registers the CVP value. Stopcocks (B) direct the flow of fluid through the systems. The dark areas and arrows show the direction of flow. The transducer system, *below*, measures pressure with sensors that transform electrical signals into waveforms that are displayed on a monitor.

Once the central line is in place, the nurse needs to ensure that equipment is available to set up the manometer. The pressure reading can then proceed (see Procedure 13–1).

Electronic Infusion Devices

An optional program available on positive-pressure electronic infusion devices measures vascular flow resistance. The internal pump sensor, which monitors for occlusion, identifies vascular resistance. Ideally, the pressure detected by an uncompromised infusion system is the CVP (Perucca, 1995).

Monitoring Pulmonary Artery Pressures

Pulmonary artery catheter (or balloon flotation catheter) pressures reflect left ventricular function and end-diastolic pressure in patients with normally functioning mitral valves (Metheny, 2000; Miller, 1995). These catheters advance through the right

Procedure
13–1

Setting Up the Central Venous Pressure Manometer

Equipment

IV pole

Venous pressure level (optional)

IV solution as ordered

Arm board with cover or commercial securement device

IV or transfusion tubing

Tape

Central venous manometer set

Action	*Rationale*
1. Wash and dry hands thoroughly.	1. Ensures a clean field
2. Close the three-way stopcock.	2. Ensures a closed system
3. Hold and squeeze the drip chamber while inserting the tubing spike into the upright IV solution container. Be sure to use Luer-lock tubing.	3. Ensures stable connection
4. Relax the hold on the drip chamber and allow the chamber to fill from one fourth to one third.	4. Equalizes pressure and thereby eliminates air bubbles
5. Assemble the manometer. If the manometer requires permanent attachment to the IV pole, tape the centimeter strip onto pole and make sure that the zero point is at mid-atrial level. Also make sure that the patient is supine and the bed flat.	5. Promotes accuracy of pressure readings
6. Measure central venous pressure.	6. Provides base reading
7. Making sure the manometer setup is taut, tape the stopcock to the IV pole at a level below the patient's right atrium.	7. Promotes consistent measurements

Action	Rationale
8. Adjust the stopcock, filling the manometer halfway.	8. Allows solution to flow into manometer
9. Adjust stopcock by turning it to the left.	9. Flushes remainder of tubing
10. Using air embolism precautions, connect manometer to catheter.	10. Prevents complications
11. Secure the catheter hub and tubing connection or use Luer-locking connections.	11. Prevents separation of device
12. Secure the catheterized arm to an arm board or apply a commercial securement device.	12. Ensures consistent pressure readings and prevents kinking of the catheter

side of the heart into the pulmonary vessels. Inflation of the balloon at a specified point in the vessel secures (wedges) the catheter in a pulmonary artery. By this means, pulmonary artery pressure can be assessed either before or after surgery to determine cardiac status. These vascular lines are also used in caring for trauma patients and those with acute respiratory and cardiac impairment. The catheters are multiluminal and can measure CVP, pulmonary artery pressure, pulmonary artery wedge pressure, cardiac output, and mixed venous oxygen saturation; this kind of line may also be used for temporary heart pacing (see Chaps. 5 and 6).

Assessing and Documenting Pressure

Central venous pressure is usually read at half-hour or hourly intervals. The patient must be quiet, not coughing or straining, and in a supine position with the zero point on the manometer at the mid-atrial level. The procedure involves turning the stopcock so that the solution flows from the container to the manometer until the manometer level reaches 30 cm, at which point the nurse turns the stopcock to stop the container flow and direct the manometer flow to the patient. The fluid level drops rapidly, reaching level in approximately 15 seconds. CVP is measured at the high point of the fluctuation. Then the nurse readjusts the stopcock to resume the infusion as follows:

1. Turn stopcock so solution flows from the container to the manometer.
2. When manometer level reaches 30 cm, turn stopcock to stop flow from the container and direct manometer flow to the patient.
3. The fluid level drops rapidly, reaching the reading level in approximately 15 seconds. Measure CVP at the high point of the fluctuation.
4. Readjust the stopcock so the infusion resumes.
5. Document readings.

Note: The catheter is presumed to be in the thoracic cavity when the manometer fluid fluctuates 3 to 5 cm during breathing and when coughing and straining cause the column of water to rise. If the catheter is inserted too far and reaches the heart, higher pressure waves synchronous with the pulse are seen (Metheny, 2000).

■ PREPARATIONS FOR CENTRAL VENOUS CATHETERIZATION

To allay fears and obtain patient cooperation, explain the reasons for the insertion and procedure (INS, 1998, 2000).

Positioning

If the catheter will be inserted by a subclavian approach, explain to the patient that he or she is positioned flat in bed with the head lowered and knees bent (Trendelenburg position). This position facilitates entry to the vein by distending the vein and increasing CVP and the venous blood supply. A rolled towel is placed under the back along the spinal cord and between the shoulders to hyperextend the neck and elevate the clavicle. For the jugular approach, the head is turned to the opposite direction and extended. This stretches and stabilizes the vein and accentuates the muscular landmarks. During a cephalic or brachial insertion, abduction of the arm may be required to pass the catheter past the shoulder area. Explaining this to the patient before the procedure promotes patient cooperation when the uncomfortable position must be maintained.

Use of Protective Gear

Explaining that the nurse and physician both wear gowns, masks, and gloves to keep normal bacteria away from the area allays the patient's apprehension. If the patient is required to wear a mask also, demonstrating how to wear one before the procedure reassures the patient that the mask will not interfere with breathing (INS, 1998, 2000; Metheny, 2000; McDonald, 1997).

Valsalva Maneuver

Practicing the **Valsalva maneuver** before the insertion also promotes the patient's cooperation when he or she is asked to hold the breath and bear down when the catheter is open to the air (INS, 1998, 2000).

Educating the Patient About the Procedure and the Device

If a tunneled catheter or implanted venous access or pump device is being inserted, seeing and touching the device that will remain in the body helps to reassure most patients. Any limitations of activity the device creates should be thoroughly discussed. If the patient will be performing any self-care, this should be completely explained and agreed to by the patient before insertion. The clinician should be thoroughly versed on the care of the specific **vascular access device** being used (see Chap. 14).

Purpose of Blood Studies

Blood studies performed before catheter insertion include platelet count, prothrombin time, and partial thromboplastin time. Any abnormal findings may require correction with vitamin K, fresh frozen plasma, or platelet concentrates before insertion is attempted.

Premedication

Depending on the type of device, insertion site, and individual patient needs, some form of sedation may be required before the procedure. This should be explained to the patient.

Informed Consent

Any central venous catheterization procedure has inherent risks. The patient's informed consent, in writing, is essential before placement of any central venous catheter device.

 SAFE PRACTICE ALERT   If peripheral veins are adequate and can be used for the desired treatment, a central venous catheter should not be inserted.

Contraindications

Contraindications to central venous catheter insertion may include

- Abnormal coagulation studies
- Septicemia
- Anomalies of the central venous vascular structures
- Thrombosis of the innominate or subclavian veins or of the superior vena cava

Importance of Catheter Tip Placement

The preferred tip placement is usually at the junction of the superior vena cava and the right atrium. If the tip lies in the right atrium, atrial arrhythmias may occur as a result of the catheter irritating the chamber. For various reasons, it is not always possible to advance the catheter far enough to achieve the desired tip location. Depending on the specific purpose of the catheter, innominate or subclavian catheter tip placement may be adequate.

Infection Control

Aseptic technique minimizes the risk of infection in the patient in whom a central line is to be placed. If the patient cannot be masked during the procedure, the head should be turned away from the insertion area. The skin should be cleansed consistent with institutional policy and guidelines issued by the Centers for Disease Control and Prevention (CDC) (CDC, 1998) and by the Intravenous Nurses Society (INS) (INS, 1998, 2000). Before using any acetone solution for defatting the skin, determine which material the catheter is made of because some materials, such as Silastic, erode from contact with acetone solutions (Hye & Stabile, 1996; INS, 1998, 2000; McDonald, Banerjee, & Jarvis, 1997). The catheter insertion site is dressed in the usual manner and catheter maintenance is performed in accord with institutional policy (see Chap. 10).

■ INSERTION OF THE LINES

Central Venous Insertion Sites

There are three basic approaches for central venous catheter insertions. The veins used for entry are the subclavian and the internal or external jugular veins for central insertion and the cephalic or basilic vein for peripheral insertion.

Subclavian Approach

The subclavian vein is typically the entry site of choice. It requires the shortest catheter because it uses the most central veins, thus creating a high blood flow around a large portion of the catheter. This results in minimal irritation or obstruction by the catheter, which lowers the risk of complications and results in a longer catheter life.

A medical act, subclavian entry can foster major complications both during and after insertion (see Complications section of this chapter). The subclavian entry may be performed by the infraclavicular or supraclavicular approach. In both approaches, the catheter is inserted under the clavicle, aiming for the jugular notch. For the infraclavicular approach, the catheter is inserted at approximately the midpoint of the clavicle. For the supraclavicular approach, the catheter is frequently inserted at the base of the triangle formed by the sternal and clavicular heads of the sternocleidomastoid muscle.

Contraindications to the subclavian approach may include

- Radiation burns at intended insertion site
- Fractured clavicle

- Hyperinflated lungs
- Malignant lesion at the base of the neck or apex of the lungs

Internal Jugular Vein Approach

The insertion of central venous catheters into the internal jugular vein is usually a medical act. Many physicians select the internal jugular vein as a site of first choice for inserting a central venous catheter. The constant anatomic location of the internal jugular vein makes it easier to catheterize than the subclavian vein. The right internal jugular vein is usually chosen because it forms a straighter, shorter line to the superior vena cava. It also avoids the higher left pleura and thoracic duct. This insertion is frequently performed by first locating the vein with a small-gauge needle. After making a small skin incision to facilitate entry, a larger-gauge catheter is inserted, following the same direction as the locator needle, aiming for the **ipsilateral** nipple.

External Jugular Vein Approach

The external jugular vein is observable and easily entered. Insertion complications are rare, so nurses with specialized skills can perform catheterization. The external jugular vein varies in size and its junction with the subclavian vein is acutely angulated. It contains two pairs of valves. The uppermost pair is 4 cm above the clavicle; the lower pair is located at the vein's entrance to the subclavian vein. Because of these factors, central catheterization can be difficult. Because a short catheter may be inserted easily, central catheterization may be achieved by using an introducer with a guidewire. Entry into the superficial vein is performed by directing the catheter toward the ipsilateral nipple. The main objections to any jugular catheterization are the following:

- Catheter occlusion is a persistent problem; it results from the patient's head movement
- Vein irritation also results from head movement; the consequence is a shorter catheter life.
- It is difficult to maintain an intact dressing on the area.
- The idea of having a catheter in the neck is aesthetically and psychologically disturbing to many patients and families.

Peripheral Insertion Sites

Technology has kept pace with demands for more sophisticated, long-term peripheral venous access devices. The peripherally inserted central catheter (PICC) line was the first product developed specifically for this clinical application. The PICC has quickly become an alternate form of access for patients who need IV therapy for more than 1 week, who have poor peripheral access, or who need vesicant medications. (Chapter 11 addresses IV equipment and provides additional information on PICC and midline insertions.)

Vein Selection

The basilic and cephalic antecubital fossa veins are the preferred sites for PICC placement. The basilic vein is usually the first choice for the peripheral insertion of a central venous catheter. It ascends obliquely in the groove between the biceps brachii and pronator teres and perforates the deep fascia slightly distal to the middle of the upper arm. With the arm held at a 90-degree angle, it forms the straightest, most direct route into the central venous system.

The median cubital vein is the second choice. Ascending on the ulnar side of the forearm, the vein may be divided into two vessels, one joining the basilic vein and the other the cephalic vein. This vein varies substantially, and the proper branch must be ascertained before venipuncture for PICC placement. The median antecubital basilic is preferred.

The cephalic vein runs proximally along the lateral side of the antecubital fossa in the groove between the brachioradialis and the biceps brachii. It becomes a deep vein at the clavipectoral fascia, ending in the axillary vein immediately caudal to the clavicle. It is much more tortuous than the basilic vein and presents a greater potential for catheter tip malposition. It is not preferred because it may also be difficult to thread. Indications for PICC placement are listed in Box 13–6. PICCs are widely accepted in the nursing and medical communities, and patients receiving a PICC benefit from sound information about the device (Box 13–7).

Advantages

The many advantages of the PICC over the short-term peripheral catheter and the centrally placed line include

- Elimination of risks associated with central venous catheter placement
- Potential reduction of catheter sepsis
- Ease of use
- Preservation of the peripheral vascular system
- Decrease in discomfort
- Reliability

BOX 13–6 **Indications for PICC Placement**

- Lack of peripheral venous access
- Infusion of vesicant or irritant drugs
- Infusion of hyperosmolar drugs
- Long-term venous access
- Infusion of antineoplastic agents, blood, or blood components
- Patient preference
- Clinician preference

BOX 13–7 Teaching Guide for Patients With PICCs

Features of an effective patient teaching plan include

- Appropriate level of information for the patient's age and language
- Purpose and rationale for PICC placement and alternatives
- Delineated responsibilities of the patient or caregivers and health care providers
- Explanation of routine risks and complications of treatment
- Discussion of prognosis (procedure-specific)

Follow-up evaluation of teaching includes

- Documented assessment of patient or caregiver comprehension
- Documentation of consent for procedure and method of consent (verbal/nonverbal/written)
- Support materials provided to patient (illustrated, audio, printed materials, as appropriate)

Tip Placement

A PICC tip may be placed in either the superior vena cava, providing true central line access, or in the subclavian (or axillary) vein. The physical landmark used for the axillary or subclavian vein is approximately 1 inch distal from the head of the clavicle.

SUPERIOR VENA CAVA

Placement of the catheter tip in the superior vena cava is preferred for all antineoplastic agents, administration of vesicants, total parenteral nutrition with a final dextrose concentration in excess of 20%, and any sclerosing agents. Measurement for tip placement is from the point of insertion, along the proposed vein track to the third intercostal space.

SUBCLAVIAN PLACEMENT

Subclavian placement is often used for the diverse IV therapies administered through a conventional short catheter. Measurement of tip placement is from the point of insertion, along the proposed vein track to 1 inch distal to the sternal notch. At this point, the catheter tip should be seated in the median segment of the subclavian vein 2 to 3 cm distal to the junction of the external jugular vein.

Role of the Interventional Radiologist in Placement

At one time, the role of radiologists in venous access was limited to preoperative venous mapping, repositioning of malpositioned catheters, and retrieval of catheter fragments. Advances in imaging (particularly in Doppler ultrasound imaging) and improved guidewire and catheter technologies have expanded the role of the interventional radiologist. Strict adherence to sterile technique has made the radiology suite an ideal clinical site in which to place CVC lines.

Radiologic imaging guidance can facilitate access to the central veins by alternative routes in patients who have limited access as a result of chemotherapy, total parenteral nutrition, trauma, surgery, radiation, or infection in the chest wall and neck area. Alternative (unconventional) access routes include inferior vena cava catheterization by direct translumbar, transhepatic, or femoral vein approach; collateral venous channels (eg, intercostal, azygous); and recanalization of occluded veins (Blum, 1999).

Catheter Selection

Many single-lumen and multilumen catheters, ports, and tunneled lines are available (Table 13–1).

Inserting the Catheter

A physician's order is needed before placing a PICC line. Before proceeding, the patient should be assessed for available venous access, clinical condition, and ability to learn procedures applicable to maintenance. In addition, the equipment should be assembled and ready. Placement of a PICC is a medical act. The procedure is discussed in Chapter 12.

T A B L E   1 3 – 1
SELECTED PICC PRODUCTS AND MANUFACTURERS

Manufacturer	Product	Special Features
Catheter Innovations	PASV Technology Valve connector is available for use with any standard Luer lock extension set	Pressure-activated safety valve—a three-way valve that is pressure and direction dependent Opens with minimal positive pressure for infusion yet requires four times as much negative pressure for aspiration
Becton-Dickinson	*First* PICC with *Introsyte* precision introducer	Peel-away design; flushable silicone catheter with hydrophilic stylet; integrated extension with oval disk to enhance patient comfort
Implemed, Inc.	OLIMPICC	Silver-based microbial technology
Johnson & Johnson	Protectiv	Safety introducer system; OCRILON II polyurethane offers flexibility and patient comfort
Luther Medical	L-CATH Peel-Away	Extended-dwell catheter preinserted into L-CATH peel-away introducer needle (siliconized to facilitate insertion)
Arrow International	Midline catheter	Trimmable; latex-free product in self-contained kit

| **KEY INTERVENTIONS:** | Steps Used in Placement of Percutaneously Inserted Central Catheters |

Placement of a percutaneously inserted, nontunneled catheter is a medical act. The nurse may assist the physician in the placement of these devices and perform routine site care, maintenance, and ongoing monitoring.

1. Wash hands with antiseptic soap.
2. Identify known patient allergies.
3. Explain the procedure and rationale to the patient.
4. Obtain consent.
5. Assess patient.
6. Assemble equipment and don personal protective gear as appropriate.
7. Observe Standard Precautions throughout the procedure.
8. Assist physician with patient positioning.
9. Cleanse intended insertion site with anti-infective soap and water as needed.
10. Remove excess hair from intended insertion site with scissors.
11. Stabilize access device after placement; suturing is the preferred method. Use of sterile surgical strips, sterile tape, or stabilizing device is also appropriate.
12. Dress access site with sterile gauze and cover with sterile, transparent, semipermeable dressing.
13. Secure connection junctions.
14. Before initiating therapy, radiographically confirm catheter placement in superior vena cava. Femoral placement is confirmed by location of catheter tip in the inferior vena cava.
15. Initiate prescribed therapy.
16. Discard used equipment in appropriate receptacles.
17. Document procedure in the clinical record.

A skills checklist may be used to determine competencies of nurses who have completed the PICC training program. Training and teaching programs are available through the INS and through the National Association of Vascular Access Networks (see Chapter 14; Fig. 13–4).

Microintroducer Alternative Technique

As with the guidewire, a modified Seldinger technique is used for inserting a central catheter with the microintroducer. A hydrophilic coating facilitates vascular access device exchanges. Disadvantages include the need for specialized training and additional components compared with standard PICC placement. Potential complications associated with this technique include venous rupture or perforation, arterial puncture, hematoma, and embolization. The clinician should consult product literature and institutional guidelines before using any PICC product.

An example of a precision introducer is one that is a component of Becton-Dickinson's Introsyte product line, Eranklin Lakes, NJ (Becton-Dickinson, 1999), and similar devices are part of the same manufacturer's midline products. Bard Access Systems, Salt lake City, UT, also offers a microintroducer, which is shown in action in the accompanying display.

1. *Didactic*	*Understanding*	*Observed Competency*
• Class attendance	☐	☐
• Policy/procedure awareness	☐	☐
• PICC post-test completion	☐	☐
2. *Practicum*		
• Explains procedure/rationale	☐	☐
• Obtains consent	☐	☐
• Site assessment	☐	☐
• Handwashing	☐	☐
• Completes measurements	☐	☐
• Skin/site preparation	☐	☐
• Use of protective attire	☐	☐
• Preparation of sterile field	☐	☐
• Guidewire preparation/trim	☐	☐
• Draping	☐	☐
• Venipuncture procedure	☐	☐
• Threading procedure	☐	☐
• Assessment blood return/patency	☐	☐
• Catheterization to predetermined length	☐	☐
• Stabilizes/removes introducer	☐	☐
• Use of breakaway device	☐	☐
• Flushing technique	☐	☐
• Dressing application	☐	☐
3. *Documentation*		
• Per protocol	☐	☐
• Patient education	☐	☐

Figure 13–4. Postinsertion skill competencies checklist.

KEY INTERVENTIONS: Using a MicroIntroducer for Catheter Insertion

The Universal MicroIntroducer (Bard Access Systems, CR Bard, Inc., Salt Lake City, UT) is one of several devices developed to assist health care professionals accomplish life-saving procedures easily and safely. Clinicians using a microintroducer to place a PICC need specialized training, but once they are sufficiently expert, they may proceed as follows:

1. Obtain the needed equipment, including the microintroducer, guidewire assemblage, a scalpel as appropriate, a sheath, and a dilator.
2. Prepare the catheter insertion site, administering an anesthetic and maintaining sterile technique in the same way as for basic peripheral insertion.
3. Insert the introducer needle into the selected vein.

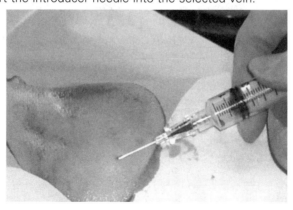

4. Unwrap the guidewire and remove its tip protector from the guidewire hoop. Insert the flexible end of the guidewire into the introducer needle and into the vein. Advance the guidewire to the desired depth.

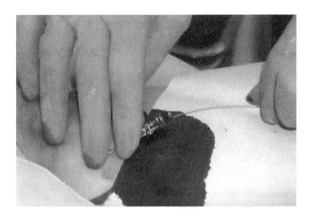

5. Gently withdraw and remove the introducer needle while holding the guidewire in position. *Caution: If the guidewire must be withdrawn while the needle is inserted, remove both the needle and the wire as a unit to prevent the needle from damaging or shearing the guidewire.*
6. If necessary and in accord with institutional guidelines, use the scalpel to make a small incision adjacent to the guidewire. This incision facilitates insertion of the sheath and dilator.
7. Using a slight rotational motion, advance the small sheath and dilator together as a unit over the guidewire.
8. Withdraw the dilator and guidewire, leaving the small sheath in place.
   Caution: Place a finger over the orifice of the sheath to minimize blood loss and risk of air aspiration. The risk of air embolism is reduced by performing this part of the procedure and having the patient perform the Valsalva maneuver.
9. Insert the catheter through the sheath. Typically, the sheath may be withdrawn after the catheter is advanced between 12 and 15 cm.
10. After removing the sheath from the vein, break the T-handle and peel the sheath apart. Apply a dressing in accord with institutional policy.

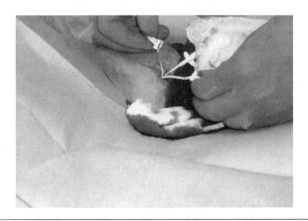

Breakaway Needle Technique

Use of a breakaway needle facilitates venipuncture with an introducer needle. The catheter, with or without a guidewire, is threaded through the introducer. The introducer is removed from the venipuncture site, broken in half, and peeled away. The U-Wing Peelaway Needle Introducer is an example of a breakaway needle. The stainless steel needle introducer offers improved access to small veins and subsequent easy removal from the catheter. The T-Peel Peelaway Plastic Sheath introducer allows catheter threading through a plastic sheath and an integrated flashback chamber to protect the clinician and confirm placement. (For a discussion of safety devices, see Chapter 11.)

Catheterization technique involves using an introducer needle to place a plastic catheter (peel-away sheath) into the vein. The catheter is then threaded through this sheath. The sheath is removed from the insertion site and peeled away from the catheter.

Ultrasonography

The use of portable ultrasound device for placing peripheral IV catheters has met with wide acceptance (LaRue, 1999; Randolph, 1996; Lin, 1998).

With ultrasonography, the IV nurse may identify arterial vessels by applying pressure with the probe against the patient's arm, and noting the relative ease of vein compression compared with artery compression. The ultrasound device also facilitates visualization of solid material in the lumen of the vessel, such as catheters or thrombus formations. Thus, a comprehensive assessment of cannulated and uncannulated veins is assured. Ultrasonography requires sterile lubricant and a sterile plastic bag to cover the ultrasound probe.

■ POSTINSERTION CARE

Once the catheter is in place, the IV nurse needs to assess the patient and indwelling devices for function and signs of complications, such as for redness, edema, pain, drainage, and a palpable venous cord. Postinsertion complications include

- Bleeding (unusual after 24 hours)
- Phlebitis
- Cellulitis (which tends to spread in a diffuse circular pattern into surrounding tissue)
- Catheter sepsis

Verification of Accurate Placement

A chest radiograph is always obtained immediately after catheter insertion to rule out pneumothorax and document tip placement. An isotonic solution is infused until tip placement is confirmed. The site should be observed for any signs of excess bleeding or swelling, and the patient's breathing should be monitored for any signs of respiratory distress. Unexpected observations should be reported to the physician immediately, as should complications associated with central line placement. PICC placement should be documented consistent with guidelines in Box 13–8.

Peripheral Port Placement and Aftercare

Some patients receive an implanted peripheral port to permit repeated venous access to the circulation. The device consists of a portal with a self-sealing septum, accessible by percutaneous needle puncture, and a catheter for the parenteral delivery of medications and fluids (see Chap. 14).

Cautions

Before placement, the patient's anatomy should be accessed for evidence of prior trauma to the veins or anatomic irregularities. After placement, certain precautions are appropriate. Blood should not be drawn from nor should medication be infused into the arm in which the implanted system is placed without using the port. Blood pressure should not be measured on this arm.

BOX 13–8 **Documenting PICC Placement**

The following are documented after completing PICC placement:

- Patient's informed consent
- Catheter information (type, composition, manufacturer, lot number, size/ original length)
- Trimmed length and method of trimming
- Actual length inserted
- External length
- Specific vein used
- Insertion technique or methodology
- Sedative or local anesthetic used
- Flush solution used and amount
- Appearance of catheter insertion site and date, time, and kind of dressing applied
- Identification of any add-on devices
- Patient's tolerance of procedure
- Patient/caregiver teaching
- Method of verifying catheter tip location
- Infusate, flow rate, and method of administration (eg, EID)
- Radiologic verification of tip placement beyond proximal portion of the extremity
- Use of ultrasonography

Potential Complications

A host of potential complications are associated with the peripherally placed port, including air embolism; artery or vein puncture; brachial plexus injury; cardiac arrhythmia; cardiac tamponade; cardiac puncture; catheter disconnection, fragmentation, and embolization; catheter occlusion or rupture; drug extravasation; fibrin sheath formation at the catheter tip; hematoma; hemothorax; implant rejection; infection; migration of the port or catheter; peripheral nerve damage; thoracic duct injury; thromboembolism; thrombophlebitis; and thrombosis.

Care and Maintenance

Care must be taken when administering solutions through the portal system because excessive pressure can be generated from all syringes. Pressure in excess of 40 psi may cause catheter rupture with possible embolization. As with any line, appropriate flushing procedures must be implemented to avoid incompatibility with heparin.

A syringe or IV administration set is attached to a 20- or 22-gauge needle, and the needle is primed. The skin is prepared and punctured directly over the septum. The nurse then advances the needle slowly through the septum until it makes contact with the bottom of the portal chamber. Without tilting or rocking the needle, the nurse flushes the device with an appropriate solution and administers the injection or infusate. The device is flushed again with 5 mL of heparinized saline solution to establish patency. Positive pressure must be maintained when withdrawing the needle to avoid reflux of blood into the catheter.

■ COMPLICATIONS OF CENTRAL VENOUS CATHETERIZATION

Among complications associated with CVC are arterial puncture, pneumothorax, hemothorax, embolisms, and infections. The IV nurse is always alert for signs and symptoms of complications and is ready to intervene as needed to prevent or ameliorate them.

Arterial Puncture

Arterial puncture, one of the most frequently reported complications of subclavian insertions, is usually not a major problem if it is recognized early. The puncture of an artery requires the immediate application of digital pressure for at least 5 minutes. If the patient has a coagulation abnormality, digital pressure must be maintained until all bleeding stops. If the artery puncture is not recognized and treated early, a massive hematoma resulting in tracheal compression or respiratory distress can occur.

Pneumothorax, Hemothorax, and Hydrothorax

Pneumothorax, another common complication of subclavian insertion, occurs as a result of pleural puncture, after which the patient may experience difficult breathing or chest pain. However, a pneumothorax that does not produce symptoms may be disclosed by radiography. A chest tube may be required to treat the complication.

Hemothorax may result if the subclavian or adjacent veins have been traumatized or transected during catheter insertion. Hydrothorax results when the IV fluid infiltrates into the chest. The symptoms and treatment of hemothorax and hydrothorax are identical to those pneumothorax.

Catheter Embolism

Catheter embolism is always a risk whenever a through-the-needle device is inserted or left in situ. During insertion, care must be taken never to withdraw the catheter back through the needle. While the through-the-needle catheter is in place, care must be taken to ensure that the needle tip is always protected with a secured tip cover. A severed catheter may require cardiac catheterization to retrieve the embolism. Breakaway needles minimize this hazard.

Air Embolism

Air embolism is always a potential danger whenever any central venous catheter is open to air. It can occur because it is always possible to have negative CVP. During insertion, placing the patient in the Trendelenburg position increases CVP. Placing a sterile gloved finger over the catheter hub, between catheter stylet removal and IV system connection, can prevent air from entering the catheter.

 SAFE PRACTICE ALERT The risk of air embolism is always present during catheter insertion because CVP can be negative. Placing the patient in the Trendelenburg position increases CVP. If possible, the patient should perform the Valsalva maneuver whenever the catheter is opened to the air. If the catheter stylet has been removed, the hub should be occluded either with a syringe or a gloved finger to prevent air entry.

Use of the PASV (pressure-activated safety valve; Catheter Innovations, Sandy, Utah,) as an add-on device may help preclude the danger of air embolism. This device reduces the risk of air embolism or bleed-out resulting from an accidental disconnection of the tubing (see Chap. 14).

Signs and symptoms of air embolism include chest pain, dyspnea, hypoxia, apnea, tachycardia, hypotension, or a precordial murmur. Immediate treatment includes placing the patient in a supine position on the left side with the feet elevated. This position is used in an attempt to trap the air in the right atrium, where it can be aspirated with an intracardiac needle.

Catheter-Related Infection

Catheter-related infection is a serious complication of central venous catheterization, occurring at the exit site, tunnel, or port pocket. Most steps taken in maintaining the IV system and site are performed to prevent IV-related sepsis.

Whenever a patient with a central venous catheter has an unexpected high fever, IV-related sepsis must be suspected. The insertion site should be inspected for signs of infection. A blood specimen may need to be drawn through the catheter and cultured. To rule out all sources of contamination, all tubings and containers should be changed immediately and sent promptly for bacteriologic culturing. Organisms that may lead to rapid progression of clinical symptoms include *Escherichia coli*, *Klebsiella* species, vancomycin-resistant *Staphylococcus*, and newer strains of antibiotic-resistant *Streptococcus* organisms (Ray, 1999). A complete "fever work-up" must be performed to rule out any other obvious source of infection. If the fever remains and no other possible source can be established, catheter removal may be necessary. See Chapter 14 for information regarding antimicrobial-impregnated catheters.

Some practitioners perform a catheter exchange with a guidewire. If the blood culture is positive or the semiquantitative culture of the catheter tip yields 15 or more colonies, the new catheter is removed and the patient is considered to have catheter sepsis. If both culture results are negative, then the catheter can be used despite the fever. In cases of septic shock, shaking chills, recent positive blood cultures for *Staphylococcus* or *Candida*, or local infection of the catheter entry site, the catheter must be removed immediately (Carlson, 1999; Hye & Stabile, 1996; Ray, 1999). In some facilities, in situ treatment of catheter-related sepsis with a combination of systemic antibiotics and local thrombolytic agents has been reported. Antibiotic lock technique has also been used (see Chaps. 11 and 12).

Of primary importance in preventing IV-related infection is maintaining strict aseptic technique during insertion, admixture, and IV line manipulations. The nurse must also perform recommended site dressing and tubing changes using aseptic technique. Figure 13–5 presents treatment algorithms for central venous access device–related infection.

Deep Vein Thrombosis

Deep vein thrombosis is not as common with the new catheter materials. The addition of 1000 U heparin per liter of infusate has been recommended as a preventive measure (Bagnall-Reed, 1998; Hye & Stabile, 1996; Ray, 1999). Thrombosis may be present without any symptoms, or arm and neck pain may suggest the diagnosis. A venogram may be necessary to confirm the diagnosis.

Signs and symptoms of pulmonary embolism in a patient with a central venous catheter strongly suggest deep vein thrombosis. Treatment consists of thrombolytic therapy with streptokinase or urokinase. In the absence of commercially available urokinase, thrombolytic agents such as alteplase (Activase; Genentech, San Francisco, CA), and reteplase (Retavase; Centocor, Malvern, PA) may prove equally effective (Blum, 1999). See the accompanying research issue box for more information on urokinase.

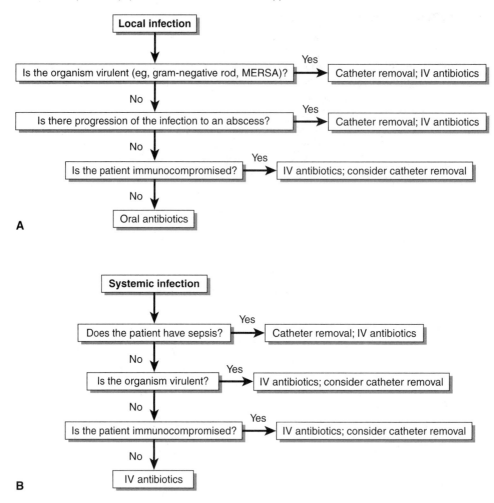

Figure 13–5. Suggested treatment algorithms for (A) local and (B) systemic infection related to central venous catheters. (Adapted with permission from Ray, C. [1999]. Infection control principles and practices in the care and management of central venous access devices. *Journal of Intravenous Nursing,* 22 [Suppl. 6], S23.)

Thrombus–Catheter Occlusion

Thrombus–catheter occlusion used to be a frequent cause for catheter removal. A fibrin sheath originates at the intimal injury, either where the catheter enters the vessel or where the catheter tip touches the intima. Within 1 to 7 days, an unorganized, unendothelialized fibrin sleeve is apparent on venography (Evidence-Based Medicine, 1998; Fitzpatrick, 1999; Holmes, 1998; Hye & Stabile, 1996; Ouriel, Veith & Sasahara, 1998). This may result in only a withdrawal occlusion. In such situations, the nurse finds it impossible to withdraw a blood sample but has no difficulty with infusion. (See Table 13–2 for an overview of possible problems.)

Research Issues: UROKINASE FOR ACUTE ARTERIAL OCCLUSION

 Ouriel K., Veith, F. J., & Sasahara, A. A., for the TOPAS investigators. (1998). A comparison of recombinant urokinase with vascular surgery as initial treatment for acute arterial occlusion of the legs. *New England Journal of Medicine, 338,* 1105–1111.

Research Question: Is urokinase safe and effective in the treatment of acute arterial occlusion?

In this randomized controlled trial (nonblinded) in an inpatient setting, 544 patients with an acute thrombotic or embolic occlusion of a leg vessel were selected at random for treatment by surgery or urokinase. The average age was 65 years. Approximately two thirds of the subjects were men. Amputation and death rates were similar between groups at 1 year. The number of open surgical procedures was significantly lower for the urokinase group (351 vs 590; P = not reported). However, major hemorrhagic complications were more common in the urokinase group (32 vs 14 patients, P = 0 .005, NNH = 15). That is, for every 15 patients given urokinase instead of surgery, one had a major bleeding episode. In addition, only 10.3% of urokinase patients had medical treatment alone by the end of the 1-year follow-up period. One final caveat: Only one patient was enrolled every $3\frac{1}{2}$ months in each study center, making a selection bias likely.

Findings: Urokinase is an alternative to surgical treatment for acute arterial occlusion, but offers few advantages.

Managing an Occlusion

In cases of thrombus–catheter occlusion when there is little or no infusion flow, the patency of the catheter can be restored by using of a thrombolytic agent; small-dose vials are available for the declotting procedure.

 SAFE PRACTICE ALERT   The following discussion is specifically about the thrombolytic agent urokinase. Other, similar agents are available and in use. For safe patient care, the clinician is urged to follow the manufacturer's recommendations for the individual product used.

PREPARE THE THROMBOLYTIC SOLUTION

When urokinase is available for use, it is packaged in a two-chamber vial. Take the following steps to prepare the solution:

1. Remove the protective cap from the vial and turn the plunger-stopper a quarter turn; press to force diluent into lower chamber.

PATIENT AND CAREGIVERS' GUIDE TO MANAGING PICC PROBLEMS

Problem	Signs and Symptoms	Action
Air enters bloodstream	Shortness of breath, coughing, chest pain	Clamp catheter.
		Patient should lie on left side with head down.
		Call Emergency Medical Services (EMS) for assistance.
Catheter breaks or is accidentally cut	Noticeable damage or leakage	Clamp catheter.
		Notify nurse or physician.
Injection cap disconnects	Blood inside cap or leakage	Clamp catheter and notify nurse.
		Apply sterile cap.
		Flush catheter as directed.
Evidence of infection	Pain, redness, swelling, fever, drainage at site	Notify nurse or physician.
		Avoid infection by using sterile technique as instructed.
		Keep dressing dry and intact.
Occluded catheter	Resistance is met when infusing drugs	Stop infusion immediately; do not force it.
		Call nurse or physician.
Central vein thrombosis	Swelling around hand, arm, or neck	Call nurse or physician.
Phlebitis	Small area of redness 8 inches in diameter surrounding insertion site; evidence of tenderness or swelling	Call nurse or physician; early treatment is necessary (may include warm, moist compresses for 20 minutes four times daily).
		If no improvement within 24 hours, contact nurse or physician.

2. Roll and tilt the vial to dissolve the components; avoid shaking the solution.
3. Sterilize stopper top with alcohol, then insert the needle through the center of the stopper until the tip is barely visible. Invert the vial and withdraw a dose.

DECLOT THE CATHETER
An aliquot of solution equal in volume to the luminal volume of the catheter is used for each injection, as follows:

- 11-French Hickman = 0.8 to 0.9 mL
- 6-French = 0.5 to 0.7 mL
- Port-A-Cath = 1.3 mL

The clinician puts on gloves before initiating the following steps to declot the catheter:

1. Using air embolism precautions, aseptically disconnect the IV tubing at the catheter hub and attach an empty 10-mL syringe.
2. Gently attempt to aspirate blood. If aspiration is not possible, remove the syringe.
3. Attach a 1-mL tuberculin syringe filled with prepared urokinase.

4. Slowly and gently inject amount equal to volume of catheter.
5. Remove syringe and connect empty 5-mL syringe.
6. Wait at least 5 minutes before attempting to aspirate drug and residual clot.
7. Repeat aspiration attempts every 5 minutes.
8. If catheter patency is not restored within 30 minutes, cap the catheter and allow drug to remain for 30 to 60 minutes.
9. A second urokinase injection may be required and may be repeated as long as systemic thrombolysis is not induced.
10. When patency is restored, aspirate 4 to 5 mL blood to ensure removal of all drug and residual clot.
11. Remove blood-filled syringe and connect 10-mL syringe with 0.9% sodium chloride solution and gently flush to ensure patency.
12. Remove syringe and aseptically reconnect sterile IV tubing to catheter hub.

■ CARE AND MAINTENANCE OF CENTRAL VENOUS LINES

Risks and complications associated with central venous catheterization may be reduced when a team of qualified nursing specialists assumes responsibility for assisting with insertions, maintaining lines, and providing ongoing IV care (INS, 1998, 2000). Astute nursing assessment and a comprehensive understanding of the vascular access device in place may avert complications such as dislodgment, migration, pinch-off syndrome, and skin erosion. Types of radiologic testing for possible catheter occlusion are given in Table 13–3.

Apparatus for Maintaining Safe Therapy

Electronic Infusion Devices

Electronic instrumentation should be used to maintain flow accuracy and catheter patency. The diversity of electronic infusion devices today ensures availability for patients with central venous access devices. When a positive-pressure instrument is

T A B L E   1 3 – 3
RADIOLOGIC CONFIRMATION OF CATHETER POSITION

Test	Evaluation	Indication for Test
Chest radiograph	Catheter placement	Suspected malposition—pinch-off syndrome, which may result from the patient's position whereby the pressure of the clavicle against the first rib pinches the catheter closed
Contrast study	Flow at distal tip of catheter	Suspected fibrin sheath formation
Venogram	Vessel patency	Suspected superior vena cava thrombosis
Duplex scan	Vessel patency	Suspected brachial, jugular, or subclavian thrombosis

(Adapted from Krzywda, R.A. [1999]. Predisposing factors, prevention, and management of central venous catheter occlusions. *Journal of Intravenous Nursing, 22* (Suppl.6), 11-17.

used, the pressure must not exceed that recommended for the type of catheter or electronic infusion device in use.

Catheter Clamps

Smooth-jaw clamps are used when tunneled silicone catheters are placed to prevent damage to the catheter material. Ideally, the clamp is applied to the distal two-thirds portion of the external catheter. If clamp damage should occur, catheter repair is easily facilitated in this area. Clamp sites should be alternated to prevent weakening an area on the catheter itself. Second-generation Silastic catheters use integral, soft-jaw clamps.

Catheter Repair

A sterile repair kit, specific to the individual type of catheter, should be readily available. Repairing the external portion of a tunneled catheter is a sterile procedure requiring surgical gloves, gown, mask, and cap. (Note that some manufacturers provide catheter repair kits that may be used for most catheters.) General directions for catheter repair are supplied in Procedure 13–2.

Once the catheter repair is achieved, taping a Luer-lock 0.2 µm Air-Eliminating Filter directly to the catheter hub reduces the risk of connection separation and air infusion that could result in a fatal embolism. If a separation occurs distal to the filter, this device prevents air infusion and an inadvertent bleed. The 0.2 µm filter can also prevent any particulate matter, fungi, bacteria, and endotoxins from entering the system through the filter.

Intravenous Containers and Admixtures

All recommendations for peripheral containers or admixtures should be strictly adhered to for central catheter usage. To prevent risks of contamination, all manipulations for admixture and container changes must be performed with strict adherence to aseptic technique.

Tubing Changes

All tubings should be aseptically changed according to INS Standards of Practice (INS, 1998, 2000). The IV nurse must always keep in mind the possibility of negative pressure with a central catheter. Therefore, the risk of an air embolism is always present when the catheter is open to the air. If the patient cannot perform the Valsalva maneuver, extension tubing with a clamp that can be closed during the tubing change may be needed. Many practitioners use this system especially for critically ill patients. Care must be taken to maintain the sterility of the extension tubing during each IV tubing change. The extension tubing is changed at least weekly.

Between changes of components, the system should be maintained as a closed system. All entries into the system should be made through injection ports that have been disinfected immediately before use.

Looping the tubing and taping it to the chest wall prevents any related stress to the connection or insertion site when the tubing is pulled or inadvertently stretched. All connections should use junction securement devices or Luer-locking connections, consistent with INS Standards of Practice (INS, 1998, 2000).

| Procedure **13–2** | **Repairing a Central Venous Catheter** |

Equipment

Sterile gear (drapes, gloves, mask or face shield, cap, gown)

Guarded hemostat

3-mL syringe

Tongue depressor

4-inch × 4-inch sterile sponges

Povidone–iodine solution

Small beaker for alcohol

Alcohol

Scalpel blades

Heparin flush solution

Iris scissors

Tape

Sterile repair kit containing replacement silicone rubber segment with Luer-lock connector; silicone rubber splice sleeve; splice segment; Luer-lock cap; tube of medical adhesive; and a blunt, 18-gauge needle

Action	*Rationale*
1. Surgically prepare catheter and create sterile field. Put on protective gear.	1. Maintains sterile environment to prevent infection
2. Use a 4 × 4-inch sponge immersed in alcohol to clean residual powder from gloves.	2. Prevents airborne contamination from powder particles
3. Load adhesive into syringe barrel, then insert plunger and attach blunt 18-gauge needle.	3. Renders apparatus ready for applying glue

Action	Rationale
4. If catheter is not clamped, clamp with guarded hemostat near chest wall, and then cut off the damaged catheter portion 15 to 20 cm from chest wall.	4. Clamping closes line to air, infection, or leakage
5. Insert splice segment into lumen of catheter (lubricate with alcohol if necessary, but be sure all alcohol is removed or evaporated before proceeding).	5. Facilitates insertion of new sound part while eliminating chance for internal contamination
6. Trim repair segment to desired length and slip onto the splice segment protruding from the implanted catheter. Do not remove the larger splice sleeve, which is now loose mounted on the repair segment.	6. Larger splice sleeve is used later.
7. Inject adhesive on the outside of the tubing in the area of the splice segment and slide the larger splice sleeve over the area of the splice segment. Inject adhesive underneath each end of splice sleeve. Roll between fingers to extrude excess adhesive and wipe excess adhesive away.	7. Ensures that adhesive does not contaminate the internal lumen
8. A sterile field is no longer required, so the repaired joint can be splinted by taping the area to a tongue depressor.	8. Once the segment is glued in place, contaminants are sealed out of the catheter line.
9. Remove clamp. Avoiding excessive pressure, gently flush the restored line with heparin solution.	9. Excessive pressure may rupture the new joint.
10. Allow the repair to cure for a few hours before using the line for infusion. Keep the tongue depressor splint in place for approximately 48 hours.	10. The catheter joint needs time to solidify, and retaining the splint in position helps the repair achieve full mechanical strength.

References and Selected Readings

Asterisks indicate references cited in

*Bagnall-Reed, H. (1998). Diagnosis of central venous access device occlusion: implications for nursing practice. *Journal of Intravenous Nursing, 21*(Suppl. 5) 115-S117.

Bard, C.R., & Bard Access Systems. (1998). Universal MicroIntroducer insertion procedure literature. UMIP1298. Bard Access Systems.

*Becton-Dickinson. (1998). Product literature: First PICC™. D12920 and MidCath™ D12911. Author.

*Blum, A.S. (1999). The role of the interventional radiologist in central venous access. *Journal of Intravenous Nursing, 22*(Suppl. 6), 32–S39.

*Carlson, K.R. (1999). Correct utilization and management of peripherally inserted central catheters and midline catheters in the alternate care setting. *Journal of Intravenous Nursing, 22*(Suppl. 6), 46–48.

Catheter Innovations. (1999). Product literature: PASV® technology. Author.

Center For Disease Control and Prevention (1999). National Surveillance System for Health Care Workers (NaSH). Atlanta, GA: Author.

Cook Critical Care. (1999). Product literature. Elletsville, IN: Author.

Darouiche, R.O., Raad I.I., Heard, S.O., Thornby, J.I., Wenker, O.C., Gabriella, A., Berg, J., Khardori, N., Hanna, N., Hachem, R., Harris, R.L., & Mayhall, G. (1999). A comparison of two antimicrobial-impregnated central venous catheters. *New England Journal of Medicine, 240*, 1–8.

*Evidence-Based Medicine. (1998). *Urokinase for arterial occlusion.* 1(7): 6. Stamford, CT: Appleton & Lange Communications and Continuing Education Group.

*Fischer, J.E. (1991). *Total parenteral nutrition* (2nd ed., pp. 36–37). Boston: Little, Brown.

*Fitzpatrick, L.M. (1999). Care and management issues regarding central venous access devices in the home and long-term care setting. *Journal of Intravenous Nursing, 22*(6S), 40–44.

Hoffman, S. (1998). Valved catheters. *Journal Vascular Access Devices,* Summer 1998. *Journal of National Vascular Access Network,* 18–19.

*Holmes, K.R. (1998). Comparison of push-pull versus discard method from central venous catheters for blood testing. *Journal of Intravenous Nursing, 21*(5), 282–285.

*Hye, R.J., & Stabile, B.E. (1996). Complications of percutaneous vascular access procedures and their management. In S.E. Wilson (Ed.), *Vascular access: Principals and practice* (3rd ed., pp. 92–103). St. Louis: CV Mosby.

*Intravenous Nurses Society. (1998). Revised intravenous nursing standards of practice. *Journal of Intravenous Nursing, 21*(Suppl. 1), 50, 64–65, 67.

*Intravenous Nurses Society. (2000, in press). Revised intravenous nursing standards of practice.*Journal of Intravenous Nursing,* (Suppl.).

JAMA. (1998). Low molecular weight heparinoid, ORG 10172 (danaparoid), and outcome after acute ischemic stroke: A randomized controlled trial. *Journal of the American Medical Association, 279,* 1265–1272. Author.

*Jensen, B.L. (1995). In J. Terry (Ed.), *Intravenous therapy: Clinical principles and practice* (pp. 318–319). Philadelphia: W.B. Saunders.

Jones, G.R. (1998). A practical guide to evaluation and treatment of infections in patients with central venous catheters. *Journal of Intravenous Nursing, 21*(Suppl.5), 134–135.

*Krzywda, E.A. (1999). Predisposing factors, prevention, and management of central venous catheter occlusions. *Journal of Intravenous Nursing, 22*(Suppl.6), 11–14.

Luther Medical, Inc. (1999) Product literature: L-CATH® Peel Away Catheter System. 39-306. Author.

LaRue, G.D. (1999). Efficacy of ultrasonography in peripheral venous cannulation. *Journal of Intravenous Nursing 23*(1), 29–32

Lin, B.S., Kong, C.W., & Tarng, D.C. (1998) Anatomical variation of the internal jugular vein and its impact on temporary haemodialysis vascular access: An ultrasonographic survey in uraemic patients. *Nephrology Dialysis Transplant, 143;* 134–8.

*McDonald, C.L., Banerjee, S., & Jarvis, W.R. (1997). Central venous catheter-associated bloodstream infections in intensive care unit patients associated with needleless access devices, CDC. Society for Hospital Epidemiology of America Annual Meeting, St. Louis (Abstract 26).

*Metheny, N.M. (2000). *Fluid and electrolyte balance* (4th ed.). Philadelphia: Lippincott Williams & Wilkins.

*Miller, T.A. (1995). In J. Terry, (Ed.), *Intravenous therapy: Clinical principles and practice* (pp. 406–409). Philadelphia: W. B. Saunders.

National Association of Vascular Access Networks. (1999). Product literature. PICC Self Study Programs. PICC Excellence. Draper, UT: Author.

*Ouriel K., Veith, F.J., & Sasahara, A.A., for the TOPAS Investigators. (1998). A comparison of recombinant urokinase with vascular surgery as initial treatment for acute arterial occlusion of the legs. *New England Journal of Medicine, 338,* 1105–1111.

*Perucca, R. (1995). In J. Terry, (Ed.), *Intravenous therapy: Clinical principles and practice* (p. 384). Philadelphia: W.B. Saunders.

Poole, S.M. (1999). Quality issues in access device management. *Journal of Intravenous Nursing, 22*(6), S26–S19.

Raad, I. , Darouiche, R., Dupuis, J., Abi-Said, D., Gabrielli, A., Hachem, R., et al. (1997). Central venous catheters coated with minocycline and rifampin for the prevention of cathete-related colonization and blood stream infections. *Annals of Internal Medicine 128,* 267–274.

Randolph, A.G, Cook, D.J, & Gonzales, C.A. (1996). Ultrasound guidance for placement of central venous catheters: A meta-analysis of the literature. *Critical Care Medicine, 24;* 2053–8.

*Ray, C.E. (1999). Infection control principles and practices in the care and management of central venous access devices. *Journal of Intravenous Nursing, 22*(6), S18–S21.

Review Questions

Note: Questions below may have more than one right answer.

1. The term *aliquot* describes which of the following?
   A. Volume of the catheter
   B. Amount of solution equal in volume to luminal volume of catheter
   C. Amount of solution greater in volume than diameter of catheter
   D. Volume of solution needed to flush the catheter

2. Which of the following statements is true of hydrothorax?
   A. Results when IV fluid infiltrates into the lung
   B. Results when IV fluid infiltrates into the chest
   C. Has signs and symptoms identical to pneumothorax
   D. Is treated the same as pneumothorax

3. Embolism may be retrieved using what procedure?
   A. Cardiac catheterization
   B. Cardiac tamponade
   C. Embolotomy
   D. Venous ligation

4. To accurately measure central venous pressure, the zero point on the manometer should be adjusted to what level?
   A. Right atrium
   B. Patient's heart
   C. Left lung
   D. Substernal notch

5. Air embolism may be avoided using which of the following procedures:
   A. PICC insertion
   B. Valsalva maneuver
   C. Pneumocentesis
   D. Fluoroscopy

6. Which of the following is an acceptable alternative to breakaway needle insertion of a PICC catheter?
   A. Cannulization
   B. Fluoroscopy
   C. Laser
   D. Guidewire

7. Radiologic imaging guidance can facilitate access to the central veins by alternative routes, including which of the following?
   A. Inferior vena cava
   B. Collateral venous channels
   C. Basilic veins
   D. Cephalic veins

8. Fibrin sheath formation originates at what site in thrombus catheter occlusion?
   A. Intimal injury
   B. Where catheter enters vessel
   C. Where catheter tip touches the intima
   D. All of the above

9. Organisms that may lead to rapid progression of clinical symptoms in the patient with a central venous access device include all of the following *except*:
   A. *Escherichia coli*
   B. *Pseudomonas pneumoniae*
   C. Vancomycin-resistant *Staphylococcus*
   D. Newer strains of antibiotic-resistant *Streptococcus* species

10. Radiologic testing for catheter occlusion includes all of the following tests *except*:
    A. Chest radiograph
    B. Air-contrast study
    C. Venogram
    D. Duplex scan

CHAPTER 14

Advanced Vascular

Access

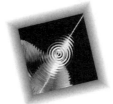

K E Y   T E R M S

Collagen Matrix
Fibrinolysis
Hemodynamic Monitoring
Intraosseous Infusion

Peel-away Sheaths
Tunneled Lines
Ventricular Reservoir

■ IMPROVEMENTS IN VASCULAR ACCESS DEVICES

Vascular access has become a highly complex area of nursing specialization. With newer and more advanced therapies available to patients with diverse clinical needs, the infusion therapy nurse specialist must remain abreast of changes in this exciting field. In all clinical settings, a working knowledge of advanced vascular access is an essential part of IV nursing care. Nowhere is this more evident than in the care of the critically ill patient, in whom central venous access is a basic component of patient care. Central line access facilitates **hemodynamic monitoring** as well as administration of fluids, blood products, medications, and nutritional solutions.

Central vascular access devices include **tunneled lines,** implanted ports, pumps, and reservoirs, and a diversity of central venous catheter products, including single-, double-, and triple-lumen catheters with and without J wires, with and without introducer needles, and with and without **peel-away sheaths.** Each product aims to simplify infusion therapy in a safe, efficient manner (see Chap. 13).

Catheter Properties, Materials, and Complications

The ideal central venous catheter would be composed of a material that inhibits thrombus formation, inserts easily, and is biocompatible and radiopaque (Box 14–1).

The deep vein thrombosis associated with central venous access has many contributing factors. Any foreign material in the bloodstream becomes coated with a protein and fibrin deposit. This in turn activates internal coagulation, causing platelet activation and platelet adherence to the catheter. Damage to endothelial cells at the puncture site also promotes platelet activation. Patients requiring central venous catheters often have activated coagulation systems because of trauma or severe disease, both of which also promote the development of central venous catheter thrombosis. Thrombosis may be limited to a fibrin sheath formation or may be severe enough to occlude the vein. It may have no clinical significance, or it may result in a fatal pulmonary embolism (Bagnall-Reed, 1998; Krzywda, 1999; Metheny, 2000).

BOX 14–1 **Catheter Materials**

Polyvinylchloride/Teflon

- Stiff
- Causes damage to the tunica intima
- Increased risk of platelet aggregation and subsequent thrombus formation
- Limited to subclavian or jugular insertion owing to lack of flexibility

Polyurethane

- Rigid during insertion but softens at body temperature
- Less thrombogenicity
- Can be used at all sites

Silicone Elastomer/Silastic

- Very flexible
- Minimal thrombus formation
- Biocompatible
- Good for long-term use
- Dramatic fibrin sheath formation when particulate matter is present; rinse gloves and catheter before insertion

Elastomeric Hydrogel

- Available in peripheral lines
- Combines stretchable polymer with hydrophilic substance (water absorbing and similar to extended-wear contact lenses)
- Rinse with normal saline solution; easier to insert

Biocompatibility

The property of biocompatibility or bioinertness in a material indicates that the tissues of the body do not react to the material as a foreign substance. Silicone is the most bioinert material in use in the manufacturing process. Most central venous catheters are made of polyvinylchloride, Teflon (DuPont, Wilmington, DE), polyurethane, or silicone.

Polyvinylchloride was the first catheter material. High incidences of thrombosis have been associated with this material (Blum, 1999; Intravenous Nurses Society [INS], 1998, 2000; Ray, 1999). Currently, most central venous catheters are made of less thrombogenic materials.

Teflon catheters are easily inserted because they are relatively stiff. However, they are associated with a high incidence of thrombus formation (INS, 1998, 2000).

Polyurethane is only moderately firm, so it is not as easily inserted. Thrombus formation is reported to be less than with Teflon, and hydromer-coated polyurethane catheters reportedly have a lower incidence of thrombus formation (INS, 1998, 2000a, 2000b).

Silicone catheters are very soft, much like a wet noodle, so they require special mechanisms for insertion. They are associated with the lowest incidence of thrombus formation and the material is suitable for multiple-lumen catheters. The silicone catheter is an excellent long-term central catheter for use in all clinical settings.

Radiopaque catheters, which can be visualized by radiologic means, are available in all materials. This property is required to confirm catheter tip placement after insertion.

Bonding to Prevent Septicemia

The most frequently occurring life-threatening complication of central venous catheterization is septicemia. Most infections derive from invasion of the catheter wound by organisms from the patient's cutaneous microflora. Studies of a bonded catheter, in which a triple-lumen polyurethane central venous catheter was impregnated with antimicrobial silver sulfadiazine and chlorhexidine, indicate that use of such catheter may substantially reduce the incidence of catheter-related infection. This improvement would extend the time that such a line may safely remain in place. Moreover, it is cost effective (Arrow, 1998; Darouiche et al., 1999; Ray, 1999).

A catheter manufactured by Arrow, Reading, PA, uses a cuff known as Vita-cuff. The cuff is composed of two concentric layers of materials: an inner silicone sleeve that secures the cuff in place around a catheter, and an outer **collagen matrix.** The collagen matrix is made from purified type I bovine tendon collagen. Silver ions are chelated to the collagen matrix. Silver possesses a broad antimicrobial spectrum and has been used extensively in topical antimicrobial preparations in burn patients. The cuff, with introducer attached, is placed around a catheter before catheter insertion. The catheter is inserted percutaneously to the desired level. Then, the cuff is placed subcutaneously with the introducer, which is then separated from the cuff. After insertion, subcutaneous tissue grows into the collagenous matrix, anchoring the catheter and creating a barrier against invasion by extrinsic organisms. Significant antimicrobial activity associated with the Arrow catheter has been demonstrated using zone of inhibition bioassays against a number of organisms.

Cook Critical Care's (Bloomington, IN) Spectrum is a central venous catheter impregnated with a unique combination of the antibiotics minocycline and rifampin. A proprietary process provides antibiotic coverage on both the external and internal surfaces of the catheter to reduce the rates of both catheter colonization and catheter-related bloodstream infection (Cook Critical Care, 1999). Studies (Raad et al., 1997) have demonstrated efficacy against *Staphylococcus aureus, Staphylococcus epidermidis, Enterococcus faecalis, Acinetobacter baumanii, Stenotrophomonas maltophilia, Klebsiella pneumoniae, Enterobacter* species, *Escherichia coli, Proteus mirabilis, Pseudomonas aeruginosa,* and *Candida albicans.* Precautions should be taken in patients with known allergy to tetracycline or its derivatives.

Research Issues: ANTIMICROBIAL-IMPREGNATED CENTRAL VENOUS CATHETERS

Darouiche, R. O., Raad, I. I., Heard, S. O., Thornby, J. I., Wenker, O. C., Gabriella, A., Berg, J., Khardori, N., Hanna, H., Hachem, R., Harris, R. L., & Mayhall, G. (1999). A comparison of two antimicrobial-impregnated central venous catheters. *New England Journal of Medicine, 340,* 1–8.

Methods: The authors conducted a prospective, randomized clinical trial in 12 university-affiliated hospitals. High-risk adult patients in whom central venous catheters were expected to remain in place for 3 or more days were randomly assigned to undergo insertion of polyurethane triple-lumen catheters (impregnated with either minocycline and rifampin on both the luminal and external surfaces or with chlorhexidine and silver sulfadiazine on the external surface only).

Findings: Of 865 catheters inserted, 738 (85%) produced culture results that could be evaluated. Catheters impregnated with minocycline and rifampin were one third as likely to be colonized as catheters impregnated with chlorhexidine and silver sulfadiazine.

Conclusions: Central venous catheters impregnated with minocycline and rifampin are associated with a lower rate of infection than catheters impregnated with chlorhexidine and silver sulfadiazine.

Catheter Designs

The design of the catheter device is frequently related to the properties of the catheter material. The design also dictates insertion methods.

Catheter With Removable Introducer

Catheters with removable introducers are frequently made of polyurethane; a wide variety of products are available from today's manufacturers. These products have been developed with safety standards in mind in an effort to minimize the incidence of needlestick injury (see Chap. 11).

COMPONENTS AND FEATURES

The unit consists of an introducer catheter or syringe and needle and a catheter with stylet.

A catheter with a removable introducer is a single-lumen catheter with a fairly easy method of insertion. Because the device is usually made of polyurethane, it is softer than Teflon and easier to thread through twists and curves. Removal of any sharp needle eliminates the risk of catheter embolism. Because thrombus formation can be a problem with polyurethane, this may not be the catheter of choice for long-term therapy. However, minimal thrombus formation has been reported with hydromer-coated polyurethane and long-term use.

INSERTION TECHNIQUE

The venipuncture is performed with the needle and syringe. The syringe is removed and the catheter threaded through the needle. The needle is withdrawn from the vein and removed from the catheter by splitting the needle into two parts.

Catheter With Introducer and Guidewire

A safety catheter with an introducer and guidewire allows for the insertion of a multiple-lumen silicone catheter.

COMPONENTS AND FEATURES

The unit consists of a syringe and needle or an over-the-needle catheter (ONC), a long central catheter, and a guidewire.

INSERTION TECHNIQUE

The venipuncture is performed with the syringe and needle or safety-type ONC. The syringe or stylet is removed. The guidewire is threaded through the short catheter or needle, and the short catheter or needle is withdrawn (usually into a self-contained locking cover to avoid needlestick injury). The puncture site may be enlarged with a no. 1 scalpel blade. The long catheter is threaded over the guidewire, which is then withdrawn, leaving the long catheter in the vein (Fig. 14–1).

Tunneled Catheters

Originally available as a Broviac catheter and later modified with a larger diameter by Hickman and associates, today's tunneled right atrial catheter is made of silicone and is available in a single-, double-, and triple-lumen configuration (Fig. 14–2). Many tunneled lines feature an integral catheter clamp and a reinforced segment of catheter to reduce the risk of silicone fatigue after repeated clamping.

COMPONENTS AND FEATURES

This single- or double-lumen catheter contains a Dacron cuff. The external end has a "ring" with a threaded Luer-lock adapter covered with a Luer-lock cap. An integral clamp may be present. One version of this catheter has a closed tip and a lateral two-

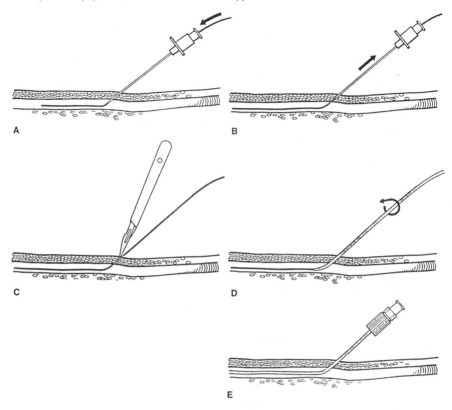

Figure 14–1. Insertion technique for catheter with introducer and guidewire. (A) The guidewire is threaded through the inserted needle. (B) The needle is withdrawn from the vein. (C) The puncture site may be enlarged with a no. 11 scalpel blade. (D) The catheter is threaded over the guidewire. (E) The guidewire is withdrawn, leaving the catheter in the vein. (Courtesy of Cook Critical Care, Bloomington, IN.)

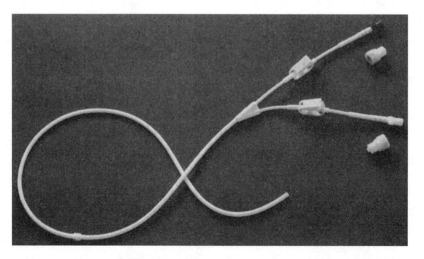

Figure 14–2. Dual-lumen Hickman catheter. (Courtesy, Davol, Inc., subsidiary of CR Bard Inc., Salt Lake City, UT.)

way valve. The valve opens outward for infusion and inward for blood sample drawing. This model does not require heparin flush to maintain catheter patency.

INSERTION TECHNIQUE

The insertion may be performed by cutdown or percutaneous puncture. This is performed under fluoroscopy, usually in a minor surgery operating room. The catheter is placed by locating the subclavian vein, forming a tunnel from the vein to an area between the sternum and the nipple, pulling the catheter through the tunnel, inserting it into the vein, and threading it until the tip is in the superior vena cava.

Tunneled Hickman

Fibrous tissue forms around the Dacron cuff of the Hickman catheter. The cuff and the tunnel anchor the catheter and help prevent infection. Because the catheter is made of polymeric silicone, it is associated with a lower incidence of thrombus formation. It is a perfect central venous catheter for home IV therapy. This catheter is also inserted for long-term inpatient use (Fig. 14–3).

Dual-Lumen Hickman

When a dual-lumen Hickman catheter is used, the lumens should be labeled to indicate the purpose and function of each. Catheter insertion is performed as a surgical procedure, through a cutdown in which the vein is isolated and the catheter is inserted. After locating the catheter tip in the central vein, the remaining portion is threaded or tunneled into the subcutaneous tissue 3 to 5 cm to an exit site outside the skin. Typical exit sites are below the nipple, in the abdomen, or in the groin. A Dacron cuff is an integral part of the tunneled line and extends from the exit site. Granulation tissue forms around the cuff in 10 to 14 days, preventing migration of microorganisms into the catheter pathway.

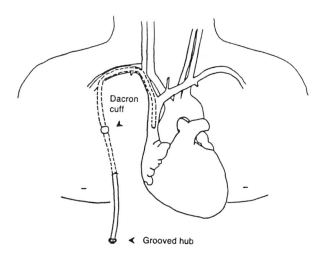

Figure 14–3. Insertion of indwelling tunneled catheter. The catheter is advanced through a tunnel formed from the vein to an area between the sternum and the nipple. The catheter tip is placed in the superior vena cava.

Groshong Catheter

Manufacturers continue to provide more advanced product options. In addition to the Hickman and Broviac catheters and their multiple-lumen styles, the Groshong catheter (Davol, Salt Lake City, UT) is distinguished by a rounded, blunt catheter tip that incorporates a three-way valve. This three-position pressure-sensitive valve remains closed at normal vena caval pressure to restrict either entry of air into the venous system or backflow of blood from the catheter.

GROSHONG VALVE

Application of a vacuum with a syringe allows the valve to open inward for blood aspiration (Fig. 14–4). Positive pressure into the catheter by the infusion forces the valve to open outward. Advantages of this type of catheter include

- Decreased risk of bleeding or air emboli
- Elimination of catheter clamping
- Elimination of the use of heparin in the catheter
- Reduction of flushing between use

For the valve to function properly, catheter tip position is critical. The tip must be situated in the mid-superior part of the vena cava. If the tip is in the right atrium, thrombus formation around the tip could result, followed by malfunction and loss of valve competence.

Occasional use of a fibrinolytic agent may restore valve function. Clamping and flushing with heparin, similar to the procedure followed with nonvalved catheters, may be needed.

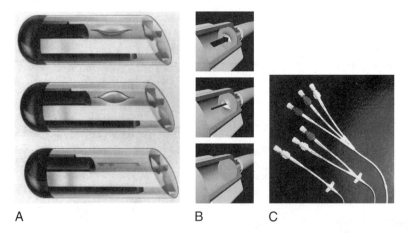

A   B   C

Figure 14–4. Valves such as (A) the Groshong (Davol, Inc., a subsidiary of CR Bard, Inc., Salt Lake City, UT) and (B) the pressure-activated safety valve (PASV; Catheter Innovations) are used in (C) single-, double-, and triple-lumen catheters to facilitate aspiration and infusion. When not at work, the valve remains closed.

PRESSURE-ACTIVATED SAFETY VALVE

Catheter Innovations, Sandy, UT, has developed a unique pressure-activated safety valve (PASV) that is applicable to vascular access products. The PASV was designed to improve patient outcomes by reducing the complications associated with vascular access. The patented valve opens with minimal positive pressure for infusion, yet requires four times as much negative pressure for aspiration. This feature reduces the risk of air embolism or bleedout resulting from an accidental disconnect. The PASV also reduces the reflux of blood into the end of the catheter during periods of increased central venous pressure. Weekly saline-only flushing is needed, and the product is consistent with needleless systems. The valve may also be used with peripherally inserted central catheters and midline catheters (see Chap. 13 and Fig. 14–4).

Ports and Pumps

Totally implanted devices for repeated venous access eliminate the need for frequent venipunctures. Implanted ports are intended for long-term use, and extreme care must be taken to maintain sterile technique while performing any manipulations.

Implanted Ports

An implanted port consists of a silicone catheter attached to a reservoir with a self-sealing septum (Fig. 14–5). The unit illustrated here is known as a Port-A-Cath (SIMS Deltec, St. Paul, MN), although several manufacturers make this type of device with either a single- or double-lumen access port. Special noncoring needles are required to access these devices.

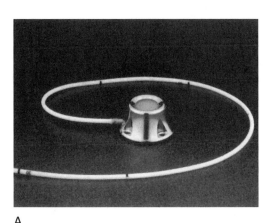
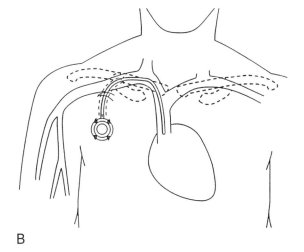

A   B

Figure 14–5. A. The Port-A-Cath Venous Access System with Poly Flow catheter (SIMS Deltec, St. Paul, MN) is an example of an implantable port positioned (B) centrally. Drug delivery through the port allows the patient greater freedom and mobility.

COMPONENTS AND FEATURES

Implanted ports are associated with a low incidence of thrombus formation from the silicone catheter. When not in use, the only care required is a monthly heparin flush. The fact that this is totally implanted, leaving no catheter exiting from the chest, makes it a favorite device with many patients. It is an "artificial vein" ideal for any patient receiving long-term periodic infusion therapy in the home or in the hospital.

Implanted ports permit repeated long-term access to the vascular system. In general, the portal consists of one or two self-sealing silicone septa, accessible by percutaneous needle puncture. As with any central venous access system, many potential complications exist, ranging from air embolism to thrombosis. For an overview of potential complications, see Box 14–2.

The implanted port may be used for arterial access or implanted into the epidural space, peritoneum, pericardium, or pleural cavity. Vascular access ports may be side entry or top entry. In a side-entry port, the needle is inserted almost parallel to the reservoir. In a top-entry port, the needle is inserted perpendicular to the reservoir.

BOX 14–2 Complications Associated With Implanted Ports

- Air embolism
- Artery or vein puncture
- Arteriovenous fistula
- Brachial plexus injury
- Cardiac arrhythmia
- Cardiac puncture
- Cardiac tamponade
- Catheter disconnection/fragmentation/embolization
- Catheter occlusion
- Catheter rupture
- Drug extravasation
- Erosion of portal/catheter through skin and/or blood vessel
- Fibrin sheath formation
- Hematoma
- Hemothorax
- Implant rejection
- Infection/sepsis
- Migration of portal/catheter
- Pneumothorax
- Thoracic duct injury
- Thromboembolism
- Thrombosis

Current advances in port technology are exemplified by the the MRI Port designed by Davol. This port is designed to eliminate interference caused by metal ports during magnetic resonance imaging or computed tomography.

INSERTION TECHNIQUE

The port is surgically placed with the patient receiving either a local or general anesthetic. The insertion technique is similar to that used for implanted-tunneled catheters. The catheter is placed in the subclavian vein and threaded into the vein until the tip lies in the superior vena cava. This position is confirmed by fluoroscopy. A pocket is made for the reservoir. The reservoir is sutured in the pocket. Because the center of the port will be punctured repeatedly, when the pocket is closed the suture line is lateral, medial, superior, or inferior to the port septum (see Fig. 14–5).

Port Needles

Only noncoring needles should be used to access a port. A noncoring needle has an angled or deflected point that slices the septum on entry. When removed, the septum reseals itself. Noncoring needles are available in straight and 90-degree angle configurations, with or without extension sets. Some clinicians recommend the use of an ONC with needleless connector for continuous access to an implanted port.

Straight safety needles are used for heparin flush, bolus injection, or blood drawing. Needles bent to a 90-degree angle are used for continuous or frequent intermittent infusions. The bent needle may also be used for heparin flush, bolus injection, or blood drawing. Noncoring needles are also available with a permanently attached extension tubing and clamp.

Needles are available with metal or plastic hubs, in gauges 24 to 19, and in lengths from 0.5 to 2.5 inches. The required needle length depends on how superficially or deeply the septum lies. The needle gauge depends on the type and rate of infusate to be given. Packed red blood cells may require a 19-gauge needle, whereas a 24-gauge needle may be adequate for flushing.

The needle must meet safety specifications; caution should be used to avoid injecting the drug into the subcutaneous tissue. An angular motion or twist of the needle must be avoided once the needle is seated in the septum to prevent cutting the septum and creating a path for drug leakage. If the heparin flush is performed without extension tubing, 3 mL heparin (100 U/mL) is used. If extension tubing is used, 5 mL heparin may be required. Again, the manufacturer's recommendations assist in developing institutional policy.

Totally Implanted Pumps

Totally implanted pumps are designed for continuous, low-volume, long-term ambulatory therapy. They may be used for arterial or venous infusion and tissue perfusion. The implanted pump provides long-term venous or arterial access, which is a safe treatment vehicle for patients who have chronic disease or who need a direct infusion targeted for a tumor or organ. Decreased infection rate and enhanced patient mobility are advantages of an implanted pumps.

COMPONENTS AND FEATURES

The implanted pump consists of two chambers separated by flexible metal bellows. One chamber is the drug–infusate compartment. The vapor pressure of the charging fluid exerts a constant pressure on the bellows, forcing the drug out of the reservoir through an outlet filter and flow restrictor into a silicone catheter (Fig. 14–6). When the pump is refilled, the increasing pressure in the drug chamber exerts a pressure on the charging fluid, causing the fluid vapor to condense to its liquid state, and thereby storing energy for the next pumping cycle.

Various models are available. The basic device has one catheter. Another model also has a direct access port that bypasses the reservoir for administering bolus injections. Yet another model has double catheters, which can be used to administer a drug to more than one site. The silicone catheter results in a low incidence of thrombus formation.

Delivering solution by pump is an excellent method for continuous long-term administration of low-volume narcotics or antineoplastic agents to patients with cancer. Because there are no external parts, the pump requires no care between refills.

Several factors influence the pump flow rate. If the catheter site is arterial and arterial blood pressure increases significantly, the flow rate can decrease by as much as 15%. Hypotension can increase the rate by as much as 6%. When the patient moves from one altitude to another, the rate can increase by as much as 38%. Fever can increase the flow rate by as much as 13%. The amount of drug in the reservoir also affects the flow rate. The pump flow rate is established with the reservoir half full. At full volume, the rate is approximately 3% faster and at low volume 3% slower than the mean flow rate.

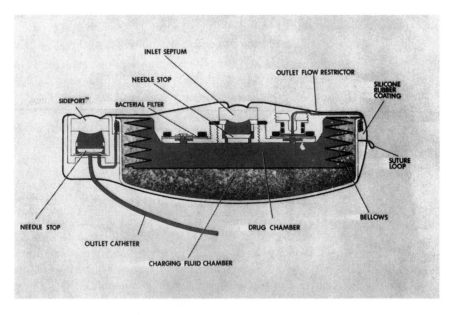

Figure 14–6. Components of the Arrow/Infusaid implanted pump. (Courtesy of Arrow International, Reading, PA.)

Criteria for using implanted pumps include histologically proven primary or metastatic hepatic cancer, absence of extrahepatic disease or malignant ascites, measurable hepatic disease, satisfactory condition for major surgery, and absence of acute infection or prolonged fever.

INSERTION TECHNIQUE

The pump is implanted in the operating room under fluoroscopic guidance. The insertion is performed during laparotomy, in which the infusion catheter is threaded through a gastric artery to a common hepatic artery. The catheter is then sutured in place and the feeding arteries are ligated. A pump pocket is prepared, usually below the umbilicus on the abdomen, and the pump is sutured to the underlying fascia. An infusate is injected into the pump reservoir and remains in place for 4 to 6 postoperative days. Then, the pump is emptied and filled with an initial dose of medication.

To activate the charging fluid, the pump must be heated for 30 minutes at 30°C to 40°C before implantation. This is done with a heating pad.

CONTRAINDICATIONS

Contraindications to the implanted pump include body size that cannot support the size and weight of the pump; severe emotional, psychiatric, or neurologic disturbances; and a lifestyle that involves extensive travel or frequent altitudinal changes. In addition, only small volumes of drugs can be delivered by an implanted pump, so the device is unsuitable for patients needing greater volumes of medication.

Intraosseous Access Devices

Intraosseous infusion may be considered when instances of venous collapse in shock, anatomic scarcity of veins, and thrombosis of venous sites preclude the ability to establish peripheral venous access. First proposed in 1922 by Drinker, intraosseous infusion of IV fluids was initiated in 1934, particularly for shock, pediatric emergencies, adults with mutilated skin, and transport of uncooperative patients. The technique has endured, despite dwindling interest after the advent of disposable needles and catheters. Commonly administered fluids were colloids, crystalline solutions, plasma, blood products, antibiotics, epinephrine, morphine, and glucose. A renewed acceptance and interest in the technique as a viable alternative to peripheral or central venous access has grown since the 1970s.

Current indications for intraosseous infusion are anaphylaxis, burns, cardiac arrest, coma, dehydration, drowning, respiratory arrest, septic shock, hypovolemia, diabetic acidosis, status epilepticus, status asthmaticus, trauma, and sudden infant death syndrome. Standard protocol calls for establishing an intraosseous line in children if percutaneous peripheral venous access cannot be established within 60 to 120 seconds. It may be the route of choice in event of cardiac arrest or hypotension.

Bones are vascular structures with dynamic circulation capable of accepting large volumes of fluid and rapidly transporting fluids or drugs to the central circulation (Fuentes-Afflick, 1990; INS, 1998, 2000a, 2000b; Metheny, 2000). Long bones consist of a shaft called the diaphysis with a very dense cortex, the epiphysis (or the rounded ends of the bone), and the metaphysis (the transitional zone). The epiphysis and the metaphysis have a much thinner cortex and contain cancellous, or spongy, bone. The iliac crest is made of a thin cortex and is filled with cancellous bone. The hollow core of the shaft of long bones and the spaces within the cancellous bone are referred to as the *medullary space,* which contains the marrow.

The marrow cavity has been appropriately called the *noncollapsible vein* (Fuentes-Afflick, 1990). Comprising a highly interconnected network of venous sinusoids, analogous to a sponge, the intramedullary space is an integral part of the vascular system. Nutrient arteries that penetrate the cortex of the bone supply the marrow. Many bone sites have been used for intraosseous infusions, including the sternum, the tibia (Fig. 14–7), the femur, and the iliac crest. In children younger than 5 years of age, the site of choice is the flat anterior medial surface of the proximal tibia just below the tibial tubercle or the distal tibia, followed by the distal femur (Fuentes-Afflick, 1990). In adults, the iliac crest or sternum is the bone of choice (INS, 2000a). Strict asepsis is essential and the skin preparation should be consistent with INS Standards of Practice (INS, 1998, 2000a). Local anesthetics may be used for conscious patients.

Intraosseous Needles: Osteoport

COMPONENTS AND FEATURES

Appropriate access needles include standard steel hypodermic, spinal, trephine, sternal, and standard bone marrow needles. The needle must be able to stand without support once the stylet is removed, and it must facilitate aspiration of blood and marrow. The standards throughout the industry for intraosseous needles have been the Kormed/Jamshidi bone marrow biopsy needle, the Osgood needle, and the Cook intraosseous infusion needle. These products come in several sizes and with various tips. A needle with a short shaft prevents dislodgment (INS, 2000a, 2000b).

The osteoport was developed by Von Hoff and colleagues, who patented the device as an intramedullary catheter (Fig. 14–8). Threads were added to the needle so that it could be placed precisely within the marrow and at the same time decrease complications of insertion. The device is made of medical implant–grade titanium,

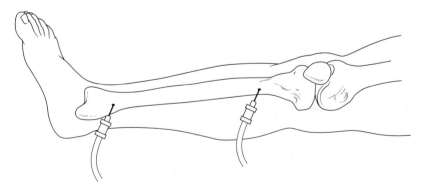

Figure 14–7. Possible insertion sites of percutaneous intraosseous infusion device in the lower extremity.

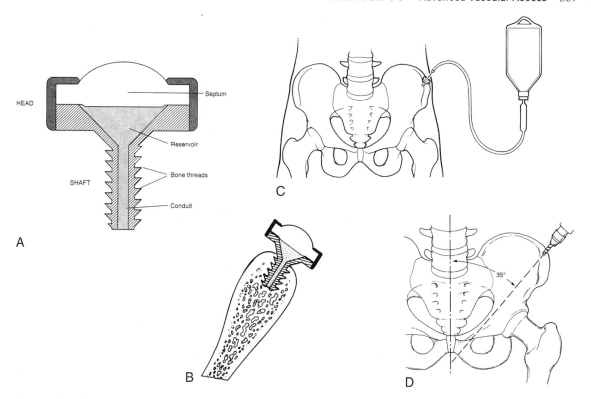

Figure 14–8. (A, B) Osteoport and osteoport in place in a bone. (C, D) are additional sites for intraosseous infusion.

with thread size and shape identical to those of commonly accepted orthopedic devices. The membrane is a medically implantable grade of Silastic (the same material commonly used in IV catheters and other implanted ports).

To decrease leakage, a cone was added to provide a tight seal between the bone and the osteoport. To decrease the rate of osteomyelitis and cellulitis, the osteoport was made implantable, thereby eliminating any direct conduit from outside the body into the bone marrow. To increase patient comfort, the osteoport has a low profile and does not require a stiff needle protruding through the skin. Rather, the port is a hollow, 1-inch titanium or stainless steel needle with a self-sealing cap. It resembles a partially threaded bolt (see Fig. 14–8). Repeated bone punctures are not required for repeated use (Blum, 1999; Fuentes-Afflick, 1990; Holmes, 1998; INS, 1998, 2000a, 2000b).

To initiate the flow of fluids, a needle attached to the IV tubing is inserted through the skin into the cap of the osteoport. The physician locates the device by feeling it under the skin. Because it is implanted in bone, the device promotes rapid absorption by the blood from the marrow cavity, eliminates clotting and lung puncture problems, and reduces the risk of infection. It is indicated for patients who require access to the vascular system but who have exhausted all other reasonable IV sites. The recommended duration of implant is less than 30 days (Fuentes-Afflick, 1990).

INSERTION TECHNIQUE

After the patient receives a local or general anesthetic, the intraosseous needle is quickly advanced through the skin to the bony cortex. With firm pressure and a rotary motion, the needle is further advanced into the marrow cavity. Insertion resistance decreases as the needle penetrates the cortex (known as the "trap-door effect"). The stylet is removed and the correct position is verified by observing the needle standing without support and the ability to aspirate blood and marrow contents. In adults, the device is usually implanted in a large bone of the hip or leg. Once the incision is closed, the device is ready for use and a continuous infusion can begin (INS, 1998, 2000a, 2000b; Metheny, 2000).

If the attempt at implantation is unsuccessful, further attempts must be undertaken in other bones. If an infusion was established in the same bone, the infused fluid would leak from the original abandoned hole in the cortex.

Ventricular Reservoirs

The implanted **ventricular reservoir** provides direct access to the cerebrospinal fluid (CSF) without performing a spinal tap. The reservoir is also used to measure CSF pressure, obtain CSF specimens, and instill medication. Implanted surgically, it is positioned in the right frontal region's lateral ventricle, sutured to the pericranium, and covered with a skin flap (see Chap. 20).

Major complications associated with ventricular reservoirs include infection, malfunction, and displacement. Infection is characterized by tenderness, redness, drainage, fever, neck stiffness, and headache with or without vomiting (Karavelis, Foroglou, Selviaridis, & Fountzilas, 1996).

Malfunction typically results when the catheter is obstructed by the distal subarachnoid blockage of CSF. This is characterized by the inability to aspirate or inject the port and slow refilling of the reservoir after manual expression of fluid.

Catheter displacement or migration is also characterized by slow or absent refilling of the reservoir after manual expression of fluid. The complication is confirmed by computed tomography and change in neurologic status. See the accompanying display for information on how to access fluid specimens and administer medication through the ventricular reservoir.

■ ADVANCES IN COMPLICATION PREVENTION

Catheter occlusion presents a serious problem, particularly if the occlusion is caused by a blood clot. In advanced practice, various techniques may be implemented by the skilled infusion nurse to prevent clotting and thereby avoid complications.

General Flushing and Commonly Used Solutions

Basic measures include injecting the heparin flush solution and clamping the catheter shut before the syringe is completely empty. Then, the syringe and needle

---

KEY INTERVENTIONS: Withdrawing and Infusing Fluids by
Ventricular Reservoir

---

1. Explain procedure to the patient and family and assemble supplies in one place.
2. Obtain the patient's vital signs.
3. Position patient comfortably. Trendelenburg position is recommended because it makes use of gravity to promote specimen collection.
4. Wash hands and put on gloves and a mask.
5. Using aseptic technique, open supply packages on a sterile field.
6. If appropriate, clip scalp hair over the port to facilitate access.
7. Swab area vigorously with povidone–iodine (Betadine) solution, in concentric circles to clean an area 2 inches in diameter.
8. Repeat skin preparation and allow skin to air dry.
9. Remove and discard gloves; then apply new sterile gloves.
10. Attach syringe to a 23- or 25-gauge winged infusion set.
11. Using the nondominant hand, palpate and stabilize the reservoir port. (Keep in mind that this hand in now no longer sterile.)
12. Puncture the reservoir obliquely with a 23- or 25-gauge needle.
13. Withdraw 3 mL of cerebrospinal fluid (CSF). Detach syringe and place it on the sterile field.
14. For syringe administration:

    a. Attach the syringe containing medication to the access needle. A $0.2-\mu m$ surfactant-free filter should be used.
    b. Administer medication as prescribed over 5 minutes. Monitor the patient's response during administration and immediately thereafter for nausea and vomiting, headache, or dizziness.
    c. Detach medication syringe and attach the syringe with 3 mL of reserved CSF.

15. For continuous infusion:

    a. Attach administration set to access needle.
    b. Administer medication as prescribed using an electronic infusion device with anti–free flow protection.
    c. Detach infusion set and attach the syringe with 3 mL of reserved CSF.

16. Flush the reservoir with the CSF.
17. Maintaining positive pressure on the syringe, withdraw the access needle.
18. Apply gentle pressure over the site with sterile gauze.
19. Instruct the patient to remain in supine position without a pillow for 30 minutes after this procedure.
20. Discard biohazardous waste in accord with institutional policy.
21. Document the intervention in the clinical record.

---

are removed while pressure is applied on the plunger. This prevents reflux of blood into the lumen that may result in catheter clotting. When the catheter is not in use, the nurse can tape the hub to the chest wall above heart level. This minimizes blood pressure at the catheter tip.

Routine flushing is also required to maintain patency of unused catheters. If the catheter has more than one lumen, the unused lumens must also be flushed. Either heparin or saline solution may be used, consistent with the manufacturer's specifications and institutional policy. An example of a product that allows the clinician to flush the catheter without changing an intermittent injection cap/needleless (latex-free) adaptor is the Tubex Injector by Wyeth (Radnor, PA; Fig. 14–9).

Flush Solutions

Most manufacturers recommend the use of saline as a flush solution. In those products in which heparin is suggested, familiarity with the internal lumen of the catheter ensures appropriate flushing technique. Implanted catheters require heparin flushing after each use and monthly when not in use. This is almost universally done with 3 to 5 mL of 100 U/mL heparin (Table 14–1).

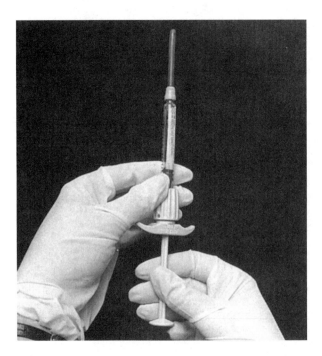

Figure 14–9   Using a flush solution injector such as the Tubex Injector (Courtesy of Wyeth Ayerst Laboratories, Radnor, PA) promotes safety and saves time. The nurse needs only a smooth-blade catheter clamp, one syringe (safety) prefilled with flush solution, one povidone–iodine swab, tape, and gloves. Once the hands are thoroughly washed, dried, and gloved, the nurse prepares the air-purged flush solution, removes the tape holding the catheter to the chest wall, cleans the rubber end of the injection port with the povidone–iodine swab for 30 seconds, and allows the site to dry. Next, while keeping the catheter hub stable, the nurse carefully inserts the connector end of the flush syringe into the center of the injection port and gently injects the solution. Then the catheter is clamped before the syringe is completely empty and the syringe withdrawn in a way that prevents air from entering the system. The clamp is removed and the catheter retaped to the chest above heart level.

TABLE 14-1

CARE OF VASCULAR ACCESS DEVICES

Type	Flush	Frequency	Set Change	Dressing Change
Percutaneous	10–100 IU heparin* = 2 times the capacity of tubing and extensions	Daily to weekly	Primary and secondary q48h consistent with institutional policy; TPN q24h; use Luer lock connections	Gauze: q48h, PRN TSM: 2–7 days or PRN Note: consistent with manufacturer's recommendations and institutional policy
PICCs	10–100 IU heparin = 2 times the capacity of tubing (1 mL) and extensions	Daily	Same as above	Same as above Gently remove existing dressing by pulling upward to avoid dislodgment
Tunneled	10–100 IU heparin = 2 times the capacity of tubing (4 mL) and extensions	Daily to weekly	Same as above	Same as above Hydrogen peroxide may be used to remove crusts; soap and water is adequate for exit site after healing occurs
	Groshong: 5 mL of 0.9% sodium chloride solution	Weekly		
Implanted port	10–100 IU heparin = 2 times the capacity of tubing (3 mL) and extensions	NA	Same as above	Same as above No dressing needed once healing has occurred; device may be secured using Steri-Strips; change noncoring needle weekly.

PRN, as needed; TPN, total parenteral nutrition; TSM, transparent semipermeable membrane; NA, not applicable; PICC, peripherally inserted catheter.

*Saline solution may be used for percutaneous catheters consistent with institutional policy and manufacturer's recommendations.

Flushing When Discontinuing Infusion

To discontinue an infusion, the nurse maintains catheter patency using a heparin flush solution and an injection, but first the catheter is flushed with normal saline solution to rinse the IV fluid from the catheter. If the catheter is made of a material that cannot be clamped without possible damage and there is no extension tubing that can be clamped, the patient must perform the Valsalva maneuver any time the catheter is open to the air.

KEY INTERVENTIONS: Safety and Clot Prevention When Discontinuing an Infusion

The following steps may be used to flush the catheter tubing when discontinuing the infusion. The intervention can also be used when connecting an injection cap and flushing the catheter with normal saline and heparin solutions consistent with institutional guidelines. The equipment needed to perform the procedure includes 1 smooth-blade catheter clamp; 3 povidone–iodine swabs; 2 to 4 Luer-lock injection ports or caps needleless connectors; 1 alcohol sponge; 1 prefilled syringe containing flush solution; a 10-mL syringe; 10 mL of 0.9% sodium chloride (normal saline) solution; a sterile 2 × 2-inch sponge; a 22-gauge, 1-inch safety needle; tape; 1 pair of sterile gloves (optional).

Procedure

1. Thoroughly wash and dry hands, then aseptically open all sterile supplies.
2. Prepare air-purged 10 mL 0.9% sodium chloride solution with the 22-gauge, 1-inch needle.
3. Prepare air-purged flush solution.
4. Shut off infusion and clamp catheter.
5. Remove existing tape from catheter filter–IV tubing connection and cleanse the connection with povidone–iodine swab for 30 seconds.
6. Place connection on sterile 2 × 2-inch sponge and allow to dry.
7. Put on gloves as preferred. Pick up connection by holding catheter hub with the sterile sponge.
8. Aseptically disconnect infusion tubing and discard.
9. Aseptically connect and lock injection port needleless connector.
10. Remove clamp from catheter.
11. Cleanse rubber end of injection port with povidone–iodine for 30 seconds and allow it to dry.
12. Carefully insert safety needle of the syringe or the needleless safety syringe containing 0.9% sodium chloride flush solution into center of injection port and inject the solution.
13. While still holding the catheter hub, remove the empty syringe/connector and reclean the injection port end with povidone–iodine for 30 seconds. Allow to dry.
14. Carefully insert needle or needleless connector of heparin or other flush solution. Do not force insertion.
15. Inject the solution and, before the syringe is completely empty, close the catheter clamp.
16. Remove syringe and needle/needleless connector while applying pressure on the plunger during withdrawal.
17. Remove clamp.
18. Secure injection port to catheter with Luer-locking device.
19. Tape catheter hub on the chest wall above heart level.

Changing Injection/Access Ports or Caps

The injection/access port or intermittent injection cap must be changed at routine intervals. The integrity of the port should be confirmed before and immediately after each use. If compromised, it should be immediately replaced. Otherwise, the port should be changed when the tubing or peripheral catheter access site is changed. It is generally recommended that injection/access ports on central, peripherally inserted central, and midline catheters be changed at least every 7 days (see Chaps. 11 and 12). Using an injection port that has a very small amount of dead space eliminates the need to preflush the port, which minimizes the risk of touch contamination. Ports vary with manufacturer, so changes should be performed in accord with the manufacturer's instructions.

If the catheter has more than one lumen, the nurse needs to change the ports/needleless connectors on all unused lumens. If the catheter is made of a material that cannot be clamped without catheter damage, the patient needs to lie flat in bed and perform the Valsalva maneuver whenever the catheter is open to the air.

Venous Sampling

Many central venous catheters are placed in patients who do not have peripheral veins available or who need minimal peripheral venipunctures. Therefore, drawing blood specimens through central catheters is common practice. Because each catheter is different, the nurse must follow the manufacturer's instructions for use and adhere to institutional policy as well. Refer to INS Standards of Practice (INS, 1998, 2000a, 2000b) and to Chapter 4. Three basic blood sampling methods are used with tunneled and nontunneled catheters. Blood specimens are drawn:

- From a continuous infusion line while maintaining the closed system
- From a continuous infusion line by opening the system
- From a catheter with an in-place injection port

If the catheter system cannot be clamped, the patient must lie flat in bed and perform the Valsalva maneuver whenever the catheter is open to the air. If this is not done, air embolism is always possible.

Preliminary Considerations

Any blood specimen drawn through a central line that has been flushed with heparin or that has heparin as a solution additive should not be used for determining prothrombin time or partial thromboplastin time. Because heparin adheres to the catheter, falsely elevated test values may result.

PATIENT IDENTIFICATION
Before any blood specimens are drawn, the patient must be accurately identified. This should be done by the patient's identification band in the inpatient setting. Asking the patient to state his or her name may supplement, but should never be substituted for some form of written identification on the patient. In some cases, patients are unable to speak or may be mentally confused.

LABELING SPECIMEN TUBES
Before drawing the blood specimen, all tubes should be labeled with the patient's full name, room number, hospital identification number, and the initials of the person drawing the blood. This is done to prevent mislabeling, which can result in inadequate or inappropriate treatment.

Care of Vascular Access Devices

Connecting Implanted Catheter to Continuous Infusion System

When a continuous infusion is to be started in a patient with an implanted device, the device is cannulated with extension tubing connected between the needle and the infusion tubing or, ideally, a needleless system. If frequent intermittent infusions are given, the needle and extension tubing are left in place and the extension tubing covered with an intermittent injection cap. This prevents the need for frequent septum punctures. The nurse should follow institutional policy and procedure.

Tubing Care and Dressing Changes

The tubing and the filter down to the extension tubing should be changed consistent with institutional guidelines and INS standards (INS 1998, 2000a, 2000b).

Additional procedures, such as venous sampling, bolus injection, and intermittent infusion may also be accomplished using needleless connectors/safety systems and current vascular access devices.

Care of Implanted Pumps and Ports

Once the pump is implanted, the surgeon should fill out the Patient Registration and Implantation Record, after which the manufacturer issues the patient a wallet-sized identification card containing information pertinent to the implanted pump. The physician should complete the section provided for any medical emergency instructions. The patient should carry this card at all times.

MONITORING
Patients should be monitored carefully after implantation to confirm proper pump performance, wound healing, and favorable response to therapy. The pump should not be used for administering drugs for several days after implantation; this permits adequate wound healing.

PATIENT EDUCATION
The patient should be instructed to

- Avoid traumatic physical activity to prevent tissue damage around the implant site.
- Avoid long hot baths, saunas, and other activities that increase body temperature and result in increased drug flow.
- Consult the physician during febrile illness to assess the effects of increased drug flow.
- Consult the physician before air travel or change of residence to another geographic location. Adjustments in drug dosage may be required to compensate for an anticipated change in drug flow.
- Avoid deep sea or scuba diving.

- Report any unusual symptoms or complications relating to the specific drug therapy or the implanted pump.
- Return at the prescribed time to refill the pump.

REFILLING THE PUMP

The pump requires refills at specific intervals. The intervals depend on the volume of the reservoir and the rate of administration. See the accompanying directions for refilling the pump.

KEY INTERVENTIONS: Refilling an Implanted Pump

---

1. Gather the necessary equipment, including

   - 1 sterile fenestrated drape
   - 1 sterile towel
   - 1 50-mL syringe with drug solution
   - 1 sterile empty 50-mL syringe
   - 1 sterile noncoring needle
   - 1 sterile extension tubing with clamp
   - 1 pair sterile gloves
   - 1 sterile 2 × 2-inch sponge
   - 3 povidone–iodine swabs
   - 1 heating pad

2. Warm the 50-mL syringe containing drug solution to 15°C to 35°C with the heating pad.
3. Identify the outer perimeter of the pump by palpating the pump. Do this to locate the pump's septum.
4. Wash hands thoroughly and dry.
5. Using sterile technique, place all sterile items on the opened sterile towel.
6. Put on sterile gloves.
7. Disinfect pump site with povidone–iodine. Use three separate preparations. Start at the center of the pump and work outward beyond the periphery.
8. Place the fenestrated drape over the prepared pump site. A sterile template may be aligned over septum at this time.
9. Securely connect barrel of empty 5-mL syringe and extension tubing to the noncoring needle.
10. Close clamp.
11. Using a perpendicular angle, insert needle into center of septum.
12. Open clamp; then lower the syringe barrel beneath the level of the patient and allow the pump to empty.
13. Close clamp and document the volume of returned drug. Add 1 mL for the amount of drug remaining in extension tubing.
14. Disconnect and discard syringe barrel.
15. Securely attach air-purged syringe with new drug solution to extension tubing and open clamp.
16. Using both hands, inject 5 mL of solution into pump. Release pressure and allow drug to return to syringe. This test confirms proper needle placement. Continue to inject and check needle placement at 5-mL increments until syringe is empty.
17. Pull needle out quickly and apply digital pressure with sterile sponge. If necessary, apply a sterile adhesive bandage.

CLINICAL OUTCOME CONCERNS

Never attempt to aspirate fluid from the pump. This causes blood to be drawn back into the catheter, resulting in occlusion. If no fluid is returned into the syringe barrel, either the septum has not been penetrated or the pump is completely empty of infusate. To test for septum penetration, remove the syringe barrel and connect a 5-mL syringe with normal saline solution. Inject the solution and release the plunger to allow the fluid to return to the syringe. If the fluid does not return, again attempt to locate and penetrate the septum, using 5 mL normal saline solution to test penetration. If this is not successful, the physician should be notified because pump failure may have occurred. Accurate fill and refill records are essential to ensure that the pump is refilled at the required intervals; these records also document appropriate pump functioning.

■ ADVANCED TROUBLESHOOTING FOR VASCULAR ACCESS DEVICES

Occlusions and Withdrawal Problems

The inability to withdraw blood through a central venous catheter even though infusion creates no difficulties is frequently encountered. It has been postulated that the formation of a fibrin sheath over the catheter tip allows infusion but inhibits blood withdrawal (Fig. 14–10). Having the patient cough or move into various positions may be helpful. Sometimes the problem is intermittent; after an hour's wait, blood specimens can be obtained without difficulty. At other times and in some patients, it may continue to be impossible to withdraw blood through the central venous catheter. Flushing the catheter with normal saline solution before blood withdrawal appears to be helpful. Figure 14–11 presents ways to manage a "stuck" catheter.

Bacterial Contamination

Preventing infection is paramount to the success of catheter management. Adherence to Centers for Disease Control and Prevention guidelines (1998) and INS Standards of Practice (1998, 2000) institutional guidelines, and the manufacturer's recommendations for the use of products helps ensure positive outcomes. Box 14–3 lists common organisms associated with central venous catheter infection (see also Chaps. 10 and 13).

Catheter Declotting

Clots develop when thrombin, an enzyme made from prothrombin, converts fibrinogen to fibrin, a collagen. The fibrin forms the clot. Activated plasminogen forms plasmin, an enzyme that dissolves the clot and keeps fibrinogen from reforming fibrin; this process is known as **fibrinolysis.**

Within the lumen of a right atrial catheter, clot or fibrin sheath occludes the line,

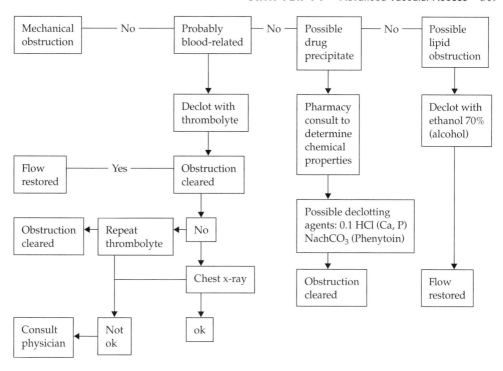

Figure 14–10. Algorithm for catheter occlusion.

and fibrinolytic agents are often used to restore patency. Thrombolytic agents dissolve clots by stimulating the conversion of plasminogen to plasmin, thereby triggering fibrinolysis. When urokinase, for example, is used as directed for IV catheter clearance, therapeutic serum levels are not observed, because only minute amounts of the drug enter the bloodstream (see Chap. 13). Studies report success in restoring patency to an occluded implantable port using a 10-mL syringe with between 0.2 and 1 mL of 0.1 N concentration hydrochloric acid solution left to dwell for 1 to 2 hours. Altepase (Genentech, Inc., South San Francisco, CA) tPA is awaiting FDA approval as an alternative thrombolytic agent (INS, 2000).

Intraluminal Precipitates

The mixing of incompatible medications in the catheter lumen may lead to precipitation and occlusion. A pharmacologic agent such as 0.1 N hydrochloric acid may be used to improve precipitate solubility related to amikacin, piperacillin, vancomycin, heparin, and calcium. Sodium bicarbonate has also been reported successfully to treat occlusions secondary to ticarcillin/clavulanate potassium, oxacillin, and phenytoin. The choice of agent is specific to the suspected source of the occlusion. In accessing occlusion, the nurse should

- Double-check catheter function
- Screen for extrinsic compression from clamps, sutures, kinked tubing

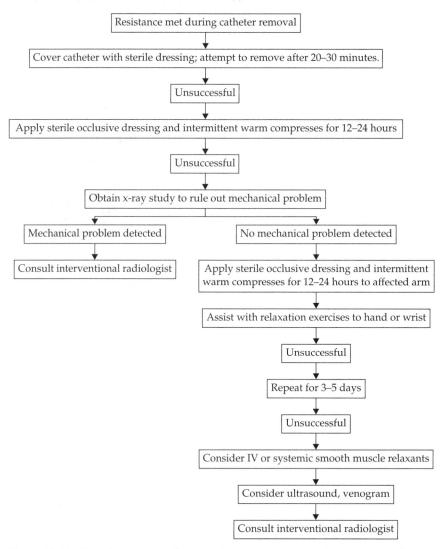

Figure 14–11. Clinical intervention for a "stuck" catheter. (Adapted from Luther Medical Products Clinical Reference [1997]).

- Assess patient's position
- Determine type of infusates/additives used
- Assess patient for signs of edema, redness, pain, or dilated vessels (Krzywda, 1999)

Intervention is initiated only after careful assessment of these factors.

Tunneled Catheter Repair

Although conventional methods of catheter repair using adhesives have been available for some time, emergency, temporary repair may be accomplished as follows:

1. Clamp the catheter between the chest wall and the tear.
2. Clean the torn area with povidone–iodine solution.
3. Using sterile scissors, cut off the damaged portion.
4. Insert a blunt needle (14- or 16-gauge) into the distal end of the catheter.
5. Insert an injection port in the hub of the needle and heparinize the catheter.
6. Secure the needle and catheter with silk suture material.
7. Release the clamp.
8. Determine patency by flushing with saline solution.

Permanent repair may be needed and is accomplished by splicing a new section of catheter with an end connector to the remainder of the line. Various manufacturers provide repair kits.

Regardless of the type of repair product used, the clinician must be familiar with the manufacturer's recommendations for use. A working knowledge of the intricacies of the catheter itself and repair methodologies ensures safe practice and return of a damaged catheter to patency.

Site Care

A regular, standardized site inspection, disinfection, and dressing change should minimize the incidence of catheter-related sepsis. Catheter site care and dressing change should be performed consistent with institutional policy and dressing material. If the dressing becomes wet, soiled, or loose, it should be changed immediately. Aseptic technique must be maintained during the procedure.

Nontunneled Catheters

Many variations are acceptable for performing site care and changing central venous catheter dressings. However, they are all based on the same principles. On a routine basis, the existing dressing must be removed; both site and catheter carefully inspected, cleaned, and disinfected; an antimicrobial ointment applied; and an occlusive dressing secured. The nurse performing the care thoroughly washes the hands and wears sterile gloves and a mask. If the patient cannot be masked, the face should be turned away from the dressing site.

BOX 14–3 Organisms Associated With Central Venous Catheter Infection

Escherichia coli
Klebsiella pneumoniae
Pseudomonas aeruginosa
Candida albicans
Staphylococcus epidermidis

Using a prepackaged dressing kit ensures the immediate availability of all required supplies. It also helps ensure that all people performing the care are using a standard procedure (see the accompanying display, Dressing Change and Site Care for Tunneled Catheters).

KEY INTERVENTIONS: Dressing Change and Site Care for Tunneled Catheters

---

1. Obtain a prepackaged dressing kit and prepare a clean table for a work area.
2. Position the patient comfortably on the bed.
3. Put on the mask, wash hands thoroughly, and dry. Put on gloves.
4. Carefully remove the old dressing. Gently lifting the tape from the outside edges inward toward the center prevents stress at the insertion site.
5. Inspect the catheter insertion site for signs of discharge or leakage. Inspect the catheter to ensure that the sutures are intact, that the length of the external portion has not increased, that any needle protective cover is in place and locked, and that the catheter and hub are intact.
6. Rewash the hands if they become contaminated during the dressing removal. If the procedure is performed with two pairs of gloves, the first pair is worn to remove the old dressing.
7. Open kit. The overlay provides a sterile field.
8. Put on the sterile gloves.
9. Clean all debris from the insertion site and from the portion of the catheter close to the site. If the catheter is polyurethane or silicone, the cleaning fluid should not be 100% acetone, which could weaken the catheter and cause leakage. Concentrated acetone may also cause skin irritation, which can increase the risk of infection. Some practitioners use a combination of dilute acetone and alcohol for cleansing. The cleansing is performed in a circular fashion, starting at the center and working outward. The cleansing agent must be allowed to dry before the disinfection is started.
10. Disinfection may be done with 1% or 2% tincture of iodine followed by a complete cleansing with alcohol or with povidone–iodine solution. Povidone–iodine must not be removed with alcohol. The skin preparation is applied in concentric circles with the nurse remembering to disinfect the catheter portion close to the insertion site and allowing the agent to dry.
11. Sparingly apply antimicrobial ointment directly to the insertion site. Povidone–iodine is recommended for central catheter sites.
12. Place a sterile 2 × 2-inch sponge directly over the ointment to ensure that the ointment stays at the site. A sterile sponge may be placed under the catheter and hub for patient comfort.
13. If the tape is likely to damage the skin, apply tincture of benzoin or similar skin protection agent to protect the exposed skin. Ensure that it dries before applying the tape.
14. Apply an adhesive cover to maintain an occlusive dressing (transparent dressings may be used). Several types are available. Foam adhesive bandage or transparent tape is frequently used. Place the sterile tape directly over the site with the catheter exiting from the bottom of the tape. This position prevents stress at the catheter hub–tubing connection when the patient moves. Be sure this connection is outside the tape to facilitate tubing changes.

15. Inspect the catheter hub–tubing connection to ensure that it is locked and taped. Then loop the tubing and tape it to the chest wall to prevent stress at the connection or insertion site when the tubing is pulled or stretched.
16. Sign and date the dressing-change label and apply it to the dressing.

Tunneled Catheters

The dressing change procedure may be modified for the tunneled catheter. If the patient is immunosuppressed or if site healing is not complete, the same care given to the nontunneled catheter may be used for this catheter. If the patient is not immunosuppressed and site healing is complete, site care may be limited to daily inspection and cleansing with soap and water while bathing.

Totally Implanted Devices

Totally implanted devices do not require any site care because the entire device is under the skin.

Catheter Patency

After using the catheter and at routine intervals, flushing with saline or heparin solution maintains catheter patency. For tunneled or nontunneled catheters, the frequency and heparin strength vary considerably depending on the agency or institution. The volume of heparin needs to be only slightly more than the volume of the catheter—2.5 to 5 mL should be sufficient. The strength of heparin may depend on the patient's condition; usually, it is 10 to 100 U/mL. Many practitioners find every-other-day flushing maintains catheter patency.

Using a prefilled syringe reduces the risk of touch contamination during preparation and ensures administering the correct heparin dose. A saline flush solution may also be used.

Whenever a flush solution—or any solution—is injected into ports or intermittent injection caps, using a short needle prevents the risk of accidental puncture of the tubing or catheter. Ideally, the system used incorporates safety standards consistent with current technology.

Competent Practice

High-quality central venous care mandates the development of policies and procedures based on INS Standards of Practice (INS, 1998, 2000a, 2000b). Competency checklists ensure safe practice (Fig. 14–12). In addition, a clinical practicum and evaluation tool should be developed to ensure safe practice by those professionals responsible for accessing and maintaining long-term venous access (INS, 1998, 2000a, 2000b) (see also Chap. 4).

Skill Set	*Understanding*	*Competency Observed*
Prepares patient for procedure	☐	☐
Confirms catheter placement/patency	☐	☐
Maintains asepsis	☐	☐
Uses needleless, safety products	☐	☐
Washes hands	☐	☐
Assembles equipment	☐	☐
Accesses catheter	☐	☐
Maintains patency	☐	☐
Exit site care	☐	☐
Recognizes complications	☐	☐
Repairs damaged catheter	☐	☐
Dressing technique	☐	☐
Manages occlusion	☐	☐
Initiates appropriate interventions	☐	☐

Figure 14–12. Long-term catheter care competency checklist.

References and Selected Readings

Asterisks indicate references cited in text.

Andris, D.A., Krzywda, E.A., Schulte, W., et al. (1997). Catheter pinch-off syndrome: Recognition and management. *Journal of Intravenous Nursing, 20*(12), 233–237.

*Arrow, Inc. (1998). Product literature: Arrow/Infusaid Pump. Author: Reading, PA.

*Bagnall-Reed, H. (1998). Diagnosis of central venous access device occlusion: implications for nursing practice. *Journal of Intravenous Nursing, 21*(5), S115–S117.

BD Medical Systems. (1999). Product literature. Author.

*Blum, A.S. (1999). The role of the interventional radiologist in central venous access. *Journal of Intravenous Nursing, 22*(6), S32–S39.

Catheter Innovations.™ (1999). Product literature: PASV™. Author: Sandy, UT.

*Centers for Disease Control and Prevention (1998). Guidelines for prevention of intravascular infection. Author: Atlanta, GA.

*Cook® Critical Care. (1999). Product literature: Antimicrobial impregnated central venous catheters C-BSG299. Author: Ellertsville, IN.

*Darouiche, R.O., Raad I.I., Heard, S.O., Thornby, J.I., Wenker, O.C., Gabriella, A., Berg, J., Khardori, N., Hanna, N., Hachem, R., Harris, R.L., & Mayhall, G. (1999). A comparison of two antimicrobial-impregnated central venous catheters. *New England Journal of Medicine, 240*, 1–8.

*Fuentes-Afflick, E. (1990, March 12). *Use and management of intraosseous infusions.* Presented at the Bay Area Vascular Access Nurses (BAVAN) Fourth Annual Conference, San Francisco, CA.

*Holmes, K.R. (1998). Comparison of push-pull versus discard method from central venous catheters for blood testing. *Journal of Intravenous Nursing, 21*(5), 282–285.

*Intravenous Nurses Society. (1998). Revised intravenous nursing standards of practice. *Journal of Intravenous Nursing, 21*(Suppl. 1), S73.

*Intravenous Nurses Society. (2000a, in press). Revised intravenous nursing standards of practice. *Journal of Intravenous Nursing,* (Suppl.).

*Intravenous Nurses Society. (2000b). *Core curriculum for intravenous nursing.* Philadelphia: Lippincott Williams & Wilkins.

*Karavelis, A., Foroglou, G., Selviaridis, P., & Fountzilas, G. (1996). Intraventricular administration of morphine for control of intractable cancer pain in 90 patients. *Neurosurgery, 39*, 57–61.

*Krzywda, E.A. (1999). Predisposing factors, prevention, and management of central venous catheter occlusions. *Journal of Intravenous Nursing, 22*(6), S11–S14.

Kupensky, D.T. (1995). Use of hydrochloric acid to restore patency in an occluded implantable port. *Journal of Intravenous Nursing, 18*(4), 198–201.

*Metheny, N.M. (2000). *Fluid and electrolyte balance* (4th ed.). Philadelphia: Lippincott Williams & Wilkins.

Poole, S.M. (1999). Quality issues in access device management. *Journal of Intravenous Nursing, 22*(6), S26–S29.

*Raad, I., Darouiche, R., Dupuis, J., Abi-Said, D., Gabrielli, A., Hachem, R., et al. (1997). Central venous catheters coated with minocycline and rifampin for the prevention of catheter-related colonization and blood stream infections. *Annals of Internal Medicine 128*, 267–274.

*Ray, C.E. (1999). Infection control principles and practice in the care and management of central venous access devices. *Journal of Intravenous Nursing, 22*(6), S18–S21.

Richardson, D. (2000). Tracking catheters: The care continuum. *Journal of Intravenous Nursing, 23*(1), 35–49.

Spivey, W.H. (1987). Intraosseous infusions. *Journal of Pediatrics, 3*, 639–643.

West, V.L. (1998). Alternate routes of administration. *Journal of Intravenous Nursing, 21*(4), 221–231.

Review Questions

Note: Questions below may have more than one right answer.

1. Which of the following flush solutions may be used for percutaneous catheters consistent with institutional policy and the manufacturer's recommendations?

   A. Saline and heparin 10 U/mL

   B. Heparin 10 U/mL

   C. Heparin 100 U/mL

   D. All of the above

2. Which of the following statements concerning central venous catheter patency is correct?

   A. Patency includes ability to infuse through and aspirate blood from the catheter.

   B. Occlusion is the most common noninfectious complication.

   C. Occlusion may occur in as many as 36% of catheters.

   D. All of the above

3. The most common cause of catheter occlusion is:

   A. Clumping of particulate matter in the infusate

   B. Catheter defects

   C. Infection

   D. Thrombosis

4. Pain with infusion is a sign of which of the following?

   A. Catheter malposition

   B. Pinch-off syndrome

   C. Fibrin sheath occlusion

   D. External compression

5. Which of the following diagnostic procedures is appropriate when fibrin sheath occlusion of a central venous catheter is suspected?

   A. Chest radiograph

   B. Contrast study

   C. Duplex scan

   D. Venogram

6. A pressure-activated safety valve is a feature specific to which catheter?

   A. Broviac

   B. Hickman

   C. PASV

   D. Groshong

7. Intraosseous access may be performed using all of the following products *except*:

   A. Bone marrow biopsy needle

   B. Laser needle

   C. Osgood needle

   D. Intraosseous port

8. Which of the following is *not* an advantage of intraosseous infusion?

   A. Fluids are rapidly absorbed.

   B. Clotting and lung puncture problems are eliminated.

   C. Fluids are absorbed slowly.

   D. The risk of infection is reduced.

9. A ventricular reservoir may be used for which of the following?

   A. Access to CSF

   B. Measurement of CSF pressure

   C. Instillation of medication

   D. All of the above

10. The most frequently occurring, life-threatening complication of central venous catheterization is which of the following?

    A. Septicemia

    B. Occlusion

    C. Thrombosis

    D. Pinch-off syndrome

CHAPTER 15

Intra-arterial Therapy

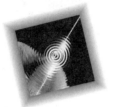

K E Y   T E R M S

Arterial Blood Gas (ABG) Analysis
Arterial Pressure Monitoring
Base Bicarbonate
Bicarbonate Excess

Hemoglobin Desaturation
Oxyhemoglobin Dissociation
Total Pressure of Atmosphere

■ ROLE OF ARTERIAL BLOOD GAS ANALYSIS

Arterial blood with all its nourishing elements supplies all body tissues; thus, arterial blood is used routinely for diagnosing abnormalities and assessing patients' conditions. Intra-arterial therapy may involve one-time or daily blood sampling to analyze the concentration of gases, such as oxygen, and other components, or it may involve inserting an indwelling catheter to obtain serial or daily samples for **arterial blood gas (ABG) analysis** and continuous **arterial pressure monitoring**.

Although venous, arterial, and capillary blood all contain comparable levels of carbon dioxide and **base bicarbonate**, the levels of oxygen in venous and capillary blood vary significantly from the level of oxygen in arterial blood.

Oxygen in Plasma

Oxygen moves through the circulatory system in plasma and hemoglobin; because the small amount of oxygen dissolved in plasma cannot be measured directly, its presence is expressed as the tension or partial pressure it exerts on plasma (Pao_2—the letter "P" symbolizes the pressure value; the letter "a" signifies that the partial pressure of oxygen measured is that in arterial blood).

Oxygen in Hemoglobin

The major portion of blood oxygen is bound to hemoglobin and measured as a percentage of the hemoglobin saturated with oxygen (SaO_2). Tissue is adequately oxygenated when the partial pressure of oxygen in arterial blood (PaO_2) ranges between 80 and 100 mm Hg and when hemoglobin saturation (SaO_2) ranges from 93% to 100% (Horne & Derrico, 1999).

Under normal circumstances, when the PaO_2 value decreases slightly, there is an incremental drop in the SaO_2 value. However, when PaO_2 falls below 60 mm Hg, the association is disturbed, and minute decreases in partial pressure cause significant drops in SaO_2, known as **hemoglobin desaturation**. The **oxyhemoglobin dissociation** curve is illustrated in Figure 15-1.

■ ACCESS SITES FOR ARTERIAL BLOOD ANALYSIS

The blood vessel of choice for obtaining an arterial blood sample is the radial artery, primarily because it is superficial and easily entered and located at the wrist, which makes it easy to stabilize for a quick entry. (See Table 15-1 for more information on choice of sites.) In addition, if thrombosis should occur, the ulnar artery will, by collateral circulation, supply blood to the entire hand, and it is easy to apply a pressure dressing after arterial puncture at this site.

Second and third site choices vary according to institution and personal preference. The brachial artery at the antecubital fossa lies deep, close to nerves and tendons, and is difficult to stabilize. If thrombosis should occur in the brachial artery, the

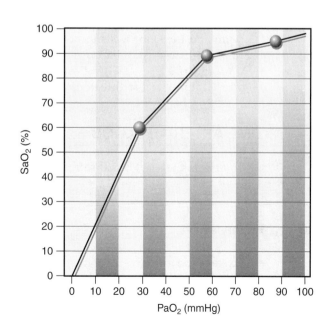

Figure 15–1. Normally, PaO_2 and SaO_2 values are closely related. When PaO_2 decreases slightly, so does SaO_2. However, when PaO_2 drops below 60 mm Hg, the close association is disrupted. The disruption is represented graphically as the oxyhemoglobin dissociation curve, which illustrates the relationship between PaO_2 and SaO_2 values known as the 30–60–90 rule. When PaO_2 measures 30 mm Hg, SaO_2 is usually 60%, and when PaO_2 is 60 mm Hg, SaO_2 is usually 90%. (Adapted from Horne, C., & Derrico, D. [1999]. Mastering ABGs: The art of arterial blood gas measurement. *American Journal of Nursing* 99 [8], 26–33.)

T A B L E   1 5 – 1

CHOOSING THE SITE OF AN ARTERIAL BLOOD SAMPLE

Site	Advantages	Disadvantages
Radial	Close to the surface Easily palpable Easy to check site	Pulsation is difficult to palpate on obese patients with short arms
Brachial artery	Largest artery in lower arm Close to surface Extension of arm stretches the artery Easily accessed Easily observed after puncture	May lie deep in muscular or obese patients Traumatic puncture may damage adjacent nerve and ligaments
Ulnar artery	Fairly close to surface and therefore accessible Good alternative to radial artery	Palpation difficult if artery is small or deep Difficulty in extending wrist if patient is uncooperative
Femoral artery	Relatively large artery Easily palpated Allows direct, perpendicular approach Incidence of arterial spasms is rare	Risk of contamination at site (groin) Possible to puncture femoral vein accidentally during procedure

blood supply to the forearm and hand may be compromised (Fig. 15-2). The ulnar artery is usually much deeper and more difficult to stabilize than the radial artery, so, although it may be larger, it is usually not the first choice as an entry site. (Most nurses agree that if the radial artery has been entered, the ulnar artery of the same arm should not be used.)

The femoral artery, located midway between the anterior superior spine of the ilium and the symphysis pubis (see Fig. 15-2), is the largest accessible artery and is easily palpated, stabilized, and entered. However, digital pressure is required for postpuncture pressure. If postpuncture thrombosis should occur in the femoral artery, a limb- or life-threatening condition may result.

■ ONE-TIME ARTERIAL BLOOD SAMPLING

To draw an arterial blood sample, the nurse needs first to assess and prepare the patient and the equipment.

Patient Preparation

To start, the nurse reviews the physician's order, which should specify the fraction of inspired oxygen (FIO_2) if the patient is receiving oxygen therapy or the fraction of oxygen in room air (21% O_2). The patient should be at this steady state continuously for 15 to 20 minutes before the blood sample is drawn. Unless a postexercise blood sample is ordered, the patient also should be at rest for this period.

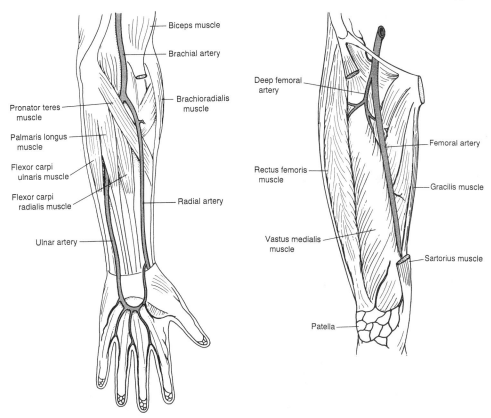

Figure 15–2. Location of radial, ulnar, and brachial arteries (*left*) and location of the femoral artery in the leg (*right*).

Next, the nurse considers the patient's position, which can affect the ABG measurement. A patient in a supine position may have more difficulty breathing than would a patient in sitting position. The position most comfortable for the patient should be used for all blood sampling procedures.

 SAFE PRACTICE ALERT While positioning the patient, the nurse fully explains the procedure to alleviate anxiety and fear, which can cause hyperventilation and hence an alteration of the blood analysis findings. Of course, the person performing the arterial puncture should be competent for the same reason. Undue trauma causes pain, often leading to hyperventilation by the patient and resulting in alteration of the blood values.

Equipment

The laboratory requisition form should have all identifying patient information plus the oxygenation status of the patient, time of day (important when drawing serial samples), and, if the patient is on a ventilator, all pertinent settings. In some institutions, the patient's temperature and hemoglobin count are also required. In any institution, the nurse follows recommended institutional policy.

Arterial blood samples can be drawn with existing equipment, such as a syringe and needle, or a prepackaged kit may be used. An ABG kit is inexpensive and the kit contains, except for ice and tape, all equipment needed to perform a one-time arterial puncture. If the kit contains a heparinized prefilled syringe, the nurse removes the syringe cap, places and secures the appropriate-size needle, wets the inner walls of the syringe with heparin (to prevent blood clotting), and expels excess heparin with the same method used for a syringe that is not prefilled. Most ABG kits contain a plastic bag for the iced blood sample.

To heparinize the syringe, the nurse attaches a needle other than the one to be used for puncture to the syringe, cleanses the top of the heparin vial or neck of the ampule with an alcohol swab, and opens vial or ampule. One milliliter (1 mL) of heparin is withdrawn into the syringe. The nurse then moves the plunger back and forth several times to coat the plunger with heparin, and rotates the plunger to eliminate dry spots. To eliminate air bubbles, the nurse holds the syringe with the needle upright and gently taps the sides of syringe, or turns the syringe with the needle pointed downward and slowly inverts the syringe upright. The needle used for heparin is discarded.

The nurse replaces the needle used for heparinization with a sterile, tightly secured needle selected for arterial puncture. Then with the syringe in inverted position, the plunger is pushed up and all excess heparin expelled. The only heparin remaining should be in the dead space of the needle and on the walls of the syringe. Excess heparin or air bubbles alter the results of the ABG analysis.

Puncture Sites and Procedure

Before performing the procedure, arterial assessment should be completed and the blood withdrawal site selected (see Table 15-1).

Radial Puncture

As with any invasive procedure, the nurse begins by putting on gloves. The site is palpated for a pulse and the condition of skin and surrounding tissues is inspected, particularly for previous arterial puncture marks. Allen's test is performed to ensure the adequacy of collateral circulation (Fig. 15-3).

A rolled towel may be placed under the wrist, causing hyperextension of the hand to stretch and stabilize the artery. The skin is prepared with iodophor by wiping the area in concentric circles and allowing at least a 30-second contact time with the intended puncture site. Again, gloves are required and Occupational Safety and Health Administration standards should be met.

A local anesthetic is not always necessary for an arterial puncture with a needle. With it, the chances for a quick, successful entry are less, and the anesthetic does not

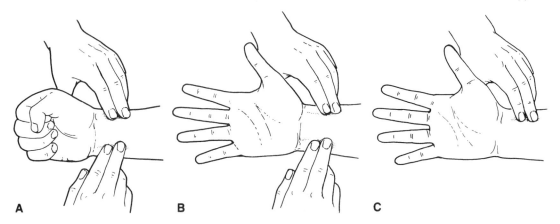

Figure 15–3. Performing Allen's test to determine circulatory adequacy. **A.** Patient clenches fist while nurse applies pressure. **B.** Patient opens hand and nurse releases pressure while watching to see how long it takes for hand to color (signifying circulation and patency of vessels). **C.** Evaluating pulse and blood return.

ameliorate the discomfort of arterial entry. However, if a difficult entry is anticipated or multiple attempts are necessary, a local anesthetic injected at the intended entry site may eliminate skin discomfort.

To perform a radial puncture, the nurse uses one hand to palpate the artery and aligns two or three fingertips along the direction the artery follows. Holding the syringe at an angle no higher than 30 degrees with the needle pointed directly toward the artery, the nurse uses the other hand to enter the skin and artery smoothly in one, quick motion. Arterial pressure usually causes the blood to pulsate spontaneously back into the syringe. If blood pressure is low or the syringe not free flowing, however, the nurse may need to pull back gently on the plunger. The plunger should be withdrawn 1 to 2 mL before the stick, for two reasons: if the sample is indeed arterial and not venous, the patient's pressure causes a brisk and often pulsatile reflux of blood into the syringe (unless the patient is severely hypotensive), and it prevents complications such as arterial spasm and blood hemolysis.

The blood return stops when the blood reaches the automatic shutoff level. If the equipment does not have a shutoff feature, a volume of 1 to 2 mL blood is a sufficient quantity for the blood gas analyzer.

Immediately after quickly withdrawing the needle and blood-filled syringe, the nurse applies digital pressure to the puncture site with a 2 × 2-inch sterile sponge folded to form a pressure point. Then, taking precautions not to encircle the entire wrist, a pressure dressing is firmly secured with tape.

If the syringe will be capped, the nurse removes the needle from the syringe and attaches the cap quickly and securely. If a rubber stopper is used, the nurse sticks the needle tip into the center of the stopper. The nurse next rolls the syringe back and forth between the hands for 5 to 10 seconds to ensure that the blood mixes with the heparin lining the syringe. The unit is then placed in an iced container and taken to the laboratory immediately for analysis. A small amount of cold water added to the ice provides for even, cold distribution and facilitates placement of the sample so that all the blood in the barrel is chilled by iced water.

SAFE PRACTICE ALERT An ABG sample that is not placed immediately on ice can produce faulty results on analysis because red blood cells continue to metabolize oxygen and give off carbon dioxide. Ice retards the process.

Femoral Puncture

The femoral artery is usually easily palpated with the patient in the supine position. If the patient is obese, assistance may be needed to hold the abdomen away, or the patient's buttocks may be placed on an inverted bedpan. A pendulous abdomen may be taped up and away to provide easier access and maintain sterility. Procedures for wearing gloves and preparing the skin are the same as for a radial artery puncture.

The following two different techniques may be used for a femoral arterial puncture:

- The artery is located and "fixed" between two fingers, allowing pulsation to be felt on both fingers but at the same time allowing enough room between them for the needle entry. The syringe and needle are held almost straight down. When the puncture is made in this manner, care must be taken not to pierce through the other wall of the artery.
- The entry may be performed with the same techniques used for a radial artery puncture. Two or three fingertips are placed along the direction of the femoral artery, and the syringe and needle are held at an angle no higher than 30 degrees. This method must be used for femoral artery catheter placement and, if used for a one-time needle and syringe sample, there is less chance of artery perforation.

Regardless of the method used, when pulsation is strong, it is relayed up through the needle and syringe as the needle touches and penetrates the artery. The walls of the femoral artery are usually thick and resistant to puncture, so feeling pulsations can be a good guide to needle tip placement. When the artery is entered, the blood usually pulsates back into and fills the syringe without any traction being applied on the plunger.

Postprocedural Patient Interventions

When the needle and syringe are removed, digital pressure is needed because a pressure dressing with tape is difficult to maintain in the femoral artery area. The pressure should be maintained for at least 10 minutes, and 20 minutes or longer in a patient who has received anticoagulant therapy. It is helpful to remember to release pressure slowly. A sudden release may cause undue pressure against the arterial wall and the patient will begin bleeding. The care of the blood sample is the same as that outlined for a radial artery puncture. Postprocedural patient care and nursing responsibilities are described in Box 15-1.

> ## BOX 15–1 **Postprocedural Patient Interventions**
>
> - Determine if the oxygen status of the patient has been altered only for the blood sampling.
> - If so, resume presampling status as soon as the blood sample is drawn.
> - Maintain pressure dressing long enough—usually between 10 and 20 minutes depending on the access site—to prevent excessive seepage of blood into the tissue. Be sure that the pressure dressing is not so tight that blanching occurs or that venous blood flow in the hand is severely restricted.
> - If the patient is receiving anticoagulation therapy, apply digital pressure. Digital pressure is also preferable to the use of a C-clamp at the femoral site because significant occult bleeding into the retroperitoneal space can occur rapidly and may result in unnecessary blood loss and discomfort for the patient.
> - Remove pressure dressing after bleeding stops.

■ USE OF AN INDWELLING ARTERIAL CATHETER

In many situations, serial or daily blood samples are needed for ABG analysis. To avoid multiple punctures, an indwelling catheter may be inserted to obtain the blood samples. The radial artery is usually the site of first choice because it is the easiest to enter, is the easiest to maintain with intact sterile dressings, and allows the patient the greatest freedom of movement. It is imperative that Allen's test be performed before placing any indwelling catheter in the radial artery because the long-term placement with decreased blood flow increases the risk of thrombosis.

 SAFE PRACTICE ALERT If at all possible, use of the brachial artery for indwelling catheter placement should be avoided because the catheter easily fractures or bends in this site, which significantly increases the chance of embolization.

The femoral artery may be a favorable site because it can accommodate a catheter of substantial diameter to achieve consistent blood sampling and monitoring. Care must be taken at all times not to leave the patient in bed at a 30-degree angle or less. Frequent pedal pulse checks for strength of pulsatile flow and color of limb should be maintained and documented. The patient's skin should be appropriately prepared and shaved before the procedure so that a sterile occlusive dressing may then be maintained intact. If the catheter is to be maintained for a substantial period, it may be prudent to suture it in place. This is also true with arterial lines to be maintained in the radial artery.

When inserting any indwelling arterial catheter, extra precautions must be taken to wash hands thoroughly. Skin preparation in this instance may include an acetone defatting as well as a complete iodophor preparation. In some institutions, sterile gloves are mandatory for this procedure and should always be used when probing is anticipated.

A local anesthetic may be injected at the insertion site, especially if an 18-gauge or larger catheter is being used. It is preferable that only experienced personnel perform this procedure; a successful entry on the first attempt is highly desired because the availability of suitable arteries is limited.

Catheter Insertion and Blood Sampling

When using a catheter with an obturator, the procedure outlined in the accompanying Key Intervention display should be followed.

KEY INTERVENTIONS: Inserting a Catheter With an Obturator and Obtaining a Blood Sample

---

Catheter Insertion

1. Put on gloves. Insert catheter at a 30-degree angle, using the same techniques as those used to perform venipuncture of a superficial vein without a tourniquet.
2. As the catheter tip touches and enters the artery, pulsation can be felt through the catheter. Keep in mind that the arterial wall is thicker and more resistant to entry than a venous wall, making this procedure painful if not performed quickly and expertly.
3. When the artery is fully entered, blood pulsates back into the stylet. The catheter then can be fully advanced.
4. To maintain a sterile field while removing the stylet and placing the obturator, place an iodophor swab or sterile 2 x 2-inch sponge under the catheter hub.
5. To facilitate the stylet–obturator change, temporarily shut off the arterial blood flow either by digital pressure at the catheter tip or by adequate placement of a tourniquet proximal to the insertion site.
6. After the obturator is removed from its protective shield, the stylet is removed from the catheter and the obturator inserted and locked by twisting in place. Pressure on the artery may now be released.
7. Dress and label the arterial entry site. Include the date and time of insertion and the initials of the person performing the procedure on the dressing.
8. Document the procedure, stating the date, time, type, and gauge catheter used, insertion site, any patient reactions, name of person performing procedure, and pertinent data regarding distal extremity, including color, pulse, warmth.

Obtaining Arterial Blood Sample for Arterial Blood Gas Analysis

1. Wearing gloves, prepare a heparinized syringe without a needle.
2. Apply digital or tourniquet pressure over the artery.
3. Place iodophor swab or sterile 2 × 2-inch sponge under the catheter hub.
4. Remove obturator.
5. Connect heparinized syringe to catheter hub.
6. Release arterial pressure.
7. Allow syringe to fill with required amount of blood.
8. Reapply arterial pressure.

9. Remove syringe from catheter.
10. Insert and lock new sterile obturator.
11. Release arterial pressure.
12. Cap syringe and treat blood sample the same way as for a one-time puncture for arterial blood gas sample.

The procedure for inserting an intermittent catheter with an injection cap, or port, is similar to inserting a catheter with an obturator, with some exceptions. For example, pressure to stop arterial blood flow is not needed because there is no stylet–obturator change. The catheter is, however, flushed with a dilute heparin solution. Dressing, label documentation at the site, and documentation in the medical record are the same as for a catheter with an obturator.

To obtain a blood sample for ABG analysis from a catheter with a heparin lock device, the nurse puts on gloves and prepares three syringes:

- A heparinized syringe with a 1-inch, 22-gauge needle
- A plain syringe with 1-inch, 22-gauge needle for withdrawal of dilute heparin from the injection port
- A syringe and needle with dilute heparin solution for flushing the catheter after drawing the blood sample

Next, the nurse cleanses the injection site of the catheter with antiseptic., securely anchors the catheter hub with the free hand to prevent excessive pressure at the insertion site, and inserts the needle of the plain syringe. Approximately 0.5 mL blood with dilute heparin is withdrawn from the catheter and discarded.

The injection port is recleansed, the needle in the heparinized syringe inserted, the syringe allowed to fill with enough blood for the analysis, and the syringe removed with the needle. Finally, the injection port is recleansed, and the nurse, still securely anchoring the catheter hub, inserts the needle of the syringe containing dilute heparin, flushes the catheter, and removes the syringe and needle. The blood sample is treated in the same manner as the sample obtained for a one-time analysis.

 SAFE PRACTICE ALERT When entering any intermittent catheter with a needle, extreme care must be taken to use a needle that is short—too short to pass beyond the catheter hub into the catheter itself. If the needle tip does enter the catheter, the catheter can be pierced and broken off by the needle tip. The result is a catheter embolus. In addition, the needle gauge must be small enough to allow postpuncture closure of the entry site. Otherwise, blood leakage and risk of contamination increase.

Close site monitoring is required after placement of any type of indwelling arterial catheter.

KEY INTERVENTIONS: Postarterial Catheter Insertion Care

1. Observe the catheter site for signs of arterial thrombosis, hematoma formation, arterial perforation, and catheter kinking or dislodgment.
2. Check the patient's hand for adequate blood supply by noting color and temperature.
3. Maintain secure, clean, and intact dressings.
4. Avoid placing undue stress at the insertion site by using the unaffected arm for blood pressure monitoring and venipunctures.

Continuous Arterial Pressure Monitoring

Continuous arterial pressure monitoring requires inserting an indwelling arterial catheter, which permits the IV nurse and other health care personnel to obtain continuous systolic, diastolic, and mean arterial pressure readings; to assess the cardiovascular effects of vasopressor or vasodilator drugs during the treatment of shock; and, at the same time, to draw arterial blood for ABG measurements.

Equipment

A cardiac monitor with a module for measuring arterial pressure is required. The monitor is connected by cable and a transducer to a special IV setup (Fig. 15-4). The IV system consists of a 500-mL bag of normal saline solution that has been heparinized (usually 500 to 2000 U/500 mL) to inhibit catheter clotting and thrombus formation at the catheter tip. *Klebsiella, Enterobacter,* and *Serratia* species and *Pseudomonas cepacia* show rapid growth within 24 hours with dextrose 5% in water. The bag is connected to IV tubing and placed inside a pressure infusor bag with a gauge and inflation bulb, the same one used to pump blood transfusions. Some institutions prefer microdrip tubings, but air bubbles are more persistent with this size drip. Other hospitals prefer macrodrip tubings; this size allows a larger volume of fluid to be infused.

The IV tubing is connected by a high-pressure extension tubing, a continuous-flush attachment, and three-way stopcocks to a transducer dome. Most of these systems deliver 3 to 5 mL of solution. The entire system is flushed. All connections must be secured and all air bubbles eliminated. The transducer is covered with the dome and secured on a plate attached to an IV pole at the level of the patient's right atrium. Each manufacturer provides detailed instructions for this setup. The instructions should be carefully followed.

General Procedure

Any indwelling catheter may be used for this procedure and the insertion procedure is the same as for serial or daily blood sample drawings. The catheter is connected to the primed IV tubing by placing an iodophor swab or sterile 2 × 2-inch sponge under the catheter hub, applying digital or tourniquet pressure over the

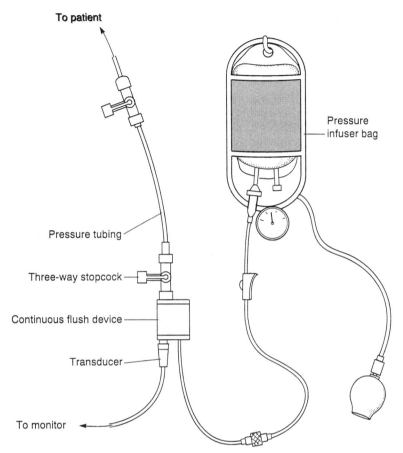

Figure 15–4. System for continuous arterial pressure monitoring.

artery distal to the site, removing the stylet, connecting and securing the tubing adapter, and releasing pressure on the artery. The pressure infusor bag is inflated to 300 mm Hg to deliver automatically a designated volume of fluid (depending on the drip size) hourly.

A sterile dressing is applied to the insertion site and taped securely. The site is labeled clearly to denote arterial access, date, time, type and gauge of catheter, and initials of person performing the insertion. A short handboard may be required to limit wrist motion. If restraints are necessary, they should be applied around the handboard, not the patient's wrist, because this could interfere with arterial pressure and thereby increase the risk of catheter kinking or dislodgment.

Aftercare

Aftercare of the insertion site is the same as that for an indwelling catheter used for drawing blood samples for serial or daily ABG analysis.

Obtaining Blood for ABG Analysis

When an ABG sample is needed, a sampling port provides an easy arterial access. Another method is to attach a three-way stopcock connection as close as possible to the site. The sampling site should be capped with a heparin lock (intermittent infusion cap). The nurse removes the cap when sampling and attaches appropriate syringe. The stopcock is turned off to pressure or to the sampling site, and the nurse gently withdraws the sample and handles it consistent with institutional policy. The port is then flushed and the stopcock turned back to pressure.

Malfunctions and Complications

Common malfunctions occurring in arterial pressure lines are listed in Table 15-2. Common complications related to arterial pressure lines include thromboses, hematomas, pseudoaneurysms, and prolonged arterial spasms. These problems may be reduced by clinical expertise during catheter insertion and by careful monitoring of insertion sites.

Infection is a serious complication as well. Arterial pressure monitoring is associated with up to 13% of reported cases of nosocomial bacteremia. Incidences of contaminated transducers, transducer domes, and flush solutions are well documented. Sterilizing the transducer after each use, using disposable domes, and changing the entire monitoring system except for the catheter every 2 days helps reduce infection rates. As with any invasive procedure, thorough hand washing before catheter insertion and maintenance of aseptic technique during setup of the system, during insertion, and during all manipulations of the line are mandatory.

Use of Swan-Ganz Catheters

Although a Swan-Ganz catheter is inserted into a vein, it is important to intra-arterial therapy because it enters the pulmonary artery and measures arterial pressures. Whereas central venous pressure lines assess only right heart pressure, Swan-Ganz

T A B L E   1 5 – 2
MALFUNCTIONS OCCURRING IN ARTERIAL PRESSURE MONITORING

Malfunction	Intervention
• Air bubbles may distort wave patterns.	• Eliminate air from system in setup; avoid entry of air in manipulation.
• Near-exsanguination has been reported.	• Secure all connections.
• "Damped" pressure tracing (almost flat) may occur if tip lies against artery wall.	• Secure catheter hub; ensure use of intact dressings.
• Catheter clotting can occur if pressure is <300 mm Hg.	• Check pressure bag to ensure that it is maintained.
• Abnormally high or low reading may occur if height of transducer is at zero reference point or is the type placed with a plate on an IV pole.	• Identify type of system used on the control switch of patient's bed.

catheters allow the heath care team to assess both right and left heart pressures. This makes a Swan-Ganz catheter suitable for diagnosing and managing heart failure resulting from myocardial infarction and cardiogenic shock. In cardiogenic shock treatment, the Swan-Ganz catheter serves many purposes. It guides the administration of IV therapy and provides the site. At the same time, it facilitates the evaluation of any therapeutic drugs given and provides information regarding the cause of shock.

Basic Swan-Ganz catheters have double or triple lumens. Catheters are approximately 110 cm long and come in sizes 5, 6, 7, and 7.5 French. Each has a balloon tip that is inflated with 0.8 to 1.5 mL air, depending on the size and manufacturer. A double-lumen catheter contains a larger port that is connected to an IV system and monitor to measure pulmonary artery wedge pressure, and a smaller port with a two-way stopcock for inflation and deflation of the balloon. Triple-lumen catheters contain a third proximal port, which is connected to another IV system and may be used to monitor right atrial pressure.

The IV system contains a heparinized bag, pressure infusor bag, pressure tubings with stopcocks, and transducer with cable connected to a monitor. This equipment is the same as that used for arterial monitoring except that for Swan-Ganz catheters, the lines may be color-coded blue to differentiate them from arterial lines, which may be color-coded red.

Insertion

The Swan-Ganz catheter may be inserted either percutaneously or by a cutdown procedure in any accessible vein large enough to allow passage of the catheter. As the catheter is threaded and the tip passes the superior vena cava, the balloon is inflated. Normal blood flow then assists catheter advancement. The tip enters the right atrium and passes through the tricuspid valve, entering the right ventricle. It then passes through the pulmonic valve into the pulmonary artery. Use of a cardiac monitor is essential during insertion because the waveform pattern defines changes with each advancement, thereby providing a guide for tip location, and simultaneously monitoring the patient's condition throughout the procedure. The catheter tip placement must be confirmed by radiography.

Pulmonary capillary wedge pressure, which reflects left heart pressure, is measured intermittently by inflating the balloon to its recommended level (Fig. 15-5). Care should be taken not to overinflate the balloon and not to inflate it too frequently. Typically, the balloon is inflated every 4 hours, with the inflation pressure maintained no longer than 1 to 2 minutes.

Complications

Possible complications include the following:

- Cardiac arrhythmias, which may occur during insertion—lidocaine hydrochloride and defibrillation equipment must be readily available. Serious dysrhythmias during insertion are rare.

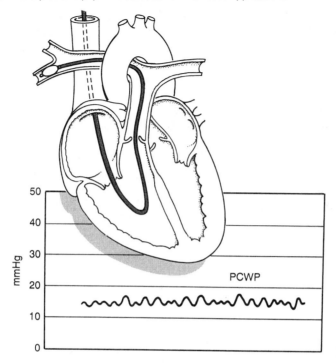

Figure 15–5. Pulmonary capillary wedge pressure.

- Catheter knotting, which may occur with the 5-French catheter when it is advanced too far for the chamber whose pressure is being registered.
- Balloon rupture, which is possible in a patient without intracardiac shunting of blood.
- Pulmonary damage, which may result from obstructed pulmonary artery blood flow caused by peripheral migration of the catheter to a wedged position. This is avoidable with constant monitoring and by following recommendations regarding balloon inflation.
- Infection, which is always a threat. The use of disposable equipment has minimized the occurrence of infection. Strict adherence to aseptic technique is mandatory.

■ INTRA-ARTERIAL PARAMETERS AND INTERPRETATION

Arterial blood gas measurements are used to detect and cope with respiratory imbalances. Specific uses include diagnosing and regulating oxygen therapy and evaluating all other therapy and metabolic imbalances. In particular, ABG levels assess the effectiveness of the therapy. To interpret ABG values, the nurse must understand the physiologic, chemical, and physical processes that influence each parameter.

pH

The pH value refers to the degree of acidity or alkalinity of the blood. It is not an absolute measurement, but gives an approximation of hydrogen ion concentration. The pH scale is as follows (numbers are inversely related to the degree of acidity): the range compatible with life is roughly 6.8 to 7.8; and the normal range lies between 7.35 and 7.45. A pH increase represents a decrease in acidity and a pH decrease represents an increase in acidity. A pH decrease of 0.3 shows a doubling of hydrogen concentration. Blood pH 7.10 has twice the hydrogen concentration of blood pH 7.40.

Blood pH is directly proportional to the ratio of carbonic acid to bicarbonate (HCO_3^-). When there is 1 part carbonic acid to 20 parts bicarbonate, the resultant pH is 7.35 to 7.45. If only carbonic acid increases or only bicarbonate decreases, the ratio becomes closer (1:5 to 16) and acidosis results. Conversely, when only carbonic acid decreases or only bicarbonate increases, the ratio widens (1:25 to 50) and alkalosis results.

Carbonic acid or bicarbonate changes themselves produce no toxic effects; it is the ratio alteration and resultant pH change that interfere severely with enzyme activity.

Hydrogen

Cell metabolism produces hydrogen, which combines with bicarbonate to form carbonic acid. This breaks down into water, which is excreted by the kidneys, and carbon dioxide, which is excreted by the lungs.

Because waste products of metabolism are mainly acidic, humans are by nature acid-producing animals. The body generates and processes 15,000 to 20,000 mEq hydrogen daily. Most (99.8%) is nonfixed or volatile acid, which means it can change into a gaseous form. The remainder (0.2%) is fixed or nonvolatile.

Body processing of hydrogen is accomplished with no appreciable change in blood concentration by elimination of volatile acid as carbon dioxide by the lungs, by excretion and reabsorption of fixed acid and bicarbonate by the kidneys, and by chemical buffering.

Buffers

A buffer is a solute that resists pH change when acids or bases are added. The buffer base consists of bicarbonate and all nonbicarbonate buffers. The bicarbonate buffer system cannot buffer volatile acids but does buffer approximately 75% of all the fixed acid generated by the body. The nonbicarbonate buffer system consists primarily of proteins, hemoglobin, and phosphate. It buffers volatile, nonfixed, acids.

Bicarbonate

The primary metabolic parameter, bicarbonate, may be reported as carbon dioxide content, carbon dioxide combining power, carbon dioxide, or standard bicarbonate, any of which refers to the same factor. Bicarbonate is measured by concentration and reported as milliequivalent per liter (mEq/L). It is universally related to the quantity of fixed acid excess and therefore is more a controlled than a controlling factor.

Sources of fixed acids include organic and inorganic dietary acids, lactic acid as a by-product of cell metabolism without oxygen, and ketoacids as by-products of cell metabolism without glucose or insulin.

The normal excretion rate of fixed acid by the kidneys is 50 mEq/day. However, the excretion and reabsorption of both hydrogen and bicarbonate can be greatly increased or decreased by body demands.

The normal bicarbonate range is 24 ± 3 mEq/L. The minimum level compatible with life is 1 mEq/L, the maximum level is 48 mEq/L.

Base Excess

The base excess (BE) parameter is the sum total in concentration of all the buffer anions (bicarbonate and nonbicarbonate) in a sample of whole blood, equilibrated with a normal P_{CO_2} (40 mm Hg). Because BE is equilibrated with a normal P_{CO_2}, it is not affected by primary respiratory imbalances.

Normal BE is 48 ± 3 mm/L but is reported as plus or minus zero, with zero representing 48 mm/L. In metabolic acidosis, BE is minus; in metabolic alkalosis, BE is plus.

Physics of Gas

The parameters discussed so far are measured by concentration. The two respiratory parameters measured by pressure (intensity) warrant a brief review of the physics of gas.

Gas has volume, which refers to the space the gas occupies and is measured in cubic centimeters (cc). Gas has pressure, which is measured mathematically as force per unit area by noting the height to which the force can support a column of mercury. This measurement is expressed in millimeters of mercury (mm Hg). Gas has temperature, which is generated by gas molecules in constant motion and is measured in degrees Celsius (°C) or Fahrenheit (°F). Dalton's law regarding the behavior of gas in a mixture, as applied to oxygen in the atmosphere (room air), indicates the following:

- The total pressure of the gas mixture equals the sum of the partial pressures of each gas, or **total pressure of atmosphere** (P_{atm}) = partial pressure oxygen (P_{O_2}) + partial pressure nitrogen (P_{N_2}) + partial pressure carbon dioxide (P_{CO_2}).
- Each gas acts independently, as if it alone occupied the total space.
- Each gas contribution to the total pressure depends solely on the percentage of the total gas it occupies. The contribution of oxygen to the total atmospheric pressure is 21%. (Other variables not discussed here can exist.)
- The partial pressure of each gas depends on the number of molecules existing in the fixed space. At high elevations the number of oxygen molecules is decreased; therefore, P_{O_2} is decreased.
- Each gas is unaffected by any changes in other gas molecules. The P_{O_2} does not increase or decrease because P_{CO_2} is increased or decreased.

Partial Pressure of Carbon Dioxide

The P_{CO_2} value reflects the adequacy of alveolar ventilation. It is the primary respiratory parameter. Carbon dioxide is eliminated by the lungs at the same rate formed by the tissues and at the same time maintains constant blood levels.

Arterial P_{CO_2} is inversely related to the level of ventilation. With hypoventilation, carbon dioxide is retained and the P_{CO_2} elevates; with hyperventilation, carbon dioxide is blown off and the P_{CO_2} decreases.

The normal range for P_{CO_2} is 40 ± 4 mm Hg. The minimum value compatible with life is 9 mm Hg; the maximum value is 158 mm Hg.

Partial Pressure of Oxygen

The P_{O_2} value is also an intensity factor, measured in millimeters of mercury. It tells how fast and for how long oxygen passes from blood into tissue. The P_{O_2} is usually not a direct influence in acid–base balance.

Normal P_{O_2} values are oxygen and age dependent. When the F_{IO_2} is 21% (room air) and the patient is 60 years of age or younger, the P_{O_2} should be at least 80 mm Hg. With each 10-year advance in age, the normal P_{O_2} decreases by 10 mm Hg. If the P_{O_2} is 50 mm Hg or lower in a patient younger than 60 years of age, respiratory failure is present. A P_{O_2} between 50 and 75 mm Hg reflects moderate hypoxemia.

Hypoxemia

Hypoxemia is insufficient oxygenation of the blood and can be measured directly by the P_{O_2}. Hypoxia—insufficient oxygenation of the tissues—cannot be directly measured but is presumed if the partial pressure of oxygen in venous blood ($P_{\overline{v}O_2}$) is 30 mm Hg or lower. To avoid hypoxia when hypoxemia is present, the cardiovascular system must increase the rate of tissue perfusion or the hemoglobin content must be elevated (Ryabov, 1995).

Shunting is a common cause of hypoxemia. Shunting is any impediment in the blood transport system that results in blood not coming in contact with oxygen. This can be seen in vascular lung tumors, a right-to-left intracardiac shunt, or capillary shunting in which pulmonary capillary blood comes in contact with totally unventilated alveoli (dead space).

Oxygen Saturation

Oxygen saturation (S_{aO_2}) is the parameter that tells the amount of oxygen taken up by hemoglobin when fully saturated. It is a quantity factor and is measured in percentage. It may also be called $P_{O_2}\%$. The normal adult values are 96% to 97% before 65 years of age and 95% to 96% in older patients. Oxygen saturation:

- Depends on P_{O_2}. When the pressure exceeds a certain value, the amount of oxygen taken in no longer increases.

- Is altered by pH. If P_{O_2} remains constant, oxygen saturation decreases when the pH decreases and increases when the pH increases.
- Is altered by temperature. If the P_{O_2} is constant, oxygen saturation decreases when the temperature increases and increases when the temperature decreases.

This indicates that hyperthermia causes metabolic acidosis and hypothermia causes metabolic alkalosis. In hypothermia, the oxygen need is decreased, but the oxygen is bound so tightly to the hemoglobin that the ability to deliver it is greatly decreased. Inhalation of carbon dioxide may be used to cause acidosis and release the bound oxygen.

Chemoreceptors and Primary Acid–Base Imbalances

Chemoreceptors located peripherally in aortic and carotid vessels and centrally in the brain play a role in body responses to abnormal P_{CO_2} and P_{O_2} values. Chemoreceptors signal the brain to stimulate or depress ventilation, according to body needs. The response to an elevated P_{CO_2} is greater than to a decreased P_{O_2} because P_{CO_2} elevation is a danger signal of respiratory failure. At high altitudes where oxygen supply is decreased, oxygen need is greater than P_{CO_2} constancy; the chemoreceptors stimulate hyperventilation to obtain more oxygen, but this hyperventilation results in a decreased P_{CO_2}. Box 15-2 summarizes normal ABG values.

Metabolic Acidosis

Metabolic acidosis results from an excess of fixed acids or a primary bicarbonate deficit. The primary causes are

- Increased production of fixed acids, including ketoacids, which are evident in diabetic acidosis or starvation when glucose and insulin are unavailable for cell metabolism, and lactic acid, which is evident in in cardiopulmonary failure when oxygen is unavailable for cell metabolism

---

BOX 15-2 **Normal Arterial Blood Gas Values**[*]

pH — 7.35–7.45
Pco₂ — 36–44 mm Hg
Po₂ — 80–95 mm Hg
Sao₂ — 95%–96%
HCO₃⁻ — 22–26 mEq/L
Base excess — ±3

---

*At sea level (Metheny, 2000).

- Failure of kidneys to excrete fixed acid
- Primary bicarbonate deficit—severe diarrhea or bowel or biliary fistula

This is a metabolic imbalance because bicarbonate is the parameter primarily affected. Acidosis is present because the carbon dioxide level has not changed, but the decrease in bicarbonate has caused the ratio to go closer than 1 part acid to 20 parts base. It can be between 1:16 and 1:5, depending on the degree of bicarbonate deficit. Because pH depends on the acid–base ratio, and this ratio has now narrowed, acidosis is present. BE is minus because there is not enough bicarbonate to buffer the fixed acid.

Arterial blood gas values in metabolic acidosis:

pH: <7.35
Hco_3^-: <22 mEq/L
Pco_2: normal (40 ± 4 mm Hg)
BE: <−3

If the metabolic acidosis is of renal origin, the kidneys cannot respond. If it is of nonrenal origin, the kidneys increase the excretion of hydrogen and the reabsorption of bicarbonate. This response is slow, but, once started, can be maintained for weeks or months.

The chemoreceptors are sensitive to the increase in hydrogen and stimulate compensatory hyperventilation to blow off carbon dioxide, decreasing the Pco_2 less than 40 mm Hg to obtain an acid–base ratio closer to normal (1:20) needed for a normal pH. This compensatory respiratory response is prompt and predictable; it occurs within minutes but becomes less effective with time. The limit of compensatory hyperventilation occurs when the Pco_2 reaches 12 mm Hg.

After the kidneys and lungs respond, bicarbonate increases to a level closer to normal. Pco_2 decreases, and the acid–base ratio comes closer to 1:20 with a resultant pH closer to normal. Compensation thus occurs.

With bicarbonate administration, the bicarbonate level reverts to normal, and the lungs stop hyperventilation. Therefore, Pco_2 reverts to normal, resulting in a 1:20 acid–base ratio and allowing a normal pH (7.35 to 7.45). Correction thereby is achieved.

Metabolic Alkalosis

Metabolic alkalosis results from a decrease in body content of fixed acids or a primary bicarbonate excess. The primary causes are

- Excessive loss of fixed acids resulting, for example, from prolonged vomiting, gastric suctioning, potassium deficit
- Primary bicarbonate excess resulting, for example, from excessive administration of sodium bicarbonate, sodium citrate, or chloride deficit, whereby bicarbonate increases to maintain cation–anion balance or sodium deficit, with bicarbonate excretion dependent on sodium

This is a metabolic imbalance because the primary parameter affected is bicarbonate. Alkalosis occurs because the acid–base ratio has widened to 1 part acid to 25 to 50 parts base. This ratio results in a pH elevation. Because there is an excess of bicarbonate, the BE is plus.

Arterial blood gas values in metabolic alkalosis:

pH: >7.45
Hco_3^-: >26 mEq/L
Pco_2: normal (40 ± 4 mm Hg)
BE: >±3

Whether the kidneys respond to metabolic alkalosis depends on several factors. An increase in bicarbonate causes bicarbonate excretion to increase, provided there is no deficit of chloride or potassium. If a chloride depletion is present, bicarbonate is reabsorbed as the accompanying anion for sodium. Because a bicarbonate increase is usually accompanied by an increase in sodium, a decrease in chloride, and a potassium deficit, bicarbonate is not excreted but reabsorbed.

Compensatory respiratory response to metabolic alkalosis is variable. The degree of hypoventilation that occurs depends on the causative factors. Regardless of the cause, hypoventilation as a compensatory response is rarely sufficient to bring the Pco_2 above 55 mm Hg because an elevated Pco_2 causes the chemoreceptors to stimulate breathing to prevent respiratory failure.

When the lungs and kidneys do respond, some compensation occurs: bicarbonate falls, Pco_2 rises, and the acid–base ratio comes closer to 1:20. The pH thus decreases to a level closer to normal.

Correction occurs with the administration of solutions containing chloride and potassium. In assessing and treating respiratory imbalances, ABG measurements are an absolute clinical necessity because ventilation is reflected in Pco_2 and oxygenation in Po_2. Furthermore, acute respiratory failure may occur with slight changes in pulse, blood pressure, or alertness until cardiopulmonary collapse occurs.

Respiratory Acidosis

Respiratory acidosis is always caused by carbon dioxide retention from hypoventilation. This is rarely seen without hypoxemia (Po_2 <60 mm Hg). The causes of hypoventilation include

- Anesthesia, narcotics
- Central nervous system disease such as polio, spinal cord lesions
- Severe hypokalemia
- Intrathoracic collection of blood, fluid, or air
- Pulmonary diseases, both restrictive (congestive heart failure, tumors, atelectasis) and obstructive (bronchitis, emphysema, asthma, or foreign body)

The acidosis process is respiratory because the P_{CO_2} is the primary parameter involved. Nonfixed, volatile acid (P_{CO_2}) is in excess but the base (bicarbonate) is normal. The acid–base ratio is closer than 1:20; it is between 1:5 and 1:20, resulting in acidosis.

Arterial blood gas values in respiratory acidosis:

pH: <7.35
P_{CO_2}: >44 mm Hg
$H_{CO_3}^-$: normal (24 ± 2 mEq/L)

Because the lungs are always the primary cause of respiratory acidosis, they cannot play a role in compensation. Renal compensation is always slow in onset but effective once started: generation and reabsorption of bicarbonate increase, excretion of hydrogen increases, and the excretion of chloride increases, resulting in a chloride deficit.

With renal response, bicarbonate rises above normal, and P_{CO_2} remains unchanged. The acid ratio comes closer to 1:20, allowing for some compensation, with a pH closer to normal.

Correction of respiratory acidosis is possible only by correction of the pulmonary cause. Chloride solutions are usually given to treat the chloride deficit.

Respiratory Alkalosis

Respiratory alkalosis is always caused by a carbon dioxide deficit due to hyperventilation. Factors causing hyperventilation include the following:

- Chemoreceptor response to hypoxemia. The chemoreceptors sense the decrease in oxygen and send a message to the brain to stimulate ventilation. This hyperventilation results in carbon dioxide being blown off, thus decreasing P_{CO_2}. This is normal at high altitudes.
- Respiratory response to metabolic acidosis. This response can persist for several hours or days after the metabolic acidosis is corrected because of higher levels of hydrogen excess in cerebrospinal fluid and the fact that chemoreceptors are more responsive to cerebrospinal fluid than to blood.
- Central nervous system malfunctions (trauma, infection, brain lesions).
- Anxiety, pain, fever, shock.
- Anemia, carbon monoxide poisoning.
- Epinephrine, salicylates, and progesterone.
- Improper mechanical ventilation. Any patient with chronic obstructive pulmonary disease who is overcorrected by mechanical ventilation so that the P_{CO_2} decreases faster than 10 mm Hg/hour will have respiratory alkalosis.

This hyperventilation process is respiratory because P_{CO_2} is the primary parameter affected. Alkalosis is present because carbon dioxide is decreased and the bicarbonate value is normal, resulting in an acid–base ratio between 1:25 and 1:50. This ratio results in a pH above 7.45.

Arterial blood gas values in respiratory alkalosis:

pH: >7.45
P_{CO_2}: <36 mm Hg
$H_{CO_3}^-$: normal (24 ± 2 mEq/L)

Because the lungs are the primary cause of respiratory alkalosis, they cannot respond for compensation. Renal response occurs after several hours or days. The kidneys decrease excretion of hydrogen and increase excretion of bicarbonate. The urine cannot become more alkaline than pH 7.0. This renal response creates some compensation. The bicarbonate value drops below 24 mEq/L. The acid–base ratio comes closer to 1:20, allowing the pH to come closer to normal.

Respiratory alkalosis can be corrected by administering chloride solutions to replace the bicarbonate ion load. However, the buffering capacity of the plasma has been compromised as a result of the alkalosis and any additional insult to the balance is poorly tolerated.

Mixed Acid–Base Imbalances

In the hospital setting, two or more primary imbalances may coexist in the same patient. The following combinations sometimes occur:

- Metabolic acidosis and metabolic alkalosis in a patient who has diabetic acidosis and who is vomiting
- Metabolic acidosis and respiratory acidosis in a patient with severe pulmonary edema, followed by cardiogenic shock
- Metabolic acidosis and respiratory alkalosis in a patient with both kidney and liver failure
- Respiratory acidosis and metabolic alkalosis in a patient who has chronic respiratory insufficiency and who is on a salt-poor diet and taking diuretics
- Respiratory alkalosis and metabolic alkalosis are usually seen as a result of mechanical overventilation.

Respiratory acidosis and respiratory alkalosis cannot coexist because a person cannot hypoventilate and hyperventilate at the same time.

References and Selected Readings

Asterisks indicate references cited in text.

American Association of Blood Banks. (1999). *Technical manual* (13th ed.). Bethesda, MD: Author.

Bennett, J.V. & Brachman, P.S. (1998). *Hospital infections* (4th ed.). Philadelphia: Lippincott Williams & Wilkins.

*Horne, C. & Derrico, D. (1999). Mastering ABGs: The art of arterial blood gas measurement. *American Journal of Nursing, 99*(8), 26–33.

Metheny, N.M. (2000). *Fluid and electrolyte balance* (4th ed.). Philadelphia: Lippincott Williams & Wilkins.

*Ryabov, G. (1995, November). *Hypoxia: Incidence, identification, and interventions.* Lecture presented at the Mount Sinai Hospital Medical Center/Finch University of Health Sciences, New York, NY.

Review Questions

Note: Questions below may have more than one right answer.

1. Which of the following tests should be performed before insertion of an indwelling catheter in the radial artery?

   A. Allen's

   B. Swan-Ganz

   C. Serial

   D. Dalton's

2. Oxygen dissolved in plasma is expressed as:

   A. Pa_{O_2}

   B. P_{O_2}

   C. P_{CO_2}

   D. pH

3. ABG values may be altered by:

   A. Bicarbonate

   B. Air bubbles

   C. Excess heparin

   D. Dry spots

4. Which of the following is true of the ulnar artery?

   A. It is deep

   B. It is difficult to stabilize

   C. It lies close to nerves

   D. A and B only

5. Mixed acid–base imbalances may coexist in the same patient. Which of the following are examples?

   A. Metabolic acidosis and metabolic alkalosis in a patient who has diabetic acidosis and who is vomiting

   B. Metabolic acidosis and respiratory acidosis in a patient with severe pulmonary edema

   C. A only

   D. A and B

6. Constant arterial monitoring is used for:

   A. Systolic, diastolic, and mean arterial pressure readings

   B. Assessment of cardiovascular effects of vasopressor or vasodilator drugs during shock

   C. Simultaneous ABG sampling

   D. All of the above

7. Blood pH is directly proportional to the ratio of:

   A. Carbonic acid to bicarbonate

   B. Bicarbonate to carbonic acid

   C. Base excess

   D. Alkalinity of the blood

8. In metabolic acidosis, base excess is:

   A. Plus

   B. Minus

   C. Zero

   D. Minimal

9. All of the following are true of the P_{O_2} value *except*:

   A. Tells how fast and for how long oxygen will pass from blood into tissue

   B. Tells how slowly oxygen will pass from blood into tissue

   C. Reflects adequacy of alveolar ventilation

   D. Is an intensity factor, measured in mm Hg

10. Impediments in blood transport system resulting in blood not coming in contact with oxygen may be seen in which of the following clinical conditions?

    A. Vascular lung tumors

    B. Right-to-left intracardiac shunt

    C. Capillary shunting

    D. Metabolic acidosis

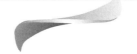

PATIENT-SPECIFIC THERAPIES

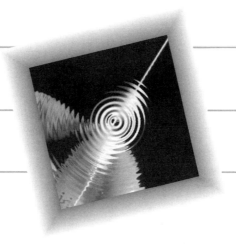

CHAPTER 16

Parenteral Nutrition

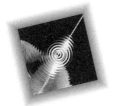

KEY TERMS

Admixture	Nutrients
Drug–Nutrient Interaction	Nutritional Screening
Enteral Nutrition	Nutritional Support
Kwashiorkor	Parenteral Hyperalimentation
Malnutrition	Protein Malnutrition
Marasmus	Total Nutrient Admixture

■ HISTORY OF PARENTERAL NUTRITION

Development of parenteral nutrition (PN), formerly known as *hyperalimentation,* began in the early 1960s in the Harrison Department of Surgical Research at the University of Pennsylvania. Dr. Stanley Dudrick devised a system of feeding by central venous routes that resulted in the normal weight gain and growth of beagle puppies that were fed only by vein (Dudrick & Wilmore, 1968). His animal experiments quickly led to human applications; he successfully used hyperalimentation to feed a severely ill infant who was unable to sustain herself with any type of gastrointestinal (GI) feeding because of small bowel atresia (Wilmore & Dudrick, 1968).

Further applications followed in the adult population. The term **parenteral hyperalimentation** was coined by Dr. Jonathan E. Rhoads and Dr. Dudrick, and defined as "the intravenous administration of nitrogen, calories, and other nutrients sufficient to achieve tissue synthesis and anabolism in patients with normal or excessive nutritional needs" (Dudrick & Wilmore, 1968). These accomplishments led to further research and application as other clinicians and researchers realized their potential. Hyperalimentation soon became a recognized specialty and nutritional support teams were formed. (Basically, **nutritional support** provides specially formulated or delivered parenteral or enteral nutrients to maintain or restore optimal nutrition status.)

JoAnne Grant became the first nurse hired exclusively for work with this new form of nutritional support at the University of Pennsylvania, in 1967. In 1976, a multidisciplinary group of professionals (physicians, nurses, dietitians, and pharmacists) was organized and the American Society for Parenteral and Enteral Nutrition (A.S.P.E.N.) held its first clinical congress in Chicago.

Hyperalimentation evolved as a science in the 1980s, and became more commonly known as total PN or simply PN, the term used throughout this chapter. Disease-specific formulas were developed to address the particular needs of patients with renal, cardiac, or hepatic disease, and became commercially available. The rehabilitation of patients surviving catastrophic illnesses by maintenance on home PN (HPN) led to the formation of support groups such as LifeLine and the Oley Foundation. Nutritional support research continued at a rapid pace. From this modest beginning, PN evolved into a sophisticated field of therapeutic intervention that has its own multidisciplinary specialists and a large body of established knowledge.

Research Issues: CURRENT INVESTIGATIONS

Current areas of ongoing parenteral nutrition research include:

- The role of amino acids such as arginine and glutamine
- Designer lipid formulations (medium-chain triglycerides and structured triglycerides) and indications for their use
- Implications of antioxidants, growth hormone, and cytokines

With the changing health care environment and emergence of managed care in the 1990s, additional changes and challenges came to the field of nutritional support. Among the challenges were a growing focus on home care, home nutritional support, and nutritional support in long-term care facilities, together with increasingly stringent restrictions on reimbursement for home nutritional support. In light of this, nutritional support teams are also moving into the outpatient setting or being eliminated.

■ INDICATIONS FOR PARENTERAL NUTRITION

Indications for PN are diverse. They depend on the patient's clinical status, the severity of the current illness, the degree of catabolism, complications and other diagnoses, and the length of time the patient will be without GI function and adequate oral intake (Curtis, 1996; Evans-Stoner, 1997; Souba, 1997).

Although the need for PN is clear in patients who have a nonfunctional GI tract and who are expected to eat in 7 to 10 days, the expense and risk of complications associated with such treatment mandate careful consideration of its use in others. The standard rule is still appropriate: "When the gut works, use it!" The enteral route is preferred whenever possible because it is more physiologic—that is, it maintains the integrity and function of the GI tract. The enteral route is also less expensive, less invasive, and easier to manage, with generally fewer complications. Some general guidelines for the appropriate use of PN are outlined in Box 16–1.

BOX 16–1 **Guidelines for Parenteral Nutrition**

Criteria

- Patient has nonfunctioning gastrointestinal (GI) tract that cannot be used safely and effectively, or it is undesirable or contraindicated to use it over a prolonged period
- Patient cannot tolerate adequate nutrition orally

Guidelines

1. Normally nourished patients who cannot eat for 7 to 10 days generally do not require PN.
2. PN should be promptly initiated as soon as it is determined that enteral starvation will persist for 7 to 10 days or more, even if the patient can take nourishment normally.
3. Moderately malnourished patients who require intensive medical or major surgical intervention should be started on PN immediately.
4. Markedly hypercatabolic patients (burns, sepsis, trauma) should be started on PN immediately, even if well nourished.
5. Severely malnourished patients should begin PN immediately.
6. Acute metabolic derangements should be corrected *before* PN is initiated (patient should be hemodynamically stable).
7. Situations in which PN may be useful include:

   - Acute pancreatitis
   - Enterocutaneous fistulas
   - Intractable vomiting, diarrhea
   - Hyperemesis gravidarum
   - Intensive cancer chemotherapy or radiation therapy
   - Inflammatory bowel disease
   - Short bowel syndrome

Contraindications

- Patients who have a functional and usable GI tract capable of absorbing adequate nutrients
- The need for PN is anticipated for fewer than 5 days
- When aggressive nutritional support is not desired by the patient or legal guardian, in accordance with hospital policy and existing law
- Prognosis does not warrant aggressive nutritional support; that is, should not be used when malnutrition is due to rapidly progressive disease that is not amenable to curative or palliative therapy (not to be used to sustain the hopelessly ill because PN may only prolong suffering)
- Periods of acute hemodynamic instability
- Surgical operations, unless it is a short procedure performed with the patient receiving a local anesthetic
- When the risks of PN are judged to exceed the potential benefit

One study showed that PN that was not indicated or that was preventable resulted annually in more than $500,000 in patient charges, not counting charges related to treatment of potentially avoidable complications of PN (Trujillo, Young, Chertow et al., 1999).

■ NUTRITIONAL ASSESSMENT

Nutritional assessment is necessary because inadequate nutrition increases complications of disease, especially infection; decreases the ability to heal wounds; prolongs length of hospital stay; and contributes to anorexia and weakness. Three major types of malnutrition have been identified. They are characterized by pathogenesis and specific clinical findings:

- **Marasmus** (caloric), a gradual wasting of body fat and muscle, with intact visceral protein stores. A patient with marasmus is emaciated. Marasmus is often associated with chronic illness and starvation.
- **Kwashiorkor** (protein), also called *hypoalbuminemia*, loss of visceral protein stores in the presence of adequate fat and muscle. Kwashiorkor is usually associated with poor protein intake in the presence of adequate calories and, in acute situations, with increased stress.
- Mixed marasmus and hypoalbuminemia, a combination of fat loss and muscle wasting with depleted visceral protein stores (Curtis, 1996).

In hospitalized patients, acute hypoalbuminemia, another clinical state, is recognized (Grant, 1992). Acute hypoalbuminemia is commonly seen with acute stress and hypermetabolism, especially in the presence of inadequate nutrition. Rapid and marked decreases in serum albumin occur, often characterized by edema or generalized anasarca. The acute fall is caused by redistribution of albumin into extravascular compartments, external losses, and, to a lesser extent, by alterations in protein synthesis to meet demands for acute-phase proteins, and increased albumin degradation.

Early nutritional intervention is recommended to avoid additional complications of malnutrition. Although not due to malnutrition, acute hypoalbuminemia is associated with increased morbidity and mortality.

Nutritional Screening and Assessment Standards

Starting in 1995, the Joint Commission on the Accreditation of Healthcare Organizations (JCAHO) standards for both hospital and home care mandated screening and nutritional assessment as part of the specific nutritional care standards. The standards emphasize an interdisciplinary approach. **Nutritional screening** is "the process of using characteristics known to be associated with nutrition problems in order to determine if patients are malnourished or at high nutrition risk for malnourishment" (JCAHO, 1999).

Many hospitals have established formal nutritional screening programs for all hospital admissions to identify those patients most at risk or already malnourished. An algorithm for nutritional screening is presented in Figure 16–1. A nutritional screening tool for use by registered nurses to classify the nutritional status of hospitalized patients appears in Figure 16–2. When indicated by nutritional screening results, a nutritional assessment should be completed.

A nutritional assessment should be included in the overall assessment of patients, particularly on admission to the hospital and periodically throughout the hospital stay. It should also be a component of nursing assessment in all health care settings, with reassessment at appropriate intervals, depending on the patient's status. Primary care, outpatient management, and the new standards have moved the role

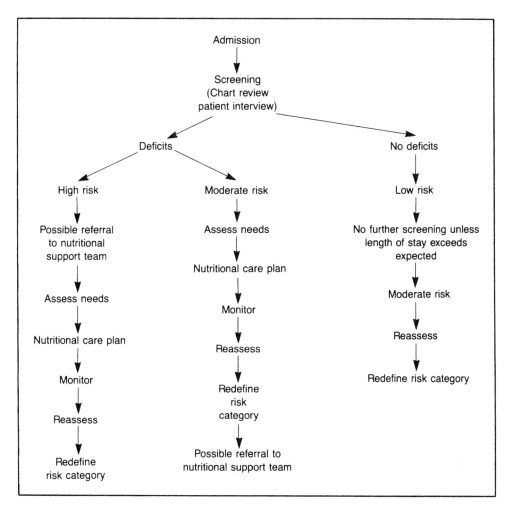

Figure 16–1. Nutritional screening (Courtesy of Grant, A., & DeHoog, S. [1999]. Nutritional assessment, support and management. Seattle: Authors).

A. Diagnosis

If the patient has at least ONE of the following diagnoses, circle and proceed to section E to consider the patient AT NUTRITIONAL RISK and stop here.

Anorexia nervosa/bulimia nervosa

Malabsorption (celiac sprue, ulcerative colitis, Crohn's disease, short bowel syndrome)

Multiple trauma (closed-head injury, penetrating trauma, multiple fractures)

Decubitus ulcers

Major gastrointestinal surgery within the past year

Cachexia (temporal wasting, muscle wasting, cancer, cardiac)

Coma

Diabetes

End-stage liver disease

End-stage renal disease

Nonhealing wounds

B. Nutrition intake history

If the patient has at least ONE of the following symptoms, circle and proceed to section E to consider the patient AT NUTRITIONAL RISK and stop here.

Diarrhea (>500 mL × 2 days)

Vomiting (>5 days)

Reduced intake (<1/2 normal intake for >5 days)

C. Ideal body weight standards

Compare the patient's current weight for height to the ideal body weight chart on the back of this form. If at <80% of ideal body weight, proceed to section E to consider the patient AT NUTRITIONAL RISK and stop here.

D. Weight history

Any recent unplanned weight loss? No _____ Yes _____ Amount (lbs or kg) _____

If yes, within the past _____ weeks or _____ months

Current weight (lbs or kg) _____

Usual weight (lbs or kg) _____

Height (ft, in or cm) _____

Find percentage of weight lost: $\underline{\text{usual wt} - \text{current wt}} \times 100 = $ _____ % wt loss
usual wt

Compare the % wt loss with the chart values and circle appropriate value

Length of time	Significant (%)	Severe (%)
1 week	1–2	>2
2–3 weeks	2–3	>3
1 month	4–5	>5
3 months	7–8	>8
5+ months	10	>10

If the patient has experienced a significant or severe weight loss, proceed to section E and consider the patient AT NUTRITIONAL RISK

E. Nurse assessment

Using the above criteria, what is this patient's nutritional risk? (circle one)

_____ LOW NUTRITIONAL RISK

_____ AT NUTRITIONAL RISK

Figure 16–2. Admission nutritional assessment tool (Reproduced with permission from Kovacevich, D. S., Boney, A. R., Braunschweig, C. L., et al. [1997]. Nutritional risk classification: A reproducible and valid tool for nurses. *Nutrition Support in Clinical Practice*, 12, 20–25.

of nutritional assessment into the physician's office and home care setting as well. Mechanisms for documenting nutritional screening and assessment should be established and monitored. Suggested goals of nutritional assessment include the following:

- To identify nutritional status and deficiencies that adversely affect health
- To obtain specific information to assist in planning and delivery of nutritional support
- To evaluate the efficacy of nutrition support and to modify the patient's care plan as needed to obtain the desired result (Curtis, 1996; Evans-Stoner, 1997)

A nutritional assessment traditionally begins with a complete history, which includes a diet history, anthropometric measurements, physical assessment, and complete medical history, including **drug–nutrient interactions,** and biochemical evaluation.

Health and Diet History

The patient's usual and current dietary intake is helpful in identifying the adequacy of **nutrients** (ie, protein, carbohydrate, lipid, vitamins, minerals, trace elements, and water) and possible nutritional deficiencies. Nutrients in the medical history should include any acute or chronic diseases that may have an impact on nutrient intake or utilization and conditions that increase metabolic needs or fluid and electrolyte losses. Surgical history, certain medications, and social factors also have an impact on nutritional status and should be evaluated. Box 16–2 lists some of the specific factors that may alter nutritional status.

Physical Assessment

A thorough physical assessment by an experienced clinician can detect signs and symptoms suggesting nutritional deficiencies. These include but are not limited to changes in hair, eyes, skin, nails, and all organ systems (Table 16–1).

Anthropometrics

Anthropometric measurements consist of simple, noninvasive, inexpensive techniques for obtaining body measurements used to evaluate a patient's nutritional status. The patient's actual height and weight should be obtained and used as a baseline. The weight should be measured periodically thereafter using the same scale, same amount of clothing, and the same time of day (Curtis, 1996).

In assessing body weight, the current weight is compared with usual body weight (UBW) and ideal body weight (IBW). Standard reference tables such as the Metropolitan Life Insurance tables, based on sex, height, and body frame, can be

---

BOX 16–2 **Factors Influencing Food Intake**

Diet

Food allergies, aversions, and intolerance
Fad diets
Diet modifications (low sodium, low fat)
Ethnic and cultural factors
Poor dentition or ill-fitting dentures
Oral sores or lesions
Alteration in taste or smell
Breathing difficulty
Inability to prepare food or feed self
Frequent fasting (NPO) status, clear liquid diet

Health Factors

Chewing or swallowing difficulty
Neurologic impairment
Malabsorption
Inflammatory bowel disease
Chronic illness (ie, chronic obstructive pulmonary disease, human immunodeficiency virus infection, liver disease, end-stage renal disease, cancer)
Increased losses from draining wounds, ostomies, fistulas, effusions, diarrhea

Surgical History

Small or large bowel obstruction
Surgical reconstruction (ie, gastrectomy, gastrojejunostomy, esophagogastrectomy, small intestine resection)
Head and neck surgery
Surgical procedure for morbid obesity

Medications

Medications may alter dietary intake or nutrient utilization:
Analgesics
Antacids
Antibiotics
Anticonvulsants
Antineoplastic agents
Diuretics
Laxatives
Oral contraceptives

Psychosocial Factors

Religion
Ethnic background
Income

(continued)

Education
Psychological or physical disabilities
Recent loss of spouse/partner
Alcohol or substance abuse
Institutionalization

used to determine IBW. Body frame can be determined by measuring the wrist circumference just distal to the styloid process (Table 16–2). Weight loss has been directly correlated to morbidity. Weight loss of 35% to 40% usually is not compatible with life. Current weight as a percentage of UBW is usually the most accurate determinant of weight loss, and can be calculated as follows:

$$\text{Usual weight} = \frac{\text{Actual weight}}{\text{Usual weight}} \times 100$$

TABLE 16 – 1
PHYSICAL ASSESSMENT FINDINGS IN NUTRITIONAL DEFICIENCIES

Physical Changes	Deficiency
Hair	
Lackluster, thin, sparse; pigmentation changes	Protein, calorie, zinc, linoleic acid
Mouth	
Angular stomatitis: cracks, redness at one or both corners of mouth	Vitamin B
Cheilosis—vertical cracks in lips	Riboflavin and niacin
Varicose veins under tongue	Vitamin C
Tongue	
May become purplish, red, or beefy red or may appear smooth and pale; one or more fissures, atrophy of taste buds	Vitamin B
Skin	
Dryness, flakiness	Vitamin A, essential fatty acids
Petechiae or easy bruising; hemorrhagic spots on skin at pressure points; may occur in presence of liver disease or during anticoagulation	Vitamins C and K
Musculoskeletal	
Muscle wasting (especially quadriceps, deltoids, and temporalis)	Protein, calorie
Kyphosis, osteoporosis	Calcium and vitamin D
Neurologic	
Confusion, listlessness	Protein malnutrition
Sensory-motor, vibratory	Thiamine and vitamin B_{12}

TABLE 16-2
DETERMINATION OF BODY FRAME

Frame	Male	Female
Large	r* = >10.4 cm	r = >10.9 cm
Medium	r = 9.6–10.4 cm	r = 9.9–10.9 cm
Small	r = <9.6 cm	r = <9.9 cm

$$*r = \frac{\text{Height (cm)}}{\text{Wrist circumference (cm)}}$$

(Curtis, S. [1996]. Nutrition assessment of adults. In K. A. Hennesy & M. E. Orr (Eds.), *Nutrition support nursing core curriculum* (3rd ed., pp. 1-1–12). Silver Spring, MD: American Society for Parenteral and Enteral Nutrition.)

Percentage of IBW may also be used, and can be determined with the preceding formula by substituting IBW for UBW, although this formula usually is not as accurate. A normally thin person, with stable weight, may be incorrectly identified as malnourished if weight is less than IBW; the obese patient with significant recent weight loss may be overlooked if weight is still above IBW (Grant, 1992) (Table 16–3). Fluid status also should be considered when evaluating weight; significant edema or ascites may contribute to significant fluid weight (Curtis, 1996; Evans-Stoner, 1997).

Other anthropometric measurements include triceps skinfold thickness, which estimates subcutaneous fat stores, and midarm muscle circumference, which estimates somatic protein stores (skeletal muscle mass). These indices are no longer as widely used because of questions concerning their validity. Reproducibility of these measurements requires strict adherence to protocol and may vary widely in the same

TABLE 16-3
EVALUATION OF WEIGHT CHANGE

Loss	Significant Weight Loss	Severe Weight Loss
1 wk	1%–2%	>2%
1 mo	5%	>5%
3 mo	7.5%	>7.5%
6 mo	10%	>10%

Values charted are for percent weight change:

$$\text{Percent weight change} = \frac{\text{Usual weight} - \text{actual weight}}{\text{Usual weight}} \times 100$$

(Reproduced with permission from Blackburn, G.J., Bistrian, B.R., Maini, B.S., Schlamm, B.A., & Smith, M.F. [1997]. Nutritional and metabolic assessment of the hospitalized patient. *Journal of Parenteral and Enteral Nutrition*, 1[1], 17.)

individual with different examiners. A more detailed discussion can be found in other resources (Elia, 1997; Evans-Stoner, 1997).

Body mass index (BMI) can also be used to assess undernutrition or overnutrition, but does not reflect changes in weight (Bray, 1992). See Box 16–3 for an interpretation of BMI. Nomograms are also available.

Biochemical Assessment

A variety of biochemical tests are used to assess nutritional status, with a broad range of cost and sensitivity. The most commonly used, and most readily available, are visceral proteins and tests to evaluate immune function.

VISCERAL PROTEINS

Depletion of visceral proteins is characteristic of **protein malnutrition,** which occurs acutely in the hospitalized patient (hypoalbuminemia). An estimate of visceral protein status can be obtained from measurements of specific serum transport proteins that are synthesized in the liver. These include albumin, transferrin, prealbumin, and retinol-binding protein (Table 16–4). Although the long half-life of albumin makes it less valuable in monitoring acute changes in nutritional status, it is still regarded as the best single test for predicting outcome in hospitalized patients. It is recommended that serum albumin measurements be included in the initial chemical profile when screening for malnutrition. Prealbumin, with a shorter half-life, seems to be a more sensitive and specific indicator to monitor the effectiveness of nutritional support. It is more expensive and may not be available in smaller hospitals. The changes in the levels of these proteins should be evaluated together because they reflect different processes in the body. Consideration should also be given to assessing nonnutritional factors that may affect these visceral proteins. Even though these tests are useful, new nutritional markers are needed that better identify malnourished pa-

---

BOX 16–3 Interpreting Body Mass Index

Formula

$$\frac{\text{Weight (in lbs)} \times 704.5}{\text{Height}^2 \text{ (inches squared)}}$$

Recommended Classification

Underweight	<18.5
Normal	18.5–24.9
Obesity	30–39.9
Extreme obesity	>40

T A B L E 1 6 – 4
VISCERAL PROTEINS

Visceral Protein	Half-Life	Normal Range	Causes of Decrease	Causes of Increase
Albumin Maintains plasma oncotic pressure Carrier protein (zinc, calcium, magnesium, fatty acids)	18–21 d	Normal: >3.5 g/dL Mild depletion: 2.8–3.5 g/dL Mod. depletion: 2.1–2.7 g/dL Severe depletion: <2.1 g/dL Reflects *chronic*, not acute change	Metabolic stress Infection, inflammation Liver disease ↑ Losses (wounds, burns, fistulas) Inadequate protein intake Fluid imbalance (ascites, edema, overhydration) Malabsorptive states	Dehydration may falsely ↑ levels Salt-poor albumin infusion
Transferrin Carrier protein for iron	8–10 d	Normal: >200 mg/dL Mild depletion: 150–200 mg/dL Mod. depletion: 100–150 mg/dL Severe depletion: <100 mg/dL	Chronic infection Inflammatory state Acute catabolic states ↑ Iron stores Liver damage Overhydration	Pregnancy Hepatitis Iron deficiency anemia Dehydration Chronic blood loss
Thyroxine-binding prealbumin (transthyretin) Carrier protein for retinol-binding protein Transport protein for thyroxine	2–3 d	Normal: >20 mg/dL Mild depletion: 10–15 mg/dL Mod. depletion: 5–10 mg/dL Severe depletion: <5 mg/dL Sensitive to acute changes in protein status Limited use in situation in which there is a sudden demand for protein synthesis	Infection Acute catabolic state Postsurgery (5–10 mg/dL drop first week) Liver disease Altered energy and protein balance Hyperthyroid	Chronic renal failure Corticosteroids
Retinol-binding protein Transport retinol (alcohol of vitamin A)	10–18 h	Normal: 3–5 mEq/dL Reflects acute change	Vitamin A deficiency Acute catabolic states Postsurgery Liver disease Hyperthyroid	Renal disease

tients and precisely monitor the effectiveness of nutritional intervention on nutritional status. Other proteins are being investigated to determine their efficacy in nutritional assessment.

IMMUNE FUNCTION TESTS

Alterations in the immune system may be influenced by stress, specific disease states, and malnutrition. The total lymphocyte count (TLC) is indicative of a patient's ability to fight infection and to maintain host integrity, and is known to decrease with malnutrition. The TLC can be derived from a complete blood count with differential, as shown in Box 16–4. Cell-mediated immunity is most frequently evaluated with delayed cutaneous hypersensitivity skin tests. The responses to intradermal injection of three or more common recall antigens are assessed at 24 and 48 hours. Plastic, disposable multiple test applicators are available, including tetanus toxoid, diphtheria toxoid, *Streptococcus*, old tuberculin, *Candida, Trichophyton, Proteus,* and a glycerin negative control. Interpretation of results and methods for measuring the results are not standardized. Results are classified as anergic if there is no response to any of the antigens, relatively anergic if only one response occurs, and normal or reactive if there is a response to two or more antigens. These results must be weighed with other findings in the nutritional assessment because non-nutritional factors, such as infection, sepsis, cancer, liver disease, renal failure, immunosuppressive diseases, and immunosuppressive drugs, may also affect immunocompetence (Elia, 1997).

Other assessment techniques include somatomedin activity, prognostic nutritional index, handgrip dynamometry, isotopic methods, imaging techniques, and whole-body conductivity and impedance measurements (Curtis, 1996; Elia, 1997; Evans-Stoner; 1997). There is no single indicator of nutritional status. A global assessment of many indices, and the patient's clinical status, is necessary to determine the incidence and degree of nutritional deficiency. Reassessment is individualized whenever the clinical status changes, and periodically throughout the course of nutritional therapy.

Once the nutritional assessment data have been collected and evaluated, the optimal method for nutritional support must be selected. This decision process is depicted in Figure 16–3.

BOX 16–4 Evaluation of Total Lymphocyte Count (TLC)

Formula

$$TLC = \frac{Percent\ lymphocytes \times white\ blood\ cells}{100}$$

Interpretation

Mild depletion	1200–2000/mm^3
Moderate depletion	800–1200/mm^3
Severe depletion	<800/mm^3

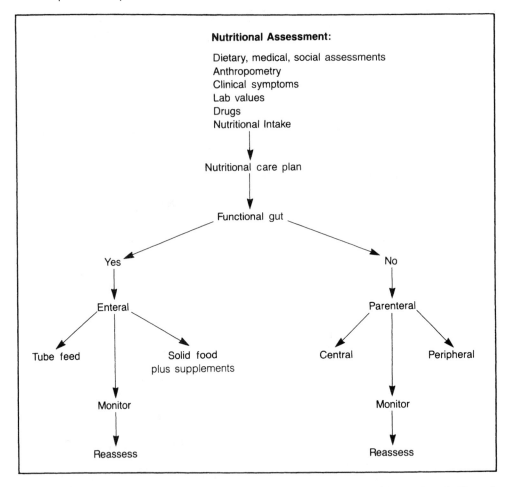

Figure 16–3. Nutritional support and decision-making process (Courtesy of Grant, J. & DeHoog, S. [1999]. Nutritional assessment, support, and management [2nd ed.]. Seattle: Authors).

■ NUTRITIONAL REQUIREMENTS

The practical outcome of the nutritional assessment is to determine the caloric and protein needs of the patient. These requirements increase in acute, catabolic illness, and in some chronic conditions.

Energy Requirements

Nutrient energy requirements are usually expressed in kilocalories (kcal). Numerous methods for determining a person's nutritional requirements are available, with varying degrees of sophistication. One of the most commonly used is the Harris-Benedict equation, which was derived from healthy individuals. It estimates basal energy expenditure (BEE) in kilocalories, using weight, height, age, and sex (Harris & Benedict, 1919), with the following equations:

BEE (male) = (66.47 + 13.75W + 5.0H) − 6.76A

BEE (female) = (655.10 + 9.56W + 1.85H) − 4.68A

where W is weight in kilograms, H is height in centimeters, and A is age in years. UBW is most commonly used, although IBW is often recommended if the patient is obese. Because the BEE does not take into consideration physiologic stress or trauma, a modification of the Harris-Benedict formula is extensively used in clinical practice. Using indirect calorimetry and nitrogen balance studies on normal patients, and those undergoing surgical stress, activity factors (AF) and injury factors (IF) were determined for a variety of stress levels (Table 16–5). Actual energy requirements are then estimated by multiplying BEE × AF × IF. An additional 10% is added to compensate for inefficient caloric utilization.

Others have proposed arbitrarily assigning degrees of catabolism or levels of stress (Cerra, 1984) to the patient's clinical state (Table 16–6). Many find these easier to use because they require no calculations. Most patients do not require more than 35 kcal/kg/day.

A third approach that is pragmatic and probably most useful to clinicians is to provide 25 to 30 kcal/kg/day and 1.5 g/kg/day of protein as a starting point. These are conservative indices; they are easy for the clinician to remember and calculate, and they will not result in overfeeding. Recommendations for nutritional requirements of patients in intensive care have also been proposed (Cerra, Benitez, Blackburn et al., 1997).

Indirect calorimetry may be used at some institutions, mainly teaching hospitals and research centers. This requires expensive equipment that directly measures oxygen consumption and carbon dioxide production to determine actual energy expenditure. The accuracy of the results is determined by the skill of the person doing the test, accurate calibration of the equipment, and the conditions under which the test is performed.

Regardless of the method chosen, it is important to avoid overfeeding. The early adage of nutritional support "the more, the better," is no longer advocated. Overfeeding, which causes hyperglycemia and has deleterious effects on respiratory and hepatic function, should be avoided, especially in the acutely ill patient (Cerra et al., 1997; McMahon, 1997; Souba, 1997). Additional calories for desired weight gain should be held until the patient recovers.

T A B L E   1 6 – 5
CORRECTION FACTORS FOR ESTIMATING NONPROTEIN ENERGY REQUIREMENTS OF HOSPITALIZED PATIENTS

Activity Factors	Injury Factors
Confined to bed 1.2	Minor surgery 1.2
Out of bed 1.3	Skeletal trauma 1.3
	Major sepsis 1.6
	Severe burns 2.1

Basal energy expenditure × (activity factor) × (injury factor) + 10%

TABLE 16-6

METABOLIC REQUIREMENTS ACCORDING TO CATABOLIC DEGREE/STRESS LEVEL

Degree of Net Catabolism	Stress Level	Clinical Type	Urinary Nitrogen Loss (g/d)	Basal Energy Expenditure Multiple	Nonprotein Calories (kcal/kg/d)	Protein Multiple (g/kg/d)	Nonprotein Calorie to Nitrogen Ratio (kcal : gN)
1	0	Non-stressed starvation	5	1.0	20–25	1.0	125 : 1–150 : 1
2	1	Elective surgery (low stress)	5–10	1.3	25	1.5	100 : 1
3	2	Polytrauma (moderate stress)	10–15	1.5	30	2.0	100 : 1–90 : 1
4	3	Sepsis (severe stress)	>15	1.75	35	2.0–2.5	90 : 1

Protein Requirements

Protein requirements for healthy people are based on the amount needed to maintain nitrogen equilibrium, assuming energy is being met by nonprotein kilocalories. The recommended daily allowance for healthy adults is 0.8 g/kg/day, although elderly adults require at least 1 to 1.2 g/kg/day for nitrogen equilibrium (Rolandelli & Ulrich, 1994). Protein requirements are increased during illness to meet stress needs for wound healing, promote immune competence, and replace losses.

Because 6.25 g protein yields 1 g nitrogen, in general, 1.5 g/kg/day of protein is required to achieve nitrogen balance with PN regimens in adults, although up to 2 to 2.5 g/kg/day may be needed.

Calorie–Nitrogen Ratio

Sufficient nonprotein calories to meet energy requirements are needed for protein synthesis. A calorie–nitrogen ratio between 90 : 1 and 150 : 1 has been most often identified, depending on the level of stress. The higher the stress, the lower the calorie–nitrogen ratio (Cerra, 1984).

Nitrogen Balance

A 24-hour urinalysis for urine urea nitrogen is obtained to determine nitrogen balance, which is an objective method of evaluating the efficacy of the patient's nutritional regimen. For the patient to be in a positive nitrogen balance or anabolic state, the amount of nitrogen taken in by the patient (IV and orally) needs to be more than that excreted. A 24-hour urine collection is needed to measure the amount of urinary urea excreted. A factor of 4 g is added (2 g for fecal losses and 2 g for integumentary losses) to measure total nitrogen excretion. The nitrogen balance formula and measures that reflect the severity of the catabolic state can be found in Box 16–5.

BOX 16-5 **Nitrogen Balance**

Formula

Nitrogen balance is calculated by subtracting the amount of nitrogen lost from the amount of nitrogen given or taken by the patient, as follows:

$$\text{Nitrogen balance} = \frac{\text{Protein intake}}{6.25} - (\text{urine urea nitrogen} + 4)$$

Interpretation

Normally at equilibrium, the following measures reflect the severity of the catabolic state:

Equilibrium	0
Mild	−5 to −10
Moderate	−10 to −15 g/dL
Severe	>−15 g/dL

Usual goal during nutritional support = +4 to 6 g nitrogen/24 h

Fluid Requirements

Individual fluid requirements vary greatly and can fluctuate on a daily basis. Fluid needs should be carefully assessed when designing the PN formula. The minimum daily requirement for healthy adults is 1 mL/kcal. Factors that may increase fluid needs include fever and increased losses from diuresis, diarrhea, vomiting, and drainage from wounds and fistulas. Environmental factors such as specialized high–air-loss beds, ultraviolet light therapy, and radiant warmers increase fluid requirements as well. Humidified air reduces insensible fluid loss and results in lower fluid requirements. Pre-existing excess or deficiency states and cardiac and renal function must also be evaluated.

Additional IV fluids may be needed to accommodate increased fluid requirements. Because fluid requirements shift rapidly with changes in clinical status in hospitalized patients, this is best done by giving additional crystalloid IV fluids, such as dextrose 5% in water (D_5W) or dextrose 5% in 0.45% sodium chloride solution, by a separate lumen or route. These can be frequently adjusted as necessary without affecting nutrient delivery. They can also be used as additional vehicles for electrolyte corrections, avoiding possible wastage of the PN solution. The PN solution can be formulated using concentrated nutrients (70% dextrose, 15% amino acids, 20% lipids) to provide adequate nutrients when fluid restriction is needed.

■ PARENTERAL NUTRITION SOLUTIONS

The complex solutions used in PN can provide all the necessary nutrients to meet requirements for growth, weight gain, anabolism, and wound healing.

Components

Solutions for PN contain **admixtures** of carbohydrates, fats, protein, electrolytes, minerals, vitamins, trace elements, and water. The proportion of each component is individualized based on the patient's clinical status, chronic diseases, fluid and electrolyte balance, and specific goals of PN.

Carbohydrates

Glucose is the primary energy source in most PN solutions. Concentrations from 10% to 70% glucose may be used with a final solution concentration of no more than 10% to 12% for peripheral infusion, and no greater than 35% for central venous infusion. A carbohydrate, parenteral glucose is hydrolyzed and provides 3.4 kcal/g. At least 150 to 200 g of glucose is needed to meet the obligate needs for glucose by the brain, central nervous system, red blood cells, white blood cells, active fibroblasts, and certain phagocytes, which normally require glucose as the sole or major energy source (Galica, 1997). No more than 5 to 7 mg/kg/minute (equals a maximum of 5 to 7 g/kg/day, which is easier to calculate) should be given, which is the maximum rate of glucose oxidation. Less is given to the diabetic, hyperglycemic, or critically ill patient—usually no more than 4 g/kg/day (Burke, Wolfe, Mullany et al., 1979; Galica, 1997; Rosmarin, Wardlow, & Mirtallo, 1996). In excess of this amount, the incidence of hyperglycemia seems to increase. Amounts exceeding this in ill and stressed patients result in conversion of excess glucose to fat, which requires energy (increased oxygen consumption and carbon dioxide production), and leads to fatty liver changes with prolonged use. From 50% to 70% of the daily nonprotein kilocalories usually are given as glucose.

Lipids

Lipids (fats) provide the second source of nonprotein for PN solutions. Lipids serve as integral structural components of cell membranes and are vital to support the synthesis of hormones and prostaglandins (Galica, 1997). IV lipid emulsions are given to prevent essential fatty acid deficiency (EFAD) and as a concentrated source of energy (each gram of fat provides 9 kcal). EFAD has been detected as early as 3 to 7 days after initiation of fat-free PN, although clinical signs of dietary inadequacy may take 3 to 4 weeks to become evident (Carpentier et al., 1993). Clinical signs include dry or scaly skin, thinning hair, thrombocytopenia, and liver function abnormalities. Prevention of this deficiency state is desirable because EFAD is associated with decreased ability to heal wounds, adverse effects on red blood cell membranes, and a defect in prostaglandin synthesis.

▲ Legal Issues: LIPID ADMINISTRATION

Legal concerns associated with the administration of lipids include:

- Prevention of essential fatty acid deficiency
- Use in patients with severe egg allergies
- Adverse reactions related to inadequate or excess amounts and too-rapid infusion rates

Use of IV lipids with glucose in a daily PN solution decreases the glucose calories and minimizes insulin requirements. Lipids should provide 30% to 50% of the nonprotein calories in PN solutions, but should not exceed 60% or 2.5 g/kg, or an infusion rate of 1.7 mg/kg/minute (Galica, 1997). IV lipids are available in 10% (1.1 kcal/mL), 20% (2 kcal/mL), and 30% (3 kcal/mL) formulations. They provide fatty acids solely as long-chain triglycerides, and contain egg phospholipid as an emulsifier. They should not be used in patients with severe egg allergies. In general, 20% and 30% solutions are used because less volume is needed. Adverse reactions may occur, although the incidence is less than 1%. Symptoms include dyspnea, cyanosis, nausea, vomiting, headache, dizziness, increased temperature, sweating, chest or back pain, pressure over eyes, and hyperlipidemia. Administration of IV fat emulsions is contraindicated in patients with disturbances in normal fat metabolism such as pathologic hyperlipidemia, lipoid nephrosis, or acute pancreatitis if accompanied by hyperlipidemia. Lipids serve as the main energy source in peripheral PN solutions, and also serve further to dilute the peripheral PN solution as it enters the vein, decreasing the final concentration and incidence of phlebitis.

The manufacturer's directions should be followed for infusion. Lipids are better tolerated and utilized if they are infused slowly, not to exceed the manufacturer's recommendations of no more than 62 mL/hour up to a maximum of 12 hours for each bottle (up to 24 hours if administering a 3-in-1 mixture). Fast infusion rates have been associated with deleterious effects on pulmonary function and impairment of the reticuloendothelial system function, potentiating the inflammatory response by altering the ability of this defense system to respond to bacterial invasion. **Total nutrient admixtures** (TNAs) are formulations consisting of carbohydrates, amino acids, lipids, vitamins, minerals, trace elements, water, and other additives in a single container.

Protein

Protein is used in PN solutions to replete muscle mass and support immune functions. Unlike the other substrates, proteins are not stored. They are in a constant, dynamic state of synthesis and breakdown that requires energy and adenosine triphosphate. In the absence of an adequate energy source, protein is used for energy. The protein or nitrogen source is provided by synthetic crystalline amino acid solutions. Whereas earlier amino acids were formulated as protein hydrolysates and were associated with toxicities, this is not a concern with the current crystalline amino acids (McMahon, 1997). These solutions contain a mixture of essential and nonessential amino acids. Special amino acid formulations for renal failure, hepatic failure, and neonates are available. There is some evidence that high–branched-chain amino acid formulas may be beneficial during sepsis and severe metabolic stress, but this remains controversial. Use of the special formulas is restricted because of the high cost and conflicting reports of efficacy (Galica, 1997).

Electrolytes

Electrolytes are essential to maintain normal metabolic function. Electrolytes are added to PN solutions to meet individual patient requirements and correct any deficiencies caused by increased loss, utilization, or requirements, or by decreased absorption. They include sodium, potassium, chloride, calcium, magnesium, and phosphorus acetate. A variety of standard electrolyte solutions are available, as well as individual electrolytes. The requirements of individual patients may vary depending on their nutritional status and underlying disease process. Table 16–7 provides standard ranges for electrolyte additions to PN solutions. The activity of electrolytes in the body is usually characterized by interrelated patterns; no one electrolyte can function, be deficient, or be overabundant in the body without affecting other electrolytes.

Vitamins

Vitamins are organic compounds essential for maintenance and growth that are not synthesized by the body (Andris, 1996). There are two main groups: fat soluble (A, D, E, K) and water soluble (B complex, C). Vitamins are sensitive to or become inactive with temperature changes and exposure to light. Therefore, they are added before administration and protected from direct light.

Parenteral multivitamins are available to meet the daily requirements set by the American Medical Association Nutrition Advisory Group. Usually, 10 mL of the multivitamins are added to the daily PN solution. Vitamin K, a fat-soluble vitamin necessary for clotting, is not included in adult multivitamins. It may be given weekly (10 mg) or daily as a trace element (1 mg/day) in the PN solution.

TABLE 16-7
DAILY ELECTROLYTE ADDITIONS TO ADULT PARENTERAL NUTRITION SOLUTIONS*

Electrolyte	Parenteral Equivalent of Recommended Dietary Allowance	Standard Intake
Calcium	10 mEq	10–15 mEq
Magnesium	10 mEq	8–20 mEq
Phosphate	30 mmol	20–40 mmol
Sodium	N/A	1–2 mEq/kg + replacement
Potassium	N/A	1–2 mEq/kg
Acetate	N/A	As needed to maintain acid-base balance
Chloride	N/A	As needed to maintain acid–base balance

N/A, nonapplicable
*Assumes normal organ function
(Reproduced with permission of National Advisory Group on Standards and Practice Guidelines for Parenteral Nutrition. [1998]. Safe practices for parenteral nutrition formulations. *Journal of Parenteral and Enteral Nutrition,* 22[2], 49–66.)

Trace Elements

Trace elements are required in small amounts and are referred to as *micronutrients.* They are essential components of metabolic pathways. Those commonly added to PN solutions include zinc, copper, chromium, manganese, and selenium. They are available individually or as multitrace solutions. Requirements for individual trace elements may be increased in certain situations (Andris, 1996; Galica, 1997).

Drugs and Medications

A variety of drugs and medications have been found to be compatible with PN solutions, although compatibility studies are lacking for many. Compatibility studies that have been done used specific PN and TNA solutions and specific concentrations of drugs tested. Compatibility results may be different if a different solution or medication dose or concentration is used. Compatibilities also differ depending on whether the medication is being added to a traditional dextrose and amino acid solution or to a TNA.

 SAFE PRACTICE ALERT The feasibility of mixing drugs with PN solutions depends on various factors, including the physical compatibility of the admixed components, the chemical stability of the drug, the retention of drug concentration over time, and the bioactivity of the components after admixture. For safety's sake, the nurse should check with the pharmacy when the compatibility of drugs and PN solutions is a concern.

The most commonly added medications are heparin, regular insulin, and histamine-2 blockers. It is preferable not to add multiple drugs to the solution. For current information about drug compatibility with PN solutions, readers are referred to Trissel's *Handbook on Injectable Drugs,* which is updated and published yearly and available in hospital pharmacies. Caution is needed to avoid drug–nutrient interactions. The responsible pharmacist should verify that the coinfusion of drugs with PN either admixed in the solution or coinfused through the same IV tubing is safe, stable, and free from incompatibilities (Rollins, 1997). If no information exists in the literature, stability and compatibility should be discussed with the manufacturer.

Because a designated port is recommended solely for PN, piggybacking medications to PN solutions usually is not recommended. A study of compatibility of medications during Y-site administration with TNA solutions found that 23 of 106 common medications were incompatible (Trissel, Gilbert, Martinez et al., 1999).

Preparation of Total Nutrient Admixtures Solution

Safe preparation of solutions requires that trained personnel admix the solution under a laminar-flow hood using strict aseptic technique. Specific protocols covering all aspects of preparation, storage, and quality assurance should be established.

Guidelines may vary from institution to institution but should meet established standards. The Board of Directors of ASPEN has recommended that the practice guidelines in the *Safe Practices for Parenteral Nutrition Formulations* document be the "standard of practice for the provision of parenteral nutrition" (National Advisory Group on Standards and Practices Guidelines for Parenteral Nutrition [National Advisory Group], 1998). Practice guidelines for labeling, formulation and nutrient ranges, nutrient prescription, compounding, quality assurance, stability and compatibility, and in-line filtration are included. These guidelines may have broad ramifications in changing clinical practice in many health care settings. Adoption of these standards should prevent future patient harm and also serve as a catalyst for future research.

Solutions may be prepared as traditional dextrose–amino acid solutions or as TNAs. If dextrose–amino acid solutions are used, the IV lipid emulsions are usually piggybacked to the PN or administered by a separate route. TNAs, also known as trimix or 3-in-1, consist of all components, including lipids, mixed together in one large bag. These solutions are used almost exclusively by home care companies and increasingly in many hospitals.

All additives should be added to the PN solution in the pharmacy under sterile conditions. Additives should not be added on the nursing unit or after the PN container has been spiked and hung. If additional additives are needed after the container is hanging, alternate methods or routes should be considered.

Total nutrient admixture solutions offer a significant advantage in the ability to provide cost effective, patient-specific nutrition support. Nursing time is saved by having only one solution container to hang each day. Pharmacy admixing is simplified by the use of computerized automixing systems, which also allow for more patient-specific formulations. Potential bacterial contamination of either the solution or line is decreased because of decreased accessing of the line. The increased use of TNA reflects the trend toward the daily use of lipid emulsions as a daily calorie source.

The stability of TNA is affected by many factors, including admixture contents, storage time and conditions, addition of non-nutrient drugs, pH of the solution, and variability in temperature (Rollins, 1997). A recent U.S. Food and Drug Administration (FDA) alert strongly advises pharmacists to use care in the compounding order of nutrients, and advocates, along with the safe practices guidelines, the use of a 1.2-μm filter during infusion to avoid problems with calcium and phosphate precipitation (National Advisory Group, 1998). A TNA solution is normally milky white and opaque, although a faint yellow hue may be evident with the addition of vitamins. The nurse should examine the solution for any signs of instability before hanging and periodically thereafter. Particulate matter is hard to detect because of the opacity of the solution. Other physical or chemical phenomena may occur and are discussed in Table 16–8. Nurses should be aware of these phenomena and be able to recognize a stable lipid emulsion or TNA solution (Rollins, 1997). A TNA solution is usually stable for 24 hours after admixing with the addition of vitamins, and for up to 7 days if vitamins are not added until the solution is ready to use. Further research is in progress.

TABLE 16-8
VISIBLE PHENOMENA IN TOTAL NUTRIENT ADMIXTURE SOLUTIONS

Phenomena	Characteristics	Considerations
Physical phenomena		
Aggregation (stratification)	Rare white "streaks" (early stages of creaming)	Not harmful
		Readily reverses with *gentle* agitation
Creaming	Dense white color at top of solution ("cream" layer)	Not harmful
		Reverses with *gentle* agitation
	Aggregates migrate to top of the solution	If creaming reappears in 1–2 h or decreases after agitation, it may indicate an unstable emulsion
		If left undistributed, may begin to coalesce (see below)
Chemical phenomena		
Coalescence/cracking (breaking/oiling out)	Oil globules on the surface of creamed emulsion coalesce or fuse to form larger oil droplets	Irreversible
		Cannot be dispersed
	May appear as an oil layer on top of the solution, as large oil globules, or streaks of oil throughout the solution	Do not hang the container
		If coalescence appears during infusion, take container down and return it to pharmacy immediately

■ ADMINISTRATION OF PARENTERAL NUTRITION

Administration of hypertonic PN solutions requires an easily placed, well-tolerated central venous access device (CVAD) that can be used for extended periods. Infusion into a large vein with high blood flow to dilute the solution rapidly is desirable to reduce phlebitis, venous thrombosis, pain, and hemolysis (Andris & Krzywda, 1997).

Vascular Access

The superior vena cava is the vein of choice for administering PN. The subclavian and internal jugular veins are the most common insertion sites for accessing the superior vena cava. Other insertion sites, such as the external jugular and femoral veins, may be used if necessary in patients with limited venous access. The desirable location for the tip of all CVADs is in the distal superior vena cava, parallel to the vessel wall, just above the right atrium (Ryder, 1996; Whitman, 1996). CVAD insertion should be performed only by an experienced physician to reduce the incidence of insertion complications.

Various CVADs are available for short-term or long-term access. Short-term access is usually obtained using single- or multiple-lumen percutaneously placed catheters. These are usually used for days to weeks in acute illness, but may be used for longer periods with meticulous care. Peripherally inserted central catheters may be used for either short- or long-term access as well.

Unlike other CVADs mentioned here, peripherally inserted central catheters can be inserted by specially skilled, registered nurses via the antecubital veins (basilic, cephalic, or median antecubital, in order of preference). They are available with single or double lumens and have become increasingly popular for PN.

Long-term central venous access is usually obtained using tunneled cuffed catheters or totally implanted venous access ports. Tunneled catheters are available with single or multiple lumens. One type of tunneled long-term catheter, the Groshong catheter, has a one-way slit valve at the distal tip. The valve eliminates the need for frequent flushing and use of heparin by preventing blood reflux into the lumen. Implanted ports are available as single- or dual-portal septa that can be accessed from either the top or side. These long-term access devices are surgically placed in the operating room and can be used for months to years. Multilumen catheters allow various medications to infuse simultaneously, but controversy still exists regarding the risk of infection with more than one lumen.

Swan-Ganz catheters usually are not recommended for infusion of PN. However, if no other access is available, the right atrium or proximal port can be used. The side arm of the introducer should not be used because it is short and located in the subclavian vein.

Nurses play a major role during the insertion and use of CVADs. They are responsible for the daily care and are held accountable for preventing or minimizing the many device-related complications, including those that are life threatening. Protocols for the insertion, care, and maintenance of CVADs should be established and followed according to current standards.

Catheter Insertion

A preinsertion evaluation of the patient should be obtained to optimize catheter insertion and reduce the risk of complications (Andris & Krzywda, 1997). Factors to be evaluated can be found in Box 16–6. A history of any prior CVAD placements, duration, and complications may identify a need for further evaluation. Risk factors for catheter insertion include previous major surgery of the neck or chest areas, prior CVAD insertion or attempts, and body size (Whitman, 1996). A chest radiograph is helpful to identify any anatomic abnormalities or mass lesions. CVADs should be placed on the side opposite to known cancer of the lung, breast, or other thoracic locations, cervical masses, or unilateral pneumonia to minimize the interaction of the CVAD with these conditions (Whitman, 1996). Venous angiography or venous duplex ultrasonography should be obtained before an insertion attempt if there is any question of vessel patency. If the patient is receiving anticoagulant therapy, warfarin or other anticoagulant medications should be withheld the night before with an international normalized ratio obtained the morning of the procedure. Heparin should be withheld 3 to 4 hours before the procedure (Whitman, 1996). A platelet count should be obtained. If the platelet count is lower than 50,000, platelet infusion within 2 hours of insertion should be considered. The only absolute contraindications to immediate insertion are a sudden clinical deterioration that changes the treatment plan, new, unexplained fevers, and absolute neutropenia that has not reached its nadir (Whitman, 1996).

BOX 16–6 Checklist: Patient Evaluation Before CVAD Insertion

☐ History of prior CVAD insertion and type, if known
☐ Number and location of insertions or attempts at insertion
☐ Duration
☐ Complications
☐ Anomalies (alternate anatomic landmarks used during insertion)
☐ Previous clavicular fracture
☐ Known venous anomalies
☐ Cervical or mediastinal adenopathy
☐ Increased risk of complications
☐ Previous major surgery in neck or chest area
☐ Body size (body mass index <20 or >30)
☐ Laboratory evaluations
☐ Platelet count and international normalized ratio
☐ Medication evaluation
☐ Medications that may affect coagulation (eg, heparin, warfarin, Ticlid, Plavix, aspirin, nonsteroidal anti-inflammatory drugs)

A thorough explanation of the procedure before insertion helps to alleviate anxiety and ensures patient cooperation. Proper teaching beforehand tends to increase patient tolerance and markedly decrease the level of pain experienced during the procedure. It is important to elicit feedback during the teaching so the nurse can assess the patient's level of understanding and eliminate fears. Sedation may be required for children and for highly anxious or combative patients. Adequate hydration is essential to dilate the central veins for successful catheterization. The nurse must gather all necessary equipment before the procedure starts and be familiar with the procedure.

Percutaneously placed catheters are inserted at the bedside using strict aseptic technique. A recent prospective study demonstrated that maximum barrier precautions—cap, mask, gown, gloves, and large drape—reduce colonization of the catheter surface at the time of insertion, with a decreased risk of catheter-related infection.

The nurse plays a key role during insertion, including instructing the patient to perform the Valsalva maneuver (ie, "Take a deep breath and hold it while bearing down and straining slightly."), observing for breaks in surgical technique, and reassuring the patient. The Valsalva maneuver is used when the needle is open to the air, before and during the threading of the catheter, to prevent possible air embolism. If the patient is unconscious or unable to do a Valsalva maneuver, the nurse can perform it by gently pressing down on the patient's sternum at the appropriate time. If the patient is intubated, the physician can time the threading of the catheter during an expiration.

A portable chest radiograph should be taken immediately after insertion to determine the location of the catheter tip and rule out potential complications. Isotonic IV solutions (D_5W, normal saline) are usually infused at a slow, keep-vein-open rate until correct placement is confirmed. Some nurses infuse 250 to 300 mL of isotonic solution before radiographic studies so that a hydrothorax can be detected and corrected before initiating PN.

Parenteral nutrition should never be initiated until catheter tip placement in the distal superior vena cava is confirmed. It is unacceptable for the tip to be located in the heart, inferior vena cava, or any extrathoracic vessel. Atrial rupture, valvular damage, myocardial irritability with arrhythmias, and cardiac tamponade are some of the complications reported when the catheter tip is located in the heart. An increased incidence of catheter-induced thrombosis and occlusion is associated with tip placement in the subclavian, jugular, inferior vena cava, or narrower extrathoracic vessels.

Complications are infrequent but the patient should be closely monitored after catheter insertion, particularly for signs of respiratory distress, pain, slowly increasing hematoma, or any unexplainable symptom. (Specific catheter-related complications are discussed later.)

Protocols and Precautions

All institutions should have specific protocols for the administration, monitoring, and discontinuation of PN, which should be reviewed annually. A.S.P.E.N. has published standards for nutritional support of hospitalized patients, hospitalized pediatric patients, home patients, residents of long-term care facilities, and nutritional support nurses. It also has similar standards for nutritional support physicians and nutritional support dietitians. In addition, the Intravenous Nurses Society has updated published standards for IV therapy, which include PN (Intravenous Nurses Society, 1998, 2000). Safe administration of PN depends on strict adherence to these protocols and the safe practices guidelines (National Advisory Group, 1998).

Normally, PN solutions are refrigerated until they are used. The recommended maximum hang time for PN solutions is 24 hours. PN solutions should be inspected for signs of precipitate or instability before hanging. The label also should be matched with the PN orders to ensure accuracy. The volume and infusion rate are usually noted on the label by the pharmacy. Published guidelines for labeling are available (National Advisory Group, 1998).

Parenteral nutrition should be infused at a constant infusion rate, as ordered, because variable infusion rates can result in wide fluctuations in blood glucose levels. Too-rapid infusion of these highly concentrated dextrose solutions can cause a hyperglycemic reaction or even hyperosmolar nonketotic coma. Rates should never be adjusted more than $\pm 10\%$, and an electronic infusion pump should be mandatory to ensure accuracy. A plethora of electronic infusion pumps is available, including small, portable pumps to enhance the patient's mobility.

The infusion is started slowly and gradually increased as fluid and glucose tolerances permit. In general, no more than 250 g glucose should be administered the first day to allow the body to adjust to the increased glucose load—100 to 200 g if the patient is diabetic or hyperglycemic (McMahon, 1997). If the blood glucose concentration is less than 200 mg/dL, the glucose can be gradually increased to the desired goal. There is usually no need to restrict protein or lipids the first day in adults.

Glucose tolerance, may, however, be compromised by sepsis, stress, shock, hepatic and renal failure, starvation, diabetes, pancreatic disease, and administration of some medications, particularly steroids and some diuretics. Age is another variable; the elderly and the very young are particularly susceptible to glucose intolerance and hyperglycemia. For these patients, administration of exogenous insulin is often necessary. It is preferable to add insulin to the PN solution because it provides a more constant serum insulin level than does periodic subcutaneous administration (McMahon, 1997). In addition, a sliding-scale, subcutaneous insulin coverage schedule should be implemented. Box 16–7 outlines steps in managing and preventing hyperglycemia in patients receiving PN. The blood glucose level should continue to be monitored closely because insulin needs may decrease as the stress or sepsis subsides, or steroids are decreased and discontinued. Blood glucose should be maintained at less than 200 mg/dL during PN administration. One study also found that dextrose infusion rates exceeding 4 to 5 mg/kg/minute increase the risk of hyperglycemia (Rosmarin et al., 1996). Avoidance of the extremes of hyperglycemia and hypoglycemia is important. Extra caution should be used when infusing PN in patients undergoing peritoneal dialysis or propofol infusions. Peritoneal dialysis can provide significant amounts of dextrose calories. The dextrose calories in dialysate solution should be calculated and a comparable amount subtracted from the dextrose ordered in the PN solution to avoid overfeeding and hyperglycemia from excess dextrose. Propofol is a lipid-based sedative that provides 1.1 kcal/mL. It is widely used in critical care units. Infusion of propofol or any other lipid-based drug must be monitored closely when given with PN to avoid the pitfalls of overfeeding and hypertriglyceridemia (Lowrey, Dunlap, Brown et al., 1996). PN solutions need to be manipulated when excessive calories are provided in these drugs. Daily calculation of dextrose or lipid calories provided by dialysate or lipid-based drugs with appropriate adjustments in the dextrose or lipids provided in PN should be mandatory.

Consideration should also be given to dextrose administered in crystalloid IV solutions. Many patients on PN need supplemental infusions of crystalloids to correct hypernatremia, or because of medication compatibility. When possible, non–dextrose-containing crystalloids should be used. If significant amounts of dextrose-containing crystalloids are needed, insulin may be added to decrease the risk of hyperglycemia.

If PN solutions are interrupted or unavailable, standing orders should be available to infuse 5% dextrose solutions at the same rate, either through the central line or peripherally if the central line is removed or lost. This prevents the sudden hypoglycemia caused by the high endogenous insulin secretion that is associated with hypertonic PN solutions. Although some institutions and physicians still prefer to use a 10% dextrose solution in these situations, it has been deemed unnecessary.

Many institutions have established standard start times for PN (eg, 4 PM) to simplify nursing management. This also allows the pharmacy to establish standard times for admixing the solutions and delivery to the nursing unit. Orders for PN are usually required in the pharmacy several hours before the established start time. A nurse should demonstrate core competencies in administering PN (Box 16–8 and Procedure 16–1).

text continues on page 384

BOX 16–7 **Managing Hyperglycemia in Patients Receiving Parenteral Nutrition**

Goals

- Maintain serum glucose levels between 100 and 200 mg/dL, with an optimal range of 100–150 mg/dL.
- Avoid overfeeding.

Initiating Parenteral Nutrition

- Limit to no more than 200 g dextrose in the first few days until glycemic control is achieved.
- If baseline fasting blood glucose level is more than 180–200 mg/dL, or if the patient is a diabetic patient previously treated with insulin or oral agent, add 0.1 U regular insulin per gram of dextrose (ie, 15 U/L 15% dextrose [150 g/L]; 20 U/L 20% dextrose [200 g/L]).
- In general, do not increase dextrose concentration in PN until serum glucose level is consistently under 200 mg/dL for 24 h.

Ongoing

- Adjust insulin accordingly whenever the concentration of dextrose increases or decreases.
- Check serum glucose level by reflectance meter every 4 to 6 h initially; every 8 h once patient's levels are stable.
- Increase regular insulin in PN by 0.05 U/g dextrose daily if serum glucose is consistently greater than 200 mg/dL in previous 24 h.
- Use subcutaneous (SQ) regular insulin to supplement PN insulin according to the following algorithm:

Glucose (mg/dL)	SQ-Regular insulin dose (units)
200–250	2–3
251–300	4–6
301–350	6–9
>350	8–12

- If serum glucose is consistently >200 mg/dL with PN insulin and adherence to the SQ insulin algorithm, a separate IV infusion may be helpful in achieving glycemic control.
- Once the patient's glucose level is stable, frequency of glucose monitoring can be decreased.
- Monitor and assess daily to anticipate effects of PN on glucose level (ie, patient's clinical status, fluid status, medication/IV profile, peritoneal dialysis, dextrose volume, and so forth).

BOX 16–8 Core Competencies for Nurses Administering Parenteral Nutrition

☐ Demonstrates appropriate use of Standard Precautions and aseptic technique
☐ Verbalizes and demonstrates knowledge of nursing policies and procedures related to administering PN
☐ States awareness of the impact of other dextrose sources (IV infusions, IV medications), lipid-based medications (eg, propofol), and dialysate on the development and exacerbation of hyperglycemia
☐ Indicates knowledge of complications associated with PN administration and their management
☐ Verbalizes knowledge of pharmacy, nursing, and hospital policies related to PN ordering (who can order, when orders need to be received in pharmacy, what to do if changes are needed, start time)
☐ Verbalizes understanding that no medications or additives can be added to PN on the nursing unit (only in the pharmacy)
☐ Verbalizes knowledge of instances when the physician should be notified
☐ Demonstrates appropriate documentation of PN administration and patient response

Cycling Parenteral Nutrition

☐ Demonstrates appropriate use of Standard Precautions and aseptic technique
☐ Verbalizes understanding of nursing policies and procedure related to cycling PN
☐ Demonstrates appropriate use of glucose monitor
☐ States knowledge of acceptable glucose monitoring parameters and management of variances
☐ Verbalizes knowledge of potential complications related to cycling, and their management
☐ Expresses knowledge of instances when the physician should be notified
☐ Demonstrates appropriate documentation of cycling and patient response

Discontinuing Parenteral Nutrition

☐ Demonstrates appropriate use of Standard Precaution and aseptic technique
☐ Verbalizes knowledge of nursing policies and procedures related to discontinuing PN
☐ States understanding of monitoring patient for signs of rebound hypoglycemia during and after discontinuation of PN
☐ Displays knowledge of need to hang 5% dextrose in water solution at same rate as PN solution if PN must stop abruptly (ie, because of no orders, signs of complications, central venous access device malfunction)
☐ Verbalizes knowledge of instances when physician should be notified
☐ Demonstrates appropriate documentation of discontinuing PN and patient response

Procedure
16–1

Administration of Total Nutrient Admixture

Equipment

Total nutrient admixture (TNA) solution

IV administration set

1.2-μg filter

Povidone–iodine wipes

Electronic infusion pump

3-mL Syringe filled with normal saline solution

Daily administration time: 1400 (2 PM)

Action	Rationale
Assemble equipment.	Gathering equipment in advance saves time
Explain the procedure to the patient.	Explanations allay anxiety
Maintain Standard Precautions and always use aseptic technique (wash hands).	Deters spread of microorganisms
Check TNA container label against physician's orders—orders may change from previous day.	Ensures accuracy (contents on label match)
• Check patient name, date, and rate of infusion. Also check expiration date on formula and time. • Notify pharmacy of any discrepancies or contact pharmacist with questions.	Ensures accuracy
Examine TNA solution for signs of instability (creaming, coalescence) and notify pharmacist if any signs of instability (cracking, particulate matter) are observed.	Avoids adverse reactions
Don clean gloves.	Prevents contamination from bodily fluids and prevents infection
Attach 1.2 μg filter to end of standard IV tubing; attach to TNA solution, then prime and clamp.	Removes air from IV tubing and filter
• Cleanse central venous access device (CVAD) lumen/IV tubing or lock connection with povidone–iodine wipe for 30 seconds; allow to dry.	Cleans any solution residue and microorganisms from catheter hub connection to prevent contamination

Clamp catheter lumen; disconnect IV tubing or lock and discard. Then flush CVAD lumen with 3 mL normal saline solution.	Cleans lumen and maintains patency
Attach new primed TNA tubing to dedicated lumen (ie, multilumen CVAD—middle lumen label, double-lumen, tunneled, long-term catheter, double-lumen peripherally inserted venous catheter. Be sure to designate a lumen for TNA and label that lumen.	Ensures safety in that the same lumen is always used for TNA and not used alternately for medications; also ensures that other fluids or blood or blood products cannot be piggybacked with TNA
Attach primed tubing to infusion pump, and set desired rate. Start pump just before opening clamp on CVAD lumen.	Accuracy in administering TNA helps to prevent fluctuations in rate and also backflow of blood into catheter hub
If TNA is interrupted or stopped or unavailable, infuse 5% dextrose in water solution at the same rate as the ordered TNA.	Prevents rebound hypoglycemia from abrupt cessation of TNA
Discard any solution left at the end of 24 hours and hang next TNA bag (1400 daily).	Maintains daily start time of 1400
Monitor patient frequently for any signs of adverse reactions or problems.	Avoids or identifies potential complications in a timely matter so that appropriate action can be taken
Document the procedure. Include problems/complications, interventions, patient response and outcomes; pertinent laboratory test findings, vital signs, intake and output, and the like.	Accurate documentation is necessary to record nursing care given and ensure continuity of care

Special notes:

- Medications cannot be added to TNA solutions on the nursing unit; they must be added in the pharmacy.
- TNA tubing and filter must be changed every 24 hours.
- TNA must be ordered daily.

Intravenous Tubing and Filters

Primary IV tubing set changes should be established in organizational policy and procedures (INS, 1998). Tubing used to administer lipid emulsions and TNA solutions should be changed every 24 hours. There is no recommendation for the hang time of non–lipid-containing PN solutions, although most adhere to 24 hours (Pearson, 1996). It is most efficient to standardize the time of tubing and filter changes to coincide with the daily start time for the day's solution. This eliminates additional breaks in the line. Luer-lock connections are optimal to avoid accidental disconnection. If not available, the tubing connection should be taped. The use of needleless systems is also encouraged.

The need for in-line filtration of PN solutions is apparent given the recommendations of the FDA and the safe practices guidelines of the National Advisory Group (1998). A 0.22-μm filter is recommended for traditional dextrose–amino acid solutions, with the lipids piggybacked below the filter. These filters effectively retain bacteria, fungi, and particulate matter. TNA solutions require use of a 1.2- or 5.0-μm filter that effectively eliminates microprecipitates, *Candida,* and some bacteria. Bacterial contamination of PN solutions is rare. The justification for use of in-line filters centers on the removal of microprecipitates rather than microorganisms. Microprecipitates are commonly not visible on inspection, particularly in TNAs.

A risk of contamination always exists when IV tubing and filters are changed. Therefore, precautions need to be taken and aseptic technique strictly followed. All connections should be swabbed thoroughly with alcohol or povidone–iodine before the tubing is changed. It is also a good idea to swab the end of the catheter hub to remove any dried blood or sticky residue. The nurse must clamp the catheter before changing the tubing to avoid the risk of air embolism. If a clamp is not available, the patient should be positioned flat in bed and advised to perform the Valsalva maneuver during the tubing change. PN should be infused through a dedicated line. PN lines should not be violated by pressure monitoring devices or transducers, stopcocks, blood drawing, or administration of blood or medications. This practice also reduces the risk of contamination and infection.

Cycling Parenteral Nutrition

Occasionally, PN may be cycled to allow the patient periods of freedom from the infusion and pump. Cyclic PN is widely used for those patients who require long-term PN support, usually over 12 to 14 hours at night. This allows for increased mobility during the day, giving the patient some time to participate in normal daytime activities and offering an improved sense of well-being and quality of life. Cycling may also benefit certain patients by allowing maximum freedom for ambulation and physical therapy. Duke University Medical Center routinely starts cyclic PN early in the clinical course for all patients expected to be on PN for more than 2 weeks.

Most patients adapt well to the fasting state. Cardiovascular status should be evaluated to ensure that the fluid volume can be accommodated over a shorter time. Most often, PN solutions are tapered during the day with all PN being infused over 12 to 14 hours at night. Cycling from 24 hours of nutritional therapy to 12 to 14 hours is usually done gradually over several days. Close monitoring is essential. Usually, the infusion rate is decreased by one half during the first and last hours of infusion to allow for tapering at the beginning and the end of infusion. Most patients tolerate this well without development of rebound hypoglycemia. Blood glucose levels during the accelerated infusion rates for cyclic PN may be up to 250 mg/dL. Normoglycemia is usually present during the hours when the patient is receiving PN. Core competencies a nurse should demonstrate before cycling PN can be found in Box 16–8.

Discontinuing Parenteral Nutrition

Parenteral nutrition should not be stopped without alternate plans for therapy so that nutritional status can be maintained or continue to improve. Nor should reductions in PN begin until an alternate source of nutritional intake, such as **enteral nutrition** (nutrition by the GI route), is initiated. As enteral or oral intake increases, PN gradually decreases. It should not be discontinued, however, until at least half of the estimated requirements are tolerated enterally or orally. Accurate calorie counts are essential to the successful transition from PN to enteral or oral intake. For more information, see Procedure 16–2 for discontinuing PN.

■ NURSING MANAGEMENT IN PARENTERAL NUTRITION

Clinical assessment and monitoring are imperative for the safe administration of PN, which should be considered in the same manner as medication administration. The nurse should be familiar with the solution composition, the expected metabolic response, and the potential complications of therapy. A good knowledge base should enable the nurse to identify patients who are at risk for metabolic complications and better to monitor the patient's response to nutrient delivery. Catheter site care, dressing changes, and monitoring PN administration are also in the domain of nursing management. The importance of clear and thorough documentation of care cannot be overemphasized. Legally, if it was not charted, it was not done. Many hospitals and nutritional support teams have developed clinical pathways for PN, allowing patient outcomes to be tracked and adequacy of therapy to be monitored. ASPEN has also developed clinical pathways for PN. Institutions should tailor PN clinical pathways to reflect their own practices. Variances should be reviewed quarterly with strategies for improvement incorporated into the pathways for the continuous improvement of patient care.

Catheter Site Care

Skin care and catheter site care is regarded as one of the most important measures for preventing catheter-related infections. The management of site care remains controversial. Use of antiseptic agents and ointments, dressing type, and frequency of dressing changes remain unresolved issues (Andris & Krzywda, 1997). General principles of site care should be used for all catheter types, with particularly strict adher-

Procedure 16–2

Discontinuing Parenteral Nutrition

Equipment
Syringe with appropriate amount of normal saline solution

Povidone–iodine wipes

Syringe with appropriate amount of heparin flush solution

Lock device (Luer lock, male adapter)

Action	Rationale
Explain procedure to patient.	Explanation allays anxiety
Maintain Standard Precautions and aseptic technique.	Deters spread of microorganisms
Follow these principles when discontinuing PN:	Avoids abrupt cessation of nutrients in absence of any other source of glucose (oral, IV, or enteral) and avoids rebound hypoglycemia
• Reduce PN infusion rate in conjunction with an increase in caloric intake by oral or enteral route.	Ensures adequacy of nutrient intake
• Be sure the patient can take half of the estimated nutrient requirements either enterally or orally before PN discontinues.	Same as above
• Fluid intake may also decrease as the PN is decreased, so provide adequate fluids by other routes.	Prevents dehydration
• Rapid weaning can be accomplished over 4 h by progressive reductions in infusion rate (ie, decrease infusion rate by half every 1 to 2 h until reaching a rate of 40 mL/h; then discontinue.	Gradual, rapid taper can deter rebound hypoglycemia
Discontinue PN before surgery: Decrease rate to 40 mL/h the night before surgery, and discontinue infusion at least 4 hours before surgery. Any 5% dextrose solution can be infused. Keep in mind that potassium shifts may occur with hyperglycemia. Also ensure adequate preoperative hydration.	Stress of surgery may increase blood glucose levels, and signs and symptoms of hyperglycemia are not easily monitored or detected in the anesthetized patient

Verify physician's order to stop infusion.	Ensures that PN is to be discontinued
Hang 5% dextrose in water at same rate as PN if PN must stop abruptly (eg, no orders, suspected infection, central venous access device [CVAD] malfunction).	Prevents rebound hypoglycemia
Cleanse CVAD lumen—PN tubing connection with povidone–iodine wipe for 30 seconds. Allow to dry.	Antibacterial and antifungal cleansing of hub deters spread of microorganisms
Disconnect PN tubing and discard. Then flush lumen per established protocol and attach lock device to end of CVAD.	Maintains patency and prevents occlusion
Document procedure in appropriate records.	Accurate and comprehensive documentation reflects nursing care given

ence to hand-washing and aseptic technique. The insertion site should be palpated daily for tenderness and observed for erythema and exudate. The catheter site should be visually inspected if the patient has a fever without obvious source or symptoms of bloodstream infection. If symptoms are present, physician notification and further evaluation are warranted.

Antiseptics and Antimicrobial Ointments

The ideal skin cleansing antiseptic remains undetermined. It should be nontoxic and nonirritating, act rapidly against most skin organisms, and provide residual activity (Andris & Krzywda, 1997). Usually, 10% povidone–iodine is used because chlorhexidine in a 2% aqueous solution, which some consider superior to povidone–iodine, is not commercially available in the United States for catheter site care. Tincture of iodine also may be superior, but is not used because it may irritate the skin. Removing the tincture of iodine with alcohol may reduce the irritation associated with its use (Pearson, 1996). A sustained-release chlorhexidine gluconate patch is available for use at insertion sites, but studies have not been published evaluating its role in site care regimens. The use of the patch at epidural catheter sites demonstrated a significant reduction in catheter colonization. Its efficacy in reducing CVAD-related infection needs to be determined (Pearson, 1996).

Using antimicrobial ointment at the insertion site remains controversial. There is a lack of conclusive research to show the benefit of ointment use, and existing studies are difficult to compare because of differences in protocol. If an ointment is to be used in patients who are considered to be at high risk, povidone–iodine products are recommended as the best for central lines because of their broader spectrum of coverage, including gram-negative bacteria and fungi (Andris & Krzywda, 1997). Routine use of ointments is not recommended (Pearson, 1996). Some practitioners think that ointment used under transparent dressings affects adherence and may provide a moist environment that supports growth of organisms resistant to the ointment.

Catheter Dressing Regimens

The favored choice of dressing material—gauze and tape or transparent—also varies. Transparent dressings allow the insertion site to be observed without disturbing the dressing. They are more comfortable for the patient and require less frequent dressing changes. Gauze and tape dressings preclude site inspection, are usually more uncomfortable for the patient, and require more frequent changes.

It is recommended that either gauze or transparent dressing be used to cover the catheter insertion site. Either dressing should be changed when the device is removed or replaced and when the dressing becomes damp, loose, or soiled, or any time the integrity of the dressing is compromised. Diaphoretic patients may require more frequent dressing changes. A careful review of the literature should be done when establishing dressing change protocols. Research is ongoing and important for establishing definitive standards and guidelines.

Dressing Change Procedures

Dressing change procedures may vary but all use the same general techniques and rationale. Prepackaged sterile dressing change kits, which include all necessary equipment, are typically used. Some kits may include instructions as well. Dressing change protocols should be maintained according to established recommendations.

Catheter Hub Care

Catheter hub care is just as important as catheter site care. The catheter hub should be cleansed with either 10% povidone–iodine or 70% alcohol before accessing the system (Pearson, 1996). Minimizing manipulation of the hub and tubing connection can also decrease the risk of infection.

Maintaining Catheter Patency

Anticoagulant flush solutions should be used to maintain catheter patency. Some controversy still exists regarding the concentration of heparin, appropriate volume, and frequency of flush. In general, however, the lowest effective concentration of heparin in a volume adequate to fill the lumen of the catheter is used. A concentration of 10 U/mL has been shown to maintain catheter patency (Pearson, 1996). Studies have found that normal saline is as effective as heparin in maintaining patency of peripheral catheters. There are no studies evaluating the use of saline in short- or long-term CVADs. It is imperative to know the specific recommendations for the catheter type being used, including catheter material, flushing volume, and pressure and syringe size limitations.

Monitoring

Nurses play a vital role in monitoring patients on PN. Patient monitoring is as important as proper administration in preventing serious metabolic complications. Accurate measurements of the patient's daily body weight, measured at the same time of day, using the same scale, and with the patient wearing the same amount of clothing, are important. A baseline weight should be obtained, then three times a week thereafter and daily in critically ill patients. Intake and output records should also be scrupulously maintained and recorded. These measures are necessary to assess fluid balance and adequacy of the prescribed nutrients.

Vital signs should be obtained and recorded at least every shift and more often if the patient is unstable or the temperature is greater than 100°F (37.7°C) orally or 101°F (38.3°C) rectally. Certain drugs and disease states suppress the normal febrile response, and affected patients must be assessed individually.

Blood glucose levels should be monitored every 4 to 8 hours depending on the level of glycemic control. This practice has become easier with the use of glucose monitors on nursing units. Most institutions have eliminated urine glucose monitoring because it is not as accurate. However, urine glucose monitoring is less invasive and useful for monitoring patients who are stable and glucose tolerant with serum glucose levels less than 200 mg/dL. A urine glucose level exceeding 2+ requires serum glucose testing for a more accurate determination.

Biochemical monitoring is also important to assess the adequacy of the PN regimen and the presence of any metabolic complications. Nutritional profiles or standing laboratory tests are recommended for routine PN monitoring. Routine laboratory tests and their frequency are outlined in Table 16–9. Ideally, a full chemical profile, including glucose, electrolytes, urea nitrogen, creatinine, albumin, transferrin, calcium, magnesium, phosphorus, liver function, prothrombin time, and complete blood count, should be obtained before initiating PN. Critically ill and unstable patients may require more frequent monitoring. Other studies may be warranted depending on the clinical status of the patient. Core competencies a nurse should demonstrate before monitoring PN are listed in Box 16–9. Refer to Procedure 16–3 for monitoring guidelines.

■ COMPLICATIONS OF PARENTERAL NUTRITION

Complications associated with PN are divided into three categories: technical, metabolic, and septic. These complications can be minimized or even avoided with the establishment of and adherence to strict protocols, and careful monitoring.

Mechanical Complications

Mechanical complications are related to the insertion or maintenance of CVADs and may be immediate or delayed. Insertion complications are infrequent when the CVAD is inserted by a physician skilled and knowledgeable about anatomy and CVAD insertion.

text continues on page 392

T A B L E   1 6 – 9
LABORATORY MONITORING OF PARENTERAL NUTRITION

Frequency	Test
Daily until stable, then Monday-Wednesday-Friday	Blood sugar
	Electrolytes
	BUN
	Creatinine
Baseline, then weekly (ie, every Monday)	Nutritional profile
	Blood sugar, electrolytes, BUN, creatinine (as above)
	Total protein
	Albumin
	Transferrin
	Calcium
	Phosphorus
	Magnesium
	Total bilirubin
	Alkaline phosphatase
	AST
	ALT
	LDH
	Cholesterol
	Triglycerides
	CBC
	PT

ALT, alanine transaminase; AST, aspartate transaminase; BUN, blood urea nitrogen; CBC, complete blood count; LDH, lactic dehydrogenase; PT, prothrombin time

---

BOX 16–9 **Core Competencies in Monitoring Parenteral Nutrition**

☐ Demonstrates appropriate use of Standard Precautions and aseptic technique
☐ Demonstrates appropriate use of blood glucose monitoring device
☐ Verbalizes knowledge and understanding of acceptable blood glucose parameters, and management of hypoglycemia and hyperglycemia
☐ Verbalizes knowledge of parameters to be monitored, and the frequency (ie, intake and output, vital signs, weight, blood analyses, central venous access device site, infusion pump)
☐ Verbalizes knowledge of when the physician should be notified
☐ Demonstrates appropriate documentation of all monitoring parameters in appropriate nursing records

Procedure
16–3

Guidelines for Monitoring Parenteral Nutrition

Equipment
Blood glucose monitor

Action	*Rationale*
Explain procedures to patient.	Patient understanding will allay anxiety
Maintain Standard Precautions.	Deters the spread of microorganisms and aseptic technique
Check vital signs every shift. If temperature exceeds 100.5°F, take vital signs q4 h and monitor blood glucose (BG) level q4–6 h. BG level should be maintained at <200 mg/dL.	Discloses signs of complications or infection during PN infusion
After 1 week, stable patients (BG <200 mg/dL) can be monitored less frequently if ordered by physician.	Determines need to increase or decrease insulin if added to PN and patient not receiving insulin
Strictly measure intake and output. • Intake includes PN, other IV solutions, IV medication volume, and any oral intake. • Output includes urine and any other output (nasogastric tube, ostomy, fistula, drainage).	Monitors fluid balance and avoids complications
Obtain baseline weight, then weigh daily if patient is in intensive care or on dialysis or weigh patient every other day if weight gain is desired or anticipated. (Stable patients on prolonged PN can be weighed weekly.)	Monitoring fluid balance points to adequacy of therapy (weight maintenance or weight gain)
Monitor blood work as ordered. Notify physician of any critically abnormal values.	Assesses need to adjust PN regimen (electrolytes, add/adjust insulin, other adjustments), and detect complications early
Observe central venous access device (CVAD) site and chest for: • Erythema, edema, exudate • Intact dressing or sutures • Pain at insertion site	Discloses complications early and establishes patency of sutures, if present

- Securely taped catheter and PN tubing that relieves tension on CVAD
- Engorged superficial chest wall vessels

Monitor infusion rate and pump for signs of possible malfunction.	Ensures ordered infusion and prevents complications
Check for possible complications and notify physician if patient's temperature exceeds 101°F, if BG exceeds 200 mg/dL, or if laboratory test values appear critically abnormal. Observe also for presence or increase in edema; weight gain ≥2 lb/week; edema over insertion site, neck, face, chest, either arm; exudate at insertion site and also greater than usual erythema at insertion site. Report any radical changes in clinical status: vital signs, mental status, convulsions, coma, increased diuresis.	Identifying and treating complications early on avoids more deleteious effects
Adhere to all polices related to PN administration and CVAD management.	Maintains established standards of care
Culture catheter tip if catheter is removed.	Identifies catheter as source of infection for suspected catheter sepsis
Accurately document all monitoring activities in appropriate nursing records. Also document any abnormal laboratory results and adverse reactions. Include actions taken and patient's response to treatment.	Documentation should be accurate and comprehensive to reflect nursing care given, actions taken, and patient's response to treatment

Complications after catheter insertion are depicted in Figure 16-4 and described in the following sections (see Chaps. 13 and 14).

Malpositioning

Catheter malpositioning can occur during insertion from coiling or misdirection, overinsertion or underinsertion, aberrant route on catheter advancement, venous thrombosis or stenosis, and venous or atrial perforation. The correct placement for

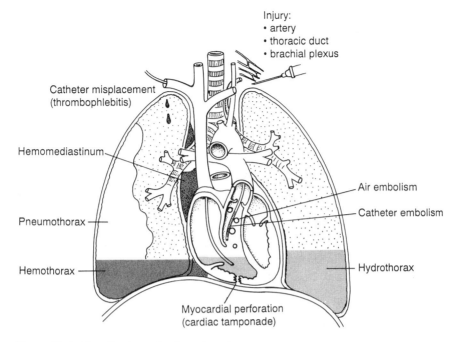

Figure 16–4. Complications of catheter insertion.

the catheter tip is in the distal superior vena cava, parallel to the vessel wall 3 to 4 cm above the junction of the superior vena cava and the right atrium (Ryder, 1996). Malposition of the catheter tip may predispose the patient to complications and can also occur spontaneously at any time after catheter insertion (eg, because of a change in intrathoracic pressure as with coughing or vomiting, a rapid infusion, or random body movement). It is imperative that a chest radiograph be done immediately after insertion and periodically thereafter to ascertain catheter tip location. Malpositioned catheters should be repositioned, most commonly with a guidewire under fluoroscopic imaging.

Cardiac Dysrhythmias

Various cardiac dysrhythmias can be precipitated by the guidewire or the catheter, causing irritation to the myocardium or carotid sinus. Retracting the guidewire (during insertion) or repositioning the catheter after insertion corrects this problem.

Pneumothorax

Pleural puncture may occur inadvertently because of the anatomic proximity of the lung to the subclavian veins. A tension pneumothorax is an emergent problem. It is most likely to occur in patients on ventilatory support, especially those requiring high inspiratory pressure or positive end-expiratory pressure (Ryder, 1996). It can be prevented by lowering positive end-expiratory pressure or removing from the ventilator and bagging during the procedure. Sharp chest pain, cough, decreased breath sounds, and hypoxia may be present, or the pneumothorax may be evident only radiologically. Treatment is based on the symptoms and the size of the pneumothorax. A chest tube is often indicated, although smaller pneumothoraces often resolve spontaneously.

Hemothorax

The subclavian vein or adjacent vessels may be traumatized during venipuncture or later by catheter erosion, causing slow, constant bleeding into the thorax. This is particularly serious if the patient has a bleeding disorder. A hematoma may form, causing respiratory distress from deviation of the trachea. Delayed bleeding, arteriovenous fistula formation, or development of a false aneurysm may occur (Ryder, 1996). Chest tube drainage may be necessary, and thoracotomy may be required in some cases.

Hydrothorax–Hydromediastinum

The vein may be perforated, either during insertion or later because of erosion of the catheter through the vein wall, causing IV solutions to be infused directly into the chest. Signs and symptoms depend on the volume and rate of extravasation. Early symptoms include low-grade fever, dyspnea, and chest pain. Hypoxia, respiratory distress, sepsis, and cardiovascular collapse may occur as the condition progressively worsens.

Inadvertent Arterial Puncture

It is possible inadvertently to enter an artery during the insertion. This can usually be determined by pulsatile or bright red blood return. Hypoxia or hypotension may mask this phenomena, with diagnosis made by reviewing the chest radiograph. The head of the bed should be elevated and direct pressure applied to the bleeding site for 5 to 10 minutes. Hematoma formation may cause deviation of the trachea and respiratory distress. PN solutions should never be infused intra-arterially.

Nerve Injury

Both the brachial plexus and phrenic nerves may be inadvertently damaged during insertion because of their proximity to the central veins. The phrenic nerve can be damaged in both internal jugular and subclavian insertions by the needle or a malpositioned catheter (Ryder, 1996). A tingling sensation in the fingers, pain shooting down the arm, or permanent weakness may occur. Hemidiaphragm paralysis can result from phrenic nerve injury.

Lymphatic Injury

Lymphatic injury or fistula or chylothorax may occur with puncture or laceration of the lymphatic trunks or thoracic duct. Lymphatic vessels are near both the jugular and subclavian veins. The thoracic duct empties into the left subclavian vein at its junction with the left internal jugular. It is enlarged in cirrhotic patients because of alterations in lymph flow. Clinical manifestations include aspiration of clear fluid on insertion or clear drainage from the insertion site. Removal of the catheter is necessary.

Catheter Embolism

Catheter embolism may occur with improper insertion technique by shearing off a portion of the catheter while withdrawing the catheter through the insertion needle. This practice should be avoided. Removal can usually be accomplished by transvenous retrieval under fluoroscopy. Newer over-the-wire techniques of catheter insertion eliminate this complication.

Air Embolism

Air embolism is fortunately rare because its occurrence is the most lethal complication of catheter insertion. Air embolism is a potential danger whenever the central venous system is open to the air, such as during insertion, IV tubing or cap changes, accidental disconnection, or through a tract left after catheter removal. This is most likely to occur on deep inspiration when the patient is in an upright position, dehydrated, or hypovolemic. Symptoms occur with an air entry rate of 20 mL/second. Death can occur with an air entry rate or 75 to 150 mL/second; a 70- to 300-mL air volume may be lethal (Ryder, 1996). Signs and symptoms vary depending on the severity; they may include dyspnea, apnea, hypoxia, disorientation, tachycardia, hypotension, pulmonary wheeze, or a precordial murmur. Severe neurologic deficits, including hemiplegia, aphasia, seizures, and coma, are associated with air embolism. This is attributed to direct access of air into the cerebral circulation in most situations.

Immediate treatment aims to prevent obstruction of the right ventricular outflow tract by air. The patient should immediately be placed on the left side in deep Trendelenburg position (right side up). This keeps the air in the right atrium and out of the pulmonary circulation. Needle aspiration of air through the catheter or by direct intracardiac approach may be necessary. Oxygen therapy should be initiated.

Precautions should be taken during catheter insertion, tubing and cap changes, and catheter removal to prevent air embolism. Tubing junctions should be properly secured. Catheter removal should be immediately followed by placement of an occlusive gauze dressing with an ointment over the site. The ointment occludes the tract and assists with healing. This dressing is usually needed for 24 to 48 hours or until the tract is totally closed.

Cardiac Tamponade–Venous Perforation

This rare but lethal complication may occur within hours of insertion or days or weeks later. Catheters can advance several centimeters during arm, shoulder, or neck movement. Perforation of the superior vena cava, right atrium, or right ventricle may occur because of the catheter tip eroding through the wall with bleeding or infusion into the precordial space. Symptoms depend on the rate and volume of fluid accumulation and pericardial compliance. Unresolved tamponade can result in death. In acute tamponade, 100 to 300 mL of excess fluid is potentially fatal. Clinical manifestations may include retrosternal or epigastric pain, shortness of breath, venous engorgement of the face and neck, restlessness and confusion, hypotension, paradoxical pulse, muffled heart sounds, or cardiac arrest. Chest radiography may reveal pleural effusions and mediastinal widening. Cardiac tamponade is immediately treatable by discontinuing the infusion, aspirating through the catheter, or performing emergency pericardiocentesis or thoracostomy. Treatment must be rapid and aggressive. A high mortality rate is associated with late diagnosis.

Catheter Occlusion

Partial or complete catheter occlusion may result from fibrin sheath formation or thrombus at the tip of the catheter, blood clots, lipid deposits, precipitates, kinking or malposition, pinch-off syndrome, and rupture or breakage of the device. Increased difficulty in infusing fluids may be the first indication of fibrin sheath formation. The fibrin sheath may cause a partial occlusion of the catheter by acting as a "flap-valve" to prevent withdrawal of blood, but allowing infusions. It may eventually encase the entire catheter, causing complete occlusion of all lumens. The sheath may also become seeded with microorganisms, serving as a nidus for infection.

Occlusion of the CVAD may also occur from drug precipitates or lipid deposition. Precipitate occlusion may occur from inadequate flushing between medications, simultaneous administration of incompatible medications or solutions, and medications admixed in concentrations exceeding that required for stability. Calcium and phosphorus precipitates are a common cause of occlusion with PN solutions. Occlusions from drug precipitates or lipid deposition typically result in sudden occlusion of the catheter either during or immediately after an infusion. Occlusion with lipid depositions is also a liability, especially with the use of TNAs.

Table 16–10 outlines the recommended interventions for treating catheter occlusions. The manufacturer's directions should be meticulously followed when using commercial products.

Catheter pinch-off syndrome can occur when a CVAD inserted through the percutaneous subclavian site is compressed between the clavicle and first rib (Andris & Krzywda, 1997). Intermittent mechanical occlusion of the catheter can occur, resulting in complete or partial catheter transection and catheter tip embolization into the central venous system. When pinch-off syndrome is identified, the catheter should be removed as soon as possible.

TABLE 16-10
MANAGING A CVAD OCCLUSION

Type of Occlusion	Treatment
Blood/fibrin	Thrombolytic agents, such as Abbokinase
	Open-Cath (urokinase)
Drug precipitate	0.1 N Hydrochloric acid
Lipid precipitate	70% Ethanol
	Sodium hydroxide

Venous Thrombosis

The development of venous thrombosis may occur with any type of CVAD secondary to injury to the vein wall during insertion, or by movement of the catheter against the vein wall after insertion. Catheter thrombogenicity may depend on the type of catheter material and the surface characteristics (Andris & Krzywda, 1997). Predisposing risk factors for venous thrombosis include hypovolemia, venous stasis, and hypercoaguable states (eg, pregnancy, cancer, hypovolemia, bone marrow transplantation). Chemically induced thrombosis can result from infusion of hypertonic solutions, including PN, and small-volume antibiotics or chemotherapy admixtures and vessicants administered through CVADs whose tips are in the upper arm, subclavian, or innominate veins. Intermittent or long-term infusion of these solutions should be delivered through catheters whose tips terminate in the superior vena cava. A lower incidence of thrombosis has been noted in catheters whose tips lie in the distal superior vena cava (Whitman, 1996).

Patients with venous thrombosis may be asymptomatic, making careful observation for early signs imperative. Signs may include increased anterior chest venous pattern, arm or neck swelling, external jugular distention, or fluid leaking from the insertion site during infusion (caused by backflow). Diagnosis may be made by arm venography, contrast studies through the catheter, Doppler duplex imaging, magnetic resonance imaging, and radionucleotide studies (Whitman, 1996). Treatment of catheter-induced venous thrombosis remains controversial, and depends on the extent of thrombus formation, the severity of the symptoms, the current clinical conditions, and the future access needs of the patient (Whitman, 1996). Conservative treatment without device removal consists of IV anticoagulant therapy followed by warfarin therapy for 3 or more months. Catheter removal followed by anticoagulant therapy may be necessary for more severe symptoms. Some advocate using low-dose warfarin to reduce the risk of thrombosis for patients who are at increased risk (Andris & Krzywda, 1997).

The major complication of catheter-associated venous thrombosis is pulmonary embolism. This complication should be treated with catheter removal plus standard therapy for that disorder, including anticoagulation or thrombolysis at the discretion of the treating physician (Whitman, 1996).

Metabolic Complications

Metabolic complications are the most frequently observed with PN and can be avoided when PN orders are written by knowledgeable physicians and laboratory studies are meticulously monitored. Frequent metabolic monitoring can ensure that potential metabolic complications are prevented or documented and treated. The nurse is in a key position to monitor for these changes and report them to the appropriate physician. Table 16–11 cites the most frequently observed metabolic complications. Only the most life threatening are discussed more fully in the following sections.

Complications Related to Glucose Level

Glucose intolerance has already been discussed. The sudden development of hyperglycemia in a patient who was previously glucose tolerant may indicate impending infection or sepsis. Hyperglycemia and glycosuria may precede clinical signs of sepsis by 12 to 24 hours.

Progressive hyperglycemia, if not detected or inadequately treated, can lead to the life-threatening complication of hyperglycemic hyperosmolar nonketotic coma. If untreated, marked hyperglycemia and glycosuria may lead to an osmotic diuresis accompanied by dehydration, electrolyte imbalance, and a decreasing level of consciousness that can result in seizures and coma and death. Reversal of this state requires immediate discontinuation of the PN solution, aggressive fluid and electrolyte replacement, correction of hyperglycemia by insulin administration, and correction of acidosis with bicarbonates. During treatment, frequent monitoring of blood glucose, electrolyte, and arterial blood gas levels and vital signs is essential (Goff, 1997).

Hypoglycemia is chemically defined as a serum glucose level of less than 50 mg/dL. Many patients may be asymptomatic at this level. Symptoms include weakness, headache, chills, tingling in the extremities or mouth, cold and clammy skin, thirst, hunger, apprehension, diaphoresis, decreased levels of consciousness, and changes in vital signs. Hypoglycemia during PN may occur with excess insulin administration. Insulin needs decrease when steroids are tapered and discontinued, and as sepsis resolves, and should be adjusted in the PN solution accordingly. Abrupt cessation of PN may also result in hypoglycemia if larger amounts of carbohydrates are used. Tapering the PN before discontinuation can eliminate this problem.

Complications Related to Electrolytes

The infusion of hypertonic dextrose results in the intracellular shift of potassium, magnesium, phosphorus, and calcium. Requirements for these electrolytes, particularly potassium and phosphorus, may be increased. Increased losses or requirements related to the patient's clinical status or treatment may also increase electrolyte requirements. Conversely, renal failure may require restriction of some or all of these electrolytes. Careful monitoring of electrolyte levels and adjustments to the PN solution are essential to maintain electrolyte balance.

TABLE 16-11
POTENTIAL METABOLIC COMPLICATIONS OF PARENTERAL NUTRITION

Cause(s)	Prevention	Treatment
Hyperglycemia		
Carbohydrate intolerance	Urine S/A q8h	Decrease PN rate or dextrose concentration/amount
Too rapid infusion of PN	Accuchecks q6h	
Too much carbohydrate load	Be aware of meds that may cause glucose intolerance (ie, steroids)	Increase proportion of calories as lipids
Insulin resistance—stress, sepsis, diabetes, steroids	Start PN infusion slowly	Add insulin to the solution or use sliding-scale insulin coverage
		Maintain blood glucose <200 mg/dL
Hypoglycemia		
Abrupt decrease or cessation of PN	Wean or slow down PN infusion when stopping	Hang D_5W at same rate of PN if unable to hang PN
Excessive insulin administration	Hang D_5W at same rate of PN if unable to hang PN	Give IV glucose STAT; 50% dextrose may be needed; maintain proper flow rate
	Maintain infusion rate; use an infusion pump	
	Monitor urine/serum glucose levels	
Hyperglycemic Hyperosmolar Nonketotic Coma		
Untreated glucose intolerance causes hyperosmolar diuresis, electrolyte imbalances, coma, death (40%–50% mortality rate)	Appropriate glucose monitoring	Monitor closely
	Frequent chemistry profiles to assess electrolytes, osmolarity	Discontinue PN
		Rehydrate with normal saline or other isotonic solution
Increased risk in elderly, diabetes malnourishment, steroid therapy, and with stress or sepsis		Correct electrolyte imbalances, especially potassium and bicarbonate
		Monitor ABGs
		Insulin as needed
Hyperkalemia		
Excessive potassium replacement	Monitor serum potassium and renal function	Stop or decrease potassium in solution
Renal disease—potassium cannot be excreted	Anticipate that a sodium deficiency may lead to hyperkalemia	Assess for other sources of potassium
		Monitor pulse for changes (bradycardia)
Leakage of potassium from cells after severe trauma	Accurate I/O to evaluate fluid balance	In severe hyperkalemia, dialysis may be necessary
Hypokalemia		
Excessive potassium losses (increased GI losses with diarrhea, fistulas)	Monitor serum potassium	Add potassium to PN solution
	Anticipate potential potassium depletion with large GI losses	May need additional IVPB potassium run over 4–6 h to correct severe deficiency
Diuretic therapy	Monitor I/O	

(continued)

T A B L E   1 6 – 1 1   (*Continued*)

Cause(s)	Prevention	Treatment
Large doses of insulin Increased requirement with anabolism	Be aware of drugs that cause excessive potassium loss Be aware that patients severely malnourished are susceptible (refeeding syndrome)	Monitor pulse for tachycardia/ arrhythmia Monitor for metabolic alkalosis (potassium loss may cause sodium retention)
Hypernatremia Dehydration Diarrhea Diabetes insipidus Excessive replacement	Maintain I/O Monitor serum sodium Be aware of drugs that cause sodium retention (ie, steroids)	Decrease sodium or provide salt-free solution until corrected Provide enough free water to meet needs Treat or correct cause
Hyponatremia Diuretics GI losses (vomiting, fistula) Congestive heart failure, renal failure, cirrhosis Water intoxication	Accurate I/O Urine specific gravity Accurate weights (assess fluid shifts)	Fluid restriction Add sodium to PN Minimize GI loss if possible Close metabolic monitoring
Hyperphosphatemia Renal failure Excessive replacement	Accurate I/O Monitor serum levels and renal status	Low or no phosphate added May need dialysis

Hypophosphatemia
 Inadequate in PN
 Insulin therapy
 Disease states:
   Alcoholism
   Respiratory alkalosis
   Renal problems
   Severe diarrhea
   Malabsorption associated with low calcium and magnesium levels
   Increased requirements
	Be aware of potential disease states that cause low phosphate levels
	 Frequent laboratory monitoring, especially if low levels/depleted
	 Be aware of medications that may lower phosphates (carafate, magnesium and aluminium hydroxide, steroids)
		Replace phosphate in PN
		 If <1.5 mg/dL—give IVPB replacement over 4–6 h
		 If <1.0 mg/dL—discontinue PN and correct by IVPB over 4–6 h before restarting PN
		 Replace calcium as needed (repletion of phosphate may cause calcium to drop)
		 Discontinue PN if patient symptomatic

Hypocalcemia Vitamin D deficiency Insufficient replacement Pancreatitis Hypomagnesemia Hyperphosphatemia Hypoalbuminemia	Monitor serum levels Be aware of disease states, medications, malnutrition that can cause hypocalcemia	Replace by adding calcium to PN May require IVPB of calcium to correct severe deficiency Correct hypomagnesemia Correct for deficiency caused by hypoalbuminemia

(*continued*)

T A B L E   1 6 - 1 1   (*Continued*)

Cause(s)	Prevention	Treatment
Hypomagnesemia		
Insufficient magnesium in PN	Monitor serum levels closely	Increase magnesium in PN
Excess GI or renal losses (diarrhea, fistula, diuretics)	Be aware of disease states or drugs that can cause hypomagnesemia	If very low, IVPB replacement
Certain drugs (aminoglycosides, diuretics, cisplatin)		Discontinue PN if patient symptomatic
		Monitor for cardiac arrhythmia
Disease states (chronic alcoholism, pancreatitis, diabetic acidosis, sepsis/infection, burns)		
Hypermagnesemia		
Excess magnesium in PN	Monitor serum levels	Decrease or delete from PN
Renal failure	Monitor renal function	Calcium salts
		Dialysis may be necessary
Metabolic acidosis		
Renal insufficiency; acute/chronic renal failure	Monitor ABGs, electrolytes	Give bicarbonate or replace some or all of chloride with acetate in PN
Diabetic ketoacidosis	Monitor renal function	Monitor vital signs
Diarrhea	Be aware of disease states that may cause metabolic acidosis	
Lactic acidosis (shock)		
Potassium-sparing diuretics		
Massive rhabdomyolysis		

ABGs, arterial blood gases; D_5W, 5% dextrose in water; GI, gastrointestinal; I/O, intake and output; IVPB, intravenous piggyback; S/A, sugar and acetone.

Hypophosphatemia is another life-threatening complication association with PN. It is caused by inadequate phosphate replacement, increased requirements due to losses, disease states, and certain medications. Severe hypophosphatemia and its associated complications can occur in malnourished patients being aggressively refed with PN and has been referred to as the *refeeding syndrome*. Severe cardiopulmonary decompensation associated with severe hypophosphatemia can lead to seizures, coma, and death. Treatment should be primarily preventive. Early detection and treatment, once cardiopulmonary decompensation occurs, is imperative. A more thorough review of this serious complication can be found in the literature (Goff, 1997) (see Chap. 17).

Complications Related to Lipids

Essential fatty acid deficiency and potentiation of inflammatory response by rapid infusion were discussed previously. Elevated liver enzyme levels may be commonly observed in patients receiving PN. Causes are multifactorial and include drugs, sepsis, shock, surgery, and anesthetics. Mild elevations may appear on days 9 to 14 of PN infusion, usually returning to normal once PN is discontinued (Goff, 1997). Overfeeding of calories is often responsible and should be avoided. Slow, continuous infusion of lipids over 16 to 24 hours has also been associated with better tolerance and clearance of lipids.

Hypertriglyceridemia usually is due to an alteration in lipid clearance and occurs most frequently in critically ill patients and those with sepsis. It has been identified as a possible etiologic factor in the development of pancreatitis, immunosuppression, and altered pulmonary hemodynamics in patients receiving PN. Although there is no consensus, lipid emulsions are in general considered safe if serum triglyceride levels are lower than 400 to 500 mg/dL and there is no serum lipemia (Cerra et al., 1997). In patients with these indices, lipid and dextrose amounts should be reduced. IV lipid emulsions should be limited to the provision of essential fatty acids (ie, 250 mL of 20% IV lipid emulsion once or twice weekly) when triglyceride concentrations rise above 400 mg/dL.

Complications Related to Protein

Azotemia can occur if excess protein is administered, causing a rise in blood urea nitrogen because of excess urea production. Adherence to current recommendations for protein eliminates this problem. Use of special renal formulas for patients in acute renal failure remains controversial. It is generally agreed that standard amino acid solutions at goal amounts can be used when dialysis is used to manage renal failure.

Infectious and Septic Complications

Catheter-related sepsis associated with PN is a serious and potentially lethal complication resulting in prolonged hospitalizations and increased morbidity and mortality. Catheter-related bloodstream infections are associated with most nosocomial infections. Short-term CVADs account for approximately 90% of all nosocomial infections. Morbidity and mortality rates of 10% to 20% have been reported in patients with CVAD-related infection (Pearson, 1996).

Reported infection rates vary in institutions, depending on the catheter type, methods of evaluation, and the patient's clinical status. Immunosuppressed and critically ill patients are the most susceptible to catheter-related sepsis. In addition, a CVAD is a foreign body that alters natural defense mechanisms and induces an inflammatory response (Andris & Krzywda, 1997; Jones, 1998; Whitman, 1996).

Catheter-related infection or sepsis may result from skin contaminants at the insertion site, the hub, or tubing. It may also result from contamination at the device's junction from the hands of health care professionals, or from homogeneous seeding from other sources (lungs, urine, abdomen, wounds). Meticulous admixing protocols make the incidence of solution contamination rare. Hub contamination is the most likely source of infection for long-term catheters (>30 days) and site contamination is most likely in short-term (<10 days) catheter-related infection (Pearson, 1996). Exit site, port pocket, and tunnel infections are localized and less common.

Definitions and treatment options for catheter-related infections can be found in Table 16–12. Semiquantitative or quantitative cultures of catheter segments should be used to diagnose catheter-related sepsis, along with peripheral blood cultures. Site cultures can also be done if signs of local infection appear (Whitman, 1996). If colony counts of the catheter segment are 5 to 10 times greater than counts from the peripheral site culture, the catheter is the likely source of infection (Pearson, 1996). The most common organisms causing catheter-related infection include coagulase-negative staphylococci (*Staphylococcus epidermidis*, 28%), *Staphylococcus aureus* (16%), *Enterococcus* (8%), and *Candida* species (3%). Catheter site infections should not be confused with catheter-related sepsis. Erythema or exudate at the site may indicate a localized infection and not necessarily a catheter infection. Conversely, patients may have sepsis without signs at the catheter site.

Catheter-related sepsis may present in the patient as fever, chills, hypotension, change in mental status, and leukocytosis. Metabolic acidosis and hyperglycemia may be early signs of sepsis in critically ill patients receiving PN. A complete fever workup is necessary. All potential sources of infection need to be cultured.

Options for managing catheter-related sepsis include exchange of the catheter over guidewire, catheter salvage, and catheter removal. The decision is determined by the patient's clinical status, culture results, and the nature of the offending organism. Catheter removal remains the treatment of choice for short-term catheters. Guidewire exchange is indicated only if the catheter is malfunctioning and there is

T A B L E   1 6 – 1 2
CATHETER-RELATED INFECTIONS

Infection Type	Description	Treatment
Insertion site infection	Erythema, induration, tenderness, and purulence localized to an area within 2 cm of the catheter insertion site	Daily site care; Warm, moist compresses; Possibly oral antibiotics
Pocket site infection	Erythema, tenderness, and induration over the port reservoir site; possibly necrosis; purulent exudate from the subcutaneous pocket	Warm, moist compresses; Oral or IV antibiotics; Port removal
Tunnel infection	Erythema, tenderness, induration or purulence extending more than 2 cm from the site, along the course of the subcutaneous tunnel	Catheter removal; Infection may respond poorly to other treatment attempts
Catheter-related bloodstream infection	Isolation of the same organism (identical species, antibiogram) from semiquantitative or quantitative cultures of the catheter tip and peripheral blood of a patient with clear signs of bloodstream infection and no other identifiable sources of infection (selected symptoms include temperature ≥101.5°F, chills, rigors, malaise, and temperature defervesence with catheter removal)	Catheter removal; Systemic antibiotics by catheter; Antibiotic lock

no sign of catheter site infection (Whitman, 1996). If infection is suspected and if there is no evidence of catheter site infection and the patient is not floridly septic, the catheter may also be exchanged over a guidewire and the catheter tip sent to the laboratory for culture. If the culture results are positive for colonization or infection, the catheter should be removed and a new catheter inserted in a different location. If the patient is floridly septic, the catheter should be removed immediately (Jones, 1998; Whitman, 1996). In either situation, empiric antibiotics are often started once all appropriate specimens for culture are obtained.

Tunneled catheters and implanted ports pose additional problems because they cannot be changed over a guidewire or readily replaced, and they often serve as lifelines for patients with limited sites for central venous access. Catheter salvage is a desired option in these instances. Many of these infections can be successfully treated with antibiotics without removing the catheter (Andris & Krzywda, 1997). The use of an antibiotic lock technique has been successful in several instances (Andris & Krzywda, 1997). Various drugs in a wide range of concentrations for varying durations have been used. Prophylactic vancomycin is not recommended, and in many institutions, *Candida* infection is automatic grounds for catheter removal, regardless of type.

Some institutions have protocols for the routine change of either catheter site or the catheter over a guidewire to prevent the incidence of catheter-related sepsis. Data show, however, that routine replacement of CVADs without a clear indication does not reduce the rate of catheter colonization or catheter-related bloodstream infections (Pearson, 1996).

Vigilant observation of protocols for insertion, use, and maintenance of CVADs is necessary to minimize the incidence of infection and catheter-related sepsis. Nurses are legally accountable for providing safe and appropriate care to patients. This includes knowledge of and adherence to established guidelines, standards of care, and institutional policies and procedures (see Chap. 9).

▲ Legal Issues: ACCOUNTABILITIES

Legal concerns and accountabilities associated with parenteral nutrition administration include:

- Adherence to established standards and guidelines
- Appropriate labeling
- Appropriate infusion rate and use of an electronic infusion pump
- Appropriate change of tubing and filters, and hang time
- Complications

Literature should be evaluated and policies and procedures reviewed annually with staff nurse participation. Schulmeister (1998) reviews a case study and subsequent legal action against the nurses and physicians by the family of a patient who died because of a complication associated with a CVAD insertion. This review discusses the nursing implications and concludes that no nurse is immune from having his or her care scrutinized at some point. The likelihood of being named in a lawsuit can be reduced by clinical competence; caring and effective communication; adherence to policies, procedures, and standards of care; and meticulous documentation.

■ HOME PARENTERAL NUTRITION

Advanced technology, managed care, and consumer demand have contributed to making HPN a successful alternative for many patients who require prolonged or life-long PN. The emergence and growth of "high-tech" home care infusion companies facilitated the safe administration of PN in the home environment. The results are shorter hospital stays, reduced costs, and improved patient well-being, both psychologically and physically. Referrals for HPN are increasingly being made from the community (ie, physician's offices, home care screening, medical clinics) as patterns of health care change. Care provided in long-term care facilities has also become increasingly complex and includes PN.

Regardless of the health care setting, all patients should be evaluated to determine their eligibility for and the appropriateness of home PN. Standards for Home Nutrition Support (A.S.P.E.N., 1999) have been established and should be used. HPN is expensive and strict policies have been established for reimbursement. The Health Care Financing Administration has published specific eligibility criteria for HPN. Permanent impairment, defined as a condition of long and indefinite duration (minimum of 3 months), is one requirement, and additional care must be taken in determining eligibility for HPN (Winkler, Watkins, & Albina, 1998).

Home PN may be provided as a continuous or a cyclic infusion. Cyclic infusion over 12 to 14 hours, as previously discussed, is preferred, especially for ambulatory patients. Most home infusion companies prefer to provide TNAs for HPN. Regardless of the method chosen for a particular patient, the teaching program should be individualized for a patient's learning needs, capabilities, and home care environment. Patients should be encouraged to assume as much responsibility for self-care as possible. Doing so enhances their sense of control.

Nurses have a primary role in preparing the patient for HPN (Evans-Stoner, 1997; Forloinses-Lynn & Viall, 1996; Winkler et al., 1998). The prospect of HPN may seem overwhelming to the patient and family or caregiver, and thorough preparation and teaching is essential because of the complexity of the procedures to be learned. Careful assessment of the patient's and caregiver's willingness and ability to perform the procedures and assume responsibility for managing this therapy should be a priority. One nurse should be selected as the primary teacher because a lack of consistency can confuse the learner and extend the learning period. Ideally, teaching should be initiated in the hospital and continued in the home if it cannot be completed before discharge. Earlier discharge of patients in the managed care environment may shift the focus for education entirely into the home setting.

Education should include verbal instructions and demonstration of all procedures. Return demonstration by the patient or primary caregiver is essential so that the instructor can assess competency. A manual of written instructions should be provided to all patients. The verbal and written instructions should include the following (Evans-Stoner, 1997; Forloinses-Lynn & Viall, 1996; Winkler et al., 1998):

- All appropriate procedures related to the administration of PN and care and maintenance of the CVAD
- Use, maintenance, and troubleshooting of the infusion pump
- Storage, management, and disposal of solutions and supplies
- Self-monitoring guidelines (Fig. 16–5) and potential complications

Managing Parenteral Nutrition at Home

Instructions

Keep a daily record, filling in the appropriate boxes. Put an X through any box that is not applicable. Your home nutrition support nurse will review this record with you on each visit. Longer comments can be written on the back of this form.

Name: _____

Date:	Sun	Mon	Tue	Wed	Thur	Fri	Sat
Weight (lbs)							
Temperature AM PM							
Blood sugar (include time)							
Urine sugar and acetone AM PM							
Rate/amount of PN/TNA infused (mL/d)							
Lipids (if infused separately)							
Antibiotics							
Oral/IV fluid intake (mL/d)							
Urine output (mL)							
Other output (mL) / type							
Stool frequency/consistency							
Dressing change/site description: C = clean/dry R = red D = drainage P = pain S = swelling L = loose							
Comments: (problems, how you feel, any food intake)							

Figure 16–5. Guidelines and form for managing home parenteral nutrition.

- Problem-solving techniques
- Emergency interventions
- Expectations of home care and follow-up plans

A social worker, discharge planner, or case manager may be helpful to patients and families who have questions and concerns about financial considerations and community resources. Psychosocial support is also essential. Principles for self-administration of TNAs are given in Box 16–10.

Arrangements for a home infusion provider should be determined as early as possible. Ideally, the home infusion nurse visits the patient and family in the hospi-

---

BOX 16–10 Principles of Self-Administration of Parenteral Nutrition

1. Patient/caregiver understand the disorder and rationale for therapy
   - Agree to home therapy and the associated benefits and risks
   - Understand alternatives, consequences if therapy not accepted, advantages and disadvantages
   - Understand short- and long-term goals and the expected duration of treatment
2. Patient/caregiver have the visual acuity, manual dexterity, cognitive ability, and mobility to perform procedures related to PN therapy
   - A backup caregiver is identified and trained in case patient needs assistance
   - Adaptive/assistive devices are available if needed
3. Patient's physical environment is safe and appropriate for home therapy
   - Adequate work area with water supply, refrigeration, storage area for supplies
   - Grounded outlets or adapters available
4. Patient/caregiver verbalize and demonstrate knowledge and understanding of PN administration
   - Aseptic technique
   - Solution storage and handling
   - Solution inspection, preparation, and addition of vitamins or other medications as ordered; attachment of administration set
   - Infusion pump operation, maintenance and troubleshooting
   - Connection and disconnection from CVAD, including appropriate flushing and locking
   - Administration schedule and importance of compliance with established schedule and protocols (including written instructions provided)
   - Self-monitoring guidelines and record keeping
   - Recognition and treatment of potential complications
   - Emergency interventions
   - When/who to call for questions or assistance
   - Identify emergency 24-hour on-call number
   - CVAD care and monitoring
5. Patient/caregiver understands and agrees to follow-up care as scheduled by the physician/nutrition support team
   - Home nursing visits
   - Follow-up in physician's office or clinic

tal to establish rapport and discuss learning needs, feelings and concerns, health status, and the regimen prescribed by the physician. In many cases, the home infusion nurse provides all the teaching in the home.

Documentation should include patient eligibility data and the indication for therapy. It should also incorporate the patient's nutritional therapy objectives into the care plan. Short- and long-term goals should be included, and updated as applicable. Patient progress and monitoring parameters, as well as any problems, should be carefully recorded. Evaluation of the nutritional prescription, readiness for transitional feeding, and periodic nutritional assessments also should be included in the documentation (Winkler et al., 1998).

An ongoing quality assessment and improvement program is important to identify variables and incorporate corrective actions to improve care and outcomes. The benefits of HPN clearly outweigh the risks, and patients today enjoy new freedoms and near-normal lifestyles as a result of this added dimension to nutritional support therapy.

References and Selected Readings

Asterisks indicate references cited in text.

*Andris, D.A. (1996). Substrate metabolism—micronutrients. In K.A. Hennessy & M.E. Orr (Eds.), *Nutrition support nursing core curriculum* (3rd ed.). Silver Spring, MD: American Society for Parenteral and Enteral Nutrition.

*Andris, D.A. & Krzywda, E.A. (1997). Central venous access: Clinical practice issues. *Nursing Clinics of North America, 32*, 719–740.

American Society for Parenteral and Enteral Nutrition (A.S.P.E.N.) Board of Directors. (1988). Standards of nutrition support, hospitalized patients. *Nutrition in Clinical Practice, 3*(1), 28–31.

American Society for Parenteral and Enteral Nutrition Board of Directors. (1996). Standards of practice: Nutrition support nurse. *Nutrition in Clinical Practice, 11*, 127–134.

American Society for Parenteral and Enteral Nutrition Board of Directors. (1996). Standards for nutrition support: Hospitalized pediatric patients. *Nutrition in Clinical Practice, 11*, 217–228.

American Society for Parenteral and Enteral Nutrition Board of Directors. (1997). Standards for nutrition support for residents of long-term care facilities. *Nutrition in Clinical Practice, 12*, 284–293.

American Society for Parenteral and Enteral Nutrition Board of Directors. (1999). Standards for home nutrition support. *Nutrition in Clinical Practice, 14*, 151–162.

*Bray, G. (1992). Pathophysiology of obesity. *American Journal of Clinical Nutrition, 55*, 488S–494S.

*Burke, J., Wolfe, R., Mullany, C., et al. (1979). Parameters of optimal glucose infusion and possible hepatic and respiratory abnormalities following excessive glucose infusion. *Annals of Surgery, 190*, 379–385.

Carpentier, Y.A., VanGossum, A., Dubin, E.Y. & Deckelbaum, R.J. (1993). Lipid metabolism in parenteral nutrition. In J.L. Rombeau & M.D. Caldwell (Eds.). *Clinical nutrition: Parenteral nutrition* (pp. 35–74). Philadelphia: W.B. Saunders.

*Cerra, F.R. (1984). Nutritional requirements. In F.R. Cerra (Ed.), *Pocket manual of surgical nutrition* (pp. 59–85). St. Louis: C.V. Mosby.

*Cerra, F.B., Benitez, M.R., Blackburn, G.L., et al. (1997). Applied nutrition in ICU patients. *Chest, 111*, 769–778.

*Curtis, S. (1996). Nutrition assessment of adults. In K.A. Hennessy & M.E. Orr (Eds.), *Nutrition support nursing core curriculum* (3rd ed., pp. 1-1–12). Silver Spring, MD: American Society for Parenteral and Enteral Nutrition.

*Dudrick, S.J. & Wilmore, D.G. (1968). Long-term parenteral feeding. *Hospital Practice, 3*(10), 65–78.

*Elia, M. (1997). Assessment of nutritional status and body composition. In J.L. Rombeau & R.H. Rolandelli (Eds.), *Clinical nutrition: Enteral and tube feeding* (3rd ed., pp. 155–192). Philadelphia: W.B. Saunders.

*Evans-Stoner, N. (1997). Nutritional assessment: A practical approach (Part 1) and Guidelines for the care of the patient on home nutrition support: An appendix (Part 2). *Nursing Clinics of North America, 32*, 637–650.

*Forloinses-Lynn, S. & Viall, C. (1996). Home care. In K.A. Hennessy & M.E. Orr (Eds.). *Nutrition support nursing core curriculum* (3rd ed., pp. 24-1–14). Silver Spring, MD: American Society for Parenteral and Enteral Nutrition.

*Galica, L.A. (1997). Parenteral nutrition. *Nursing Clinics of North America, 32*, 705–718.

*Goff, K. (1997). Metabolic monitoring in nutrition support. *Nursing Clinics of North America, 32*, 741–754.

Grant, A. & DeHoog, S. (1999). Nutritional assessment and support. In A. Grant & S. DeHoog (Eds.), *Nutritional assessment, support, and management*. Seattle: Authors.

*Grant, J.P. (1992). *Handbook of total parenteral nutrition* (pp. 15–47, 107–136, 171–201). Philadelphia: W.B. Saunders.

Hammond, K.A. (1996). Transitional feeding. In K.A. Hennessy & M.E. Orr (Eds.), *Nutrition support nursing core curriculum* (3rd ed., pp. 25-1–8). Silver Spring, MD: American Society for Parenteral and Enteral Nutrition.

*Harris, J.A. & Benedict, F.G. (1919). *A biometric study of basal metabolism in man* (Publication No. 279). Washington, DC: Carnegie Institute of Washington.

*Intravenous Nurses Society. (1998). Standards of practice. *Journal of Intravenous Nursing, 24*(1) (Suppl.).

*Joint Commission on Accreditation of Healthcare Organizations. (1999). Comprehensive Accreditation Manual for Hospitals. Oakbrook Terrace, IL: Author.

*Jones, G.R. (1998). A practical guide to evaluation and treatment of infections in patients with central venous catheters. *Journal of Intravenous Nursing, 21* (Suppl. 5), S134–S142.

Kovacevich, D.S., Boney, A.R., Braunschweig, C.L., et al. (1997). Nutritional risk classification: A reproducible and valid tool for nurses. *Nutrition in Clinical Practice, 12*(1) 20–25.

Krzywda, E.A. & Andris, D. A. (1995). Treatment of Hickman catheter sepsis using antibiotic lock technique. *Infection Control and Hospital Epidemiology, 16*(10), 596.

*Lowrey, T.S., Dunlap, A.W., Brown, R.O., et al. (1996). Pharmacologic influence on nutrition support therapy: Use of propofol in a patient receiving combined enteral and parenteral nutrition support. *Nutrition in Clinical Practice, 11*(4), 147–149.

*McMahon, M. (1997). Management of hyperglycemia in hospitalized patients receiving parenteral nutrition. *Nutrition in Clinical Practice, 12*, 35–41.

*National Advisory Group on Standards and Practice Guidelines for Parenteral Nutrition. (1998). Safe practices for parenteral nutrition formulations. *Journal of Parenteral and Enteral Nutrition, 22* (2), 49–66.

Nutrition Advisory Group. (1979). Multivitamin preparations for parenteral use: A statement by the Nutrition Advisory Group. *Journal of Parenteral and Enteral Nutrition, 3*, 258.

*Pearson, M.L. (1996). Guidelines for prevention of intravascular device-related infections. *Hospital Epidemiology, 17*, 438–463.

*Rolandelli, R.H. & Ulrich, J.R. (1994). Nutritional support in the frail elderly surgical patient. *Surgical Clinics of North America, 74*, 79–92.

*Rollins, C.J. (1997). Total nutrient admixtures: Stability issues and their impact on nursing practice. *Journal of Intravenous Nursing, 20*, 299–304.

*Rosmarin, D.K., Wardlow, G.M., & Mirtallo, J. (1996). Hyperglycemia associated with high continuous infusion rate of total parenteral nutrition dextrose. *Nutrition in Clinical Practice, 11*(4), 151–156.

*Ryder, M.A. (1996). Vascular access devices. In K.A. Hennessy & M.E. Orr (Eds.), *Nutrition support nursing core curriculum* (3rd ed., pp. 23-1–23-32). Silver Spring, MD: American Society for Parenteral and Enteral Nutrition.

*Schulmeister, L. (1998). A complication of vascular access device insertion: A case study and review of subsequent legal action. *Journal of Intravenous Nursing, 21*, 197–202.

Shuster, M.H. (1996). Parenteral nutrition. In K.A. Hennessy & M.E. Orr (Eds.), *Nutrition support nursing core curriculum* (3rd ed., pp. 22-1–12). Silver Spring, MD: American Society for Parenteral and Enteral Nutrition.

*Souba, W.W. (1997). Nutritional support. *New England Journal of Medicine, 336*, 41–48.

*Trissel, L.A., Gilbert, D.L., Martinez, J.F., et al. (1999). Compatibility of medications with 3-in-1 parenteral nutrition admixtures. *Journal of Parenteral and Enteral Nutrition, 23*(2), 67–74.

*Trujillo, E.B., Young, L.S., Chertow, G.M., et al. (1999). Metabolic and monetary costs of avoidable parenteral nutrition use. *Journal of Parenteral and Enteral Nutrition, 23*(2), 109–113.

*Whitman, E.D. (1996). Complications associated with the use of central venous access devices. *Current Problems in Surgery, 33*(4), 311–378.

*Wilmore, D.W. & Dudrick, S.J. (1968). Growth and development of an infant receiving all nutrients exclusively by vein. *Journal of the American Medical Association, 203*, 860–864.

*Winkler, M.F., Watkins, C.K., & Albina, J.E. (1998). Transitioning the nutrition support patient from hospital to home. *Infusion, 4*(7), 39–44.

Review Questions

Note: Questions below may have more than one right answer.

1. Which of the following visceral proteins is most useful in monitoring the effectiveness of nutritional support because of its shorter half-life and sensitivity to acute changes in protein status?

   A. Albumin

   B. Transferrin

   C. Prealbumin

   D. Total protein

2. What is the minimum amount of glucose needed to meet the obligate needs for glucose by the brain, central nervous system, red blood cells, white blood cells, active fibroblasts, and certain phagocytes?

   A. 50–75 g

   B. 150–200 g

   C. 250–300 g

   D. 350–400 g

3. All of the following are adverse reactions to IV lipids *except:*

   A. Dyspnea

   B. Chest pain

   C. Headache

   D. Leg cramps

4. As a general rule, the higher the stress, the lower the calorie-to-nitrogen ratio. Which of the calorie-to-nitrogen ratio ranges below is most often considered appropriate for the highly stressed patient?

   A. Between 60:1 and 90:1

   B. Between 90:1 and 100:1

   C. Between 90:1 and 150:1

   D. Between 100:1 and 150:1

5. Which of the following complications is not associated with placement of the central venous catheter tip into the heart?

   A. Thrombosis

   B. Cardiac tamponade

   C. Valvular damage

   D. Cardiac dysrhythmias

6. During parenteral nutrition administration, the serum blood glucose level should be maintained at less than

   A. 50 mg/dL

   B. 80 mg/dL

   C. 100 mg/dL

   D. 200 mg/dL

7. If symptoms of an air embolism occur, the patient should be placed in which of the following positions?

   A. On the back in semi-Fowler's

   B. On the left side, in deep Trendelenburg

   C. On the right side, in deep Trendelenburg

   D. On the left in semi-Fowler's

8. Symptoms of hyperglycemic hyperosmolar nonketotic coma include all of the following *except:*

   A. Glycosuria

   B. Seizures

   C. Coma

   D. Anuria

9. During parenteral nutrition administration, the refeeding syndrome is associated with which of the following electrolyte abnormalities?

   A. Hypophosphatemia

   B. Hypermagnesemia

   C. Hypercalcemia

   D. Hyponatremia

10. Mechanical complications associated with central venous access devices include all of the following *except:*

   A. Malposition

   B. Pneumothorax

   C. Dysrhythmia

   D. Sepsis

Transfusion Therapy

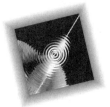

K E Y   T E R M S

Adverse Effects
Immunohematology

■ TRANSFUSION THERAPY IN THE 21ST CENTURY: AN OVERVIEW

As a new century begins, expectations are for the field of transfusion therapy to progress beyond the monumental events of the past 100 years, when the two most important systems, ABO and Rh, were discovered. Many historical markers since the beginning of the 20th century influence today's practice. Prevention against hemolytic disease of the newborn, technology of freezing components, establishment of internationally recognized standards and governing agencies for transfusion medicine, component transfusion therapy, and the ability to test for many transmittable diseases are just a few examples of the accomplishments scientists and physicians made during the 20th century. The future is wide open for more complex informational technology, automation technology, the need for an alternative to allogeneic blood, the eradication of transfusion reactions, and the ability to better preserve the blood supply. Or will human blood and its components even be used? Ongoing work involves producing a product that can replace or substitute for blood. The industry is actively developing emulsions derived from perfluorocarbons, human hemoglobin, animal hemoglobin, and recombinant human hemoglobin, which may serve as blood substitutes (Stowell & Tamasulo, 1998).

As nurses cope with the numerous changes that have sprung from today's managed health care model, it is certainly anyone's guess what health care will become. It is probably safe to assume that transfusion medicine will become even more customized for some patients than it is today. Almost certainly, the health care industry will strive to improve transfusion therapy for recipients.

With the increase in acuity in medical facilities and the reduced length of stay

411

that patients are experiencing, quality improvement programs are necessary to monitor quality measures surrounding all aspects of transfusion therapy. In this way, health care workers can feel confident that standards are met and policies and procedures are followed. The U.S. Food and Drug Administration (FDA), Clinical Laboratory Improvement Act of 1988 (CLIA), Occupational Safety and Health Administration (OSHA), Joint Commission on Accreditation of Healthcare Organizations (JCAHO), and American Association of Blood Banks (AABB) have established rules and regulations governing quality programs and the procurement, storage, and administration of transfusion therapy. The AABB sets standards that represent accepted performance guidelines for the provision of safe transfusion, transplantation, and work environments for personnel. In addition, state and local governing bodies may require additional practical issues. Patients are more likely to inquire about various aspects of this integral part of their treatment. The administration of blood and its components is associated with serious problems and potentially fatal complications that can result in litigation. Only personnel with documented qualifications and who demonstrate continued competence should perform administration of blood.

Nurses share with the blood transfusion service the responsibility for providing the safest transfusion therapy. Nurses must incorporate the fundamental principles of immunohematology into their daily nursing care; the indications, advantages, and disadvantages of a large variety of components; proper procedures for safe administration; and the ability to recognize early symptoms of transfusion reactions and to perform appropriate interventions. Being knowledgeable and maintaining the skills of administering blood and components help decrease the risks of this important therapy.

▲ Legal Issues: CONCERNS OF TRANSFUSION THERAPY

- Incorporation of American Association of Blood Banks and Food and Drug Administration standards and guidelines into practice settings: All written policies and procedures should include the standards and guidelines.
- Documentation: The entire transfusion should be documented according to institutional practice.
- Exposure to bloodborne pathogens: Standard Precautions should specify how to draw blood samples and administer the transfusion. Latex-free equipment should be available for latex-sensitive patients and personnel.
- Disposal of equipment: Policy is established to prevent accidental blood exposure and needlestick injury.
- Physician accountability: The Medical Director should review and approve all policies and procedures.

■ BASIC IMMUNOHEMATOLOGY

Immunohematology is the science that deals with antigens of the blood and their antibodies. An antigen is a substance capable of stimulating the production of an antibody and then reacting with that antibody in a specific way. People who have been exposed to the red blood cells or leukocytes of other people through transfusion, transplantation, or pregnancy (maternal–fetal hemorrhage) may produce antibodies to the foreign antigens carried on those cells. An antibody is a protein in the plasma that reacts with a specific antigen. Antibodies are named for the antigen that stimulated their formation and that with which they react. For example, an antibody against the D antigen formed after the transfusion of an Rh (D)-positive unit to an Rh (D)-negative recipient is called *anti-D*. Antibodies formed in response to exposure to foreign antigens are called *immune antibodies*.

The ABO system, discovered by Karl Landsteiner in 1901, is the most important group of antigens for transfusion as well as transplantation. The synthesis of these antigens, which are located on the surface of red blood cells, is under the control of the A, B, and O genes. In the presence of the A gene, a person makes A antigen and is classified as group A. Group B people have B antigens on their red blood cells, group AB people have both, and group O people have neither (Table 17–1). These antigens, inherited genetically, determine the person's blood group.

Some blood group antibodies are formed without exposure to allogeneic red blood cells. The most important of these so-called naturally occurring antibodies, or isoagglutinins, are anti-A and anti-B. During the first few months of life, infants make immunoglobulin M (IgM) antibodies to whichever of the ABO antigens they lack. For example, a group A infant makes anti-B. These isoagglutinins can produce rapid hemolysis of red blood cells with the corresponding antigen, forming the basis of ABO incompatibility.

The Rh system, discovered in 1940 by Stetson and Levine, is the second most clinically important system for transfusion. The antigens of the human Rh system are of great clinical significance because they often are responsible for transfusion incompatibility and hemolytic disease of the newborn. Approximately 80% to 85% of the white population has the D antigen on their red blood cells and is classified as D or Rh positive. In approximately 10% to 15% of the population, the D antigen is missing; these people are classified as Rh negative and can readily form anti-D after exposure to the antigen. Severe hemolytic reactions and hemolytic disease of the newborn result from this antigen–antibody reaction. Other common antigens in the system are C, E, c, and e.

Approximately 50 other known blood group antigen systems containing approximately 500 antigens are known. Fortunately, only a few systems, such as Kell, Duffy, and Kidd, are encountered commonly. Leukocytes also carry antigens on their surfaces. The most important group is human leukocyte antigens (HLA).

T A B L E   1 7 – 1
ABO CLASSIFICATION OF HUMAN BLOOD

	Cell Antigens		Plasma Antibodies		
Group	A	B	A	B	% U.S. Population
O	–	–	+	+	45
A	+	–	–	+	40
B	–	+	+	–	10
AB	+	+	–	–	5

Mechanism of Immune Response

When a patient is transfused with allogeneic blood bearing "foreign" (ie, nonself) antigens, the immune system may respond by producing antibodies. Phagocytic cells called *macrophages* play an important role in the body's defense system. One of their roles in the immune response is to capture and process foreign antigens. The macrophages then present the processed antigens to other members of the immune system, namely, the T and B lymphocytes. B lymphocytes, with help from T lymphocytes, begin to produce antibodies specific for the antigens that the macrophages presented. Stimulated by the appropriate foreign antigen, the B cell swells, changes its internal structure, and differentiates into plasma cells to produce antibodies (Stroup & Tracey, 1982). Each plasma cell produces large quantities of antibodies of the precise specificity and immunoglobulin class genetically programmed into the cell. The cells secrete the antibodies into a variety of body fluids, including the blood plasma. The T lymphocytes act as helpers or suppressors to B-lymphocyte function. The intertwined relationship between B and T lymphocytes regulates the type and sensitivity of the immune response.

Mechanism of Red Blood Cell Destruction

Two mechanisms of red blood cell destruction are known: intravascular hemolysis and extravascular hemolysis. Intravascular hemolysis occurs within the vascular compartment. This mode of red blood cell destruction results from the sequential binding of antibody to a red blood cell with a foreign antigen on its surface. This antibody then fixes complement. If the entire complement cascade is triggered, a lytic complex forms on the red blood cell membrane, which leads to rupture of the red blood cell and the release of hemoglobin into the intravascular compartment.

Antibodies that activate complement often agglutinate in vitro and can cause intravascular hemolysis in vivo. The most frequent cause of this type of red blood cell destruction is transfusion of ABO-incompatible blood. Anti-A and anti-B are mostly IgM antibodies capable of engaging the complement, coagulation, and kinin systems when they bind with their corresponding antigens. The consequences of this type of hemolysis are usually immediate and severe and are often fatal.

The other mechanism of red blood cell destruction, extravascular hemolysis, is more commonly seen as a result of incompatibilities in blood group systems other than the ABO. Antibodies to these other blood group antigens are usually IgG and bind to red blood cells with the corresponding antigen. Phagocytic cells of the reticuloendothelial system, particularly in the spleen, bind the IgG-coated red blood cells, ingest them, and destroy them extracellularly—hence the term, *extravascular hemolysis*. These IgG antibodies also may fix some amount of complement, but not enough to lyse the red blood cells. Instead, the phagocytic cells of the liver, the Kupffer cells, clear the complement-coated red blood cells from the circulation and destroy them intracellularly. The consequences of extravascular hemolysis are less severe than those of intravascular hemolysis, but are recognizable by a drop in the hematocrit, an increase in the bilirubin level, and perhaps the clinical signs of fever or malaise.

Blood Group Systems

The ABO system is the only system in which the reciprocal antibodies are consistently and predictably present in the sera of normal people whose red blood cells lack the corresponding antigen(s). The ABO system is the foundation of pretransfusion testing and compatibility.

The Rh system is so called because of its relationship to the substance in the red blood cells of the rhesus monkey. Because of the ease with which antibody D is made, grouping is done on all donors and recipients to ensure that D-negative recipients receive D-negative blood, except for reasonable qualifying circumstances. D-positive recipients may receive either D-positive or D-negative blood. Antibodies to the Rh antigens are not present unless a person has been exposed to D-positive red blood cells, either through transfusion or pregnancy. People who develop Rh antibodies have detectable levels for many years. If undetected, subsequent exposure may lead to a secondary immune response. Occasionally, weak variants of the Rh D antigen are found, which are identified by special serologic tests. These people are termed weak D or Du positive, but they are considered Rh positive both as donors and recipients.

Other blood group systems have been defined on the basis of reaction of cells with antibodies. Antibodies to antigens in the Kell, Duffy, Kidd, and Lewis systems are encountered frequently enough to be clinically important. Antibodies to the blood group antigens in most other systems are found so infrequently that they do not cause everyday problems. When present, these antibodies may produce hemolytic reactions. Once demonstrated, precautions must be taken to ensure that the patient receives compatible blood lacking the corresponding antigen. When difficulty arises in crossmatching or when a transfusion reaction occurs, these systems acquire special significance.

Today, systems to identify, validate, and ensure ABO and Rh groupings are set up on computer databases. Confirmatory testing must be in place according to AABB guidelines.

■ PRETRANSFUSION TESTING

The Donor

A donor may donate blood no more than every 8 weeks. A donation shall be no more than 10.5 mL/kg body weight. In addition to ABO and Rh group determination and a screen for unexpected antibodies, several other tests are performed on donor blood before it is released for patient use. Donated units are to be negative for antibodies to hepatitis B surface antigen (HBsAg), human immunodeficiency virus (anti-HIV), hepatitis C virus (anti-HCV), hepatitis B core antigen (anti-HBc), human T-cell lymphotropic virus (anti HTLV-I/II), HIV antigen (HIV-1-Ag), antibodies to HIV-1, HIV-2, and a serologic test for syphilis (STS). No blood component is issued unless test results are negative (Box 17–1). Alanine aminotransferase (ALT), an enzyme that is released from damaged cells in a person with liver injury or inflammation, is no longer considered an appropriate test to qualify blood donations for transfusions (American Red Cross, 1999).

BOX 17–1 **Donor Testing Requirements**

Allogenic Donor

ABO group
Rh type
Hepatitis B surface antigen
Anti-hepatitis B core antigen
HIV-1 antigen
Anti-HIV-1 and 2
Anti-hepatitis C virus
Serologic test for syphilis
Anti-human T-lymphotropic virus-I and II
Unexpected antibodies

Recipient Testing Requirements

ABO group
Rh type
Unexpected antibodies to red cell antigens
Crossmatch against donor red cells

HIV, human immunodeficiency virus.

The Recipient

Tests performed on the intended transfusion recipient include ABO and Rh group determination and screening for unexpected antibodies. Before the administration of whole blood or red blood cell components, a major crossmatch (combining donor red blood cells and recipient serum or plasma) is performed to detect serologic incompatibility.

The AABB requires that if a patient has been transfused in the preceding 3 months with blood or a blood component containing red blood cells, has been pregnant within the preceding 3 months, or the history is uncertain or unavailable, the sample must be obtained from the patient within 3 days of the scheduled transfusion (AABB, 1999a). This requirement is made to rule out the possibility of missing a newly formed antibody.

In situations in which delaying the provision of blood may jeopardize life, blood may be issued before completion of routine tests according to AABB standards (AABB, 1999). Recipients whose ABO group is not known must receive group O red blood cells. Physicians must indicate in the record that the clinical condition is sufficiently urgent to release blood before the completion of compatibility testing. The tag or label must conspicuously indicate that compatibility testing is not completed, and standard compatibility tests should be completed as promptly as possible. Recipients whose ABO group has been determined by the transfusing facility without reliance on previous record may receive ABO group-specific whole blood or ABO group–compatible red blood cell components before other compatibility tests have been completed.

Directed Donations

Risk of transfusion-transmitted diseases has generated programs whereby prospective patients may designate their own blood donors. Blood centers and hospitals have increased the availability of this program, known as *directed donation*, for the public. Each donor enters the same process as any other, but the blood is labeled for a specific recipient provided screening tests are appropriate and the unit is compatible. Units are specifically labeled for the intended recipient.

The primary benefit of the program may be to reduce the fear of disease transmission in recipients, who feel reassured knowing who their donors are. If the donor is a blood relative of the recipient, the cellular components must be irradiated (AABB, 1999). All these programs must incorporate finances, staffing, quality assessment measures, and legal considerations.

Autologous Donation

Autologous transfusion is the collection, filtration, and reinfusion of a person's own blood; thus, the donor and recipient are the same individual. There are several types of autologous donation, all of which eliminate risk of disease transmission as well as immunosuppression, although other mechanical and nonhemolytic reactions can occur. *Autologous transfusion* takes on several different meanings and methods and is accepted practice for appropriate candidates in a setting based on the patient's clinical condition. Autologous transfusion is a conservative approach. The primary reasons for the increased use of this procedure include technologic advances, blood conservation, public awareness, and the need to decrease the transmission of bloodborne diseases. All products of autologous donation must be labeled "For Autologous Use Only."

Receiving one's own blood is the safest transfusion, and these modalities are increasingly encouraged. Careful administration of autologous blood is still required. To avoid any errors, those administering the blood must verify all aspects of the component, including proper identification. Verification procedures should be identical to those for giving homologous transfusions.

The goals of these programs are to conserve blood and prevent reactions, isoimmunization, and disease transmission (Maffei & Thurer, 1988). The public continues to become more aware of the hazards of disease transmission by transfusions, even though testing is quite sensitive. Health care workers should be able to offer therapies to patients that might benefit their overall care. The AABB endorses all modalities of blood conservation, including the goals of autologous transfusions. Autologous transfusion can be accomplished by preoperative donation, acute normovolemic hemodilution, intraoperative salvage, and postoperative blood salvage.

Preoperative Autologous Donation

This technique is best used when a patient is planning an elective surgical procedure that normally would cause the loss of a significant number of units of blood. The patient may plan periodic visits to a donor center for phlebotomies to store his or her own blood for later use. Autologous transfusions account for an average of 5.7% of collected blood, and in some donor centers as much as 20% (Gould & Forbes, 1995; Heaton, 1994).

Acute Normovolemic Hemodilution

In this procedure, the patient's blood is collected, stored at room temperature for up to 8 hours in the operating room, and returned to the patient at the time of blood loss. Deterioration of platelets and coagulation factors is minimal. The benefit of this technique is that it reduces the patient's hematocrit before surgical blood loss so that the patient loses a smaller red cell mass. The patient receives infusions of a crystalloid or colloid solution to maintain plasma volume. Frequently used in cardiac surgery, hemodilution may be limited by the patient's blood volume and hemodynamic considerations. Because the hematocrit is reduced, patients with lung disease or hypooxygenation require close monitoring.

Intraoperative Blood Collection

This frequently used method of autologous transfusion involves recovering blood during surgical procedures associated with significant blood loss from clean wounds. Blood is aspirated from the operative site, washed by using cell-washing machines, and reinfused back to the patient. The process may be performed completely in the operating room. It is most frequently used in cardiovascular, thoracic, orthopedic, neurologic, and hepatic surgery, including transplantations. The technique makes large volumes of blood immediately available when bleeding occurs in a clean operative procedure. The procedure is contraindicated in patients with malignancy or infection because reinfusion of contaminated cells may disseminate the tumor cells or infectious organism.

Sterile technique is mandated to prevent infectious agents from entering the system. Initial equipment and personnel costs can be high, but improved medical care outweighs the disadvantages. The program's success requires (1) availability of responsible staff 24 hours a day, (2) preferably dedicated operators for each machine, (3) a quality improvement program, and (4) physician support and public awareness programs. Some hospitals have developed programs that have established a "break-even" point for using this method of autologous transfusion. Others may hire outside agencies to do "traveling" intraoperative autologous transfusions.

Postoperative Blood Collection

This technique involves collecting shed blood from surgical drains after cardiac, trauma, orthopedic, and plastic surgery. Other clinical conditions also may be appropriate. The advantage of this technique is that it can be done for planned surgery or emergency operations and trauma. Postoperative shed blood is collected through special equipment and reinfused. If the blood in the sterile canister is not initiated for reinfusion with 6 hours, it must be discarded. This technique is safe, simple, and cost effective. Combined with other methods of autologous transfusions described, the goal of avoiding homologous blood transfusions is closer.

■ ANTICOAGULANTS—PRESERVATIVES

Blood is routinely collected in plastic bags that may contain different anticoagulants–preservatives. Whole blood collected in citrate–phosphate–dextrose (CPD) or citrate–phosphate–double dextrose (CP2D) has an expiration date not exceeding 21 days after phlebotomy. The difference in the solutions is that CP2D has twice the amount of dextrose. The anticoagulant–preservative system of CPD-adenine (CPDA-1) may be stored for 35 days. The duration for storage is based on the standard that a minimum of 75% of the transfused red blood cells (stored for 35 days) must be present in the bloodstream of the recipient 24 hours after the transfusion. Providing a nutrient biochemical balance to red blood cells during storage is important to maintain viability and function of the components in the blood and to prevent physical changes. To minimize bacterial proliferation, specific temperatures must be maintained.

Each ingredient in the solution has a function. The phosphate acts as a buffer, slowing the drop in pH of the stored cells and improving viability. Sodium citrate, by combining with ionized calcium, inhibits clotting, thus serving as an anticoagulant. Dextrose (glucose) prolongs the life of the red blood cells by providing a nutrient source. Adenine is a substrate from which red blood cells can synthesize adenosine triphosphate (ATP). The red blood cell depends on ATP to maintain cell surface ion pumps.

A second group of anticoagulant–preservative systems is similar to CPDA-1. They differ, however, in that, once the platelet-rich plasma is removed from the unit within 8 hours, an additive solution of 100 mL containing saline, dextrose, and adenine is added to the packed red blood cells. These additive systems permit storage for up to 42 days. FDA-approved solutions are AS-1 (Adsol), AS-3 (Nutricel), and AS-5 (Optisol).

Solutions such as pyruvate and other compounds have been licensed and may be added to stored red blood cells nearing the end of their shelf life. Following the addition of these solutions, the red blood cells are called rejuvenated cells. These additives allow units to be stored even longer.

■ WHOLE BLOOD

Whole blood contains cells (red blood cells, white blood cells, and platelets), plasma (blood proteins, antibodies, water, and waste), and electrolytes. Transfusions of whole blood are infrequent and may be indicated only when an acute, massive blood loss has occurred. *Massive* transfusion indicates that a patient has received an amount of blood approximating the total blood volume within 24 hours (AABB, 1999). The goal is to restore intravascular blood volume to prevent hypovolemic shock. The patient requires both the oxygen-carrying capacity of the red blood cells and plasma for volume replacement. It is imperative quickly to restore the blood volume to improve oxygen delivery. Crystalloid and colloid solutions correct hypovolemia only temporarily. Patients should be monitored closely for dilutional coagulopathies. Labile coagulation factors deteriorate in whole blood within 24 hours after collection.

Whole blood, stored less than 4 to 5 days, may be indicated for an exchange transfusion in a newborn. The blood may ensure electrolyte concentration limits tolerable for infants. These units of blood should lack hemoglobin S (AABB, 1999a). Autologous donated whole blood is frequently returned to the patient (donor) as a whole-blood infusion.

Whole blood has many disadvantages. Patients must receive from their own blood group, which eliminates ABO compatibility between blood groups (Table 17–2). With the continuous metabolic changes of red blood cells, definite changes occur in stored blood. Potassium leaks out of the cell and into the plasma. Studies have shown that the potassium level rises to approximately 21 mEq/L by day 21 after collection. Infusions of stored whole blood could potentially cause complications to patients with compromised cardiac status or patients undergoing exchange transfusion. Another problem is the formation of microaggregates. As cells break down, this cellular debris may be detrimental to patients with lung disease, although physicians differ in opinion on the significance of microaggregates. Special filters are available and are designed to protect against the infusion of this particulate matter.

Whole blood is stored at a temperature of 1°C (34°F) to 6°C (43°F). Expiration depends on the anticoagulant–preservative. The rate of administration for whole blood should be as rapid as necessary to correct and maintain hemodynamic status. In massive hemorrhage, one or more large-gauge catheters, such as 14 or 16 gauge, allows a free-flow infusion of blood. Electronic infusion devices do not deliver high enough rates to meet the needs of this clinical crisis. In this instance, pressure cuffs applied to the bag of blood may be required for rapid infusion.

Whole Blood, Modified

Whole blood, modified is prepared by removing the plasma, collecting the platelets or cryoprecipitate, and then returning the plasma back to the red blood cells. This product may be used for patients with hemorrhage and other clinical conditions

TABLE 17–2
ABO COMPATIBILITY FOR WHOLE BLOOD

Recipient	Donor
A	A
B	B
AB	AB
O	O

when whole blood is warranted. Although this component has the same hemostatic properties as whole blood, a patient may also require separate components.

Fresh whole blood, defined as being less than 24 hours old, has no valid indications. Although it contains viable platelets and other coagulation factors, a patient's deficit of these components should be specifically replaced with the component to correct the underlying problem. In addition, processing of donor blood is difficult to complete within 24 hours.

Whole Blood, Irradiated

Whole blood, irradiated is a unit that has been exposed to gamma irradiation to prevent or minimize the proliferation of transfused T lymphocytes in recipients at risk for development of transfusion-associated graft-versus-host disease (TAGVHD) (AABB, 1999b). Patients at risk for TAGVHD are recipients of donor units from blood relatives, recipients undergoing bone marrow transplantation, select immunocompetent or immunocompromised patients, and fetuses receiving intrauterine transfusion. Because irradiation may damage and reduce the viability of red blood cells, the original expiration date of the component prevails.

■ RED BLOOD CELL COMPONENTS

Packed Red Blood Cells

Packed red blood cells are prepared by removing approximately 225 to 250 mL of platelet-rich plasma from a unit of whole blood, either by centrifugation or sedimentation. This process packs the red blood cells and separates most of the platelet-rich plasma. The red blood cell concentrate contains the same red blood cell mass as whole blood, 20% to 30% of the original plasma, and some leukocytes and platelets. Packed red blood cells usually have a hematocrit between 70% and 80%; thus, the viscosity of the unit is increased. One unit of packed red blood cells provides the same amount of oxygen-carrying red blood cells as a unit of whole blood, but at a reduced volume.

The major indication for packed red blood cells is to restore or maintain oxygen-carrying capacity. Because of the reduced volume of the unit, the danger of circulatory overload is decreased—a definite advantage in patients with renal failure or congestive heart failure and elderly or debilitated patients (AABB, 1999b). When approximately two thirds of the plasma is removed, the patient is not subjected to infusions of additional potassium, citrate, or sodium.

Each unit of packed red blood cells is expected to raise the hematocrit 3% and the hemoglobin level 1 g/dL in the average 70-kg person. In infants, the hemoglobin level is expected to rise by 1 g/dL when administered at 3 mL/kg. The expiration time of packed red blood cells is 35 to 42 days, depending on the anticoagulant–preservative used.

Because most of the plasma is removed, thereby reducing the amount of anti-A or anti-B agglutinins (or both), group O may be given to other blood groups. In emer-

TABLE 17-3
ABO COMPATIBILITIES FOR RED CELL COMPONENTS*

Recipient	Donor		
	First Choice	Second Choice	Third Choice
O+	O+	O−	
A+	A+	O+, A−	O−
B+	B+	O+, B−	O−
AB+	AB+	AB−, A+, B+	O+, A−, B−, O−
O−	O−	O+	
A−	A−	O−	A+, O+
B−	B−	O−	A+, O+
AB−	AB−	A−, B−, O−	AB+, A+, B+, O+

*Not whole blood, which must be administered ABO *identical*.

gencies, when time does not permit ABO determination, group O red blood cells may be given (Table 17–3).

Red Blood Cells, Leukocytes Reduced

Red blood cells, leukocytes reduced can be produced by (1) leukocyte-absorption filtration of red blood cells; (2) frozen deglycerolization of red blood cells; (3) microaggregate filteration of red blood cells; (4) washing of red blood cells; or (5) buffy coat depletion of red blood cells. Thus, the removal of leukocytes from red blood cells requires either centrifugation, washing, or filtration. Prestorage leukocyte removal by filtration is the most effective method, achieving a 2- to 3-log reduction in leukocytes, and is the method of choice (AABB, 1999b).

Red blood cells, leukocytes reduced are used to restore red blood cells to patients who have previously experienced two or more nonhemolytic febrile reactions and who may have developed antibodies against transfused leukocytes. Leukocyte reactions may be extremely uncomfortable and may last for several hours. The component also may be considered for patients with diseases such as leukemia and aplastic anemia for which multiple transfusions are anticipated. These patients are at risk of becoming refractory to platelet transfusions because of the formation of antibodies to leukocyte antigens, such as HLA, which also are found on platelets. Patients who have a history of allergic transfusion reactions and are IgA deficient are also candidates for this component.

This component of red blood cells must be administered within 24 hours after preparation. Increasingly, special high-efficiency leukocyte removal filters are being used at the bedside. The rate of infusion and ABO compatibility are the same as for packed red blood cells.

Red Blood Cells, Rejuvenated

Red blood cells prepared from whole blood and collected in CPD or CPDA-1 can be rejuvenated at any time during storage or up to 3 days after expiration. The FDA-approved rejuvenating solution consists of pyruvate, inosine, phosphate, and adenine, which restores 2,3-diphosphoglycerate and ATP to normal levels. If not administered within 24 hours, these red blood cells must be glycerolized and frozen (AABB, 1999). They must be washed before infusion to remove the inosine, which may be toxic (American Red Cross, 1999).

Red Blood Cells, Deglycerolized

This component undergoes cryopreservation and is prepared by adding a cryoprotectant, such as glycerol. Initially, plasma is extracted from the whole blood. The red blood cells are then coated with glycerol and may be frozen at $-85°C$ for up to 10 years. At the time the unit is needed, it is thawed and the glycerol is removed by a variety of washing procedures. After thawing, the component should be administered within 24 hours of the washing process. The finished product has virtually all the plasma and anticoagulant removed. It contains less than 5% of the original donor platelets and leukocytes and has a hematocrit of approximately 80%.

This red cell component is not used as a routine red cell replacement, but is useful to preserve blood from donors with rare blood groups. It is also useful to patients who are sensitized to IgA or other plasma proteins because the cellular components have been removed. It also serves as an alternative method to reduce cytomegalovirus (CMV) transmission for selected patients. It also is used as a red blood cell replacement for patients who have recurrent febrile nonhemolytic reactions to decrease HLA alloimmunization (AABB, 1999b). Because of the growing concerns over disease transmission, the increase in autologous donations may produce an increase in the number of units frozen if blood is donated more than 35 to 42 days before being needed. The major disadvantage is the substantial additional cost related to the process of preparing and storing the component and the cost of personnel involved. The rates of infusion and ABO compatibility are the same as for packed red blood cells.

KEY INTERVENTIONS: Administration of Whole Blood or Red Blood Cell Components

1. Assemble equipment: whole blood or red blood cell component; blood recipient set; blunt cannula if connecting to primary IV; alcohol prep pad; electronic infusion device, if needed; equipment for performing IV access if patient does not have an IV line.
2. Verify written order for transfusion.
3. Verify signed transfusion consent form.
4. Verify the blood component for donor/recipient ABO and Rh compatibility.
5. Confirm that blood numbers on the component match those on transfusion requisition.
6. Check expiration date of the component.
7. Make positive patient identification.
8. At bedside, set up equipment for transfusion. Clamp on blood recipient set should be closed.

9. Open one tab port of component bag and insert the spike of the blood recipient set into this port.
10. Invert and hang the component bag on IV pole.
11. Prime filter and fill drip chamber of blood recipient set half full. Prime entire surface of filter for best flow rates. Open clamp and flush all air from the line. Close clamp.
12. Attach appropriate blunt cannula to blood set if blood will be infusing by primary IV. Sodium chloride 0.9% should be used to flush any set that may contain a drug incompatible with red blood cells.
13. Scrub the injection site with alcohol and attach the blunt cannula into the injection site. Secure catheter tightly.
14. Regulate component to prescribed rate or set pump to desired rate. All transfusions must be infused within 4 hours.
15. Document vital signs 1 hour before the start of and within 1 hour after transfusion. Note "pre" and "post" vital signs. Record date, time, and signature on blood requisition that accompanies the blood component. Place in appropriate part of patient's record. Document the patient's immediate response to initial administration of red blood cells.

Procedure can be converted for institutions using multilead blood administration sets. This procedure also may be modified for the administration of plasma and single-donor platelets.

■ PLATELETS

Platelets are available in two preparations: random donor concentrates made from units of whole blood and concentrates obtained by plateletpheresis of a single donor. Platelets contain factor III, a phospholipid that enhances the conversion of prothrombin to thrombin, which forms one of the most important steps in the coagulation process (Guyton, 1986).

Platelets, Pooled

Clinical conditions that adversely affect platelet function include sepsis, diseases of the liver and kidney, drugs, cardiopulmonary bypass, and certain bone marrow disorders (AABB, 1999b). Platelet transfusions are indicated for thrombocytopenia caused by massive loss of blood, chemotherapy, and leukemia. The decision to transfuse platelets must be based on the clinical condition of the patient, the etiology of the thrombocytopenia, and the ability of the patient to produce platelets. Platelet transfusions should not be given on the basis of the number of red blood cells infused, but by the platelet count and signs and symptoms of hemorrhage. Platelets are not indicated for patients with thrombocytopenia secondary to TTP and idiopathic thrombocytopenic purpura (ITP).

Platelet concentrate prepared from whole blood contains a minimum of 5.5×10^{10} platelets in at least 75% of the units tested (Goodnough, Brecher, Kanter, & Aubuchon, 1999). Each unit contains approximately 40 to 70 mL and is expected to increase the platelet count by 5,000/L to 10,000/L in a stabilized patient. Routinely, random donor platelets (usually 6 units) are pooled and transfused. Patients are subjected to multiple allogeneic donors.

Platelet concentrates do not require crossmatching before infusion. Incompatibility between donor plasma and recipient red blood cells is usually clinically insignificant unless large numbers of platelet transfusions are required or if the patient is a small child. Then, ABO compatible platelets should be sought. D-negative patients should receive compatible platelets, if available. An acceptable rate of transfusion is 5 mL/minute.

Platelets, Leukocytes Reduced

Specific leukocyte removal filters for platelets are available for effective leukocyte removal at the bedside. They are indicated for preventing recurrent febrile nonhemolytic transfusion reactions and are not subject to quality-control testing. The manufacturer's guidelines for priming the filter must be adhered to for effective administration.

Platelets, Pheresis

Because of immune or nonimmune mechanisms, some patients become sensitized and develop platelet-specific and HLA antibodies. These patients are called *refractory:* they fail to achieve a satisfactory elevation in their platelet count. Causes of refractoriness to platelets include disseminated intravascular coagulation (DIC), drug therapies, ITP, and sepsis (AABB, 1999b). These patients are more likely to benefit from single-donor platelets. Obtained by the process of plateletpheresis, these platelets may be produced from HLA-matched donors if necessary (AABB, 1999b). Obtained from a single donor, the platelet infusion volume may be between 100 and 500 mL. One unit of pheresis platelets can be expected to raise the platelet count of the average adult by 30,000 to 60,000/μL if tested within 1 hour (American Red Cross, 1999). Reactions to platelets may include disease transmission, graft-versus-host disease, alloimmunization, febrile or allergic effects, and circulatory overload.

■ GRANULOCYTES

Granulocytes, administered infrequently, are obtained by the process of leukapheresis. Previously prescribed for gram-negative sepsis, new antibiotic regimens, new recombinant growth factors, and improved management of infections have greatly decreased the use of this component. Patients with chronic granulomatous disease or profound neutropenia may be candidates for granulocyte transfusion when they have not responded to antibiotic therapy and their recovery is expected. These transfusions only temporarily improve the patient's condition.

Granulocytes are stored at room temperature (20°C to 24°C [68°F to 75°F]) for no more than 24 hours, and preferably less than 6 hours. Granulocytes are contaminated with donor red blood cells, which must be ABO compatible with the recipient's plasma.

Patients undergoing granulocyte transfusions are acutely ill, and adverse effects are not uncommon. Febrile and pulmonary reactions may occur, and CMV transmission and TAGVHD are of particular concern. Patients who are CMV negative should not receive CMV-positive granulocytes. As a cellular product, granulocytes may be irradiated to prevent TAGVHD.

Granulocytes, usually suspended in 200 to 300 mL of anticoagulant and plasma, are administered through a set containing the standard blood filter (80 to 170 μm) over a 4-hour period for adult and pediatric patients. Granulocytes should not be administered through depth-type microaggregate and leukocyte reduction filters.

■ PLASMA

Plasma is the liquid content remaining after the red blood cells have been removed from a unit of whole blood. It contains water, electrolytes, proteins (principally albumin), globulin, and coagulation factors.

Liquid Plasma

Single-donor liquid plasma is stored at 1°C to 6°C for no more than 26 days in CPD or 40 days in CPDA-1, or 5 days after the expiration of whole blood (AABB, 1999b). Plasma plays an important role in the treatment of burns by supplying plasma proteins that are lost from the wound. Some of the clotting factor activity is lost during storage, limiting its use in patients with coagulation problems.

Under ordinary circumstances, single-donor plasma should be compatible with the recipient's red blood cells. Because it lacks anti-A and anti-B agglutinins, AB plasma may be used for all ABO groups and in emergencies when the patient's blood group is unknown.

Fresh Frozen Plasma

Fresh frozen plasma (FFP) contains all the normal components of blood plasma, including the clotting factors, in addition to 200 to 400 mg fibrinogen. It has a shelf life of 1 year when stored at a temperature of −18°C, or 7 years at −65°C. The plasma is separated from the cells and frozen within 8 hours of collection. Kept frozen until the time of transfusion, FFP is then thawed in a water bath at 37°C (98.6°F) and optimally should be administered within 6 hours, but no more than 24 hours after thawing, to minimize the loss of the most labile clotting factors, factor V and factor VIII. To provide factors V and VIII, the component should be used within the first year of storage for treatment of coagulation disorders. After 12 months, FFP may be frozen provided it is relabeled "plasma" because it should not be used for correcting coagulation disorders. If cryoprecipitate has been removed from the plasma, the remaining unit must be labeled as such.

Fresh frozen plasma is beneficial to patients with demonstrated multiple coagulation deficiencies or inherited or acquired bleeding disorders and, on occasion, to treat active bleeding due to vitamin K deficiency. Because FFP is an isotonic volume expander, patients receiving multiple units should be monitored closely to prevent fluid overload. FFP should never be used for volume expansion; this is more safely treated with crystalloid or colloid solutions that are less expensive than FFP and lack the risk of transmitting disease. Other, safer volume expanders are albumin and plasma substitutes, which do not carry the risk of viral disease transmission. FFP should not be used as a nutrient supplement.

The rate of administration may be 200 mL/hour (the approximate volume of each unit), or lower if circulatory overload is a potential complication. The pediatric rate of infusion should be approximately 1 to 2 mL/minute. Although a crossmatch is not required, the component should be compatible with the recipient's red blood cells (Table 17–4).

Solvent–Detergent-Treated Plasma

Somewhat controversially, a newly licensed plasma component is available. Referred to as PLAS + SD (pooled plasma, solvent–detergent treated) or SDP, this plasma component is prepared from ABO blood group–specific donor pooled plasma. The solvent–detergent process inactivates the viruses by stripping away their lipid coating (AABB, 1999b). It is the only human blood plasma product treated to inactivate HIV, HCV, and hepatitis B virus (HBV). It is thought that the process used to treat the plasma adds another layer of protection to the public for safety from disease transmission. Clinical indications include treating patients with clotting factor deficiencies when factor concentrates are not available. The two disadvantages of SDP are cost and a potential greater risk of nonenveloped virus transmission such as hepatitis A virus (HAV) and parvovirus because of pooling of plasmas. An alternative to SDP is nonpooled FFP, donor-retested. This method requires the donor to be retested after a minimum of 90 days after collection. Used extensively in Europe, advantages and disadvantages are still being weighed in the United States because, to date, the risk/benefit and cost/benefit ratios are not favorable compared with a single unit of FFP.

TABLE 17–4
ABO COMPATIBILITY FOR FRESH FROZEN PLASMA

Recipient	Donor
A	A or AB
B	B or AB
AB	AB
O	O, A, B, or AB

Hetastarch

Hetastarch (hydroxyethyl starch) processed for viral inactivation is an artificial colloid in 0.9% sodium chloride composed almost entirely of amylopectin. As a plasma expander, it approximates 5% human albumin, draws in interstitial water in a way similar to albumin, and is used as an adjunct therapy in the treatment of shock resulting from burns, hemorrhage, sepsis, surgery, or trauma. The risk of circulatory overload should be monitored. Its effect appears to last approximately 3 to 24 hours. It is not a substitute for blood or plasma. The product is administered IV undiluted, in doses of 20 mL/kg body weight, with a typical dose being 500 to 1000 mL/day for a 70-kg patient. Dosage depends on the amount of blood or plasma lost and resultant hemoconcentration.

Adverse reactions have been associated with the use of hetastarch, although life-threatening situations are rare. This product should not be used in patients with renal disease with oliguria or anuria that is not related to hypovolemia (Dupont Pharma, 1997).

Cryoprecipitate Antihemophilic Factor

Cryoprecipitate is a concentrate containing factor VIII (antihemophilic factor [AHF]) extracted from cold-thawed plasma. It is the cold-insoluble portion of plasma after FFP has been thawed. It contains 80 to 120 U factor VIII, 40% to 70% of plasma von Willebrand factor (vWF), and 150 to 250 mg fibrinogen in a 20- to 30-mL volume. The component is frozen at $-18°C$ for up to 12 months. It should be administered within 6 hours after thawing. Once thawed, the vWF and fibrinogen remain stable, but factor VIII is labile.

In the past, this concentrate was predominantly used to treat hemophilia A and revolutionized the treatment of this sex-linked bleeding disorder. However, it is associated with the transmission of viral agents and should be used only for specific clinical conditions such as von Willebrand's disease. These patients have a platelet dysfunction and partial deficiency in the ratio of factor VIII to vWF, and benefit from infusions of cryoprecipitate. Cryoprecipitate should not be used if viral-inactivated factor VIII concentrates are available (American Red Cross, 1999).

For factor VIII replacement, repeated transfusions are required because the half-life of factor VIII is 8 to 12 hours in the circulation. Single units may be pooled into one container and administered at a rate of 1 to 2 mL/minute. Because cryoprecipitate contains few red blood cells, it should be administered under the same guidelines as plasma when large volumes are transfused.

Plasma Derivatives and Plasma Substitutes

Normal Serum Albumin and Plasma Protein Fraction

Albumin comprises approximately 40% of the plasma protein and is prepared from pooled human plasma by cold ethanol fractionation followed by heating at 60°C for 10 hours. This process inactivates viruses including HIV, HBV, and HCV. It replaces plasma in many clinical conditions. Albumin is available in two concentrations: 5% in 250 mL saline and 25% in 50 mL saline.

Albumin 5% is isotonic, being osmotically equivalent to an approximately equal volume of citrated plasma. It may be used to provide volume and colloid in the treatment of shock and burns. Initially after a burn, large volumes of crystalloid solution are needed to correct extracellular fluid losses because of fluid leakage into the intracellular compartment. Smaller amounts of colloid are required at this time. After 24 hours, large amounts of albumin are required to maintain intravascular volume and avoid hypoproteinemia, whereas smaller amounts of crystalloid are infused.

Albumin 25% is hypertonic and depends on additional fluids, either drawn from the tissues or administered separately, for its maximal osmotic effect; 50 mL of 25% albumin is osmotically equivalent to 250 mL citrated plasma. It must be administered with caution because a rapid infusion may cause an increase in intravascular oncotic pressure, resulting in circulatory overload or interstitial dehydration particularly in severely dehydrated patients without adequate amounts of supplemental fluid. Controversy exists over its use for protein replacement in severe hypoalbuminemia. Albumin 25% needs to be infused at a slow rate of 2 to 3 mL/minute, adjusted to the patient's condition. Albumin may also be beneficial in newborns with hyperbilirubinemia because it binds with additional bilirubin and reduces the incidence of kernicterus (Petz, Swisher, Kleinman et al., 1995). Other uses that depend on patient condition include therapeutic apheresis, large-volume paracentesis, and diuresis, as well as in patients with subarachnoid hemorrhage. Inappropriate uses include for hypovolemia unless accompanied by also hypoalbuminemia; malnutrition; chronic nephrosis or hepatic failure; and peripheral edema.

Administration of 5% and 25% albumin requires strict aseptic and antiseptic handling. Once the container is entered, it must be used immediately or discarded because albumin has no preservatives. Drugs should not be added to albumin, nor should albumin be added to IV solutions. Albumin is a good culture medium and although bacterial contamination is rare, the product should be held, the lot number recorded, and the manufacturer and the FDA notified if reactions are suspected. More frequently, adverse reactions are caused by improper administration. Both products have been heat treated to eliminate transfusion-transmitted diseases.

KEY INTERVENTIONS: Administration of Albumin

1. Assemble equipment: albumin 5% or 25%; vented administration set; blunt cannula, if connecting to primary IV; alcohol prep pad; equipment for performing IV access if patient does not have an IV line.
2. Verify written order for transfusion.
3. Verify signed transfusion consent form. Some health care facilities do not require a consent for albumin.
4. Make positive patient identification.
5. Remove closure disk from the albumin bottle and prepare entry port with an alcohol pad.
6. Squeeze the drip chamber of the albumin set and insert spike of the set into the center of the stopper of the albumin bottle. Clamp of albumin set should be closed.
7. Suspend the albumin bottle from the IV pole, release the drip chamber, and flush all air in line. Close clamp.

8. Attach appropriate blunt cannula to the albumin set. Do not administer through any IV containing any medications.
9. Scrub the injection site with alcohol and attach the blunt cannula into the injection site. Secure tightly.
10. Regulate albumin to prescribed rate: 25% albumin = 2 to 3 mL/minute; 5% albumin = 5 to 10 mL/minute.
11. Document vital signs 1 hour before the start of and within 1 hour after transfusion. Note "pre" and "post" vital signs. Record date, time, and signature on blood requisition that accompanies the blood component. Place in appropriate part of patient's record. Document the patient's response. Record volume of infusion on intake record.

Procedure can be converted for institutions using multilead blood administration sets. This procedure also may be modified for the administration of plasma and single-donor platelets.

Plasma protein fraction (human) 5% is an isotonic solution of protein consisting of 83% albumin and 17% alpha- and beta-globulins. Similar to albumin, it is used for emergency treatment of shock due to burns, trauma, and surgery and for the prevention of marked hemoconcentration in trauma, surgery, and certain infections (Salama, David, Wittmann et al., 1998). Plasma protein fraction is given IV without dilution. Each 100 mL contains 5.0 g of selected plasma proteins. If plasma protein fraction is administered to patients with normal blood volume, rates should not exceed 1 mL/minute to prevent fluid overload. Rapid infusion of greater than 10 mL/minute may produce hypotension. For treatment of shock, the minimum effective dose is usually 250 to 500 mL, depending on the patient's condition and response.

Neither albumin nor plasma protein fraction has any clotting factors, and neither should be considered plasma substitutes. There is no ABO or Rh matching for albumin or plasma protein fraction.

Antihemophilic Factor (Human)

Antihemophilic factor (human) is a sterile, purified, dried concentrate prepared from the cold-insoluble fraction of pooled FFP by a variety of methods, including fractionation by physiochemical techniques to provide factor VIII concentrates, and extraction and purification from plasma using monoclonal antibodies to factor VIII. These newer techniques offer a higher activity of AHF and are less likely to transmit disease. The levels of AHF vary depending on the technique used to make the component, but are usually too low to be useful for treating von Willebrand's disease. Various processes used to inactivate viruses have yielded a safer product and greatly decreased the incidence of viral infection after transfusion.

The clinical use of AHF concentrate is the treatment of hemophilia A, a hereditary bleeding disorder characterized by deficient coagulant activity. Infusions offer a temporary replacement of the deficient clotting factor to prevent bleeding episodes or provide coagulant activity when emergency or elective surgery is performed on hemophiliac patients. The stability of the component allows patients to treat themselves at home and maintain a more normal lifestyle than in the past.

Supplied as a lyophilized powder, preparations are labeled in international units per bottle. The concentrate is provided with a sterile diluent and should be administered within 3 hours after reconstitution. Preparation cautions include gently rotating vials to dissolve the concentrate, rather than shaking the vials. Users should adhere to guidelines supplied by the manufacturer. Direct injection with a syringe is preferred as the rate of administration; 5 to 10 minutes for the entire dose is usually well tolerated, but timing should be adapted to individual patient response (Bayer Corporation, 1998). No ABO or Rh matching is required.

Factor IX Concentrate

Several preparations of factor IX concentrate are available; two products are discussed in this section. BeneFix (Genetics Institute, Cambridge, MA) is a purified protein produced by recombinant DNA technology free from the risk of transmission of human bloodborne pathogens such as HIV, hepatitis viruses, and parvovirus. The product is not derived from human blood and contains no preservatives or animal or human components (Genetics Institute, 1998). The second, Profilnine SD (Alpha Therapeutics, Los Angeles, CA), is a nonactivated factor IX preparation made from pooled human plasma and is processed by a solvent–detergent treatment to reduce risks of transmission of viral infection. The manufacturer states that no treatment method has been shown totally to eliminate all potential infective virus in preparations of coagulation factor concentrates (Alpha Therapeutics, 1995). The clinical indication for factor IX concentrate is the prevention and control of bleeding in patients with hemophilia B, also known as Christmas disease. This disorder resembles hemophilia A. The cause of the deficiency of factor IX is an abnormal gene that leads to defective synthesis of factor IX, or an acquired factor IX deficiency. To achieve therapeutic levels of factor IX, large volumes of FFP would be required. Factor IX concentrate is the only concentrated source available for patients with this deficiency. The product, in conjunction with activated factor VIII, results in the conversion of prothrombin to thrombin. Thrombin then converts fibrinogen to fibrin, with clot formation as the end result. The concentrate is provided with a sterile diluent and should be administered within 3 hours after reconstitution. Preparation cautions vary from one product to another. It is important for users to gently rotate vials to dissolve the concentrate, rather than shaking the vials, and to adhere to other guidelines supplied by the manufacturer. The number of units of factor IX is printed on each vial.

The rate of administration is determined by the patient's condition, and the concentrate may best be infused by a push method not exceeding 10 mL/minute.

Intravenous Immune Globulin

Intravenous immune globulin (IVIG) is a highly purified solution of human IgG for IV use. It is prepared by cold fractionation from large pools of plasma or solvent–detergent process, and contaminants such as bacteria and viruses are removed. Many preparations are available and need to be specifically ordered. One brand should not be substituted for another. Most contain over 90% IgG antibodies and have an approximate half-life of IgG in the circulation of patients with normal levels.

The primary use of IVIG is to supply sufficient amounts of IgG antibodies passively to patients who are unable to produce their own antibodies. Disease states most commonly requiring immune globulin are congenital agammaglobulinemia, selected autoimmune peripheral neuropathies, severe combined immunodeficiencies, and some clinical situations of acute or chronic ITP.

Intravenous immune globulin preparations (ie, the diluent and the lyophilized product) should be at room temperature before reconstitution. It is recommended that the infusion kit supplied with the product be used, or the contents transferred to a sterile vacuum bottle. IVIG contains no preservatives and should be administered promptly after the vial is reconstituted. Dosage varies depending on the patient's response, and may be repeated every 3 to 4 weeks. IVIG is not an irritant or a vesicant and may be administered by peripheral or central venous access by an electronic infusion device. The recommendation for initial infusion is 0.01 to 0.02 mL/kg/minute for the first 30 minutes (Dalakas, 1999). If tolerated, the rate may be increased until the maximum infusion rate is achieved. Most reactions are rate related, so caution is necessary. Other reactions are mild and self-limiting. The manufacturer's guidelines for the specific component being used should be followed. IVIG should not be mixed with other medications or IV solutions, and filtration is not required.

KEY INTERVENTIONS: Administration of Intravenous Immune Globulin (IVIG)

---

1. Assemble equipment: IV immune globulin; vented IV administration set; infusion pump, if needed*; alcohol prep pad; blunt cannula.
2. Allow product to warm to room temperature.
3. Verify written order for transfusion.
4. Make positive patient identification.
5. Calculate dosage based on weight of patient.
6. If product is not pooled, spike the bottle with IV tubing.

Techniques to administer:

7A. If infusion by gravity:
   a. Hang container on IV pole and half-fill drip chamber. Open clamp, flush air from the line. Close clamp.
   b. Scrub the injection site with alcohol and attach the blunt cannula into the injection site. Secure cannula tightly.
7B. If infusion with IV pump:
   a. Insert spike of IV pump set into bottle. Prime as directed.
   b. Secure catheter to injection site closest to IV site.
8. Initiate infusion of 0.01 mg/kg/minute. Rate of infusion will be 0.01 to 0.02 mL/kg/minute for 30 minutes. If well tolerated after 30 minutes, gradually increase to a maximum of 0.08 mL/kg/minute by increments of 0.02 mL/kg/minute.
9. Record date, time, and signature on requisition, which accompanies the blood component. Place in appropriate part of patient's record. Document patient's response. Record volume of infusion on intake record.

---

*Most adverse reactions are rate related.

Intravenous Cytomegalovirus Immune Globulin (Human)

Intravenous CMV immune globulin (CMV-IVIG) is a purified pooled plasma product containing a standardized amount of antibody to CMV. It is derived from plasma selected for high titers of the antibody and is primarily indicated for renal transplant recipients who are seronegative for CMV and receiving a kidney from a CMV-seropositive donor (Werner, Snydman, Freeman et al., 1999). The risk of viral transmission of this pooled product is considered low because of a solvent–detergent viral inactivation process. The maximum recommended dosage per infusion is 150 mg/kg administered by a 16-week post-transplantation schedule. After initial doses of CMV-IVIG are administered, later treatments can be administered at home after assessment of the patient's ability to understand the necessary education on safe constitution and administration.

Because the product contains no preservatives, infusion should begin within 6 hours after preparing the dose and be completed within 12 hours after entering the vial. The recommended initial rate of infusion is 15 mg/kg/hour, increasing to a maximum of 60 mg/kg/hour if the patient experiences no adverse reactions. No infusion should exceed 75 mL/hour (Massachusetts Public Health Biological Laboratories, 1996). Use of an electronic infusion pump is usually necessary to maintain a constant infusion.

Most reactions are rare and are usually rate related. When flushing, chills, muscle cramps, nausea, back pain, fever, or hypotension are observed, the infusion should be slowed or temporarily stopped. Vital signs should be monitored on a scheduled basis.

Rh Immune Globulin

Rh immune globulin (RhIG) is a concentrate of IgG anti-D derived from plasma. It is used to prevent Rh immunization of Rh-negative individuals exposed to the D antigen by transfusion or pregnancy. The Rh antibody produced by the Rh-negative mother of an Rh-positive infant is the cause of Rh hemolytic disease of the newborn. RhIG has decreased the incidence of pregnancy-associated immunization from approximately 13% to 1% to 2% (AABB, 1999b). RhIG is also given antepartum at 28 weeks and again postpartum. This prophylaxis reduces the risk of immunization to 0.1% (AABB, 1999b). Mothers are not candidates for RhIG if the fetus is Rh negative or there is evidence of immunization to D antigen not related to antepartum RhIG therapy (AABB, 1999b). Use of RhIG may be appropriate when an Rh-negative recipient receives Rh-positive red blood cells or components, such as platelets or granulocytes, which may contain sufficient cells to cause immunization. One vial contains 300 μg of anti-D, which counteracts 15 mL of transfused Rh-positive red blood cells (AABB, 1999b). In some situations, the volume of fetomaternal hemorrhage may be higher and require more than one dose of RhIG to prevent immunization (Salama et al., 1998).

Individual situations dictate prophylaxis for red blood cell transfusions because the dose required is extremely large and causes discomfort. The preparation available, RhoGAM (Ortho Diagnostics, Raritan, NJ), should be administered within 72 hours after delivery and for other outcomes of pregnancy (abortion, miscarriage) or amniocentesis, when a fetomaternal hemorrhage could occur. It is administered by intramuscular injection. An IV preparation has been approved by the FDA and is suitable for patients who are at high risk for hematoma from intramuscular injections (AABB, 1999b). Use of RhIG is not associated with viral transmission (AABB, 1999).

■ BLOOD ADMINISTRATION

Worldwide, approximately 90 million units of whole blood are collected (Stowell & Tamasulo, 1998). In the United States, nurses are mainly responsible for the administration of blood components and derivatives. It is particularly important that they be well versed in every phase of therapy. Nurses not only should be knowledgeable about the administration of components and monitoring patients during and after the transfusion, but qualified to perform ABO and Rh certification of the components. The patient's safety depends on adherence to specific rules regarding safe administration. Some institutions have delegated the administration of blood and blood components to a restricted group of specially trained personnel. Strict aseptic technique and universal precautions apply for all aspects of handling blood and blood components.

Blood Samples

Mislabeled specimens account for approximately one third of transfusion-related deaths (AuBuchon & Kruskall, 1997). The intended recipient must be identified positively at the time of blood sample collection at the patient's bedside. Labeling requirements are aimed at preventing a potentially tragic outcome in patient care, and significantly decrease errors in blood grouping (Lumadue, Boyd, & Ness, 1997). Labels must be affixed to the blood tubes and contain institutional required information related to the recipient, including the date of sample collection and identification of the person drawing the specimen. Although an institution may define the length of time samples may be used, the general ruling is that samples intended for use in crossmatch should be collected no more than 3 days before the intended transfusion. This ensures that the sample reflects the recipient's current immunologic status (AABB, 1999a).

Issue and Transfer

Patient and blood identification is of paramount importance in preventing reactions from incompatible blood. The risk of identification errors is reduced by the use of triplicate requisitions or an on-line ordering system. Such requisitions, identifying the patient and indicating the amount and kind of blood and time needed, are usually sent to the blood bank with the blood sample.

The mode of transfer of blood components to the nursing unit depends on institutional policy. It may involve a pneumatic tube system, a messenger service, hospital personnel, or the person who will administer the blood. One of the most common causes of hemolytic reaction is the accidental administration of incompatible blood from the wrong container to the patient. To prevent administration of incompatible blood, only 1 unit should be transported by a person at a time.

Patient and Blood Identification

ABO-incompatible transfusions kill as many as 24 patients each year because of misidentification of crossmatch samples or recipients, a higher fatality rate than from HIV transmission. Omission of any of the validation steps can allow for misidentification (AuBuchon & Kruskall, 1997). Absolute and positive identification of the donor blood and the patient must be made. All personnel handling the blood should be responsible for checking patient and blood identification. The nurse makes the final check and must decide whether to administer the blood or question it. ABO and Rh compatibility identification is made by comparing (1) the patient's previous ABO and Rh determination with patient's and donor's ABO and Rh on the compatibility tag; and (2) the blood identification number on the blood container with the identification number on the blood tag and the blood unit itself. Many health care facilities have incorporated computer information and validating systems to tie the patient to the blood bank for more reliable checking.

Patient identification is made by checking the name and hospital identification number on the blood tag against the admitting sheet in the patient's clinical record. The patient then must identify himself or herself by complete name. Identity should never be made by addressing the patient by name and awaiting a response. Errors can occur from faulty response of medicated patients. Patients unable to respond should be identified by the primary or attending nurse. Hospital numbers on the identification bracelet must match hospital numbers on the tag to prevent errors in cases of similar names. Any discrepancy must be investigated and corrected before the blood is administered. Blood must never be administered to a patient who has no identification bracelet.

In summary, the person performing the transfusion is responsible for the verification of information regarding the component, proper patient identification, administration, and documentation. Transfusion information is part of the patient's permanent record (Box 17–2).

Reducing Blood Exposure and High-Risk Injuries

Needleless Devices

Health care workers are at risk for acquiring bloodborne infections from blood and body fluid exposures by blood-filled hollow-bore needles commonly used for vascular access and blood sampling. Of greatest concern are HIV, HBV, and HCV (Green, Berry, Arnold, & Jagger, 1996). Shielded or self-blunting needles for vacuum tube phlebotomy, shielded butterfly needles, automatically retracting fingerstick/heelstick lancets, and plastic capillary tubes should be used for blood sampling. Catheter stylets are the primary cause of blood-related needlesticks

---

BOX 17–2 **Responsibilities of a Transfusionist**

- Verifying the presence of a written physician's order for the transfusion
- Verifying that documented informed consent has been obtained from the patient
- Verifying ABO and Rh compatibility between donor and recipient
- Performing procedures relevant to patient and blood identification
- Inspecting the unit before administration
- Explaining the procedure to the patient
- Taking pretransfusion vital signs
- Selecting and using proper technique and equipment
- Observing the patient for 5 to 15 minutes at the beginning of the transfusion
- Notifying the attending nurse to monitor the patient throughout the transfusion and for 1 hour after the transfusion
- Documenting the transfusion according to established policy
- Taking post-transfusion vital signs

(Jagger & Bently, 1997). When the nurse needs to obtain IV access for the administration of the transfusion, IV catheters designed to prevent stylet injuries should be used. When connecting the transfusion to a primary line, blunted or integrated safety devices designed to reduce injury should be used (see Chap. 11).

Barrier Protection

Barrier protection must be used when exposure to blood may occur. Minimal protection consists of gloves for handling any blood component; liquid-resistant gowns and protective eyewear may be advisable in emergency and trauma settings. In addition, electronic infusion devices used to administer blood and blood components should have tight, Luer-locking connections to prevent high-pressure rupture to avoid risk of blood exposure.

Latex-free gloves and equipment are strongly recommended, and required for any patient with a history of latex sensitivities (see Appendix I).

Handling Blood

To prevent excessive warming, blood should be administered within 30 minutes of the time it leaves the bank. If blood is not maintained at 1°C to 10°C (34°F to 50°F) while outside the control of the blood bank, it cannot be reissued. Banked blood stored at 1°C to 6°C (34°F to 43°F) will exceed 10°C (50°F) in approximately 30 minutes at room temperature; blood that cannot be administered immediately should be returned to the blood bank within this time. Blood should never be placed in the patient care unit refrigerators because they are not controlled and contain no alarms to warn of temperature fluctuation.

If warmed blood is ordered, an FDA-approved blood-warming device that maintains a controlled temperature should be used to warm the blood. Equipment should have a visible thermometer and, if possible, an audible warming alarm. Temperatures must not rise above 37°C. These warming devices should be available in emergency departments, where it is common to administer blood rapidly. Patients receiving cold blood rapidly (ie, 100 mL/minute) reportedly have increased incidences of cardiac arrest. Hot water and standard microwave ovens must never be used to warm blood.

Before the blood component is administered, the expiration date should be noted to avoid infusion of an outdated component. Sodium Chloride Injection, USP 0.9% (normal saline), may be used to initiate the infusion and flush administration sets at the completion of the transfusion of red blood cells, whole blood, platelets, or leukocytes. Hypotonic or hypertonic solutions should not be used to dilute blood. Extreme hypotonicity causes water to invade the red blood cells until they burst (ie, hemolysis). Hypertonic solutions dilute blood, resulting in reversal of this process with shrinkage of the red blood cells.

No medication or IV fluid (with the exception of 0.9% sodium chloride) should be added to blood or administered simultaneously through the same set unless it has been approved for this use by the FDA, and available records show that the addition is safe and does not adversely affect the blood component (AABB, 1999a).

Venipuncture

Peripheral veins with an adequate diameter should be used to ensure the flow of viscous components. The lower extremities are avoided in adults because thrombosis and blood pooling may occur. Areas of joint flexion should also be avoided.

The peripheral IV site should be checked frequently during the infusion for early detection of extravasation. Red blood cells and whole blood can usually be administered through an 18- or 20-gauge catheter, although smaller gauges may be used for other components. A 22- or 23-gauge catheter often is used for pediatric patients.

Blood and blood components may be administered through centrally placed catheters. Increasing numbers of peripherally inserted central catheters and midline catheters are being placed in patients receiving long-term IV therapy. In most situations, components infuse in a timely manner through 20-22-gauge or larger peripherally inserted central catheters. If a dual-lumen catheter has been placed, the larger lumen should be reserved for transfusions. It is necessary adequately to flush the catheter with normal saline at the conclusion of the transfusion. Subclavian and tunneled catheters or implanted ports are also suitable for the administration of blood and blood components. Use of an electronic infusion device is recommended.

Rate of Infusion

The rate of infusion is governed by the clinical condition of the patient and the viscosity of the component being infused. Nurses have an important role in assessing the patient's clinical condition and ensuring proper rate of administration.

Macrobore IV administrations sets should be used and changed after every unit or every 4 hours. Infusions should be set at a slow rate for the first 15 minutes to avoid infusion of a large quantity of blood in case of an immediate reaction.

Most patients can tolerate infusions of 1 unit of red blood cells over 1 to 1.5 hours. Patients in congestive heart failure or in danger of fluid overload require infusions given over a longer time, but not to exceed 4 hours. External-pressure devices and large-gauge catheters should be used when it is necessary to infuse blood rapidly. Physicians need to be readily available because certain risks are inherent to rapid volume replacement. Electronic infusion devices for the administration of blood and its components are frequently required and especially important for slow rates of infusion to elderly, pediatric, and neonatal patients.

Blood Filters

A standard (usually 170 to 260 μm), sterile, pyrogen-free blood filter designed to remove debris, including clots, is acceptable for administration of most blood components. For best flow rates, the entire surface area of the filter should be filled with the component. A single filter may be used to infuse 2 to 4 units of blood, although some institutions have a policy that a new filter be used with each component. Filters need to be added to dedicated infusion pump sets. Once the blood filter contains debris, it should be discarded. Continued use of such filters may result in bacterial contamination, a slowed rate of infusion, or hemolysis of the blood at room temperature.

Microaggregate Filters

The demonstration of microaggregates, composed of leukocytes, platelets, and fibrin, led to the manufacture of microaggregate filters in the early 1960s. Over time, the filters evolved into depth filters with high efficiency. Pore size is 20 to 40 μm, and they are used for the administration of red blood cells. The volume required for priming is significant; thus, it is recommended to flush the set with isotonic saline at completion of the transfusion (AABB, 1999b). Pediatric microaggregate filters are useful because of the small priming volume, rather than the removal of debris (AABB, 1999b).

Leukocyte Removal Filters

Red blood cell and platelet leukocyte removal filters are available to reduce a number of transfusion-associated complications: HLA alloimmunization and platelet refractoriness, transmission of cell-associated viruses (CMV), and febrile nonhemolytic reactions (Holme, Adres, Goermar, & Giordano, 1999). Clinical conditions where benefit is realized include patients with cancer and those with renal disease, who may become immunocompromised and are at risk of alloimmunization. These filters, which remove approximately 98% of leukocytes, are quick and convenient to prime and are increasingly being used for filtration at the bedside. Some institutions prefilter the transfusion before dispensing it from the blood bank, a practice that seems to be growing. The filters are efficient and effective, and provide a convenient method of removing leukocytes. Filters designed for either red blood cells or platelets may not be interchanged. These filters have no effect on the shelf life of the unit. Filters are not required for the infusion of albumin or immune globulin.

Patient Monitoring and Education

A review of the medical record is necessary to determine if any premedication is required before the transfusion. The patient should be informed of the steps involved in having a transfusion to lessen any anxiety. The length of time of the transfusion, expected outcome, and symptoms that could reflect a reaction should be included as patient teaching.

After initiation, the nurse–transfusionist should observe the patient for the initial 5 to 15 minutes of the infusion. Many of the fatal incompatible transfusion reactions produce symptoms early in the course of the infusion. Primary nurses also share a responsibility for safe transfusion administration. They must be familiar with the various transfusion reactions, be able to recognize adverse reactions, and know what procedures to follow.

If venous spasm occurs from infusion of cold blood, a warm pack applied to the vein through which the blood is being infused relieves the spasm and increases the rate of flow.

 SAFE PRACTICE ALERT

Patient transfusion history

- Previous reactions may trigger need to premedicate the patient.
- Goal: lessen potential reactions, relieve anxiety

Latex sensitivity

- Use only latex-free equipment.
- Goal: eliminate any progression of reaction

Signed transfusion consent form from patient

- All patients must be informed of administration of transfusion. The patient or parent must sign forms, which a physician must witness. Some institutions grant approval to witness to nurse practitioners.
- Goal: Patient awareness and participation in course of therapy

Documenting the Transfusion

All data relevant to the transfusion should be recorded in the patient's clinical and transfusion records. The time the transfusion was complete, the volume of fluid infused, and the condition of the patient should be noted. Observation of the patient for 1 hour after the transfusion is recommended. Post-transfusion monitoring of vital signs and laboratory values ensures that the clinical goal was achieved. Latex sensitivity or any other comments about the transfusion should be noted.

Disposal of Equipment

Sharps must be disposed of in specially designed, puncture-resistant, leak-proof containers located near the area of use. All transfusion-related equipment should be placed in biohazard containers. Administration sets used to infuse blood components should be discarded within 24 hours after use. Bacterial growth may occur on the trapped proteins and debris contained in the set. Institutional guidelines for observing universal precautions should be followed.

■ TRANSFUSION REACTIONS

Significant improvements in collection and storage methods, together with growing knowledge in the field of immunohematology, have increased the safety of transfusion therapy. An inherent risk still exists, however, with every unit of transfused blood. Both the transfusionist and primary nurse should be aware of this and alert for symptoms of untoward events. ABO and Rh compatibility testing cannot eliminate all reactions to administered blood.

Whenever a transfusion reaction is suspected, the transfusion should be terminated and the IV line kept open for possible therapy. Vital signs should be taken, the physician should be notified, and a 10-mL blood sample should be sent to the blood bank with the blood container and a completed transfusion reaction report (except in the case of a urticarial reaction). When a hemolytic reaction is suspected, urine also should be sent to the laboratory for urinalysis. Urinary output should be monitored and all urine saved and observed for hemoglobin or bilirubin. Complete documentation of the reaction is important.

KEY INTERVENTIONS: Suspected Transfusion Reactions

Any sign or symptom experienced by the patient receiving a transfusion should be considered serious and the transfusion should be discontinued. The following signs and symptoms are reportable: fever, chills, hives, rash, nausea, anxiety, dyspnea, lumbar pain, chest pain, pain along the vein, generalized bleeding or oozing, pink/red urine, oliguria/anuria, and hypotension. Urticarial reactions usually are not worked up, but should be reported to the Transfusion Service.

1. Assemble equipment: blood-drawing equipment; 250 mL 0.9% sodium chloride; IV administration set; plastic bag with tie; suspected transfusion reaction form, completed and signed by physician; any residual blood, attached set, and filter.
2. At initial sign of suspected transfusion reaction, STOP the transfusion.
3. Immediately set up a 250-mL infusion of 0.9% sodium chloride. Flush all air in the set.
4. Disconnect the blood recipient set from the hub of the catheter and replace with the set primed with sodium chloride. If using Y-tubing blood set, DO NOT OPEN lead infusing sodium chloride because this causes more blood to be infused.

5. Begin infusion of sodium chloride solution.
6. Draw blood samples as directed by institutional protocol. Samples are necessary to determine the cause of the reaction.
7. Confirm that blood component set is tightly clamped and distal end is covered to prevent leakage of blood.
8. Place component bag with any residual fluid, attached administration set, and filter in a plastic bag.
9. Secure bag and send to Transfusion Service with suspected transfusion reaction report. Report must be on the outside of plastic bag.
10. Send a urine sample for hemoglobinuria.
11. Continue to monitor patient closely for any further signs and symptoms of reaction.
12. Document any signs and symptoms observed and the time of recognition. Note type of component, amount infused, amount remaining, and nursing interventions performed. Record that remaining component and suspected transfusion reaction report were sent to Transfusion Service.

Transfusion reactions may be divided into two main classes: immediate and delayed. Both may be further divided into immunologic and nonimmunologic.

Immediate Effects

Immediate **adverse effects** of transfusion usually occur during or within 1 to 2 hours after the completion of an infusion. Therefore, the patient must be closely monitored during and after the transfusion to assess and identify signs and symptoms of impending reactions. Most immediate adverse effects are preventable and caused by improper administration, failure to comply with standards, or lack of knowledge of the procedure or impact of the therapy. Thoroughly following written procedures and complying with policy are crucial for safe transfusion therapy.

Immunologic

Antigen–antibody reactions from red blood cells, leukocytes, or plasma proteins are responsible for adverse effects in the recipient. They are usually produced by the body's response to foreign proteins.

ACUTE HEMOLYTIC REACTION

Acute hemolytic transfusion reactions occur when an antigen–antibody reaction occurs in the recipient as the result of an incompatibility between the recipient's antibodies and the donor's red blood cells. Incompatibilities in the ABO blood group system are responsible for most deaths from acute hemolytic transfusion reactions.

The interaction of the isoagglutinins and ABO-incompatible red blood cells activates the complement, kinin, and coagulation systems. The entire complement system is activated in the ABO mismatch, causing intravascular hemolysis. If the amount of free hemoglobin released from the destruction of red blood cells exceeds the quantity that can combine with haptoglobin in the plasma, the excess hemoglobin filters through the glomerular membrane into the kidney tubules, and hemoglobinuria occurs.

The kinin system is activated by the antigen–antibody complex and produces bradykinin, which increases capillary permeability, dilates arterioles, and decreases systemic blood pressure. The coagulation system activates the intrinsic clotting cascade, causing small clots in the circulation, and may trigger DIC, which in turn can cause formation of thrombi in the microvasculature. Intravascular hemolytic reactions are often fatal. Investigation of fatal hemolytic transfusion reactions shows that the most common causes are clerical or other errors in the identification of the recipient sample sent to the blood blank, of the blood unit, or of the recipient. Hemolytic transfusion reactions may be accompanied by chills, fever, facial flushing, a burning sensation along the vein in which the blood is being infused, lumbar or flank pain, chest pain, frequent oozing of blood at the injection site and surgical areas, or shock. When reactions occur, the transfusion must be stopped at once and the vein kept open with 0.9% sodium chloride. When Y-tubing is used, a new setup (container of fluid and a new administration set) should be connected directly to the catheter. The flow to the normal saline hanging with the Y-tubing should not be opened; to do so could result in the patient receiving additional incompatible blood cells contained in the Y-tubing.

Vigorous treatment of hypotension and promotion of adequate renal blood flow are imperative. Therapy may consist of administration of volume, diuretics, and volume expanders to promote diuresis and to minimize renal damage. Urinary flow rates in adults should be maintained at or over 100 mL/hour for at least 18 to 24 hours (AABB, 1999b). Vasopressors, such as dopamine in low doses, dilate the renal vasculature while increasing cardiac output. Their use requires careful monitoring of the patient's urinary flow, cardiac output, and blood pressure. A diuretic agent such as furosemide is recommended to be given concurrently with adequate IV fluid replacement. The drug improves renal blood flow, thus minimizing the possibility of renal tubular ischemia and renal failure. Mannitol is infrequently used because, if ineffective, it may cause hypervolemia and pulmonary edema. The use of heparin therapy for the resulting DIC remains controversial and is addressed after evaluation of all consequences of the acute hemolytic reaction. Prevention is the hallmark of therapy for this severe reaction.

FEBRILE NONHEMOLYTIC REACTION

Febrile nonhemolytic reactions are usually the result of transfusion of cellular components in the absence of hemolysis, whereby anti-leukocyte antibodies in the recipient are directed against the donor's white blood cells. Even though some leukocytes break down rapidly during storage, the membrane fragments are still capable of sensitizing patients in the same manner as intact leukocytes. Patients who have been sensitized by numerous transfusions or multiple pregnancies are more likely to have a febrile nonhemolytic reaction, defined as a rise in temperature of 1°C and usually occurring within 1 to 6 hours after initiation of the transfusion. Febrile reactions, which occur in 0.5% to 1.5% of transfusions, may be accompanied by facial flushing, palpitations, cough, tightness in the chest, increased pulse rate, or chills (AABB, 1999b). As the name implies, no red blood cell hemolysis occurs. Antipyretics are used for treatment. Antihistamines are not indicated because most febrile nonhemolytic reactions are not caused by release of histamine (AABB, 1999b). Documentation of the reaction is important for possible prevention of future adverse effects. This reaction can be prevented by use of leukocyte-reduced components, which usually are produced by filtration techniques. Deglycerolized red blood cells and washed red blood cells are also relatively depleted of leukocytes. All febrile responses should be clinically monitored because other reactions may occur.

ANAPHYLACTIC REACTIONS

Fortunately, anaphylactic reactions are rare, estimated to occur in 1 of 170,000 transfusions. They may occur in patients who are IgA deficient and who have developed anti-IgA antibodies. The two classic signs that an anaphylactic reaction is imminent are symptoms after only a few milliliters of blood or plasma have been infused, in the absence of fever. Bronchospasm, respiratory distress, abdominal cramps, vascular instability, shock, and perhaps loss of consciousness characterize the reaction. This medical emergency requires immediate resuscitation of the patient along with administration of epinephrine and steroids. Close observation during the first 15 minutes of the transfusion and continuing surveillance throughout and for 1 hour after completion of the transfusion are important to monitor for signs of this reaction.

Prevention includes the use of autologous transfusions or obtaining units from donors who lack IgA. Reducing the plasma content of red blood cell and platelet transfusions may also be effective in reducing the severity of this reaction.

URTICARIA

These reactions are relatively uncommon, occurring in 1% to 3% of transfusions, and are based on a hypersensitivity response, probably to protein in donor plasma. Urticarial reactions are usually mild and characterized by local erythema, hives, and itching. Occasionally, fever may be present. The transfusion usually is interrupted and may be continued after the patient has responded to antihistamine therapy. If the patient has extensive urticaria, total-body rash, or fever, the transfusion may have to be discontinued. In these situations, washed or frozen, thawed, and deglycerolized red blood cells may be indicated for future therapy.

TRANSFUSION-RELATED ACUTE LUNG INJURY

Although transfusion-related acute lung injury occurs infrequently, it can provoke severe symptoms. The usual etiology is a reaction between donor high-titer anti-leukocyte antibodies and recipient leukocytes. The reaction can result in leukoagglutination. The leukoagglutinins may become trapped in the pulmonary microvasculature. The reaction causes severe respiratory distress unassociated with circulatory overload and without evidence of cardiac failure. The severity of the respiratory distress is usually disproportional to the volume of blood infused (AABB, 1999b). Chest radiography reveals bilateral pulmonary infiltrates consistent with pulmonary edema but without other evidence of left heart failure. Clinical signs and symptoms other than respiratory distress include chills, fever, cyanosis, and hypotension. Treatment begins by discontinuing the transfusion and providing respiratory support measures. Once a donor has been implicated in such a reaction, that person's plasma should not be used for any plasma-containing components.

Nonimmunologic

Immediate nonimmunologic adverse effects are caused by external factors in the administration of blood: bacterial infection of the patient, contamination of the donor blood, improper handling of blood, and administration of a hypertonic fluid with the transfusion. An antigen–antibody reaction is absent.

CIRCULATORY OVERLOAD

Circulatory overload may occur when blood or its components are infused at a rate exceeding the recipient's cardiac output. The consequence is hypervolemia. Patients more prone to this adverse effect are the young and elderly and those with cardiac or renal disease. Symptoms include a pounding headache, dyspnea, constriction of the chest, coughing, and cyanosis. The transfusion must be stopped and the patient placed in a sitting position. Rapid-acting diuretics and oxygen usually relieve the symptoms. If the condition is severe, a therapeutic phlebotomy may be indicated. Prevention consists of frequent monitoring of those susceptible to congestive heart failure and the administration of concentrated components slowly. This adverse effect is preventable.

AIR EMBOLISM

The use of plastic bags has dramatically reduced this complication of transfusion therapy, which may result from faulty technique in changing equipment or plastic bags, careless use of Y-type administration sets, or air infused from one of the containers when fluid and blood are being pumped together. If air does enter the patient, acute cardiopulmonary insufficiency occurs. Symptoms are the same as those for circulatory collapse: cyanosis, dyspnea, shock, and occasionally cardiac arrest. The infusion should be stopped immediately and the patient turned on the left side, with the head down. This position traps air in the right atrium, preventing it from entering the pulmonary artery; the pulmonic valve is kept clear until the air can escape gradually. It may be necessary for the physician to aspirate the air with a transthoracic needle. This adverse effect is preventable.

CITRATE TOXICITY

Patients at risk for development of citrate toxicity or a calcium deficit are those who receive infusions of plasma, whole blood, or platelets at rates exceeding 100 mL/minute, or lower rates in patients who have liver disease. The liver, unable to keep up with the rapid administration, cannot metabolize the citrate, which chelates calcium, reducing the ionized calcium concentration. Hypocalcemia may induce cardiac arrhythmia. This adverse effect occurs infrequently but may be encountered in emergency departments and operating rooms when large amounts of blood (1 U every 5 minutes) and components have been administered. Symptoms of hypocalcemia include tingling of the fingers, muscular cramps, convulsions, hypotension, and cardiac arrest. Treatment consists of slowing the rate of infusion and the administration of calcium chloride or calcium gluconate solution. However, the calcium must never be added to any IV administration set infusing blood.

HYPOTHERMIA

Hypothermia occurs when large volumes of cold blood are infused rapidly. Rapid infusions may cause chills, hypothermia, peripheral vasoconstriction, ventricular arrhythmias, and cardiac arrest. Clinically, it is important to be certain that central catheters, if placed, are not positioned in the right atrium, a situation that can stimulate arrhythmias if rapid infusions are given. In many situations, warming blood to 37°C with automatic blood warmers during rapid, massive replacement prevents hypothermia. However, time does not always permit the setting up of equipment.

BACTERIAL CONTAMINATION

Bacterial contamination of blood may occur at the time of donation or in preparing the component for infusion. In addition to skin contaminants, cold-resistant gram-negative bacteria may contribute to this untoward event. Organisms such as *Pseudomonas* species, *Citrobacter freundii*, and *Escherichia coli* are potential causes. These organisms, capable of proliferating at refrigerator temperatures, release an endotoxin that initiates this rare, potentially fatal reaction. Inspecting the unit before administration can prevent this complication. Observation of any discoloration of the blood or plasma or obvious clots should be reported. Clinical manifestations of a septic reaction include high fever, flushing of the skin, "warm" shock, hemoglobinuria, renal failure, and DIC. These signs and symptoms are similar to those of an acute hemolytic reaction, so diagnosis must be made quickly. The transfusion should be discontinued; immediate therapy, including aggressive management of shock and administration of steroids and antibiotics, is required. Cultures obtained of the patient's blood, the suspected component, and all IV solutions determine whether the blood or an IV-related infection caused the bacteremia.

Many of the reactions discussed thus far are preventable. It is thought that the incidence of bedside transfusion errors (ie, those happening when blood products have left the blood bank) is underestimated because many are medically treated and not reported as transfusion reactions. Quality improvement and monitoring measures can assist in avoiding other errors, as may computerized methods of verifying necessary data.

Delayed Effects

These complications occur days, months, or years after the transfusion and usually are the result of alloimmunization or transmitted disease.

Immunologic

DELAYED HEMOLYTIC REACTION

Delayed hemolytic reactions, caused by an immune antibody created in response to a foreign antigen, are classified as primary and secondary. The primary or initial reaction usually is mild and may occur a week or more after the transfusion. Known as *primary alloimmunization*, it rarely produces symptoms and may be clinically insignificant. The degree of hemolysis depends on the quantity of antibody produced. The secondary reaction occurs in a patient previously immunized by transfusion or pregnancy. These patients have formed a red blood cell alloantibody, but the level of this alloantibody has become so low that it is serologically undetectable. On a later occasion, when donor red blood cells possessing the corresponding antigen are infused, they provoke a rapid increase in the specific antibody. The incompatible red blood cells survive until sufficient antibody is present to initiate a rejection response. The reaction is called a *secondary* or *anamnestic* ("memory") response and is caused by re-exposure to the same antigen. These reactions are rarely caused by ABO incompatibility. Manifestations of a delayed hemolytic reaction include fever, mild jaundice, and an unexplained drop in hemoglobin. Treatment is usually not necessary. These coated cells are removed from the body by the reticuloendothelial system (extravascular hemolysis). A direct antiglobulin test may detect the antibody, and future donor units are selected that lack the corresponding antigen to the antibody formed.

TRANSFUSION-ASSOCIATED GRAFT-VERSUS-HOST DISEASE

Transfusion-associated graft-versus-host disease is a complex, rare, and often fatal immunologic reaction. The usual cause appears to be the transfer of immunocompetent T lymphocytes in blood components to a severely immunocompromised patient. It may also occur from transfusion from first-degree family members (American Red Cross, 1999). The donor lymphocytes engraft and multiply in a severely immunodeficient recipient. These engrafted cells react against the foreign tissue of the host recipient, causing bleeding and infectious complications (AABB, 1999b).

The onset of TAGVHD is usually 4 to 30 days after transfusion and begins with a high fever. Generalized erythroderma, profuse diarrhea, hepatocellular damage, and pancytopenia follow. TAGVHD is associated with a mortality rate of at least 90% of affected patients (Mori, Matsushita, Ozaki et al., 1995). Bone marrow suppression and infection are the causes of death.

Two suggested methods to prevent or reduce the incidence of TAGVHD are irradiation of components and administration of blood that has been stored for more than 7 days (Yasuura & Matsuura, 1998). Pretransfusion inactivation of lymphocytes by irradiating cellular components reduces the risk of TAGVHD in the following situations: (1) fetuses receiving intrauterine transfusions; (2) selected immunoincompetent or immunocompromised recipients; (3) recipients of donor units known to be from a blood relative; and (4) recipients who have undergone bone marrow or peripheral blood progenitor cell transplantation (American Red Cross, 1999).

Nonimmunologic

HEPATITIS

Hepatitis often presents clinically with self-limiting fever, fatigue, and jaundice, but may lead to progressive inflammation of the liver, resulting in cirrhosis or hepatic cancer. The clinical outcome of hepatitis, manifested by elevated liver enzyme test results, anorexia, fatigue, malaise, dark urine, fever, and jaundice, usually resolve within 4 to 6 weeks. Some patients demonstrate few symptoms, whereas others may become extremely ill and die of fulminant hepatic failure. Post-transfusion hepatitis (PTH) has been recognized as a complication of receiving blood since the 1940s, and potentially can be caused by HAV, HBV, HCV, hepatitis D virus (HDV), and hepatitis E virus (HEV). HAV and HEV are exceedingly rare causes of PTH, largely because the virus is present only during the acute phase of the disease and there is no carrier state. HDV needs HBV to replicate and must be transmitted at the same time as HBV into a person already infected with HBV. HDV usually is transmitted through IV drug use or sexual contact with an infected person and, as a superinfection, may worsen the course of chronic hepatitis B infection. The viruses predominantly responsible for PTH are HBV and HCV, although the risk of these infections from transfusions has been substantially reduced. The incidence of PTH has decreased dramatically since 1995 because of the screening of donors and the use of more sensitive laboratory tests to identify at-risk donors. The national rate of PTH in the 1960s was approximately 33%, dropped to 10% to 12% in the 1980s, and at present is in the range of 1 in 30,000 to 150,000 units (Goodnough et al., 1999).

Hepatitis B Virus. Hepatitis B virus accounts for only a small proportion of cases of PTH. The primary reasons for this low incidence are screening of donors for behaviors that expose them to viral hepatitis and the testing of all donations for HBsAg and anti-HBc. The prevalence of the HBsAg carrier state in blood donations in the United States is approximately 0.02% to 0.04%. The frequency of PTH attributed to HBV is 1 in 30,000 to 250,000 units transfused (Goodnough et al., 1999).

The average incubation period for HBV infection is 90 days, with a range of 30 to 180 days. Although most patients clear the virus, a proportion remains chronically infected although asymptomatic. Becoming an HBsAg carrier is age dependent, with 5% of adults infected with HBV becoming carriers, compared with more than 90% of infants infected becoming carriers (AABB, 1999b). Hepatitis B can be transmitted directly by percutaneous needle inoculation or by transfusion of infected blood. It can be transmitted indirectly by percutaneous introduction of infectious serum, saliva, or semen through minute cuts or abrasions on the skin or mucosal surfaces. Health care workers are strongly advised to be immunized with hepatitis B vaccine to reduce the risk of acquiring HBV infection.

Hepatitis C Virus. Hepatitis C virus is the major etiologic agent of PTH. Approximately 50% of HCV carriers have evidence of chronic liver disease. Screening blood donors for antibody to HCV has been in place since 1998. An enzyme immunoassay (EIA) for antibodies to HCV is used to identify blood donors who have been exposed. Donors found to be repeatedly active by EIA are deferred. A supplemental test, the recombinant immunoblot assay, may be used to determine which reactive EIA results are true positives because the EIA screening test is extremely sensitive but not completely specific for HCV. Before the test for antibody to HCV was available, surrogate tests (serum ALT and anti-HBc) were used to eliminate donors whose blood might transmit HCV.

The modes of transmission of HCV appear to be similar to those of HBV; however, the route of HCV infection in many infected people is unknown. The incubation period for HCV is approximately 50 days, with a range of 15 to 180 days. The initial and acute illness is usually milder than in HBV, and is often subclinical. Approximately 75% of patients are anicteric. Liver abnormalities persisting after 1 year indicate chronic hepatitis, and progression to cirrhosis and liver failure occurs in 20% of patients. Chronic HCV infection also predisposes patients to hepatocellular carcinoma.

HUMAN IMMUNODEFICIENCY VIRUS

Human immunodeficiency virus is a retrovirus that infects and kills CD4-positive lymphocytes (helper T cells), thereby disabling the cellular immune system. It produces a severe cellular immunodeficiency and renders the infected person vulnerable to opportunistic infections. HIV-2 (type 2) is similar to HIV-1 (type 1), but the incubation period appears to be longer and transmission is less efficient than for HIV-1 (AABB, 1999b). HIV-1 and HIV-2 can both be transmitted by transfusions. Their existence has necessitated aggressive work to safeguard the blood supply. The first test for HIV antibody was developed and testing initiated in 1985. Since then, very few cases of HIV transmission by transfusion have occurred. The post-transfusion HIV risk in the United States ranges from approximately 1 in 200,000 to 2,000,000 units transfused (Goodnough et al., 1999). Donated blood is tested for antibody to the virus (anti-HIV-1 and anti-HIV-2) using an EIA (Sullivan, Guido, Metler et al., 1998). The confirmatory test for repeatedly reactive anti-HIV EIA tests is the Western blot. Of concern are donors who may have been recently infected with HIV and are able to transmit the disease, but have not yet seroconverted. Since 1996, donated blood has also been tested for HIV-associated antigen p24, which appears sooner than HIV antibodies. This test reduces the phase known as the *infectious window* period. Today, sensitive screening tests have closed the seronegative interval from 45 days in 1992 to 6 days in 1996. These techniques have virtually eliminated transmission of enveloped viruses, such as HBV, HCV, and HIV, by plasma derivatives. Techniques also have been developed to inactivate viruses in plasma derivatives, such as antihemophilic factor, albumin, IVIG, and others.

HUMAN T-CELL LYMPHOTROPIC VIRUSES

Both HTLV-I and HTLV-II can be spread through viable lymphocytes in blood. Plasma, which contains no lymphocytes, is not infective. The lymphocytes that transmit the virus are prone to degradation, so that red cell components stored for 10 days or more are less likely to transmit the virus than are fresher units. Testing for HTLV-I has been ongoing since 1988, and seropositive people have been removed from donor pools. Testing for antibodies to HTLV-II began in 1997. The frequency of transfusion-transmitted HTLV is quite low in the United States, with estimates ranging from 1 in 250,000 to 2,000,00 units transfused (Goodnough et al., 1999). The Western blot is confirmatory for a positive EIA screening test result for anti-HTLV-I and II.

Human T-cell lymphotropic virus type I is associated with adult T-cell lymphoma–leukemia and a neurologic disorder called HTLV-associated myelopathy or tropical spastic paraparesis (AABB, 1999). Transmission is by breast milk, sexual contact, and exposure to blood. The prevalence of this disease varies widely geographically, and is most common in Japan and other Pacific regions, Central and South America, and parts of Africa.

The only disease known to be associated with the retrovirus HTLV-II is HTLV-associated myelopathy. The virus is prevalent in some native American populations and among IV drug users in the United States (AABB, 1999b).

SYPHILIS

Serologic testing for syphilis is required on all donations, although refrigerated storage of red blood cell components has nearly eradicated the transmission of syphilis because temperatures of 4°C (39°F) have a spirocheticidal effect. Most likely, only components stored at room temperature or those administered within 72 hours after donation could transmit the disease. Positive STS results also may denote immunologic abnormalities unrelated to syphilis or inadequately treated syphilis, a fact that may be more helpful to the donor than the recipient (AABB, 1999b). There have been no reports of transfusion-transmitted syphilis in several decades.

CYTOMEGALOVIRUS INFECTION

Recognized to be present in blood and transmitted by transfusion, CMV poses little problem to most immunologically intact recipients. CMV is in the herpes virus family, and white cells are the major reservoir of CMV transmitted by blood (Larsson, Soderberg-Naucler, Wang et al., 1998). Patients most at risk for serious consequences of the infection are those who have not been previously exposed and are immunoincompetent. These include low–birth-weight neonates, patients with malignancies who are immunosuppressed as a result of therapy for their disease, patients with acquired immunodeficiency syndrome, and recipients of bone marrow and solid organ transplants. Many of these patients have depressed cell-mediated immunity and are at risk for development of systemic CMV infections, including pneumonia, hepatitis, and retinitis. To reduce CMV infection in specific patient populations, use of blood from CMV-seronegative donors or those with depleted leukocytes is effective.

MALARIA

Nearly eradicated in the United States and Canada, malaria is still prevalent in other parts of the world. The number of cases of transfusion-transmitted malaria reported in the United States is 0.25 cases per million units of blood collected (Petz et al., 1995). Monitoring for this complication of transfusion is ongoing because of increased travel, immigration, and the continued presence of malaria in many areas of the world. No laboratory test is used widely to screen blood donors for malaria, and diagnosis still is made routinely by identifying the organism on a blood smear. The patient may have a high fever, which reflects the lysis of infected red blood cells as they release the parasites into the bloodstream (Petz et al., 1995). Blood transfusion can transmit malaria parasites. Prevention is accomplished by excluding donors from regions of the world where malaria is prevalent.

Prospective donors who have actually had malaria are deferred for 3 years after becoming asymptomatic (AABB, 1999a). Travelers who have visited an endemic area are deferred for 1 year. Immigrants, refugees, and citizens from endemic countries may be accepted as blood donors 3 years after departure from the area if they are asymptomatic (Petz et al., 1995). Donors with a history of babesiosis or Chagas disease are deferred permanently.

References and Selected Readings

Asterisks indicate references cited in text.

*Alpha Therapeutics Corporation. (1995). Profilnine SD. Los Angeles: Author.

*American Association of Blood Banks. (1999). *Standards for blood banks and transfusion services* (19th ed., pp. 18, 32, 58, 62, 68). Arlington, VA: Author.

*American Association of Blood Banks. (1999). *Technical manual* (13th ed., pp. 91, 168, 171, 175–177, 181, 378, 455, 457–458, 487, 505, 521, 583, 585–588, 596, 603, 611, 616–177, 624). Arlington, VA: Author.

*American Red Cross, Council of Community Blood Centers, American Association of Blood Banks. (1999). *Circular of information for the use of human blood and blood components* (pp. 2, 6, 14, 21, 26). Washington DC: American Red Cross.

*AuBuchon, J.P. & Kruskall, M.S. (1997). Transfusion safety: Realigning efforts with risks. *Transfusion, 37,* 1211–1213.

*Bayer Corporation. (1998). Antihemophilic Factor (Human). Elkhart, IN: Author.

*Dalakas, M.C. (1999). *Current concepts in autoimmune peripheral neuropathies: Pathogenesis and treatment.* Lincoln, NE: University of Nebraska Medical Center.

*Dupont Pharma. (1997) Hetastarch. Wilmington, DE: Author.

*Genetics Institute, Inc. (1998) Benefix, Coagulation Factor IX (Recombinant). Cambridge, MA: Author.

*Goodnough, L.T., Brecher, M.E., Kanter, M.H., & Aubuchon, J.P. (1999). Medical progress. *Transfusion Medicine, 340,* 438–445.

*Gould, S.A. & Forbes, J.M. (1995). Controversies in transfusion medicine: Indications for autologous and allogeneic transfusion should be the same. *Pro Transfusion, 35,* 446.

*Green, E.S., Berry, A.J., Arnold, W.P., & Jagger, J. (1996). Percutaneous injuries in anesthesia personnel. *Anesthesia and Analgesia, 83,* 273.

*Guyton, A.C. (1986). *Textbook of medical physiology* (7th ed., pp. 76–77). Philadelphia: W.B. Saunders.

*Heaton, W.A.L. (1994). Changing patterns of blood use. *Transfusion, 34,* 365.

*Holme, S., Adres, M., Goermar, N., & Giordano, G.F. (1999). Improved removal of white cells with minimal platelet loss by filtration of apheresis platelets during collection. *Transfusion, 39,* 74.

*Jagger, J. & Bently, M.B. (1997) Injuries from vascular access devices: high risk and preventable. *Journal of Intravenous Nursing, 20,* S33–S37.

*Larsson, S., Soderberg-Naucler, C., Wang, F.-Z., et al. (1998). Cytomegalovirus DNA can be detected in peripheral blood mononuclear cells from all seropositive and most seronegative healthy blood donors over time. *Transfusion, 38,* 272.

Liu, W., Smythe, J.S., Scott, M.L., et al. (1999). Site-directed mutagenesis of the human D antigen: Definition of D epitopes on the sixth external domain of the D protein expressed on K562 cells. *Transfusion, 39,* 17.

*Lumadue, J.A., Boyd, J.S., & Ness, P.M. (1997). Adherence to a strict specimen-labeling policy decreases the incidence of erroneous blood grouping of blood bank specimens. *Transfusion, 37,* 1169.

*Maffei, L.M. & Thurer, R.L. (1988). *Autologous blood transfusion: Current issues.* Arlington, VA: American Association of Blood Banks.

*Massachusetts Public Health Biological Laboratories. (1996). Cytomegalovirus immune globulin intravenous (human). Boston: Author.

*Mori, S., Matsushita, K., Ozaki, K., et al. (1995). Spontaneous resolution of transfusion-associated graft-versus-host disease. *Transfusion, 35,* 431–435.

*Petz, L.D., Swisher, S.N., Kleinman, S., et al. (1995). *Clinical practice of transfusion medicine* (3rd ed., pp. 625, 670, 896–897). New York: Churchill Livingstone.

Rottman, G. & Ness, P.M. (1998). Acute normovolemic hemodilution is a legitimate alternative to allogeneic blood transfusion. *Transfusion, 38,* 477–479.

*Salama, A., David, M., Wittmann, G., et al. (1998). Use of the gel agglutination technique for determination of fetomaternal hemorrhage. *Transfusion, 38,* 177.

*Stowell, C.P. & Tamasulo, P. (1998). *Red blood cell substitutes: Basic principles and clinical applications.* New York: Marcel Dekker.

*Stroup, M. & Tracey, M. (1982). *Blood group antigens and antibodies* (pp. 29–30). Raritan, NJ: Ortho Diagnostics System.

*Sullivan, M.T., Guido, E.A., Metler, R.P., et al. (1998). Identification and characterization of an HIV-2 antibody-positive blood donor in the United States. *Transfusion, 38,* 189.

*Werner, B.G., Snydman, D.R., Freeman, R., et al. (1993). Cytomegalovirus immune globulin for the prevention of primary CMV disease in renal transplant patients: Analysis of usage under treatment IND status. *Transplantation Proceedings, 25,* 1441–1443.

*Yasuura, K. & Matsuura, A. (1998). High risk of transfusion-associated graft-versus-host disease with nonirradiated allogeneic blood transfusion in cardiac surgery. *Transfusion, 38,* 1117–1118.

Review Questions

Note: Questions below may have more than one right answer.

1. The antigen in the ABO system that denotes a person's blood group is located:
   A. On the red blood cell
   B. In the plasma
   C. In the serum
   D. On body tissue

2. Which of the following may stimulate a reaction?
   I. Antigen A combining with anti-A antibody
   II. Antigen AB combining with anti-AB antibody
   III. Antigen B combining with anti-A antibody
   IV. Antigen D combining with anti-D antibody
      A. I and II
      B. III and IV
      C. I, II, and IV
      D. All of the above

3. Methods to reduce febrile nonhemolytic transfusion reactions include:
   A. Washed red cells with a standard 80- to 170-μm filter
   B. Packed red cells with a leukocyte filter
   C. Packed red cells with a standard 80- to 170-μm filter
   D. All of the above

4. The most important intervention for patients with IVIG-associated nonallergic reactions is:
   A. Slow the infusion rate
   B. Discontinue the infusion
   C. Continue rate because reaction will resolve
   D. Stop the infusion for 4 to 8 hours; then resume therapy

5. A patient, group O, may receive red blood cells from a donor who is:
   A. Group A only
   B. Group O only
   C. Group A or O
   D. Any group

6. A patient, group AB, may receive plasma from a donor who is:
   A. Group A, AB, or O
   B. Group AB or O
   C. Group AB only
   D. Any group

7. Intravascular hemolytic reactions are potentially caused by:
   A. ABO incompatibility
   B. Rh incompatibility
   C. ABO and Rh incompatibility
   D. None of the above

8. The primary cause of post-transfusion hepatitis is:
   A. HAV and HBV
   B. HBV and HCV
   C. HAV and HDV
   D. HBV only

9. A patient experiences the following signs and symptoms 1 hour after a unit of packed red blood cells has been infused: chills, increased pulse rate, fever, and facial flushing. Which of the following adverse reactions is suspected?
   A. Citrate toxicity
   B. Congestive heart failure
   C. Febrile nonhemolytic reaction
   D. Anaphylaxis

10. The cause of most reactions to the administration of IVIG is:
    A. Crystallization of fluid
    B. Too rapid a rate
    C. Pain along infusion site
    D. Hypersensitivity reaction

Drug Administration

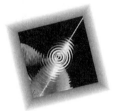

K E Y   T E R M S

Compartment Models	pH
Double Decomposition	Pharmacokinetics
Drug Concentration	Plasma Concentration
Half-life	Precipitation
Hydrolysis	Receptor Site
Incompatibility	Reduction
Laminar Flow	Therapeutic Index
Oxidation	

■ ADMINISTERING DRUG THERAPY BY THE INTRAVENOUS ROUTE

The nurse whose patients receive IV drug therapy needs to be well versed in the advantages and disadvantages of drug therapy delivered by the IV route. The nurse also needs to be a skilled practitioner who can administer IV drugs safely, prevent potential hazards, and monitor the patient's response to therapy.

■ ADVANTAGES OF THE INTRAVENOUS ROUTE

The IV route of drug administration offers pronounced advantages, particularly for patients who cannot take medications orally or for medications that cannot be absorbed by any other route. The IV route allows drugs to be administered to a patient who cannot tolerate fluids and drugs by the gastrointestinal route, and the capacity for slow administration permits drug delivery to be stopped at once if sensitivity reactions occur.

In some cases, the large molecular size of some drugs prevents absorption by the gastrointestinal route, whereas other drugs, unstable in the presence of gastric juices, are destroyed. The IV route is also appropriate for certain drugs that, because of their irritating properties, cause pain and trauma when given intramuscularly or subcutaneously. The vascular system affords a method for providing rapid drug action because the drug bypasses processing in the gastrointestinal system and circulates directly in the bloodstream. Moreover, the IV route offers better control over the rate of administration of drugs; prolonged action can be provided by administering a dilute infusion intermittently or over a prolonged period.

To understand how the IV route offers rapid drug action and better control over the duration of drug action, the nurse must understand the basics of pharmacokinetics, pharmacodynamics, and pharmacotherapeutics.

Pharmacokinetics and Selected Parameters for Intravenous Drugs

The pharmacokinetic basis of therapeutics relies on various factors, such as the drug's route and frequency of administration, to achieve and maintain a proper **drug concentration** at the **receptor site** wherever that site may be in the body. If an insufficient amount of drug reaches this site, the drug's action may appear to be ineffective, and therapy may therefore be discontinued. Conversely, what seems to be the right amount of drug may produce toxicity, and therefore therapy may be discontinued simply because excessive amounts are in the body. An awareness of how drug **pharmacokinetics** (the way a drug is absorbed, distributed, metabolized, and eliminated by the body) affects the body is an essential part of reducing and preventing potential toxicity through excess drug dosages. Factors influencing the pharmacokinetics of drugs are found in Box 18–1.

Therapeutic Index

Some aspects of pharmacokinetics that are particularly relevant to IV drug administration are the therapeutic index, plasma concentration, and drug distribution. The **therapeutic index** is the margin between a drug's therapeutic and toxic concentra-

---

BOX 18–1 **Factors Influencing the Pharmacokinetics of Drugs**

Patient Characteristics

Age, sex, body weight, dietary habits, smoking habits, alcohol consumption, coingestion of other drugs

Disease States

Hepatic disease, renal disease, congestive heart failure, infection, fever, shock, severe burns

tions at the receptor site. Pharmacokinetic models describe and predict drug amounts and concentrations in various body fluids and the changes in these quantities over time.

Plasma Concentrations

Plasma concentration is a measurement representing drug that is bound to plasma protein plus drug that is unbound or free. Two factors determine the degree of plasma protein binding. The first is the binding affinity of the drug for the plasma proteins; the second is the number of binding sites available or the concentration of plasma protein. An acidic drug, such as salicylate or phenytoin, may be bound to albumin. A basic drug, such as lidocaine or quinidine, may be bound to serum globulins. Calculated plasma concentrations may assist the physician in evaluating effectiveness of therapy. Figure 18–1 shows concentration–time curves after IV drug injection at three different rates.

Distribution and Compartment Models

Knowledge of **compartment models** enables the nurse to better understand pharmacokinetic distribution principles. The one-compartment model states that when a drug is introduced into the body, it is rapidly and homogeneously distributed throughout the entire space or "compartment." Precise anatomic sites of drug distribution can be determined only by direct analysis of tissue concentrations, which is possible only in animal studies.

According to the two-compartment model, the body can be divided into two compartments, a "central" and a "peripheral" compartment. These compartments

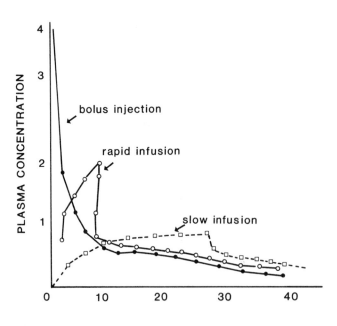

Figure 18–1. Concentration–time curves after IV injection at three different rates.

also may be given anatomic designations, such as the "plasma" and the "tissue" compartments. The central compartment may correspond approximately to the vascular system, together with rapidly perfused lean tissues such as heart, liver, lung, kidneys, brain, and endocrine organs. The peripheral compartment corresponds to body fat, together with poorly perfused lean tissues (ie, skin and muscle). The drug concentration levels we monitor are assessed through the central compartment (ie, blood). Drug behavior in the body depends on *both* distribution and elimination. (American Society of Health-System Pharmacists [ASHP], 1998)

Therapeutic Concentration and Loading Dose

The drug concentration level may be calculated after the dosage regimen is initiated to ensure that the selected dosage produces the drug concentration desired. It may also be measured periodically to ensure that the dosage continues to produce the desired target concentration or to determine if the therapeutic regimen is failing. Table 18–1 highlights therapeutic drug concentrations and toxic values.

The loading dose is the initial dose of drug ordered. Designed to produce an immediate target concentration, this dose is not always practical or safe. An initial dose of lidocaine, calculated to achieve an average target concentration, may produce toxicity after administration as a bolus because it reaches high concentrations in the heart and brain (toxic sites of action) before it is diluted by distribution elsewhere in the body.

Drug Half-Life

The term **half-life** denotes the time required for the plasma concentration of a drug or the total amount of drug in the body to decline by one half. The half-life of a drug depends on its volume of distribution (the distribution between the plasma and the various other fluids and tissues, and the actual nature of distribution and clearance). During drug administration, it takes one half-life to reach 50% of steady state, two half-lives to reach 75%, three half-lives to reach 87.5%, and four half-lives to reach 93.75%. On discontinuation of a drug or after a drug dose, one half-life is required for the plasma concentration to fall to 50% of its initial level.

TABLE 18–1
SELECTED THERAPEUTIC DRUG CONCENTRATIONS AND TOXIC VALUES

Drug	Therapeutic Concentration	Toxic Value
Amikacin (Amikin)	25–35 μg/mL (peak level) or 43–60 μmol/L	>35–40 μg/mL or >60–68 μmol/L
Nitroprusside (Nipride)	0.5–1.5 μg/mL or 2.7–4.1 μmol/L	>10 μg/mL or >27.0 μmol/L
Procainamide (Pronestyl)	4–10 μg/mL or 17–42 μmol/L	10–12 μg/mL or >42–51 μmol/L
Theophylline (Slo-Phyllin)	9–20 μg/mL or 44–111 μmol/L	>20 μg/mL or >111 μmol/L
Tobramycin (Nebcin)	8–10 μg/mL (peak level) or 17–21 μmol/L	>10 μg/mL or 21–26 μmol/L
Vancomycin (Vancoled)	20–40 μg/mL (peak level) or 14–28 μmol/L	>80–100 μg/mL or 55–69 μmol/L

■ DISADVANTAGES OF THE INTRAVENOUS ROUTE

Despite the advantages of the IV route, certain potential or other hazards arise. They include:

- Incompatibilities when one or more drugs are added to the IV solution
- Speed shock (an adverse systemic reaction to a substance rapidly injected into the bloodstream)
- Vascular irritations and subsequent problems
- Rapid onset of action, with inability to recall a drug once it enters the bloodstream
- Precipitate formation, which may occur when one or more drugs are added to parenteral solution. The precipitate does not always form when the solution is prepared, which increases the challenge of IV administration. Some drugs, which are stable for a limited time, degrade and may or may not precipitate as they become less therapeutically active. If administered IV, fluids containing insoluble matter carry the potential danger of embolism, myocardial damage, and effect on other organs such as the liver and the kidneys.
- Medication errors. Medication systems in hospitals are complex and multilayered, involving many steps and many people. According to the Institute for Safe Medication Practices, this complexity increases the probability of problems (Cohen, 1999; American Hospital Association, 1999). Errors may occur at any stage—prescribing, ordering, dispensing, administering, or monitoring the effects of medication. Common sources of medication errors in health systems may be found in Box 18–2. Table 18–2 identifies the collaborative roles of health care personnel involved in IV drug therapy.

Incompatibilities

The number of possible drug combinations is overwhelming, as is the potential for **incompatibility.** Manufacturers provide an ever-increasing number of new drug products for the treatment of disease processes. Compounding drugs for IV administration is usually performed by an IV admixture service as a component of a hospital-based or home infusion pharmacy. Today, admixture programs have expanded their service base to provide compounding services for extended care, ambulatory care, and any clinical setting in which infusion therapies are delivered.

All people responsible for mixing and compounding IV drugs must be alert to the hazards involved. Compatibility charts are provided through admixture services to alert the nurse to potential problems, particularly when additions to infusions in progress are made on a nursing unit or added in a patient's residence.

A factor related to compatibility is the composition of the solution container. Box 18–3 lists drugs affected by increased adsorption (adhesion to the surfaces of substances with which they are in contact) when infused in polyvinyl chloride containers (Trissel, 1998). Factors affecting the compatibility of drugs include order of mixing, quantity of the drug and solution, room temperature, and light. Incompatibilities

BOX 18–2 **Common Sources of Medication Errors**

Unavailable Patient Information

The patient's clinical record lacks critical patient information (laboratory values, allergies).

Unavailable Drug Information

Clinical pharmacy expertise is not provided onsite.

Miscommunication

Failed communication due to illegible handwriting, confusion of drugs with similar names, confusion of metric and apothecary systems, ambiguous or incomplete orders is a common cause of error.

Problems With Labeling, Packaging, and Nomenclature

Unit dose medications may not be available throughout the health care institution, and drug administration procedures do not ensure that medications remain labeled until they reach the patient.

Poor Storage Procedures

Stocking multiple concentrations or storing drugs in look-alike containers may contribute to error.

Inconsistent Standards

Drug device acquisition, use, and monitoring may be inadequately standardized, leading to use of unsafe equipment or errors.

Workplace Stress

Excessive interruptions and *excessive workload* may lead to error.

Limited Staff Education

Inservice training should alert and remind staff to potential for errors.

Insufficient Patient Education

Patient education is essential to good patient outcomes. Patient engagement and participation in care promotes good care and helps prevent errors.

Flawed Quality Improvement Processes and Risk Management

Quality systems should include methods for identifying, reporting, analyzing, and correcting errors as well as measurement systems for tracking the effect of system changes.

RESPONSIBILITIES FOR INTRAVENOUS DRUG ADMINISTRATION

Institution	Nurse	Pharmacist	Physician
Provide written policies	Adhere to five "rights" of drug administration	Maintain a drug incompatibility profile	Provide written drug order
Issue approved drug list			
Offer continuing education	Assess and monitor patient during drug administration	Implement admixture process	Act as overall gatekeeper
Provide institutional review board approval of investigational drugs	Participate in continuing education	Perform safe compounding	Administer drugs not on approved list
	Keep current knowledge base of drug delivery systems	Act in clinical pharmacy role	Participate in continuing medical education
	Educate patients	Participate in continuing education	
	Update knowledge of antidotes		

are not always obvious to the naked eye. They may be classified as physical, chemical, or therapeutic, and are described in Box 18–4.

Chemical

The most common incompatibilities are the result of certain chemical reactions (Baldwin, 1995)—for example, **hydrolysis** is the process in which water absorption causes decomposition of a compound. In preparing solutions of salt, the nurse should understand that certain salts, when placed in water, hydrolyze, forming a strong acid and a weak base or a weak acid and a strong base. Because pH is a significant factor in the solubility of drugs, the increased acidity or alkalinity from hydrolysis of a salt may result in an incompatibility if another drug is added. For example, the acid salt sodium bicarbonate when placed in water hydrolyzes to form a strong alkali (sodium hydroxide) and a weak and unstable acid (carbonic acid). Many organic acids are known as weak acids because they ionize only slightly.

BOX 18–3 **Drugs With Increased Adsorption When Infused Using Polyvinyl Chloride Containers**

Hydralazine (Apresoline)
Insulin
Nitroglycerin
Phenothiazine tranquilizers (Thorazine, Compazine)
Vitamin A acetate (nonpalmitate form)
Warfarin (Coumadin)

BOX 18–4 **Types of Incompatibilities**

Physical — Those in which an undesirable change is physically observed, such as sodium bicarbonate and calcium chloride forming an insoluble precipitate (Baldwin, 1995).

Chemical — Those occurring in the molecular structure or pharmacologic properties of a substance (note: They may or may not be physically observed), such as penicillin and ascorbic acid lowering the pH.

Therapeutic — Those in which an undesirable reaction results from the overlapping effects of two drugs given together or closely together, such as penicillin and tetracycline inhibiting the bactericidal effect of penicillin.

Reduction is the process whereby one or more atoms gain electrons at the expense of some other part of the system (ASHP, 1998)

Oxidation is the corresponding loss of electrons occurring when reduction takes place. Antioxidants are often used as preservatives to prevent oxidation of a compound.

Double decomposition is the chemical reaction in which ions of two compounds change places and two new compounds are thus formed (ASHP, 1998). A great many salts act by double decomposition to form other salts, and this process probably accounts for the greatest number of incompatibilities. For example, calcium chloride is incompatible with sodium bicarbonate; the double decomposition results in the formation of the insoluble salt, calcium carbonate.

Physical

Precipitation may occur in some parenteral solutions because some commonly prescribed drugs precipitate when added to IV solutions. Differences in the physical and chemical properties of each of these solutions may affect the stability of any drug introduced.

Moreover, a compound that is soluble in one solution may precipitate in another. Sodium ampicillin deteriorates in acid solutions. This drug, when added to isotonic sodium chloride at a concentration of 30 mg/mL, loses less than 10% activity in 8 hours. However, when it is added to 5% dextrose in water, usually a more acid solution, its stability is reduced to a 4-hour period.

pH AND STABILITY

Because pH plays an important role in drug, solubility, stability, and compatibility, a definition is in order. The symbol **pH** stands for the degree of concentration of hydrogen ions or the acidity of the solution. The weight of hydrogen ions in 1 L pure water is 0.0000001 g, which is numerically equal to 10^{-7}. For convenience, the negative logarithm is used. Because it is at this concentration that the hydrogen ions balance the hydroxyl ions, a pH of 7 is neutral. Each unit decrease in pH represents a 10-fold increase in hydrogen ions.

The greatest number of drug incompatibilities may be produced by changes in pH (ASHP, 1998). For example, precipitation occurs when a compound is insoluble in solution. The degree of solubility often varies with the pH. A drastic change in the pH of a drug when added to an IV solution suggests an incompatibility or a decrease in stability.

Solutions of a high pH appear to be incompatible with solutions of a low pH and may form insoluble free acids or free bases. A chart denoting the pH of certain drugs and certain solutions to be used as a vehicle is helpful in warning of potential incompatibilities. A broad pH range (3.5 to 6.5) of dextrose solutions is allowed by the *United States Pharmacopeia*. A drug may be stable in one bottle of dextrose 5% in water and not in another (Baldwin, 1995).

Again, whereas one drug may be compatible in a solution, a second additive may alter the established pH to such an extent as to make the drugs unstable (Box 18–5). Buffers or antioxidants in a drug may cause two drugs, however compatible, to precipitate.

For example, ascorbic acid, the buffering component of tetracycline, lowers the pH of the product and therefore may accelerate the decomposition of a drug susceptible to an acid environment.

Preservatives in the diluent may lead to problems as well. Sterile diluents for reconstitution of drugs are available with or without a bacteriostatic agent. The bacteriostatic agents usually consist of parabens or phenol preservatives.

DILUTION AND SOLUBILITY

Solubility often varies with the volume of solution in which a drug is introduced. For example, tetracycline hydrochloride, mixed in a small volume of fluid, maintains its pH range over 24 hours. However, when added to a large volume (1 L), it degrades after 12 hours, becoming less therapeutically active.

Other Factors

- The order in which drugs are added to infusions often determines their compatibility.
- Light may provide energy for chemical reactions to occur. Certain drugs, such as amphotericin B and nitrofurantoin, once diluted, must be protected from light.
- Room temperature may effect incompatibility. Heat provides energy for reactions, which is why reconstituted or diluted drugs are refrigerated to prolong stability.

Vascular Irritation

Vascular irritation is a significant hazard of drugs administered IV. Any irritation that inflames and roughens the endothelial cells of the venous wall allows platelets

Precipitation of Parenteral Solution

- Some commonly prescribed drugs precipitate when added to IV solutions.
- Differences in the physical and chemical properties of each of these solutions may affect the stability of any drug introduced.
- A compound soluble in one solution may precipitate in another. Sodium ampicillin deteriorates in acid solutions. This drug, when added to isotonic sodium chloride at a concentration of 30 mg/mL, loses less than 10% activity in 8 h. However, when it is added to 5% dextrose in water, usually a more acid solution, its stability is reduced to a 4-h period.

pH

- A broad pH range (3.5–6.5) of dextrose solutions is allowed by the United States Pharmacopeia (USP). A drug may be stable in one bottle of dextrose 5% in water and not in another.

Additional Drugs

- One drug may be compatible in a solution, but a second additive may alter the established pH to such an extent as to make the drugs unstable.

Buffering Agents in Drugs

- Presence of buffers or antioxidants, which may cause two drugs, however compatible, to precipitate. For example, ascorbic acid, the buffering component of tetracycline, lowers the pH of the product and therefore may accelerate the decomposition of a drug susceptible to an acid environment.

Preservatives in the Diluent

- Sterile diluents for reconstitution of drugs are available with or without a bacteriostatic agent.
- The bacteriostatic agents usually consist of parabens or phenol preservatives.
- Certain drugs, including nitrofurantoin, amphotericin B, and erythromycin, are incompatible with these preservatives and should be reconstituted with sterile water for injection.

Degree of Dilution

- Solubility often varies with the volume of solution in which a drug is introduced. For example, tetracycline hydrochloride, mixed in a small volume of fluid, maintains its pH range over 24 h. However, when added to a large volume (1 L), it degrades after 12 h, becoming less therapeutically active.

Length of Time Solution Stands

- Decomposition of substances in solution is proportional to the length of time they stand. For example, sodium ampicillin with the high pH of 8–10 becomes unstable when maintained in an acid environment over time.

continued

> ### Order of Mixing
>
> - The order in which drugs are added to infusions often determines their compatibility.
>
> ### Light
>
> - Light may provide energy for chemical reactions to occur.
> - Certain drugs, such as amphotericin B and nitrofurantoin, once diluted must be protected from light.
>
> ### Room Temperature
>
> - Heat provides energy for reactions.
> - After reconstitution or initial dilution, refrigeration prolongs the stability of many drugs.

to adhere to the wall and promote the formation of a thrombus. Thrombophlebitis is the result of the sterile inflammation. When a thrombus occurs, the inherent danger of embolism is always present.

If aseptic technique is not strictly followed, septic thrombophlebitis may result from bacteria that is introduced through the infusion catheter and then trapped within the thrombus. This is much more serious because of the potential dangers of septicemia and acute bacterial endocarditis. Strategies for avoiding vascular irritation are found in Box 18–6.

■ SAFEGUARDS TO MINIMIZE HAZARDS OF ADMINISTERING INTRAVENOUS DRUGS

Various safeguards are in place to diminish the potential hazards of IV drug administration. They include lists of drugs approved for IV use by an institution's pharmacy, laws regulating the use and availability of potentially dangerous drugs (controlled substances), standards and protocols for admixture preparation, safety improvements in drug delivery systems, standards for monitoring and documenting patient responses to drugs, resources for accurate dosage calculation, drug expiration dates, patient education programs, and so forth.

Approved Drug Lists

Lists of drugs approved for administration by nurses in all clinical care settings must be readily available. In the inpatient setting, the institution's pharmacy and therapeutics committee is the group that usually approves such lists. IV nursing professionals are often members of this committee, and protocols are brought to this group for approval before a drug is added to the list. Ideally, the committee provides a list of approved drugs for administration by nurses, a list of drugs approved for addition

---

BOX 18–6 **Measures for Preventing Vascular Irritation**

Select Most Appropriate Site

- Use veins with ample blood volume.
- Avoid veins in lower extremities.
- Start at most distal location.

Select Most Appropriate Catheter

- Select a catheter that is appreciably smaller than the lumen of the vein so that smooth blood flow can provide adequate hemodilution.

Infuse Drug Carefully

- Administer isotonic solutions after administering hypertonic solutions to flush irritating substances.
- Infuse slowly; slow administration provides greater dilution of the drug in a large vein.
- Adhere to recommendations for the following: use of filters, inspection of solution for clarity, proper reconstitution, and dilution of additives.

Monitor Regularly

- Change insertion site at designated intervals and as needed because prolonged catheter insertion increases risk of phlebitis.

---

to infusions in progress, and a list of investigational agents approved for administration (ASHP, 1998; Spath, 2000). In the alternative care environment, home health agencies and clinics may also develop lists that are subsequently approved by their medical directors before acceptance by the nursing community.

Controlled Substances Act

This act established five categories of controlled substances, known as schedules, based on their potential for abuse, the medical indications, and the potential for dependence on the drug. Many of the drugs administered for pain control are Schedule II drugs. Their safe use is regulated by specific prescription and record-keeping requirements.

Safe Admixture Preparation

Intravenous additives and solutions are best prepared in an IV additive station of the institution's pharmacy. Aseptic technique is observed and enhanced by a "clean-room" approach. A laminar-flow hood, proper illumination, and hand-washing facilities are readily available in such a setting.

Use of Laminar-Flow Hood

Laminar flow is airflow that is confined to a specific area. The entire body of air within that area moves with uniform velocity along parallel flow lines (ASHP, 1998). Laminar-flow hoods play a vital role in eliminating the hazard of airborne contamination of IV solutions and admixtures. Nurses should be familiar with the general operating guidelines of the hood. Vertical and horizontal hoods are available. Laminar-flow hoods should be used according to state and federal guidelines as well as the recommendations of the ASHP. In addition, extreme care in preparing solutions always diminishes the risk associated with IV therapy.

Admixture Preparation Policies and Procedures

The IV policies and procedures addressing admixing should define potential hazards, compatibility, stability requirements, and the types of admixtures in the scope of practice. The following are some safeguards that may be implemented to protect both patients and health care personnel from potential health hazards associated with the admixing of medications:

- Aseptic technique is imperative. Bacterial and fungal contamination of drug products and parenteral solutions must be avoided.
- Proper dilution of lyophilized drugs is essential. Two special cautions to ensure complete solubility in the reconstitution of drugs must be observed: the specific diluent recommended by the manufacturer should be used, and the drug should be initially diluted in the volume recommended.
- Introduction of extraneous particles into parenteral solutions must be avoided. Fragments of rubber stoppers are frequently cut out by the needles used and accidentally injected into solutions. Large-bore (15-gauge) needles are practical for use in the nurses' station and appear to have fewer disadvantages than smaller needles, for several reasons. Smaller needles may deposit particles that may be difficult to see on inspection of the solution. The particles may be so small that they can advance through the indwelling catheter. Using filtered aspiration needles when preparing admixtures can remove extraneous particles.
- Any solution that contains visible fragments of rubber must be discarded.

See the accompanying Key Intervention for more information on compounding and administering medications in parenteral solutions.

Improved Drug Delivery Systems

Manufacturers have kept pace with demands for improved drug delivery systems for use in all clinical settings in which infusion therapy is administered. Standard methods of drug delivery and terminology still apply (see Chap. 11).

Intermittent infusion allows drugs to be administered on an intermittent basis

KEY INTERVENTIONS: Compounding and Administering Parenteral Medication

Preparations

1. Check and recheck the order with the drug label.
2. Inscribe order for drug additive directly from original order to medication label or submit electronically to pharmacy.
3. Substantiate drug orders with the drug product and the parenteral solution.
4. Inspect solution for extraneous particles.
5. Check drug product:
   - Expiration date—do not use outdated drugs, which may have lost potency or stability. Check the expiration dates of the drug and of the diluent.
   - Method of administration—intramuscular (IM) preparations are seldom used for IV administration because they may contain components, such as anesthetics or preservatives, not meant for administration by the vascular route. In addition, some are packaged in multidose vials, which may contribute to contamination, and the dosage recommended for IM administration may be inappropriate for IV administration.
   - Clarify any questions or doubts with the patient's physician
6. Clean injection site of both the drug product and the diluent with an accepted antiseptic.
7. Use sterile syringe and needle.
8. Reconstitute medication according to manufacturer's recommendation.
9. *Make sure diluted drug is completely dissolved* before adding to parenteral solution.
10. After adding to solution, invert solution container to mix the additive completely.
11. Clearly and properly label solution container with the
    - Name of patient
    - Drug and dosage
    - Date and time of compounding
    - Expiration date
    - Preparer's signature
12. As an added precaution to prevent errors, recheck label with used drug ampules before discarding ampules.

Administering

1. Inspect solution for precipitates. If any precipitates are present, discard the solution.
2. Make sure that the drug is compatible with the IV solution if it is administered through a primary line. If incompatible, clamp the set and flush the injection port with compatible fluid. Do not use sterile water. (Note: Electronic infusion devices may be set to automatically flush the line following medication administration.)
3. Also make sure the drug is compatible with heparin when a heparinized lock is used. If incompatible, flush the lock with a compatible fluid before and after the IV injection.
4. Substantiate identity of patient with solution prepared.
5. Wear gloves when preparing medications and administering IV therapy. (If latex allergy is a concern, keep in mind that glove manufacturers have developed alternative materials to lessen this concern.)
6. Perform venipuncture consistent with institutional policy and standards of the Intravenous Nurses Society (INS, 1998, 2000).

7. Ensure placement within lumen of the vessel.
8. Ensure first-dose delivery of drug in a clinically monitored environment and administer the medication at an evenly divided rate over the length of time recommended by the manufacturer, using a watch with a second hand.
9. Observe patient for a few minutes after the initial IV administration of any drug that may cause anaphylaxis.
10. Use added caution in administering any drug whose fast action could produce untoward reactions.

---

through a slow, keep-vein-open infusion using a secondary container, single-dose additive, or multidose admixture connected to a controlled-volume set. The intermittent infusion may also be given through a self-contained administration system such as an elastomeric pump. Intermittent infusions are typically given through an intermittent infusion device (heparin lock) to conserve veins, allow freedom of motion between infusions, and provide a minimal amount of infusate for the patient whose intake may be restricted.

Peripheral and central IV catheters are adaptable as intermittent infusion devices by the addition of a catheter plug or resealable adapter. Patency of these lines is maintained by administering an amount of flush solution sufficient to fill the internal diameter of the line in use. Dilute heparin solution (hence, heparin lock) is most often used. Saline solution is being used more frequently today, and use of antibiotic flush solutions in the immunocompromised patient continues to grow.

Intravenous push is the direct injection of a medication into the vein. It may be administered through the distal Y-site of an administration set, through the intermittent infusion device, or by catheter. The terms *IV push* and *bolus* may be confusing. Substances such as radiopaque dye (contrast media) used to visualize the cardiac chamber must be injected as a bolus (defined as a discrete mass). Most medications ordered for IV push or bolus administration must be administered slowly (up to 30 minutes), depending on the drug itself. Rapid injection increases the drug concentration in the plasma, which may reach toxic proportions, flooding the organs rich in blood—the heart and the brain—and resulting in shock and cardiac arrest. The rate of administration, included with the order for the medication, can reduce any misconceptions and prevent the potential risk of a life-threatening reaction from too-rapid administration of the drug.

Because delivery of drugs by IV push instantly increases the drug levels in the blood, IV push offers immediate relief to the patient. Nurses in many special care units are trained and authorized to administer specific IV pushes. In the past, the IV push was restricted to the intensive care unit, where the patient was monitored and where a potential crisis might arise requiring its immediate use in the absence of a physician. Today, nurses frequently administer IV push injections.

Many drugs given as IV injections can be potentially dangerous to the patient. The nurse must understand the action of the drug and assess the patient's condition before administering the medication (see Box 18–7 and next section, Monitoring Response to Treatment).

Continuous administration is the term applied to medications mixed in a large volume of infusate and infused over a time in excess of 2 hours (Baldwin, 1995). De-

---

BOX 18–7 Important Checkpoints in Intravenous Drug Administration

The Drug

- Understand the expected therapeutic effect of the medication.
- Know the recommended dosage range and the length of time required for administration.
- Understand the side effects and toxic symptoms that can occur.
- Be skilled in using proper antidotes and have appropriate antidotes readily available.

The Patient

- Ensure positive identification of the patient (check identification band). Do not rely on the patient's verbal identification of himself or herself.
- Ascertain allergy history (food and drug).
- Assess the patient's condition and be aware of any factors that can affect the drug action.
- Know what other medications the patient is receiving; be aware of therapeutic incompatibilities that may occur between any other medication the patient is receiving and the IV medication.
- Watch for the patient's response during and after injection of medication.

---

creased tolerance to the drug can result from various factors in the patient's condition:

- Decreased cardiac output
- Reduced renal flow or poor glomerular filtration
- Diminished urinary output
- Pulmonary congestion
- Systemic edema

Greater dilution of the drug and a longer injection time can prevent drug accumulation, reduce venous irritation caused by a low pH, and allow time to assess the patient's response and detect early reactions. Use of the manufacturer's recommended diluent is most important because different drugs require different diluents.

Monitoring Response to Treatment

Knowing the expected therapeutic effects of the medication, the recommended dosage range, the side effects, and symptoms of toxic reactions is essential. Side effects may be manifest as gastrointestinal distress, including nausea, vomiting, and diarrhea; as allergic skin reactions; and as central nervous system dysfunction (Karch, 2000).

BOX 18–8 **Untoward Drug Responses**

Accumulation — Increased concentrations of drug in circulation when the rate of administration is greater than rate of drug metabolism

Dependence — The need for continued drug administration to prevent withdrawal symptoms

Allergic reaction — Hypersensitivity resulting from previous exposure to a drug and manifested by symptoms as mild as itching or hives or as serious as life-threatening anaphylaxis

Idiosyncratic reaction — Unpredictable response not attributed to hypersensitivity

Tachyphylaxis — Rapidly developing drug tolerance

Major reactions may consist of respiratory distress, anaphylaxis, cardiac dysrhythmias, and convulsions. Reactions must be detected and reported at once so that proper treatment can be administered. Untoward responses are described in Box 18–8.

Nurses who administer IV medications should have a knowledge of various antidotes and their use. Emergency supplies of antidotes should be readily available. Many are prepared in prefilled syringes for emergency use. Sterile cartridge needle units, with accurately machine-measured doses, provide a closed-injection system ready for instant use.

Accurate Calculations

An integral component of IV nursing practice is the ability to perform the mathematical calculations required to administer correct doses of medication and solution to patients. Accuracy is a priority when medications are administered IV. Guidelines to ensure safety in calculating doses may be found in Box 18–9.

BOX 18–9 **Dosage Calculation**

When to calculate base dose:

- At the start of your shift
- When titrated medications are started and when a transferred patient is receiving titrated medications

Consider patient's fluid replacement and duration of infusion
Stronger concentrations may be needed to avoid fluid overload
Titrate the drug to the patient's condition and note the response
Use an electronic infusion device to ensure delivery of the prescribed dose

---

Flow Rate Calculations

Flow rate calculations require the following basic information:

- Amount of solution to be infused
- Duration of the administration
- Drop factor of the set to be used

First, the amount of solution to be administered is determined, and then that number is divided by the delivery time:

$$\frac{1000 \text{ mL}}{8 \text{ h}} = 125 \text{ mL/h}$$

Next, the drop factor of the set being used is noted. A macrodrip set takes 10, 15, or 20 drops to deliver 1 mL of solution:

$$\frac{\text{No. drops/mL of set}}{60 \text{ (minutes in an hour)}} \times \text{total hourly volume} = \text{no. drops/min}$$

$$\frac{\text{mL/h} \times \text{drop factor of set}}{60} = \text{drops/min}$$

For microdrip or pediatric systems, the equation is:

$$\frac{\text{mL/h} \times \text{drop factor}}{60} = \text{drops/min}$$

Drug Dosage Calculations

Ratio and proportion or "desired over have" (D/H) may be easily applied to calculation of drug dosages for infusion therapy. Rate of administration of IV drugs may be calculated in units per hour. For example, there are 12,500 U heparin sodium in 250 mL IV solution. The dose ordered is 800 U/hour:

$$X = \frac{250}{12,500}$$

$$X = 0.02$$

Then, calculate the rate of the prescribed dosage:

$$0.02 \text{ mL} \times 800 \text{ U} = 16 \text{ mL/h}$$

In this example, the nurse has 200 mg drug in 500 mL of 5% dextrose in water, and wants to know the number of milligrams of drug the patient is receiving per hour. The amount of drug per milliliter of solution is determined by placing D/H, or:

$$\frac{500}{20} = 25$$

$$\frac{200}{25} = 8 \text{ mg/h}$$

Percent Solutions

The relationship between the amount of solute and the total quantity of solution is expressed as a percentage or ratio. Percentage strength of solution may be calculated in one of three ways:

- Percent weight in weight (w/w)—the weight of the solute (drug) compared with the weight of the solution (g drug/100 g solution)
- Percent weight in volume (w/v)—the weight of the solute compared with the volume of the total solution (g drug/100 mL solution)
- Percent volume in volume (v/v)—the volume of the solute compared with the volume of the total solution (mL drug/100 mL solution)

Expiration Dates

To ensure safe and effective drug therapy, drug containers are labeled with expiration dates that identify when a medication or product is no longer acceptable for use. Institutional policy and procedure should state that medications must not be administered beyond their expiration dates. Expiration dates should be verified by the nurse before drugs and infusates are given to patients.

Regulation of Investigational Drugs

Administration of investigational agents is governed by state and Federal regulations. Signed informed consent is required before patients can participate in the investigation (Box 18–10). An informed consent must be written by the investigator, approved by the institutional review board, signed by the subject, and witnessed.

BOX 18–10 Elements of Informed Consent Regarding Investigational Therapy

---

- Written by the investigator
- Approved by the institution's review board or ethics committee
- Signed by the subject (patient or volunteer) or authorized representative
- Witnessed

BOX 18–11 **Phases of Clinical Drug Trials**

Phase I: Clinical Pharmacology and Therapeutics

- Evaluate drug safety.
- Determine an acceptable single dosage or levels of patient tolerance for acute multiple dosing of drug.

Phase II: Initial Clinical Investigation for Therapeutic Effect

- Evaluate drug efficacy.
- Conduct pilot study.

Phase III: Full-Scale Evaluation of Treatment

- Evaluate the patient population for which drug is intended.

Phase IV: Postmarketing Surveillance

- Provide additional information about the efficacy or safety profile.

Before approval by the U.S. Food and Drug Administration, drug studies are conducted in four phases (Box 18–11). Policies and procedures should be developed pertaining to the administration of investigational agents, regardless of the clinical setting in which care is provided.

Patient Education

Not to be overlooked is the responsibility for patient education. A number of patient information resources are available to facilitate this process. Education is a primary nursing responsibility in the acute care as well as other clinical settings (Table 18–3). Moreover, education helps prevent hazards associated with IV drug administration.

T A B L E 1 8 – 3
RESOURCES FOR PATIENTS AND EDUCATION PROGRAMS

Brochure	Source	Website
Your Role in Safe Medication Use: A Guide for Patients and Families	Massachusetts Hospital Association	www.mhalink.org
Partners in Quality: Taking an Active Role in Your Health Care	Hospital and Health System Association of Pennsylvania	www.hap2000.org
How to Take Your Medications Safely	Institute for Safe Medication Practice	www.ismp.org
Just Ask!	U.S. Pharmacopeia	www.usp.org

References and Selected Readings

Asterisks indicate references cited in text.

Ahmed, D.S. & Hamran, P.M. (1999). Similar name, different diagnosis. *American Journal of Nursing, 99*(5): 11–12.

*American Hospital Association. (1999; December). *Quality advisory: Improving medication safety.* Chicago: Author.

*American Society of Health-System Pharmacists. (1998). *American hospital formulary service.* Bethesda, MD: Author.

*Baldwin, D. (1995). Pharmacology. In J. Terry (Ed.), *Intravenous therapy: Clinical principles and practice* (p. 191). Philadelphia: W.B. Saunders.

*Cohen, M.R. (Ed.). (1999). *Medication errors.* Washington, DC: American Pharmaceutical Association.

Corrigan, J. (1999). *To err is human: Building a safer health system.* Washington, DC: National Academies Press.

*Intravenous Nurses Society. (1998). Revised intravenous nursing standards of practice. *Journal of Intravenous Nursing, 21*(Suppl. 1).

*Intravenous Nurses Society. (2000). Revised intravenous nursing standards of practice. *Journal of Intravenous Nursing, 21*(Suppl. 39), 40.

*Karch, A.M. (2000). *Lippincott's nursing drug guide.* Philadelphia: Lippincott Williams & Wilkins.

Leape, L. (1998). *Reducing adverse drug events.* Boston: Institute for Healthcare Improvement.

Richards, J.F. & Creamer, L. (1999). Med errors: Solving the microgram/kilogram puzzle. *American Journal of Nursing, 99*(10): 11–12.

*Spath, P.L. (2000). *Error reduction in health care.* Chicago: Health Forum, Inc.

*Trissel, L.A. (1998). *Handbook on injectable drugs* (9th ed.). Bethesda, MD: American Society of Health-System Pharmacists.

Review Questions

Note: Questions below may have more than one right answer.

1. Responsibilities for drug administration are shared by which of the following?

   A. Nurse and pharmacist

   B. Institution and physician

   C. A only

   D. A and B

2. Common sources of error in drug administration include all of the following *except:*

   A. Packaging

   B. Workplace stress

   C. Readily available drug information

   D. Miscommunication

3. Which of the following disease states influences pharmacokinetics of drugs?

   A. Hepatic and renal failure

   B. Congestive heart failure

   C. Presence of infection

   D. Burns

4. Potential hazards of vascular irritation can be minimized by all of the following *except:*

   A. Using veins with ample blood volume

   B. Selecting a large catheter

   C. Slowing administration

   D. Changing insertion site

5. Before preparing medication, the nurse should implement which of the following measures?

   A. Question patient regarding sensitivity

   B. Check and recheck order with drug label

   C. Use manufacturer's diluent

   D. Clarify order with the pharmacist

6. Untoward drug responses include which of the following?

   A. Dependence

   B. Allergic reaction

   C. Accumulation

   D. All of the above

7. Drugs with increased adsorption when infused via polyvinyl chloride containers include:

   A. Insulin and hydralazine

   B. Vitamin A acetate and warfarin

   C. A only

   D. A and B

8. The term "half-life" refers to which of the following?

   A. Time of initial dose of drug administered

   B. Target concentration of drug divided by two

   C. Time for plasma concentration of drug to decline by one half

   D. Time for distribution to occur

9. Quality improvement processes in drug administration include which of the following?

   A. Identifying

   B. Reporting

   C. Analyzing and correcting measurement systems

   D. All of the above

10. Which of the following is true of the Controlled Substances Act?

    A. It classifies drugs based on potential for abuse.

    B. It classifies drugs according to medical indications and potential for dependence.

    C. A only

    D. A and B

C H A P T E R   1 9

Antineoplastic

Therapy

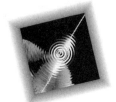

K E Y   T E R M S

Adjuvant	Cytotoxic
Alkylating Agents	Extravasation
Alopecia	Investigational Protocol
Anticancer	Nadir
Antimetabolite	Plant Alkaloids
Antineoplastics	Toxicity
Bolus	Vesicant
Cell Cycle	

■ ROLE OF THE INTRAVENOUS NURSE IN CHEMOTHERAPY EDUCATION

Chemotherapeutic agents, which include **antineoplastics** used in cancer treatment, present a real challenge to nurses responsible for their administration. Many nurses point to the reputation of antineoplastics as intimidating and express anxiety about administering them. Success with these substances usually is ensured, however, for nurses with refined IV skills, sensitive patient preparation practices, and keen awareness of how and why chemotherapy works.

Approximately 85% of all patients with cancer receive chemotherapy in the course of treatment. Successful administration of a chemotherapeutic regimen depends on the depth of patient preparation and education, the competence and skill of the nurse, mutual understanding of patient and nurse on the current goal of therapy (control or palliation), and, finally, a healthy respect for the powerful chemicals themselves. In fact, there seems to be a direct relationship between the IV therapy skills of the nurse and the "tolerability" of a patient's cancer experience. A new opportunity awaits the professional who chooses to participate in this aspect of cancer care.

Education in Administering Antineoplastic Drugs

The privilege of administering antineoplastic agents is preceded by extensive exposure to standardized educational preparation and practical experience. To provide consistently safe, appropriate, and high-quality patient care, many centers mandate comprehensive training programs leading to credentialing in chemotherapy administration.

The Oncology Nursing Society (ONS) provides a standardized framework for this credentialing through *Cancer Chemotherapy Guidelines,* a series of modular professional education resources (ONS, 1999). The guidelines provide structured recommendations for a combined theoretic and clinical curriculum, specific to acute, outpatient, or home care settings. Each module calls for a didactic core curriculum followed by a clinical practicum.

The didactic component includes basic information on the biology of cancer, pharmacology and principles of cancer chemotherapy, specific antineoplastic agents, the major principles governing chemotherapy administration, and patient assessment and management. The information is applied during the practicum phase, where clinical skills are exercised and evaluated. Successful candidates are credentialed as qualified to administer chemotherapy safely and confidently.

Box 19–1 presents a sample course outline of the major subject areas needed to prepare for chemotherapy credentialing, whether to practice in a specific institution or to prepare for professional certification through the ONS (ONS, 1999).

Safe delivery of IV antineoplastic agents is only one part of caring for patients on chemotherapy. A nurse who specializes in oncology needs a solid foundation of special knowledge. See Box 19–2 for a list of suggested areas of special emphasis in a basic education program for oncology nurses.

Clinical Challenges

The remarkable progress of antineoplastic agents as a major treatment modality poses a growing series of challenges to administering nurses. Ongoing and vigorous clinical investigations from cooperative groups are dedicated to drug development and discovering new therapeutic methods of delivering **cytotoxic** (cell-killing) drugs. Nurses who specialize in oncology have a responsibility to maintain their up-to-date expertise through study of current professional literature along with continuing education programs. The ONS recommends development of an institutional mechanism for annual evaluation of knowledge and skills relative to chemotherapy administration. The ONS offers general and advanced national certification for oncology nurses. Certification is renewed every 4 years (ONS, 1999).

text continues on page 478

BOX 19–1 **Credentialing Competencies: Course Outline**

Major subject areas to be mastered by nurses who administer chemotherapy are based on Oncology Nursing Society credentialing guidelines for credentialing in chemotherapy.

I. Audiovisual Component
    A. Historical overview of cancer chemotherapy
    B. Cell cycle
    C. Cellular kinetics
    D. Indications for antineoplastics use
    E. Drug actions and classifications
    F. Drug development and investigative trials
    G. Therapeutic intent with combined-modality therapy
    H. Side effects associated with cytotoxic agents
    I. Drug calculations, handling, preparation, storage, and disposal
    J. Normal dosage ranges
    K. Drug administration techniques

II. Didactic Component
    A. Individual facility policy statement and legal aspects
    B. Pharmacology of antineoplastics
    C. Drug calculation and reconstitution
    D. Drug administration principles and techniques
    E. Management of side effects and common problems
    F. Education materials and teaching strategies for patients and families
    G. Documentation
    H. Patient and family resources

III. Individual Handout Materials
    A. Nursing qualifications
    B. Policies and procedures
    C. List of drugs approved for administration by nurses
    D. Samples of written education tools for patients
    E. Nomogram to calculate body surface area
    F. Math test
    G. Pretest
    H. Class evaluation
    I. Bibliography

IV. Clinical Practicum
    A. Drug calculation
    B. Drug preparation and handling
    C. Drug storage and transport
    D. Drug administration techniques
    E. Complications management
    F. Appropriate documentation
    G. Patient and family teaching and follow-up

BOX 19–2 Suggested Emphases in Basic Education for Oncology Nurses

Patient Evaluation and Medical History

- Performance status
- Nutritional status
- Hematologic assessment
- Psychosocial assessment (coping skills and support systems)
- Systems review (cardiac, renal, hepatic, pulmonary, GI), comorbidity, and staging
- Diagnostic evaluation

Treatment Selection

- Histology (special studies, DNA, S-phase fraction, tumor markers)
- Tumor location, size
- Prior therapy and response
- Therapeutic intent: cure, control, palliation
- Treatment type: primary, adjuvant, neoadjuvant, combined modality
- Drug calculation, scheduling, and dosage modifications
- Treatment response

Principles of Cancer Chemotherapy

- Pharmacology
- Drug classifications
- Cellular kinetics
- Drug interactions
- Drug delivery: route and rate

Complications and Toxicities

- Short-term: alopecia, GI reactions, bone marrow suppression, dermatologic and cutaneous disturbances, allergic reactions, phlebitis and extravasation, psychosocial changes
- Long-term: genetic, oncogenetic, immunosuppression, reproductive alterations, psychosocial changes
- Specific organ toxicities: cardiac, renal, pulmonary, hepatic, GI, neurologic, dermatologic, reproductive

Nursing Care

- Early detection and prevention of complications
- Delivery of expert care
- Patient and family education
- Psychosocial support throughout the continuum of care (newly diagnosed, remission, recurrence, terminal)
- Follow-up support needs: complete remission, disease control, hospice

---

GI, gastrointestinal.

Legal Considerations Related to Education

A thorough understanding of legal responsibilities and implications is an essential element of professional education for the nurse administering antineoplastic agents. Nurses need to know the specific regulations related to chemotherapy administration in their own state's Nurse Practice Act. General legal considerations pertinent to cancer chemotherapy include the following:

- Clinical education: Before treating any patient, the nurse's successful training in IV fluid and drug administration should be documented and available in personnel files.
- Lines of supervision: The nurse should have a clear, written statement of the lines of supervision.
- Standards of care. The nurse should have a clear, written statement of the employing facility's standards of care, including a definition of reasonable care in each pertinent area of practice. Facility-specific policies and procedures should be based on nationally established standards from professional organizations, including but not limited to the Intravenous Nurses Society (INS), ONS, and American Nurses Association (ANA).
- Patient and family education: The nurse should initiate and complete patient and family education regarding treatment goals, all medications in the treatment regimen, side effects, length of therapy, and follow-up restaging. Evaluation of the patient's understanding and response to teaching should be documented.
- Informed consent: Patients who are participating in clinical drug trials must sign an informed consent form before administration of the **investigational** (experimental) **protocol.** Specific regulations regarding written informed consent for noninvestigational protocols vary from state to state. Although obtaining informed consent is a physician's responsibility in most states, a nurse should make sure that consent has been granted before administering chemotherapy. The hospital or institution may be held liable if treatment is administered without the informed consent of the patient or responsible parties. Failure to obtain a patient's consent may constitute battery, defined as any physical contact of a patient without his or her permission.

It is in a nurse's best interest to request a written definition of the institution's scope of practice and to explore details of medical liability insurance covering the practice. Many employers provide adequate coverage for care administered when the nurse is on duty. All nurses—especially independent practitioners, instructors, or those working in physicians' offices—may opt for personal malpractice coverage. Nurses who assume greater responsibility in administering cancer chemotherapy are at greater risk for litigation.

Meticulous adherence to the details of defined statutes and standards of care may minimize that risk. The ANA, individual departments of professional regulation for the state's Nurse Practice Act, INS, and ONS can provide more details on legal statutes that govern nursing practice pertaining to administration of chemotherapeutic agents.

Because a patient's clinical record is a legal document that can be used as evidence in a lawsuit, it is a crucial nursing responsibility to ensure that documentation is accurate, comprehensive, and current. The essentials of adequate documentation include time of a significant incident, a thorough and objective description of the care provided, the patient's status, and the exact nature of physician involvement.

The expert oncology nurse frequently practices more autonomously than nursing colleagues in other specialties, which implies increased legal vulnerability. For example, because extensive telephone contact is common with patients with cancer, the nurse should therefore be mindful of the accepted "scope of practice" when responding to patient needs.

The nurse commonly is a key clinician involved in clinical trials that call for take-home investigational drugs. By law, only a pharmacist or physician may dispense medication. Therefore, packaging and delivering investigational drugs are not usually legal functions for nurses.

Finally, knowledge of common dosing and scheduling of each common chemotherapeutic agent is the best protection (for patient and nurse) from delivering an incorrect and possibly lethal drug dose.

Patient Education

Experience indicates that treatment acceptance and response usually are more favorable when the patient is actively involved in the therapy program. The patient and significant others should be educated in all aspects of the disease process and treatment methods. When administering cytotoxic agents, the nurse should invite open communication with the patient in all phases of care, even to the extent of actively soliciting patient assistance in clinical functions such as assessing vein status. The wise nurse listens to, and is guided by, patient statements like: "The nurse tried that vein two times last week, and it didn't work." In addition to providing a sense of patient involvement and control, the nurse can capitalize on a patient's intimate knowledge of his or her own body.

It is wise to inform a patient that, as IV solutions are infused, it is normal to detect a sense of coolness along the venous pathway. Likewise, it is prudent to alert a patient to early signs of **extravasation** (pain, burning, stinging, a feeling of tightness, tingling, numbness, and any other unusual sensations) when **vesicant** (caustic) agents are infused because patients can usually detect them before they are apparent to the nurse.

Some antineoplastics can be associated with localized and generalized anaphylactic reactions. When signs and symptoms are reported early and treated properly, their course can be reversed or minimized. Particularly with these agents, patients should be encouraged to report unusual symptoms of generalized tingling, chest pains or sensations, shortness of breath, or light-headedness. The sensitive nurse assesses the patient's overall anxiety level in deciding the best way to impart this information.

As levels of patient participation increase, there is always the risk that some patients will aggressively seek to direct their own care. Patient statements like these are not uncommon: "This is the vein we'll use today," or "I'll give you one try, but then you'll have to find someone else." Professional nurses know that such patient behaviors can be traced to understandable anxiety. They do not allow it to undermine their self-confidence. Several minutes spent explaining the rationale and process of vein selection may eliminate the problem. Patients with a cancer diagnosis experience dramatic life changes and loss of control. It is therapeutic for the nurse to allow the patient control when appropriate.

Once a working rapport is established, the nurse usually finds that patient behavior shifts to implicit trust in the skill and judgment of the nurse with whom he or she is most familiar. In fact, personal attachment to a particular nurse often begins during the patient education phase of treatment, even before drugs are administered. It is in the patient's best interest for the nurse to encourage a wholesome and balanced professional relationship from the outset, before any unwholesome dependence develops.

Patients are best served when encouraged to tap their own resources and empowered to endure therapy without inordinate focus on the personality of the treatment provider. Ideally, a healthy partnership develops in which the patient is a valued contributor to the nurse's plan of care.

Nurses administering chemotherapy have a tremendous opportunity to minimize treatment-related morbidity (and thus to enhance their patients' quality of life) through competent patient education. Patient, family, and caregiver education is as integral to the cancer treatment regimen as is optimum selection of veins for agent infusion.

The primary focus of this chapter is, of course, the technique of chemotherapy administration. At the same time, it is important to recognize that safe, skilled, efficient craftsmanship in delivery of antineoplastics is only half the job of contemporary IV therapy nursing professionals. The more sensitive (and sometimes more influential) part of the art revolves around intuitive patient and family education, fashioned to address a particular patient's situation. Some key individual teaching plan guidelines include the following:

- The nurse assesses and identifies what the patient and family need and want to know about the disease and treatment, and takes steps to ameliorate the informational impact.
- The nurse and patient (and family) agree on learning outcomes based on the patient's needs (not the nurse's convenience or habit).
- The nurse selects educational methods and materials consistent with the patient's (and family's) learning needs and abilities.
- The nurse considers how, when, and by whom teaching will be done.
- The nurse continuously evaluates the patient's and family's learning level, with reference to original learning outcomes.
- The nurse conscientiously documents all components of the education process. An organized and systematic form in the medical record is an efficient and effective way to ensure that this phase of therapy is up to date and critical components are not missed.

Multiple psychosocial, emotional, and physiologic barriers come into play because of the nature of the disease and public perceptions of cancer and cancer therapy. A nurse's primary concern is that the patient not only has adequate information but has absorbed sufficient information to provide legitimate "informed consent."

Some barriers to patient learning (Table 19–1) can be overcome by such simple means as teaching in a physical environment that reduces anxiety, including the family in the educational process, and providing patient-appropriate materials. Often it is wise to allow a span of time between a scheduled teaching session and treatment itself so that the patient has time to assimilate important information and form questions concerning areas that are unclear. Certainly patient education is an ongoing process, from the outset and for the duration of therapy. The process may sort itself into a natural division of three phases, with the common outcome of all phases an increased patient understanding of chemotherapy. Table 19–2 summarizes the essential components of the education process. The following guidelines are for nurses involved in patient education. They can be used to evaluate teaching content and technique by assessing the degree to which expected patient outcomes are achieved:

1. Patient demonstrates knowledge related to diagnosis and disease process.

   - States diagnosis and explains disease process
   - Describes previous experience with cancer and treatments
   - Acknowledges need for treatment
   - States alternatives to prescribed treatment

TABLE 19–1
POTENTIAL BARRIERS TO SUCCESSFUL EDUCATION

Type of Barrier	Examples
Emotional	Anxiety related to cancer diagnosis, anticipation of cancer therapy, concern over cost issues
	Depression related to disease process and treatment
	Denial, used as coping mechanism
	External locus of control—learned helplessness and powerlessness
Physiologic	Biochemical imbalances causing nausea and vomiting, fatigue, restlessness, irritability
Psychosocial	Altered consciousness caused by disease process or medications
	Cultural attitudes, beliefs, roles, or values contributing to unwillingness to learn ("My wife/husband takes care of this kind of thing").
	Refusal to claim ownership of self-care; attention to self perceived as selfish and culturally unacceptable
	Lack of inquisitiveness in effort to be perceived as a "good patient"
Functional	Compromised literacy level or language differences
	Being overwhelmed by new information, names of drugs, disease jargon, personnel names, schedules, sequence, and so forth
	Age, *undeveloped or* decreased data retention or memory
Environmental	Busy, rushed, and distracting facility
	Unusual or foreign, high-tech, frightening or threatening surroundings
	Restrictive and depersonalized surroundings in close proximity to personnel and other patients

T A B L E   1 9 – 2

EDUCATIONAL ESSENTIALS FOR PATIENTS RECEIVING CHEMOTHERAPY

Outcomes	Nursing Actions
Pretreatment Phase • Presentation of sufficient information for the patient to give valid informed consent • Provision of a nonthreatening environment conducive to learning and to accepting chemotherapy confidently	• Provide written, patient-appropriate educational materials explaining specific chemotherapeutic agents and their effects before treatment begins. Allow for extended learning period, if necessary. • Thoroughly discuss expectations of therapy. • Discuss anticipated procedures and administration technique, including need for central venous access, potential side effects, and planned interventions for symptom management. • Encourage patient involvement in decision making regarding care and treatment plan. Have patient bring pretreatment question list to clinic or office. • Conduct patient teaching in a quiet, comfortable, and private environment. • Offer opportunity for the patient and family to tour treatment area. • If possible, introduce patient to IV nurse assigned to patient. • Provide nutritional counseling. • Encourage patient to express fears, concerns, and comprehension of situation. • Emphasize variability and reversibility of side effects such as alopecia and offer patient assistance and alternatives. • Be absolutely honest with patient. • Review drug and food allergy history (document this before first treatment).
Treatment Phase • Provision of sufficient and enabling information allowing the patient to cope effectively with immediate effects of chemotherapy • Enhancement of the patient's sense of participation in and control over care	• Explain how chemotherapy works (eg, cytotoxic effect of drugs). • Instruct patient to report immediately any discomfort, pain, or burning during the administration of chemotherapy. • Review antiemetic schedule, foods to avoid, and hydration requirements. • Identify known side effects of each drug in use. • Discuss precautions to take against potential adverse effects. • Assess potential for multiple drug therapy complications-incompatibilities, and caution patient to take only medications ordered by physician. • Instruct patient in oral hygiene and use of non–alcohol-based mouth rinses. • Provide calendar with schedule of treatments, appointments with physicians, laboratory tests, and expected time line for neutropenia or thrombocytopenia. • Assist patient in energy conservation program and in setting realistic goals for work and social activities. • As appropriate, discuss contraceptive measures, potential for infertility, and sperm banking.

T A B L E   1 9 - 2 (*Continued*)

Outcomes	Nursing Actions
Post- or Ongoing-Treatment Phase	
• Provision of sufficient information to allow patient to demonstrate self-management strategies to control side effects and to promote functioning at maximum realistic potential	• Explain self-care measures to use in managing side effects of each drug treatment.
	• Explain reasons for follow-up studies to evaluate disease response.
	• Remind patient not to travel alone immediately after treatment in most cases.
	• Instruct patient to report temperature exceeding 101.0°F (38°C) and other signs and symptoms of complications, such as increased bruising, blood in urine or stool, bleeding gums, rashes, fatigue, shortness of breath, sore throat, oral lesions, change in bowel habits, numbness or tingling in fingers or toes.
	• Stress importance of good personal hygiene and hand washing; and avoidance of rectal thermometers, enemas, anal sex, and people with known communicable diseases.
	• Encourage patient to call for assistance with any new or unusual signs or symptoms.
	• Provide information on how to reach appropriate health care personnel 24 hours a day.
	• Confirm return appointments and assist with patient transport services, if needed or possible.
	• Phone patient after first and subsequent treatments, when there is a potential for problems.
	• Solicit questions from patient and caregivers.
	• Review and reinforce previous information related to diagnosis, disease, and treatment.

2. Patient demonstrates knowledge related to rationale for chemotherapy.

   • Verbalizes need for chemotherapy
   • Expresses attitude toward and expectations about cancer treatment
   • States understanding of use of chemotherapy alone or with other treatment modalities, if applicable
   • Identifies treatment protocol

3. Patient demonstrates knowledge related to potential therapeutic side effects of chemotherapy.

   • States diagnosis and expected response to treatment
   • Identifies specific effect of treatment with chemotherapeutic agents

4. Patient demonstrates knowledge of treatment plan and schedule.

   • Identifies drugs to be given
   • States frequency and duration of treatment

- Identifies studies, tests, and procedures required before treatment
- Identifies follow-up tests, studies, and procedures needed to evaluate treatment results

5. Patient demonstrates knowledge of potential drug side effects.

- States mechanism of drug action
- Defines reason for side effects
- Identifies specific side effects that may occur with each drug
- States self-management interventions to control side effects
- Verbalizes signs and symptoms reportable to health care professionals
- Identifies procedures for reporting signs and symptoms

6. Patient demonstrates knowledge of techniques to manage chemotherapy treatment.

- Maintains nutritional status to best of ability
- Follows oral, body, and environmental hygiene measures
- Maintains optimal rest and activity pattern
- Uses safety precautions to prevent injury
- Seeks and uses resources as necessary
- Verbalizes reduced anxiety related to chemotherapy
- States intention to comply with treatment plan

7. Patient demonstrates knowledge relative to various access devices, if applicable.

Wise oncology nurses are encouraged to refer to the comprehensive works of colleagues who have provided outlines of nursing responsibilities to ensure patient and family education in the disease process, treatment, toxicities, and symptom management (Groenwald, Frogge, Goodman, & Yarbro, 2000; McCorkle, Grant, Frank-Stromborg, & Baird, 1996; Murphy, Lawrence, & Lenhard, 2000).

■ SAFE PREPARATION, HANDLING, AND DISPOSAL OF CHEMOTHERAPEUTIC AGENTS

Administering cancer chemotherapy carries some occupational risks. Adherence to recommendations for safe handling of these agents minimizes risks such as skin, mucous membrane, and eye irritation, light-headedness, facial flushing, headache, nausea, and **alopecia** (hair loss). These manifestations appear in direct relationship to the time, amount, and method of exposure to specific classes of antineoplastics. Until more definitive information is available, prudent health care professionals can minimize their own potential health risks by strict adherence to guidelines in antineoplastic policy and procedure development, along with cautions during drug preparation and handling (Fig. 19–1) (Groenwald et al., 2000; McCorkle et al., 1996; ONS, 1999). Because of the teratogenic, mutagenic, and carcinogenic properties of antineo-

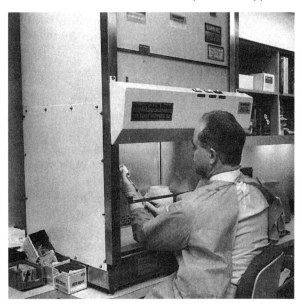

Figure 19–1. An oncologic pharmacist prepares the drug, using aseptic technique, in a class II biologic safety cabinet, also known as a vertical laminar airflow hood.

plastic agents, these guidelines should be followed strictly, especially by nurses who are pregnant, planning pregnancy, or breast-feeding (Box 19–3) (Itano & Taoka, 1998).

Managers should keep an individual staff chemotherapy exposure log as a monitoring tool to document unintentional exposure. Successful administration of chemotherapy calls for seasoned and keen judgment based on scientific evidence. It is not safe to administer these agents without a clear understanding of why they are used and how they work. Expert technical skills aside, a basic understanding of indications for use and mechanisms of action is pivotal to the quality of patient care an IV nurse provides.

text continues on page 488

BOX 19-3 **Safe Handling and Disposal of Antineoplastic Agents**

Drug Preparation

All antineoplastic drugs should be prepared by specially trained personnel in a centralized area to minimize interruptions and risks of contamination.

- Prepare drugs in a Class II biologic safety cabinet (vertical laminar-airflow hood) with vents to the outside, if possible. The blower remains on at all times. The hood is serviced regularly according to the manufacturer's recommendations.
- Never eat, drink, smoke, chew gum, or apply cosmetics in the drug preparation area.
- Cover the work surface with a plastic absorbent pad to minimize contamination. Change the pad immediately in the event of contamination and at the completion of drug preparation each day or shift.

(continued)

- Use aseptic preparation technique and mix according to the physician's order, other pharmaceutical resources, or both.
- Use unpowdered, disposable, surgical latex (or appropriate substitute) gloves when handling the drugs. Change gloves hourly or immediately if torn or punctured.
- Wear a disposable long-sleeved gown made of lint-free fabric with knitted cuffs and a closed front during drug preparation.
- Wear a thermoplastic (Plexiglas) face shield or goggles and a powered air-purifying respirator if a biologic safety cabinet is unavailable.
- Protect yourself from a potential chemical contaminant by priming all IV tubing under the protection of the laminar airflow hood before adding chemotherapy to the IV fluid. This prevents chemical exposure when connecting IV tubing.
- Take other measures to guard against drug leakage during drug preparation, such as venting the vial and using large-bore needles, Luer-lock fittings, and sterile gauze or sponge around the neck of the vial during needle withdrawal. Minimize contact with aerosol spray by attaching an aerosol protection device (CytoGuard; Bristol-Myers, Princeton, NJ) to the vial of drug before adding the diluent.
- After reconstituting the drug, label it according to institutional policies and procedures. Include the drug's vesicant properties and antineoplastic drug warning on the label.
- Transport antineoplastic drugs in an impervious packing material, such as a zippered bag, and mark the bag with a distinctive warning label.
- Be informed on procedures to follow in the event of drug spillage.

Drug Administration

Chemotherapeutic agents are administered by registered professional nurses who have been specially trained and designated as qualified according to specific institutional policies and procedures.

- Ensure that informed consent has been given before administering any chemotherapeutic agent; also clarify any misconceptions the patient may have regarding the drugs and their side effects.
- Review laboratory test results (eg, complete blood count, renal and liver function values) for acceptable levels. Drug dosages may need to be adjusted by the physician according to laboratory values.
- Implement measures to minimize side effects of the drugs before drug administration. Provide hydration, antiemetics, antianxiety agents, and patient comfort measures.
- Review the physician's order.
- Wear personal protective equipment, including nonpowdered latex disposable gloves and an optional disposable gown made of a lint-free, low-permeability fabric with a closed front, long sleeves, and elastic or knit closed cuffs.
- Protect the work surface with a disposable absorbent pad.
- Administer the drug or drugs according to established institutional policies and procedures and physician's order.
- Flush tubing with 100 mL normal saline solution through distal part to remove chemotherapeutic agent before disconnection.

- Document drug administration, including any adverse reaction, in the medical record.
- Establish a mechanism for identifying the patient receiving antineoplastic agents for the 48-h period after drug administration.
- Put on disposable, nonpowdered latex gloves when handling body secretions such as blood, vomit, or excrement from patients who received chemotherapeutic drugs within the previous 48 h. Wear a disposable gown if potential splash contamination is a concern.
- In the event of accidental exposure, remove contaminated gloves or gown immediately and discard according to official procedures.
- Wash the contaminated skin with soap and water.
- Flood an eye that is accidentally exposed to chemotherapy with water or isotonic eyewash for at least 5 min.
- Obtain a medical evaluation as soon as possible after exposure and document the incident according to institutional policies and procedures.

Drug Disposal

Regardless of the setting (hospital, ambulatory care, physician office, or home), all equipment and unused drugs are treated as hazardous and disposed of according to the institution's policies and procedures.

- Discard all contaminated equipment, including needles, intact to prevent aerosolization, leaks, and spills.
- Dispose of all contaminated materials used in drug preparation in a leak-proof, puncture-proof container with a distinctive warning label. Label and place the materials in a sealable 4-mm polyethylene or 2-mm polypropylene bag.
- Put linen contaminated with bodily secretions of patients who have received chemotherapy within the previous 48 h in a specially marked laundry bag and place the bag in an impervious bag marked with a distinctive biohazard warning label.
- Put on a double pair of nonpowdered latex gloves, face shield, and tightly closing disposable gown to dispose of a large spill exceeding 5 mL.
- Clean up small amounts of liquids with gauze pads; use absorbent pads for large spills exceeding 5 mL.
- Clean up small amounts of solids or powder with damp cloths or absorbent gauze pads.
- Clean the spill area three times with a detergent followed by a clean water rinse.
- Place broken glassware and disposable contaminated materials in a leak-proof, puncture-proof container. Then place the container in a sealable 4-mm polyethylene or 2-mm polypropylene bag marked with a distinctive biohazard warning label.
- Keep in mind that contaminated reusable items are washed by specially trained personnel wearing double unpowdered latex gloves.
- Document the spill according to established institutional policies and procedures.

(From Oncology Nursing Society. [1999]. Fishman, M. & Orlowski, M. [Eds.]. *Cancer chemotherapy guidelines: Modules I–IV.* Pittsburgh: Author.)

■ OVERVIEW OF CHEMOTHERAPY

Nitrogen mustard was the first modern chemical used therapeutically to treat the uncontrolled cellular proliferation that characterizes cancer. This lucky discovery resulted from scientific observation that bone marrow depletion (hypoplasia) occurred in soldiers exposed to mustard gases during World War II. In years that immediately followed, patients with leukemia and lymphoma were treated with nitrogen mustard; short-term but significant antitumor activity resulted. Various analogues of nitrogen mustard have been synthesized and are included in most cancer treatment regimens.

Indications for Use

Before cancer-fighting chemicals were discovered, surgery and radiation therapy were the primary cancer treatment techniques. These modalities remain useful in treating localized tumors that can be surgically removed or destroyed by radiating the genetic material in the cancer cells.

In many cases, cancer is a systemic disease that requires systemic therapy. By nature, cancer cells deviate from normal cells in structure, function, and production; therefore, a characteristic of cancer is the cells' ability to invade surrounding tissue and blood and lymphatic vessels and spread beyond the localized region of the primary disease site (DeVita, Hellman, & Rosenberg, 2000). The ability of these aberrant cells to metastasize forms the basis for systemic **anticancer** therapy. Although immunotherapy is a promising systemic approach to cancer, chemotherapy is the primary systemic modality in clinical use today.

Mechanisms of Action

Chemotherapy controls cancer with cytotoxic (cell-killing) chemical agents designed to kill rapidly dividing cancer cells with minimal impact on cells with normal, healthy mitotic characteristics. Chemotherapy is responsible for cure in approximately 12% of human cancers and has a significant effect on improved survival in another 40% to 50% (Box 19–4). Remaining cancers are less responsive to chemotherapeutic intervention as a curative modality (DeVita et al., 2000).

BOX 19–4 **Tumor Responsiveness to Chemotherapy**

Tumors Curable in Advanced Stages by Chemotherapy

Acute lymphocytic leukemia
Acute myelogenous leukemia
Burkitt's lymphoma
Diffuse large cell lymphoma
Follicular mixed lymphoma
Lymphoblastic lymphoma (in children and adults)
Choriocarcinoma (in children and adults)

Embryonal rhabdomyosarcoma
Ewing's sarcoma
Hodgkin's disease
Neuroblastoma
Ovarian cancer
Peripheral neuroepithelioma
Small cell cancer of the lung
Testicular cancer
Wilms' tumor

Tumors Curable with Adjuvant Chemotherapy

Breast cancer
Colorectal cancer
Osteogenic sarcoma
Soft tissue sarcoma

Tumors Responsive in Advanced Stages but Not Curable by Chemotherapy

Adrenocortical carcinoma
Bladder cancer
Breast cancer
Carcinoid tumors
Cervical carcinoma
Chronic myelogenous leukemia
Chronic lymphocytic leukemia
Endometrial cancer
Follicular small cleaved-cell lymphoma
Gastric carcinoma
Glioblastoma multiforme
Hairy cell leukemia
Head and neck cancer
Insulinoma
Medulloblastoma
Multiple myeloma
Polycythemia rubra vera
Prostate cancer
Soft tissue sarcoma

Tumors Poorly Responsive in Advanced Stages to Chemotherapy

Carcinoma of the vulva or penis
Colorectal cancer
Hepatocellular carcinoma
Non-small cell lung cancer
Melanoma
Osteogenic sarcoma
Pancreatic cancer
Renal cancer
Thyroid cancer

Palliation is a legitimate chemotherapeutic goal for patients with advanced or incurable disease. Even when there is no real hope of complete cure, cancer cells often remain somewhat sensitive to antineoplastic agents, so disease progression can be slowed. Agents often can control pain caused by tumor pressure, ease fluid obstruction and edema, and control hypercalcemia and other organic carcinoid processes. Agents are grouped according to their specific effect on cancer cell chemistry and the cell cycle phase in which they interfere. The **cell cycle** refers to the time required for a single cell to reproduce itself (McCorkle et al., 1996).

Antineoplastic agents fall into two categories: cell-cycle phase-specific agents are active only during a particular phase in the cell replication cycle; cell-cycle phase-nonspecific agents are active at any point of the cell replication cycle. Regardless of whether the chemotherapy is cell-cycle specific or cell-cycle nonspecific, the basic mechanism of antineoplastic action is the same: to inhibit DNA synthesis. This disables cell reproduction, so the cancer cells die. Chemotherapy is most effective when the cell is actively dividing.

Chemotherapeutic agents are further categorized into major groups as **alkylating agents, antimetabolites, plant alkaloids** (the forerunner of the plant alkaloids are the vinca alkaloids), antitumor antibiotics, hormones, miscellaneous, taxanes, and, most recently, topoisomerase I inhibitors. Within each of these categories is a spectrum of agents of various toxicities all of which relate to their antineoplastic properties.

Unfortunately, chemotherapy affects healthy cells along with malignant cells. Drug toxicities can be appreciated by understanding that these agents are designed to destroy rapidly dividing cells. It is logical, therefore, that toxicities are seen in other cells that divide rapidly, such as bone marrow, hair follicles, gastrointestinal mucosa, and reproductive tissues. Therefore, the most frequent side effects of these drugs include cytopenia, alopecia, mucositis, nausea, vomiting, and infertility.

Table 19–3 provides a quick reference guide for basic drug preparation, handling, and administration, plus frequently experienced toxicities. Comprehensive tables are available and should be used for more detailed information on indications for use, routes of delivery, pharmacokinetics, and dosing, which vary extensively as new protocols indicate the use of new combinations of existing drugs (DeVita et al., 2000; McCorkle et al., 1996).

Combined Modality Therapy

Although any treatment modality can be used alone, usually chemotherapy regimens rely on drug combinations. Frequently chemotherapy is used as **adjuvant** treatment to assist in curing or controlling disseminated disease. Combining the available modalities aims to optimize cancer cell kill while minimizing associated toxicities (McCorkle et al., 1996).

With the exception of oral alkylating agents used for chronic leukemias, single-agent chemotherapy regimens are rare in contemporary practice. Simultaneous multiagent use capitalizes on synergistic drug actions on the cell cycle to maximize their antitumor effects. Combining agents also modifies dose-limiting toxicities. Box 19–5 lists common combinations of cytotoxic agents. A classic example of com-

text continues on page 506

QUICK REFERENCE TO COMMONLY ADMINISTERED PARENTERAL CHEMOTHERAPEUTIC AGENTS

Drug	Amount/ Vial	Diluent	Final Concentration	Usual Dose	Usual Administration Technique	Comments and Major Toxicities
Asparaginase Enzyme Nonchemotherapeutic agent	10,000 IU	5 mL SWI 2 mL SWI	2000 IU/mL 5000 IU/mL	15–25,000 IU/kg as a single dose 200 IU/kg/day for 28 days	IVP 30 min IVPB (D_5W, NS) $\leqslant$1000 mL IM	Acute liver dysfunction Nausea and vomiting Hypersensitivity Depression, lethargy, drowsiness
Bleomycin Antibiotic	15 U	7.75 mL NS	2 U/mL	10–20 U/m² qwk or twice weekly IM, IV or SQ. Constant infusions over 3–7 days at 20 U/m²/day	IVP, IM, or SQ IVPB (rare)	Pulmonary fibrosis Hypersensitivity, fever and chills (premedicate with Tylenol) Pruritic erythema common Alopecia Mucositis, stomatitis, nausea and vomiting
Carboplatin Plant alkaloid	450 mg 150 mg 50 mg	45 mL SWI 15 mL SWI 5 mL SWI	10 mg/mL	360–400 mg/m² q4wk	IV infusion ONLY (D_5W, NS) May dilute to as low as 0.5 mg/mL	Nadir at day 21; recovery by days 28–30 Nausea and vomiting Increase in creatinine and blood urea nitrogen DO NOT USE ALUMINUM NEEDLES
BCNU (carmustine) Alkylating agent	100 mg	3 mL of provided diluent, then 27 mL SWI	3.3 mg/mL	150–200 mg/m² q6wk	IVPB ONLY (D_5W, NS) Infuse in 100–250 mL over 1–2 h	Delayed nadir 4–5 wk after administration and lasting 1–2 wk Nausea and vomiting 2–6 h after administration and lasting 4–24 h Painful venous irritation during administration Pulmonary fibrosis Renal failure

(continues)

491

T A B L E   1 9 – 3 (Continued)

Drug	Amount/ Vial	Diluent	Final Concentration	Usual Dose	Usual Administration Technique	Comments and Major Toxicities
Cisplatin Plant alkaloid	50 mg aqueous solution 100 mg aqueous solution	Already in solution	1 mg/mL	20–40 mg/m² day × 3–5 days q3–4 wk 20–120 mg/m² given as a single dose q3–4 wk	IV infusion ONLY (D₅W, NS) 250–1000 mL Infuse over 1–8 h Prehydrate	Severe nausea and vomiting—1 h after treatment and lasting 24 h Nephrotoxicity Ototoxicity Nadir on day 18–23 and recovery by day 39 Alopecia Electrolyte imbalances USE 5-µm FILTER FOR SOLNS CONTAINING MANNITOL DO NOT USE ALUMINUM NEEDLES
Cladribine (Leustatin) 2-CdA Antimetabolite	10 mg/ 10 mL	100–500 mL 0.9% sodium chloride solution	0.1 mg/mL 0.02 mg/mL	0.09 mg/kg/d × 7 days	24-h continuous infusion for 7 days	Hairy cell leukemia Unstable in D₅W Side effects: neutropenia with nadir at 7–14 days, fever, rash with pruritus, fatigue related to anemia, diarrhea, or constipation, cough, nausea
Cyclophosphamide (Cytoxan) Alkylating agent	1000 mg 500 mg	50 mL SWI 25 mL SWI	20 mg/mL	500–1500 mg/m² q3–4 wk	IVP over 5–10 min (doses <750 mg). IVPB (D₅W, D₅NS) infuse in 100–150 mL over 15–30 min	Acute hemorrhagic cystitis Leukocyte nadir 8–14 days and recovery in 18–25 days; nausea and vomiting 6 h after treatment and lasting 8–10 h Alopecia Pulmonary toxicity Cardiac necrosis with high dose Nail and skin hyperpigmentation Nasal stuffiness Testicular atrophy and amenorrhea

Drug/Class				Dose	Administration	Toxicity/Comments
Cytarabine (Ara-C) Antimetabolite	1000 mg 500 mg	10 mL SWI 10 mL SWI	100 mg/mL 50 mg/mL	100–150 mg/m² IV or SQ for 5–10 days 20–30 mg/m² intrathecally High dose: 3 g/m² q12h for 6 days	IVP (low dose) over 1–2 min IVP (D₅W, NS) in up to 1000 mL fluid for high-dose therapy	Mesna for high doses Frequent voiding; hydrate to prevent cystitis Nadir in 5–7 days Nausea and vomiting Pulmonary toxicity Stomatitis Diarrhea Lethargy Keratoconjunctivitis with high doses (use dexamethasone eye drops for prevention) Alopecia Cerebellar toxicity
DTIC (dacarbazine) Alkylating agent	200 mg 100 mg	19.7 mL SWI 9.9 mL SWI	10 mg/mL	75–125 mg/m²/d for 10 days repeated q4wk 50–250 mg/m²/d for 5 days repeated q3wk 650–1450 mg/m² as a single dose q3–4wk	IVP over 1 min IVP (D₅W, NS) in up to 250 mL Infuse over 30 min	Nadir at 21–25 days Severe nausea and vomiting common; occurs 1–3 h after treatment, lasts up to 12 h Anorexia Flu-like symptoms with high doses Alopecia Facial flushing IRRITANT: Avoid extravasation. Local pain at injection site. Slow rate of infusion to decrease pain from venous spasm.
Dactinomycin Antibiotic Vesicant	0.5 mg	1.1 mL SWI	0.5 mg/mL	*Adults* 10–15 µg/kg/d q3wk or 15–30 µg/kg/d × 5 days q3–4wk *Children* 10–15 µg/kg/d × 5 days; not to exceed 0.5 mg/d	IVP slowly over 2–3 min IVPB (D₅W, NS) in 50–100 mL over 20–30 min	PROTECT FROM LIGHT Nadir at 7–10 days with approx. 3 wk to recover. Severe nausea and vomiting immediately or delayed, lasting 4–20 h Erythema, hyperpigmentation, and alopecia Stomatitis, dysphagia, proctitis, and diarrhea

(continues)

493

TABLE 19–3 (Continued)

Drug	Amount/Vial	Diluent	Final Concentration	Usual Dose	Usual Administration Technique	Comments and Major Toxicities
Daunorubicin (Cerubidine) Antibiotic Vesicant	20 mg	4 mL SWI	5 mg/mL	30–60 mg/m²/d for 2–3 days q3–4wk	IVP slowly over 2–3 min; Continuous infusion; IVPB (D_5W, NS) in 50–100 mL to infuse over 20–30 min	Skin irritation, erythema, or necrosis in previously irradiated areas ("radiation recall"); Nadir between 1–2 wk, recovery in 2–3 wk; Nausea and vomiting 1 hr after dose and lasting for several hours; Diarrhea and stomatitis; Rash, alopecia; Cumulative cardiotoxicity at max. lifetime dose of 500–600 mg/m² (aggravated by concurrent radiation); Fever; Red urine—advise patient
Dexrazoxane (Zinecard) Cardioprotectant Antidote	250 mg, 500 mg	0.167M (M/6) Sodium lactate	10 mg/mL 0.3–0.9 mg/mL, final concentration <0.9 mg/mL	Dosage ratio of 10:1 of dexrazoxane:doxorubicin	Slow IVP, rapid IV infusion (NS, D_5W) In final conc. of 1.3–5 mg/mL	Give doxorubicin after completing dexrazoxane, but no later than 30 min from start of dexrazoxane dose; Dexrazoxane may add to myelosuppression
Docetaxel (Taxotere, Taxane)	80 mg/2 mL 20 mg/0.5 mL 40 mg/mL	Accompanying diluent 13% ethanol in SWI; further dilute with 250 mL D_5W or 0.9% sodium chloride solution		60–100 mg/m² q1–3 wk	IV over 1 h q1–3wk	Premedicate with corticosteroid; Side effects: hypersensitivity or anaphylaxis, neutropenia with nadir on day 9, fluid retention due to capillary leak syndrome in patients after cumulative dose of 400 mg/m², rash, palmar-plantar syndrome, alopecia, peripheral neuropathy, nausea and vomiting, diarrhea, stomatitis

Drug	Supplied	Preparation	Concentration	Dose	Administration	Adverse Effects
Doxorubicin (Adriamycin) Antitumor Antibiotic Vesicant	200 mg multiple-dose vial	Already in solution	2 mg/mL	30–75 mg/m² as a bolus injection of a continuous infusion over 2–4 days q3–4wk 30 mg/m² daily for 3 days q3–4wk	IVP slowly over 20–30 min IVPB (D$_5$W, NS) in 50–100 mL over 20–30 min Continuous infusion over 24–96 h via IV fluid or electronic infusion device	Nadir at 10–14 days and recovery in 21 days Alopecia, hyperpigmentation of nailbeds and dermal creases Nausea and vomiting, anorexia, stomatitis—especially with daily schedule Radiation recall: irritation of previously irradiated areas Cardiotoxicity: CHF, ECG changes Lifetime cumulative dose 550 mg/m² May enhance cyclophosphamide cystitis Red urine up to 24 h after administration Erythematous streak up the vein ("Adria flare") Incompatible with heparin and 5-FU
Doxorubicin Liposomal (Doxil) Anthracycline	20 mg	Liposomal dispersion	2 mg/mL	20 mg/m² q3wk	IVPB (D$_5$W). Infuse in 250 mL over 30 min	Same toxicities as doxorubicin HCl, but less frequent fever and nausea Acute infusion reaction: rate-related: flushing, shortness of breath, facial swelling, chest tightness, hypotension—decrease rate or stop
Etoposide (VP-16) Plant alkaloid	100 mg	Already in solution	20 mg/mL	50–100 mg/m²/d × 5 days 75–200 mg/m²/d × 3 q3–4 wk	IVPB (D$_5$W, NS) ONLY in 250 mL over at least 30 min to 1 h	Leukopenia; nadir within 7–14 days and recovery within 20 days; thrombocytopenia uncommon Mild alopecia Nausea and vomiting: mild; anorexia Elevated bilirubin and transaminase levels

(continues)

T A B L E   1 9 – 3 (Continued)

Drug	Amount/ Vial	Diluent	Final Concentration	Usual Dose	Usual Administration Technique	Comments and Major Toxicities
						Peripheral neuropathy
						TRANSIENT HYPOTENSION ASSOCIATED WITH RAPID ADMINISTRATION: INFUSE OVER 30 MIN TO 1 H
						Discontinue infusion if hypersensitivity/bronchospasm occurs.
Fludarabine (Fludara) Antimetabolite	50 mg	2 mL SWI	25 mg/mL	25 mg/m^2/d for 5 consecutive days May repeat course q28d	IVPB, IV infusion (NS, D$_5$W) Infuse in 50–125 mL, in a glass container	Dose-dependent central nervous system toxicity—delayed blindness, coma, death—can occur up to 21 to 60 days after the last dose
						Pancytopenia
						Nausea, vomiting, diarrhea, anorexia
						Tumor lysis syndrome associated with large tumor burdens
						Cough, pneumonia, dyspnea Chills, fever, malaise
Fluorouracil (5-FU) Antimetabolite	500 mg	Already in solution	50 mg/mL	300–450 mg/m^2/d IVP × 5 days q28d 300–750 mg/m^2 IVP weekly or every other week 1000 mg/m^2 infused over 24 h × 4–5 days Intraocular 1 mg/0.1 mL in preservative-free NS	VP at any convenient rate Continuous infusion (D$_5$W, NS) CADD pumps over 5 days Intraocular	Nadir at 9–14 days, with recovery in 21–25 days; less common with continuous infusion
						Dermatitis, nail hyperpigmentation, alopecia, and chemical phlebitis with long-term infusion
						Nausea, vomiting, and anorexia; diarrhea can be dose limiting
						Stomatitis (more common with 5-day infusion)
						Pharyngitis
						Cerebellar ataxia and headache

Drug/Classification	How supplied	Diluent/Reconstitution	Final concentration	Dose	Administration	Side effects/Notes
Gemcitabine (Gemzar) Antimetabolite	200 mg/10 mL, 1 g/50 mL	0.9% sodium chloride solution	5 mL 0.9% sodium chloride solution to 200 mg vial or 25 mL to 1-g vial, final concentration is 40 mg/mL	1000 mg/m² every week × 7 wk, then 1-wk break, then every week × 3 wk	IV over 30 min	First-line treatment for advanced adenocarcinoma of the pancreas. Side effects: myelosuppression with recovery within 1 wk, nausea and vomiting, diarrhea, stomatitis, flu-like symptoms, elevation of liver function test values, alopecia, rash with pruritus, edema
Idarubicin (Idamycin) Antitumor Antibiotic Vesicant	10 mg, 5 mg	10 mL NS, 5 mL NS	1 mg/mL	12 mg/m²/d for 3 days; 8–15 mg/m² as a single dose q3wk sometimes used	IVP over 10 to 15 min; IVPB (D₅W, NS) in any convenient volume	Myelosuppression, dose limiting; Nausea, vomiting, diarrhea, and stomatitis; Alopecia, extravasation reactions, and rash; Transient arrhythmias, decreased left ventricular ejection fraction, and CHF
Ifosfamide (Ifex) Alkylating agent	1 gm, 3 gm, 200 mg	20 mL SWI, 60 mL SWI, Already in solution	50 mg/mL, 100 mg/mL	1–1.2 g/m² over 5 consecutive days q3–4wk; Higher doses have been given over 2–3 days	IVPB ONLY (D₅W, NS, D₅NS) in 250–1000 mL over 30 min or more; IVP over 5 min.	Leukopenia, thrombocytopenia (dose limiting); anemia; Nausea, vomiting, anorexia, constipation, and diarrhea; Alopecia, rash, and urticaria; Increased ALT, AST, and bilirubin; Hemorrhagic cystitis and hematuria; HYDRATION OF >2 L/D TO MAINTAIN URINARY OUTPUT, FREQUENT VOIDING. MESNA RECOMMENDED. Somnolence, lethargy, disorientation, confusion, dizziness, and malaise
Mesna Uroprotective agent (nonchemotherapeutic)				20% of ifosfamide dose given just before and at 4 and 8 h after	IVPB (D₅W, NS) 50–100 mL	Chemical thrombophlebitis; Nausea, vomiting, diarrhea, abdominal pain, altered taste; Rash and urticaria; Lethargy, headache, joint or limb pain, fatigue

(continues)

TABLE 19–3 (Continued)

Drug	Amount/Vial	Diluent	Final Concentration	Usual Dose	Usual Administration Technique	Comments and Major Toxicities
Irinotecan (Camptosar, Camptothecan 11) Topoisomerase I inhibitor		D_5W is preferred but can be mixed in 0.9% sodium chloride solution to a final concentration of 0.12–1.1 mg/mL		ifosphamide 125 mg/m² every week × 4, then 2-wk rest and repeat cycle; dose escalation to 150 mg/m²	IV over 90 min	Treatment of metastatic colon Irritant Side effects: dose-limiting toxicities are diarrhea and myelosupression Flushing may occur during administration; nausea and vomiting
Leucovorin, Calcium Tetrahydrofolic acid derivative Nonchemotherapeutic agent	350 mg 50 mg	17.5 mL SWI 5 mL SWI	20 mg/mL 10 mg/mL	Methotrexate rescue: 10–25 mg/m² q6h × 6–8 doses To potentiate the effect of 5-FU: 20–500 mg/m² dose	IVP at any convenient rate IM Oral IVPB (D_5W, NS) 50–250 mL over 15 min	Rare hypersensitivity reactions
Mechlorethamine (Nitro Mustard) Alkylating agent Vesicant	10 mg	10 mL SWI	1 mg/mL	Hodgkin's disease: 6 mg/m² on days 1 and 8 (MOPP regimen) Up to 0.4 mg/kg as a single agent monthly	IVP over 1–3 min into the tubing of a rapidly running IV	Leukopenia and thrombocytopenia within 24 h, with a nadir at 6–8 days to 3 wk Severe nausea and vomiting beginning 1–3 h after treatment and lasting approx. 8 h, diarrhea Discoloration of infused vein and phlebitis Alopecia and stomatitis Vesicant: antidote sodium thiosulfate if extravasation occurs Metallic taste Amenorrhea and impaired spermatogenesis

Drug / Classification	Dose	Reconstitution	Concentration	Dosage	Administration	Comments / Side Effects
Methotrexate Antimetabolite	200 mg 50 mg 1 g	Already in solution, preservative free 19.4 mL SWI	25 mg/mL 50 mg/mL	Solid tumors: 20–40 mg/m² 1–2 wk Leukemias and lymphomas: 200–500 mg/m² q2–4wk Intrathecal: Usually 12 mg in preservative-free NS	IVP (<100 mg) at any convenient rate IVPB (D₅W, NS) in up to 500 mL over 30 min to 1 h Intrathecally IM	Incompatible with other antineoplastic agents Short stability Leukopenia and thrombocytopenia with high dose Stomatitis, sore throat, and pruritus with high dose Severe diarrhea with melena Hematemesis Nausea and vomiting Renal toxicity Hepatotoxicity Encephalopathy with multiple intrathecal doses Confusion, ataxia, tremors, irritability, seizures, and coma Hypersensitivity reactions associated with fever, chills, and rash Skin erythema, depigmentation or hyperpigmentation, alopecia, and photosensitivity Doses >80 mg/wk should be accompanied by leucovorin rescue
Mitomycin C Antibiotic Vesicant	20 mg 5 mg	50 mL SWI 10 mL SWI	0.5 mg/mL	10–20 mg/m² q6–8wk	IVP over 1–5 min IVPB (D₅W, NS) in up to 250 mL over 30 min	Leukopenia and thrombocytopenia: delayed, cumulative, and dose limiting; anemia Leukopenia nadir at day 25, recovery by days 32–39; thrombocytopenia nadir at day 28, recovery by days 42–49

(continues)

499

T A B L E   1 9 – 3 (*Continued*)

Drug	Amount/Vial	Diluent	Final Concentration	Usual Dose	Usual Administration Technique	Comments and Major Toxicities
						Stomatitis, alopecia, dermatitis, and pruritus
						Nausea, vomiting, anorexia, and diarrhea
						Hepatotoxicity
						Paresthesias, fatigue, lethargy, weakness, and blurred vision
						Interstitial pneumonitis
						Bronchospasm
						Nephrotoxicity at doses >50 mg/m^2
						Pain on injection and phlebitis
Mitoxantrone Antibiotic	20 mg 25 mg 30 mg	Already in solution	2 mg/mL	10–12 mg/m^2/d $\times$ 5 days for induction therapy for ANLL Other: 12 mg/m^2 q3–4wk	IVP has been used (over $\geq$3 min), but IVPB preferred route IVPB (D$_5$W, NS) in at least 50 mL over not less than 3 min	Nadir at 10–12 days, with recovery on day 21
						Alopecia (mild), pruritus, and dry skin
						Nausea, vomiting, diarrhea, and stomatitis (mild)
						Cumulative cardiomyopathy
						Hypersensitivity: hypotension, uticaria, and rash
						Blue-green urine, stool, and sclerae for 24–48 h after treatment; vein may be discolored.
						Fever, conjunctivitis, phlebitis, and amenorrhea

Drug	Supplied	Reconstitution	Concentration	Dosage	Administration	Side Effects/Comments
Paclitaxel (Taxol) Plant alkaloid	30 mg	In solution	6 mg/mL	Ovarian: 135–175 mg/m^2 q3wk Breast: 175 mg/m^2 q3wk	IV infusion (NS, D_5W, D_5NS, D_5 Ringers) Ovarian: over 24 h Breast: over 3 h Conc. of 0.3–1.2 mg/mL in glass Avoid contact of the undiluted Taxol with plasticized polyvinyl chloride equipment Use in-line filter of 0.22 μm or less, and a polyethelene-lined administration set	Pancytopenia Premedicate to avoid hypersensitivity reaction, with dexamethasone, diphenhydramine, and ranitidine (or cimetidine) Hypotension and bradycardia—monitor vital signs during 1st hour; ECG abnormalities Infection Peripheral neuropathy, arthralgia/myalgia Nausea, vomiting, diarrhea, mucositis Alopecia, rash, flushing Dyspnea
Plicamycin (Mithracin) Antibiotic	2500 μg	4.9 mL SWI	500 μg/mL	Testicular tumor: 25–30 μg/kg day for 8–10 days Hypercalcemia: 25 μg/kg/d for 3–4 days	IV infusion (NS, D_5W) in 250 to 1000 mL over 4–7 hr Premedicate with antiemetics if using shorter infusion time IVP, through a running infusion over 5 min	Anorexia, nausea, vomiting, diarrhea, stomatitis Dose-related hemorrhagic syndrome: epistaxis, thrombocytopenia Nephrotoxicity Hypocalcemia Parenteral irritant—avoid extravasation
Streptozocin Antibiotic Nitrosourea	1000 mg	9.5 mL NS	100 mg/mL	500 mg/m^2/d × 5 days q3–4wk 1–1.5 g/m^2 weekly	IVP over 15 min or more IVPB (D_5W, NS) in up to 250 mL over 1–2 h Continuous infusion × 5 days	Anemia (common); leukopenia and thrombocytopenia Eosinophilia Nausea and vomiting, anorexia, diarrhea, abdominal cramps Nephrotoxicity with proteinuria Vein irritation during administration; slow infusion to minimize pain

(continues)

T A B L E 1 9 – 3 (*Continued*)

Drug	Amount/Vial	Diluent	Final Concentration	Usual Dose	Usual Administration Technique	Comments and Major Toxicities
						Transient increases in ALT, AST, alkaline phosphatase and LDH.
						Glucose intolerance and glycosuria
Teniposide (VM-26)	50 mg	In solution	10 mg/mL	165 mg/m^2 2 × wk for 8–9 doses	IV infusion (NS, D$_5$W)	Contains 30 mg benzyl alcohol/amp—use with caution in premature infants
				250 mg/m^2 weekly for 4–8 wk	Infuse in concentration of 0.1, 0.2, 0.4 or 1 mg/mL, over 30–60 min or longer	Anaphylaxis may occur
						Mucositis, nausea, vomiting, diarrhea
						Refractory to cytarabine regimen
						Refractory to vincristine/prednisone regimen
Thiotepa Alkylating agent	15 mg	1.5 mL SWI	10 mg/mL	Nontransplant: 12–16 μg/m^2 q1–4wk	IVPB (D$_5$W, NS) in 50–100 mL over 10 min	Nadirs at 14 days and recovery after 2–4 wk
				Transplant: 900 mg/m^2	Bladder instillation: in 50 mL NS	Anemia
				Intrathecal: 1–10 mg/m^2 q1–2wk		Alopecia
				Bladder instillation: 30–60 mg q1–4wk		Hypersensitivity reactions: hives, rash, and pruritus
				Intracavitary: 0.6–0.8 mg/kg		Nausea, vomiting, anorexia, and stomatitis
						Headache, dizziness, and weakness of lower extremities
						Paresthesias associated with intrathecal administration
						Azoospermia and amenorrhea
						Pain at site of injection

Topotecan hydrochloride (Hycamptin)	4 mg/vial	Reconstitute with 4 mL SWI	2.5 mg/mL; further dilute in 0.9% sodium chloride solution or D_5W immediately	1.5 mg/m^2 × 5 consecutive days q21d	IV over 30 min	Indicated for treatment of relapsed or refractory metastatic ovarian primary tumor
						Minimum of four courses needed to see clinical response
						Patients with moderate renal compromise require a dose adjustment
						Side effects: neutropenia grade 4 with nadir on day 11, which may require granulocyte colony-stimulating factor support; thrombocytopenia grade 4 with nadir on day 15; nausea and vomiting, diarrhea, abdominial pain, some liver enzyme elevation in 5% of patients, especially those with hepatic dysfunction
Trimextrexate (Neutrexin) Antimetabolite	25 mg/vial	Dilute with 2 mL SWI	Final concentration 12.5 mg/mL; further dilute with D_5W Do not use chloride-containing solutions to reconstitute or dilute, or a black precipitate will form	45 mg/m^2 × 21 days and repeat q3–4wk	May be given by IV push but is more often administered by infusion diluted in 50 mL D_5W over 15–60 min or as a continuous infusion	Inhibits parasitic infective agents that cause *Pneumocystis carinii* pneumonia and toxoplasmosis Flush line with D_5W to clear line
Vinblastine (Velban) Plant alkaloid Vesicant	10 mg	10 mL NS	1 mg mL	6–10 mg/m^2 or mg/kg q2–4wk	IVP over 1 min IVPB not recommended; stable in NS at a concentration of 20 mg/mL	Marked leukopenia with early nadirs Thrombocytopenia and anemia Alopecia Extravasation: treat with SQ injections of hyaluronidase and application of heat

(continues)

TABLE 19 – 3 (*Continued*)

Drug	Amount/Vial	Diluent	Final Concentration	Usual Dose	Usual Administration Technique	Comments and Major Toxicities
					Continuous infusions 96 h through a central catheter	Rash and photosensitivity Nausea, vomiting, and constipation; abdominal pain, anorexia, diarrhea, and stomatitis Peripheral neuropathy, myalgias, headache, seizures, depression, dizziness, and malaise Acute bronchospasm, especially when administered with mitomycin C Severe jaw pain Phlebitis and vein discoloration Azoospermia and amenorrhea
Vincristine (Oncovin) Plant alkaloid Vesicant	1 mg	Already in solution	1 mg/mL	0.5–1.4 mg/m^2 q1–4wk Usually the maximum dose is 2 mg	IVP over 1 min Occasionally given as a continuous infusion (D$_5$W, NS) over 96 h via a central line	Leukopenia (mild and rare), thrombocytopenia (rare) Alopecia; if extravasated use SQ hyaluronidase and application of heat; rash Nausea, vomiting (rare); constipation; abdominal pain, anorexia Intrathecal administration is fatal Peripheral neuropathy, parasthesias, constipation, paralytic ileus, and myalgias Acute bronchospasm when administered with mitomycin C

| Vinorelbine (Navelbine) Mitotic inhibitor | 10 mg, 50 mg | In solution | 10 mg/mL | $30 \text{ mg/m}^2/\text{wk}$ | IV syringe (NS, D_5W), IV bag (0.45 NS, NS, D_5W, D_5 0.45 NS, Ringer's, lactated Ringer's)

Syringe: conc. 1.5–3 mg/mL, IV bag: conc. 0.5–2 mg/mL, infuse over 6–10 min into side port of a free-flowing IV, flush with 75–125 mL of solution | Myelosuppression: dose limiting

Acute shortness of breath, especially with concurrent mitomycin therapy, severe bronchospasm

Alopecia, injection site erythema, pain, phlebitis

GI: mild nausea, constipation, diarrhea, stomatitis

Hepatic: transient elevated LFTs

Neurologic: peripheral neuropathy |

ALT, alanine aminotransferase; ANLL, acute nonlymphocytic leukemia; AST, aspartate aminotransferase; CHF, congestive heart failure; D_5W, 5% dextrose in water; ECG, electrocardiographic; IM, intramuscular; IVP, intravenous push; IVPB, intravenous piggyback; LDH, lactate dehydrogenase; LVEF, left ventricular ejection fraction; MDV, multiple-dose vial; NS, normal saline; rxn(s), reaction(s); SQ, subcutaneous; SWI, sterile water for injection.

The information here is provided as guidance only. Nurses should always consult the manufacturer's current prescribing information before administering drugs.

(As revised by Jane Leung-Vega, RPH, MS, Merck-Medco Managed Care. Prepared by Christopher Charlton, RPH, and M. M. McCluskey, RN, OCN, CRNI, St. Joseph Hospital, Chicago IL [1992]. From: Dorr, R., & Fritz, W. [1980]. *Cancer chemotherapy handbook.* New York: Elsevier; Hubbard, S. M., Seipp, C. A., & Duffy, P. L. [1992]. Administration of cancer treatments: Practical guide for physicians and oncology nurses. In V. T. DeVita, S. Hellman, & S. A. Rosenberg [Eds.]. *Cancer: Principles and practice of oncology* [3rd ed., pp. 2371–2375]. Philadelphia: J. B. Lippincott; ECOG drug information sheets [1992]. [4th ed.]. Madison, WI: Eastern Cooperative Oncology Group.)

BOX 19–5 **Anticancer Drug Combinations**

ABVD	doxorubicin + bleomycin + vinblastine + dacarbazine
CHOP	cyclophosphamide + doxorubicin + vincristine + prednisone
CMF	cyclophosphamide + methotrexate + fluorouracil
COPP	cyclophosphamide + vincristine + procarbazine + prednisone
CVP	cyclophosphamide + vincristine + prednisone
CY-VA-DIC	cyclophosphamide + vincristine + doxorubicin + dacarbazine
FAC (CAF)	fluorouracil + doxorubicin + cyclophosphamide
FAM	fluorouracil + doxorubicin + mitomycin
MOPP	mechlorethamine + vincristine + procarbazine + prednisone
MPL + PRED	melphalan + prednisone
MTX + MP + CTX	methotrexate + mercaptopurine + cyclophosphamide
VAC	vincristine + dactinomycin + cyclophosphamide
VBP	vinblastine + bleomycin + cisplatin
VP-L-asparaginase	vincristine + prednisone + asparaginase

---

bination chemotherapy is the MOPP regimen—mechlorethamine (Mustargen), vincristine (Oncovin), procarbazine, and prednisone—used to treat Hodgkin's disease (McCorkle et al., 1996).

The specific and fixed sequence in which drugs are administered yields specific and predictable toxicities. Figure 19–2 illustrates this regimen's depletion of bone marrow, which results in neutropenia. The **nadir** refers to the lowest drop of the blood count between cycles. Chemotherapy regimens are usually repeated every 21 to 28 days, depending on the protocol. This allows for recovery of the bone marrow. The nadir is considered in adjusting the next dose. If the white blood cell count does not drop below 3 ng/dL, the dose is usually increased. When the nadir falls below 1.5 ng/dL or the patient experiences infection, the dose is reduced for the next cycle (Groenwald et al., 2000; McCorkle et al., 1996).

Combining cytotoxic agents, then combining them with one or more additional therapeutic modalities, potentially provides the greatest collective benefit of each therapy and thus the greatest likelihood of cure. A combination of therapies, either for cure or control, may expose a patient to significant **toxicity.** Most patients (especially those who have been cured) report that the discomfort caused by these toxicities was well worthwhile (DeVita et al., 2000).

The importance of the nurse's own positive attitude when educating patients about the dramatic potential benefits of chemotherapy in balance with its toxicities and side effects cannot be overemphasized. The nurse also offers hope to patients and their families and helps to relieve fear of therapy by reassuring the patient that every effort will be made to control side effects.

Routes and Modes of Administration

Proper pretreatment evaluation can have an enormous impact on the efficacy of the nurse's care plan and on the patient's chemotherapy experience. The nurse should ascertain answers to the following questions before proceeding with treatment:

- Does the patient understand enough to provide fully informed consent?
- Is the patient being treated with chemotherapy for the first time? If not, is the record complete regarding previous chemotherapy experience, physical and emotional response, experience with and management of side effects, and successful intervention?
- Is assessment of the patient's and family's ability to manage at home complete? Is the patient familiar with resources to assist with sequelae of chemotherapy?
- Has the nurse assessed and reviewed the patient's physical history before administering treatment? Have all compromised organ systems been considered in dose calculation, especially liver and kidneys, which metabolize and clear the agents?
- Has the patient mobilized available coping mechanisms? Is the patient "ready for therapy?"
- Is the patient prepared for potential hair loss?
- Has an antiemetic regimen, both medical and dietary strategies, been explained and initiated, and does it include both immediate and delayed nausea and vomiting?
- Does the patient have special hydration and electrolyte replacement needs? Have replacements been ordered? Does the patient understand the need to continue supplementing fluids after treatment? Is the patient capable of fulfilling this requirement?
- In the past 48 hours, have laboratory values been obtained to include appropriate studies of complete blood counts, platelets, blood urea nitrogen, creatinine, and liver function studies? Are they within normal limits? Has the dose been adjusted depending on the nadir?
- Does the nurse have a therapy protocol or a written/signed physician order that specifies patient name, drug name(s), dosage per square meter of body surface area, total dose, and rate, frequency, and route of administration?
- Is the patient as physically comfortable as possible, with easy access to a nurse call light?
- Are all necessary treatment supplies at hand, such as safe handling equipment, IV therapy materials, and hazardous waste containment? Is light adequate to facilitate venipuncture and patient observation? Is the environment conducive to privacy, especially in the event of emesis (Fig. 19–3)?
- Is the nurse prepared for anaphylaxis or extravasation? Is proper emergency equipment readily available (Tables 19–4 and 19–5)? Are necessary professional staff and supplies available in the event of patient emergency?
- Does the patient have adequate venous access?

Successful chemotherapy treatment relies on proper preparation in these areas. Individual patients often require extended pretreatment evaluations for special needs, such as those who are exceptionally anxious, lack family or social support, are cognitively challenged, or are scheduled to receive investigational antineoplastic agents. When chemotherapeutic protocols change, any or all of these steps must be

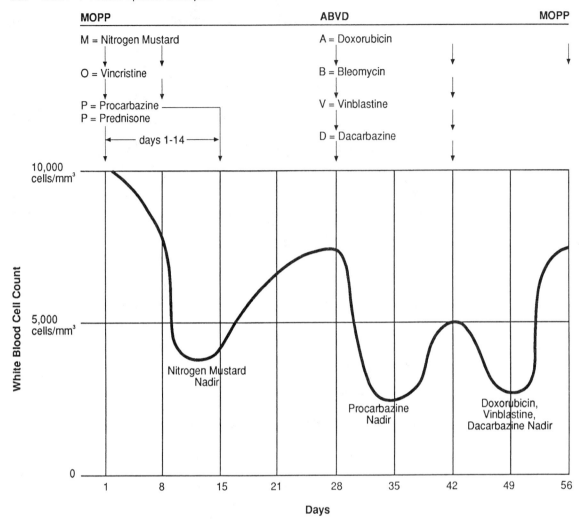

Figure 19–2. MOPP/ABV ± D administration schedule and corresponding white blood cell count nadirs. (From Goodman, M.S. [1986] *Cancer: Chemotherapy and care.* Evansville, IN: Bristol-Myers).

repeated or modified to update patient education. When the nurse and patient have combined their resources to satisfy these questions, administration of chemotherapy may begin.

■ SYSTEMIC DRUG DELIVERY TECHNIQUES

Although chemotherapy can be administered through a variety of routes, oral and IV continue to be most common. Antineoplastic agents are delivered orally if they can be tolerated and absorbed by the gastrointestinal tract. Only a few agents fall into this category. IV administration is far more common. Successful IV administration demands careful vein selection and venipuncture.

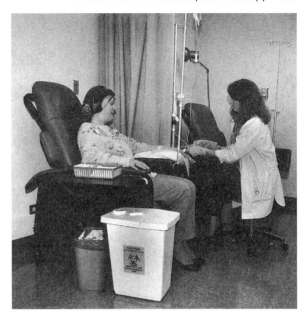

Figure 19–3. An environment conducive to successful chemotherapy administration is pleasant and well lit and contains the necessary equipment, including adjustable infusion chair with arm rests, easily reached IV therapy equipment and materials, biohazard waste container, safe handling materials, emesis basin, sphygmomanometer, emergency and extravasation equipment, and available nurse call system.

Vein Selection

Vein selection depends on the purpose and length of infusion and the vesicant and irritant properties of the drugs. Peripheral veins may be used for bolus or short-term infusion. Central venous access is preferred for patients scheduled for long-term infusions or those at risk of extravasation caused by vein fragility or inaccessibility. Most patients receive chemotherapy for a minimum of 3 to 6 months, with most reg-

T A B L E   1 9 – 4
EMERGENCY DRUGS AND EQUIPMENT

Drugs	Strength	Volume
Epinephrine	1 : 1000 (1 mg/mL)	10 mL
	1 :10,000	
Anhydrous theophylline	400 mg	100 mL
Diphenhydramine	50 mg	1 mL
Hydrocortisone	2 mL	100 mL
Dopamine	(200 mg) 800 mg	250 mL
Levarterenol bitartrate	2 mg	500 mL
Sodium bicarbonate	8.4%	50 mEq/50 mL
Furosemide	40 mg	4 mL
Diazepam	10 mg	2 mL
Lidocaine	100 mg	5 mL
Naloxone hydrochloride	0.1–0.4 mg	5 mL
Nitroglycerin	0.15 mg	Sublingual

T A B L E   1 9 – 5
EXTRAVASATION KIT: ITEMS AND QUANTITIES

Needles	18 gauge (2)
	25 gauge (2)
	Filter needle (1)
Tape	1-in. paper
Telfa pads	4 × 4 in. (4)
Sterile gauze dressing	4 × 4 in. (2)
Alcohol wipes	(4)
Syringes	Tuberculin
	3 mL
	5 mL
	10 mL
	20 mL
Local anesthetic	Ethyl chloride
Diluent	Sterile saline solution: 10 mL (1) preservative free
	Sterile water: 10 mL (1)
Steroid cream	1% Topical lotion (optional)
Antidotes	Drug-specific antidote
Latex gloves	Several
Hot pack	
Cold pack	
Policy and procedure for extravasation management	
Extravasation record	
Camera	1

Note: *Restock kit after each use.* Kit should be available wherever vesicant drugs are being administered.

imens repeated every 21 to 28 days. Patients with widespread metastatic disease may require years of chemotherapy, and therefore a central line placement should be considered early in the treatment plan.

For peripheral venous access, patients should be positioned comfortably in a chair with extended arm rests and hand and arm stabilizers. Successful IV nurses allow ample and unhurried time to assess both arms and hands to avoid areas of sclerosis, thrombosis, hematoma, or phlebitis. The examination of both arms also gives the nurse a baseline reference should changes occur during treatment.

If veins are obscure, comfortably warm, moist compresses may be applied to the patient's hands and forearms. Clothing can be loosened to allow full view of the IV site. Watches and tight jewelry should be removed if they constrict the venous pathway or impede the smooth flow of drugs along the venous network.

Alternating arms, from treatment to treatment, may help minimize vascular irritation and phlebitis associated with IV administration of chemotherapy drugs; it also allows time for healing. Documentation should specify which arm and location was used for each treatment. If not informed of this procedure, and if treated by various nurses, a patient may unwittingly prefer to have all treatments in one arm, increasing the risk of phlebitis.

 Safe Practice Alert Aseptic techniques, including sterile venipuncture procedures, universal precautions, and safe handling of antineoplastics, require a nurse's constant vigilance, especially because of the susceptibility of these patients to systemic infection resulting from leukopenia.

A nurse should follow a pattern for venipunctures, using the most distal veins first and moving proximally with successive venipunctures up the forearm. For example, if a forearm venipuncture was unsuccessful, or if blood was drawn earlier, cytotoxic agents administered to the same arm might leak into tissue surrounding the recent proximal puncture. With vesicant therapy, necrosis could result.

Large veins along the distal forearm (cephalic, median, and basilic) are easy to access and may provide safe, convenient venipuncture sites. Using these larger veins diminishes the risk of chemical phlebitis from the caustic properties of antineoplastic drugs, especially with **bolus** (IV push) administration (DeVita et al., 2000). In the event of extravasation, this area also offers a greater mass of soft tissue than the hand and may be more easily grafted, thereby avoiding functional impairment.

Because IV solutions often contain admixtures incompatible with cytotoxic drugs (eg, heparin sodium combined with doxorubicin), there is a potential for precipitates to develop, which can result in vein irritation and phlebitis. Compatibility issues are imperative to consider, not only with antineoplastics but with adjunctive drug therapies, such as those involving antiemetics or corticosteroids.

Vesicant chemotherapy should not be administered using previous IV sites. Ideally, vesicants should be administered through a central line. The following precautions must be considered if an existing IV line is the only available site for chemotherapy administration:

- Ensure venous patency before treatment and use transparent dressings that allow the site to be seen without disturbing the dressing.
- Flush the line before and after treatment.
- When establishing a new IV line, avoid joint flexion areas (eg, wrist, antecubital fossa) whenever possible. The chosen vein should feel smooth and resilient, not hard or cord-like.

Several factors contraindicate the use of the antecubital fossa. This area includes the important anatomic structures of the median nerve and brachial artery. Serious complications—sometimes even amputation—may ensue if necrosis occurs. At a minimum, extensive tissue necrosis could require complicated, costly, and psychologically difficult reconstructive efforts.

In addition, phlebotomists favor antecubital fossa veins for drawing blood specimens. If repeated needle insertions and infusions trigger tissue fibrosis, future blood sampling may become difficult. Moreover, prolonged infusions restrict arm mobility because elbow function is limited during infusion and the area's fat and tissue volume make it difficult to visualize and detect early subcutaneous infiltration.

Despite the nurse's technical competence, usable veins sometimes are difficult to locate and access. An arbitrary limit of two to three unsuccessful venipunctures is suggested before a nurse seeks assistance from a coworker. Repeated venipunctures increase anxiety levels for both patient and nurse and may decrease the likelihood of successful vein catheterization.

The lower extremities or an arm with impaired circulation should not be used for infusing cytotoxic agents. Stagnant or sluggish blood flow delays the agent's flow into the general circulation, and the agent also can potentiate any local reaction. Impaired circulation in the extremities can result from an invading neoplasm, existing phlebitis, varicosities, axillary node dissection on the side of a mastectomy, an immobilized fracture, or even extensive hematomas or inflamed areas.

 SAFE PRACTICE ALERT   Perform a thorough examination of the extremity before inserting the catheter into the vein. Avoid using phlebitic, bruised, inflamed, or sclerotic areas. A useful and often overlooked peripheral infusion site is the basilic vein on the medial aspect of the forearm.

Administration Techniques

Most chemotherapeutic regimens can be administered on an outpatient basis. When treating an outpatient for a bolus or short infusion in a peripheral site, a stainless steel winged infusion needle is preferred. Often nurses must catheterize veins in elusive areas, such as between the knuckles, or the cephalic vein at the arch over the radial wrist bones. The nurse may choose to tape the tube (rather than the wings) securely to the skin in difficult areas like these to ensure needle stability in the vein.

Bolus (IV push) administration of some medications may threaten insertion because of the needle's short bevel. Tape should be applied so that the needle insertion site and immediate surrounding area are clearly visible. A common extravasation site is just above the insertion site. If obscured, subtle infiltration evidence may go unnoticed. Tubing should be taped independently, then looped so that blood return can be checked during administration. When the needle is securely in place, the remainder of the IV set should be arranged to remain intact and functional, even in the event of sudden movements like vomiting.

Before cytotoxic drug administration, an IV fluid flush should be given to test and ensure venous patency. If a fragile vein bursts, or if a needle has perforated its wall, conventional IV fluids are absorbed without damaging surrounding tissue. A patient with a peripheral lock or permanent central venous catheter requires a flush solution infusion before chemotherapy administration to avoid drug incompatibilities. At least 10 mL IV of fluid between drugs avoids inopportune chemical interactions. Likewise, a final flush clears the line and vein after antineoplastic administration is complete.

Bolus (IV push) administration calls for slow, even pressure. Small-gauge needles offer greater resistance than larger needles. Any unusual resistance calls for cessation of infusion to investigate the cause. If the bevel of the needle is resting against the vein wall, careful repositioning may resolve the problem. If the nurse applies too much force, the patient may experience pain or venous spasm. A fast, forceful infusion may even cause nausea or exaggerated hypersensitivity sensations (eg, nasal congestion with Cytoxan). Most adverse reactions can be avoided when there is even push pressure and constant supervision of all administration process.

Figure 19–4 illustrates standard procedure for drug delivery using a butterfly needle. Short-term chemotherapy may also be delivered with a conventional mini-infusion piggyback approach. When injecting vesicants, needle stability and adequate blood return must be checked approximately every 1 to 2 mL. Immediate cessation

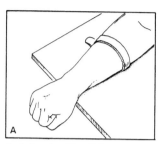

Apply tourniquet to mid-forearm, palpate radial pulse and loosen tourniquet if pulse cannot be felt. Have patient open and close fist for venous distention.

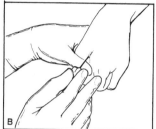

Cleanse injection area and hold patient's hand, using thumb to keep skin taut and anchor vein. Place needle in line with vein, bevel up, about one-half inch below proposed entry site.

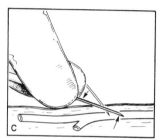

Insert needle through skin and tissue at 45° angle, relocate vein, decrease needle angle slightly and slowly enter vein with a downward then upward motion.

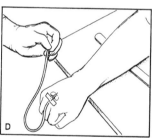

Remove tourniquet and tape scalp vein tubing.

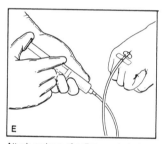

Attach syringe of saline, aspirate to remove air and irrigate.

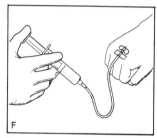

Remove saline syringe, attach chemotherapy syringe and inject slowly, checking for blood return and swelling.

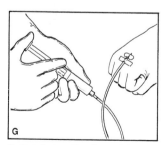

Flush catheter with saline solution.

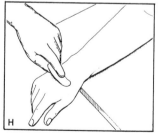

Remove needle, apply pressure to prevent bleeding and apply Band-Aid.

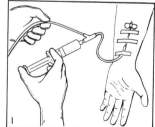

If administering agent via sidearm of continuously running IV, establish intravenous access and freely dripping fluid. Cleanse sidearm, insert needle of chemotherapy syringe and administer drug, maintaining even pressure.

Figure 19–4. Venipuncture and peripheral administration of chemotherapeutic drugs.

of drug administration is required if there is any doubt about venous patency. With vesicants, the complicated site should be treated as an extravasation; with nonvesicants, treatment can be resumed with a new catheter site.

After chemotherapy, the catheter tubing is flushed with normal saline solution to remove all drug from the system and the catheter is removed with a dry sterile sponge. The extremity is elevated and pressure applied until bleeding stops. Then a dressing is applied to the site. Because thrombocytopenia is a common sequel of chemotherapy, blood leakage into subcutaneous tissues can result in hematomas that are painful and unsightly, and, until reabsorbed, preclude use of the site. Patients also should be cautioned not to handle heavy items with the treated extremity immediately after chemotherapy.

Venous Access Devices

Nonperipheral venous access devices may be required for patients with a vesicant in their treatment programs or with impaired peripheral venous vasculature (McCorkle et al., 1996; Murphy et al., 2000). Tunneled, nontunneled, or implanted subcutaneous devices can be used for either long- or short-term treatment plans. They can be percutaneously inserted, either centrally or peripherally, eventually to dwell in the superior vena cava or above the junction of the right atrium. They have become the state of the art in chemotherapy administration because of their ease of placement, convenience, and safety benefits. Central lines eliminate peripheral venipuncture for drawing blood specimens, and dramatically enhance patient serenity and comfort. As other advantages, the central line

- Preserves the peripheral venous system
- Serves also as line for blood and nutritional products, antibiotics, analgesics, antiemetics, as well as cytotoxic agents
- Allows home infusion of vesicants and multiple-drug therapies that otherwise can be administered safely only in acute care settings
- Is cost effective

Potential disadvantages include costs of insertion and maintenance, thrombus consequent to improper or inadequate irrigation, infection or sepsis, air embolism, and catheter severance or migration. Before discharge, patients and families need meticulous training in device maintenance, and they also should receive written instructions for later reference.

Vascular access devices afford dramatic quality-of-life advantages, but they demand extraordinary patient responsibility and maintenance activities. If improperly instructed, patients may experience catheter occlusions caused by inadequate irrigation, infections, or catheter breakage, or air embolism caused by line mismanagement, poorly stabilized or improper connections, or mishandled clamps. Device removal may be the only option if the patient or caregiver cannot properly care for the access device.

Box 19–6 lists various devices for long-term venous access. Device selection depends on frequency of access, treatment, duration, administration mode, venous integrity, and patient preference (Murphy et al., 2000). Criteria for patient assessment are featured in Box 19–7. Common placement sites are discussed in Chapters 13 and 14.

BOX 19–6 **Selected Venous Access Devices and Their Uses**

Silastic Atrial Catheters

Frequent venous access for blood sampling, delivery of blood products, and therapy
Bone marrow transplantation
Multiple transfusions, such as for treating patients with leukemia
Single bolus injections of chemotherapy
Infusion of total parenteral nutrition, fluids, pain management, and antibiotic therapy
Short- or long-term, inpatient or outpatient chemotherapy infusions, vesicant or nonvesicant

Note: Patient or responsible caregiver must be capable of caring for this device.

Small-Gauge Central Venous Catheters

Short-term infusion of chemotherapy or vesicant or nonvesicant chemotherapy, total parenteral nutrition, blood, fluids, pain management and antibiotic therapy
Inpatient or outpatient infusion therapy
Single bolus injections of chemotherapy
Frequent venous access needed for chemotherapy
Frequent blood sampling
Brief life expectancy

Note: Patient or responsible caregiver must be capable of caring for this device.

Implanted Ports

Infrequent venous access
Single bolus injections of chemotherapy
Inpatient or outpatient infusion of chemotherapeutic agents
Short- or long-term chemotherapy
Total parenteral nutrition, blood sampling, blood transfusions, fluid replacement, antibiotic therapy, pain management
Alternative for patients physically unable to care for other access device
Young children (when frequent venous access is not required)
Cosmesis or patient preference

In fact, these venous access devices are so simple and reliable that there is a real risk of complacency for nurses treating these patients. Individual manufacturer recommendations for care and maintenance should be followed strictly, particularly because specific diameters, volumes, lumen sizes, and clamping procedures vary among models. Although IV therapy is the primary use of these devices, they also can be placed intra-arterially for organ profusion or intraperitoneally for "belly baths."

Implanted ports offer an alternative to percutaneously inserted central venous lines. Advantages include reduced infection risk, no care requirements for external catheters, and diminished risk of drug infiltration or vein sclerosis from irritating

---

BOX 19–7 **Patient Assessment Criteria for a Central Vascular Access Device**

General assessment guidelines for assessing whether a central vascular access device (VAD) is appropriate for the patient include the frequency of venous access, longevity of treatment, mode of drug administration, venous integrity, and the patient's preferences. Priorities for central VAD placement are compared below.

Low Priority	High Priority
Infrequent venous access	Frequent venous access
Short-term therapy	Long-term, indefinite treatment period
Intermittent single injections	Continuous infusion of chemotherapy
Administration of nonvesicant, nonirritating drugs	Administration of vesicant, irritating drugs
No previous IV therapy	Venous thrombosis or sclerosis from previous IV therapy
Both extremities available	Venous access limited to one extremity
Venous access with two or fewer venipunctures	Multiple (>2) venipunctures to secure venous access
Patient does not prefer central VAD	Patient prefers central VAD
	Home infusion of chemotherapy
	Prior tissue damage due to extravasation

---

drugs administered peripherally. Implantable devices are available from a variety of manufacturers; an example appears in Figure 19–5.

Implanted ports carry a risk of needle dislodgment and consequent extravasation when long-term infusions of vesicant drugs such as doxorubicin (Adriamycin), mitomycin (Mutamycin), or vincristine (Oncovin) are administered through implanted devices. Proper needle placement must be assessed and documented at least every 8 hours with these vesicants. A patient with an implanted device receiving a continuous infusion of a vesicant requires inpatient care. This is not the case with vesicant administration through indwelling Silastic central venous catheters, such as the Hickman, Broviac, or Groshong devices. Complications are rare and usually avoidable when professional standards and chemotherapy administration practices are observed. When complications do occur, however, they are severe and often life threatening.

Infusion Systems

Venous access devices provide another key benefit to patients requiring continuous or intermittent chemotherapy; they allow treatment at home. External ambulatory infusion systems for antineoplastics reduce inpatient admissions and costs and allow patient autonomy in familiar home surroundings.

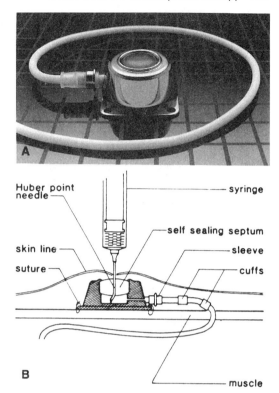

Figure 19–5. (**A**) PORT-A-CATH Implantable Access System (Courtesy of Sims-Deltec, Inc., St. Paul, MN). (**B**) A subcutaneously implanted port with Huber point needle penetrating the skin and the injection septum.

All external ambulatory infusion systems are self-powered independent of household electrical current; they may or may not be mechanical. Usually they are battery powered, lightweight, and reusable. They infuse either through a piston–valve (Autosyringe) or a peristaltic mechanism (Fig. 19–6). Administration rate is controllable. Mechanically powered pumps feature alarm systems that detect any back-pressure that might occur with occlusion or infiltration. These pumps also detect air in the line, and an alarm sounds when the fluid reservoir is empty. The Travenol Infuser system, on the other hand, exerts positive pressure when its balloon, containing the drug, deflates into the venous access device. Infusion rate is determined by the amount of fluid that exerts the balloon pressure.

Any list of ambulatory infusion systems products and technologies might be obsolete within weeks of publication. IV nurses are better served to keep abreast of manufacturer-provided instructional materials, patient education information, and trouble-shooting support services of the devices currently favored in their own clinical setting.

Nurses also must be intimately familiar with system operations to educate patients and families in early detection of complications, including line occlusion, thrombosis, infiltration or extravasation, and system failure. The ONS provides course contents and clinical practicum recommendations for nursing education and practice, which nurses may find helpful in preparing patients to succeed with these systems (ONS, 1999).

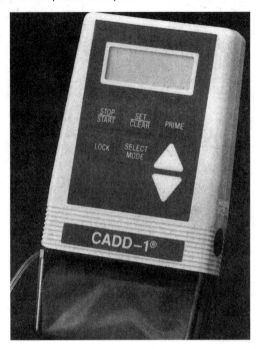

Figure 19–6. CADD-I Ambulatory Infusion pump, model 5100 HFX. (Courtesy of Sims-Deltec, Inc., St. Paul, MN).

Following is a list of assessment factors to consider when recommending use of an ambulatory infusion system:

- Level of patient and family understanding of pump and alarm features and functions; degree of patient and family compliance, reliability, dexterity, and comfort with the device; patient or family visual acuity keen enough to see pump function clearly
- 24-Hour availability or proximity to health care provider in the event of pump failure or occlusion
- Drug regimen that matches device capacities and features
- Insurance coverage of unit rental or purchase costs

Infusion systems can be attached by belt or shoulder strap to ease patient movement. Mechanical systems usually call for hands-on programming and reprogramming, requiring an on-site visit from a nurse when changes are needed. The same is true for replenishing fluid and drug reservoirs. Upcoming developments to ease ambulatory infusions (eg, pump reprogramming by computer and over phone lines, without hands-on human intervention) are promised for the near future.

Regional Drug Delivery

Although systemic IV administration of chemotherapy is most common, some tumors respond better to local exposure to antineoplastics. Alternative methods of drug administration have been established to deliver high concentrations of chemotherapeutic agents locally, into a body cavity or into the organ site of the tumor. A drug can be directed into the area of known disease, such as intraperitoneally to treat malignant ascites or metastatic seeding of peritoneum from ovarian carcinoma. Intravesical administration of chemotherapy and biologic response modifiers is frequently used to treat bladder cancer. Intrathecal or intraventricular administration is used for cancers known to have invaded the central nervous system; intrapleural is beneficial for malignant effusions and sclerosing purposes; topical application can be used for early malignancies of the integumentary. Intra-arterial administration provides higher concentrations for the regional delivery of chemotherapy. Primary and metastatic disease of the liver is the most frequent indication for intra-arterial chemotherapy, but other organs can also respond to this therapy (Murphy et al., 2000).

Another advantage of the regional delivery of these infusions is that they can "bathe" the affected body cavity or organ with decreased toxic effects on the whole system.

Intra-arterial Delivery

The most likely alternative route of antineoplastic administration involving the IV nurse is the intra-arterial infusion, which may use a percutaneously inserted catheter or a totally implanted infusion pump (see Chaps. 11,14, and 15 for more information). This route usually is used to treat primary hepatic tumors or hepatic metastases, colorectal, gastric, esophageal, pancreatic, breast, or lung tumors, or malignant melanoma. Intra-arterial infusion is also is used to treat large, localized disease in primary head and neck tumors, brain tumors, and widespread metastatic disease in the pelvis. Large drug concentrations are administered through arteries that supply these areas (Groenwald et al., 2000).

The Infusaid Pump (Infusaid Corp., Sharon, MA) is the most common totally implantable drug delivery system. The U.S. Food and Drug Administration approved its commercial use for 5-fluorouracil (5-FU), methotrexate, floxuridine (FUDR), heparin, morphine sulfate, insulin, and some aminoglycosides. Volatile fluorocarbon vapor pressure powers the pump, which uses bellows to force the fluid from the drug chamber at a specific rate. Vapor pressure is influenced by changes in body temperature, atmospheric pressure, and drug viscosity. Because the pump's flow rate increases by roughly 10% for each degree Celsius increase in body temperature, patients must agree to report any fever so that pump refill schedules can be assessed and adjusted. Because infection and thrombosis are the most common complications, patients also are instructed to report pain, changes in temperature, color, or sensation of the skin over the pump, or fluid leakage (DeVita et al., 2000).

About every 1 or 4 weeks, the pump is refilled by percutaneous injection with either active antineoplastics or saline to maintain constant perfusion to the area and patency of the catheter. The device's side port may be used for direct intra-arterial access. The nurse must be intimately familiar with techniques and risks of this route of drug delivery, and adhere strictly to details available from manufacturer data and institutional policy and procedures when attempting pump accessing or filling. These devices also support effective pain management when used to infuse low-dose narcotics through intrathecal or subcutaneous delivery modes.

Intrathecal Delivery

Intrathecal therapy is another alternative route of cancer chemotherapy that might call for IV nurse involvement. A cerebrospinal access device, like the Ommaya reservoir, is subcutaneously implanted into the ventricle to avoid repeated lumbar punctures in treating meningeal carcinomatosis, the infiltration by cancer of the cerebral leptomeninges. The reservoir provides access to the cerebrospinal fluid through a bur hole in the skull (Fig. 19–7).

First, the reservoir is pumped several times to fill the device with cerebrospinal fluid (CSF). Then, the skin is prepared and the reservoir is obliquely punctured, using sterile technique, with a 25- to 27-gauge scalp vein needle. Sufficient CSF is removed for laboratory studies and to keep exchanges isovolumetric. Then, a chemotherapeutic agent is injected slowly through a scalp vein needle into the reservoir, which next is flushed with Elliott's B solution, an electrolyte and dextrose solution used as a diluent in intrathecal administration of methotrexate and cytarabine. After the needle is removed, the reservoir is pumped to distribute the drugs into the intraventricular space. Preservative-free morphine sulfate also can be administered into an Ommaya reservoir for prolonged pain relief.

Controversial Issues

Some aspects and techniques of antineoplastic therapy have earned unanimous consensus, whereas others are handled in various ways, depending on contradicting studies, personal experience, preference, opinion, and talent. Some controversy will probably always remain in a few areas of chemotherapy theory and practice. The ONS acknowledges the controversies among practicing nurses. For a summary of selected controversies, see Box 19–8.

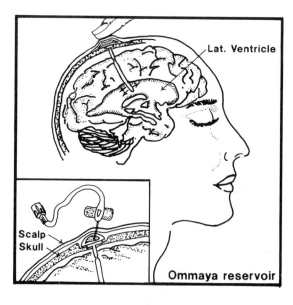

Figure 19–7. Cerebrospinal fluid reservoir (Ommaya type) vacilitates repeated intraventricular administration.

BOX 19–8 **Controversial Issues**

Several issues that require further investigative studies are summarized, without judgment, in the following:

Use of the Antecubital Fossa for Administration of Antineoplastic Agents

- Arguments in favor focus on the fact that larger veins promote greater hemo-dilution and thus permit more rapid drug infusion and administration, thereby permitting potentially irritating agents to reach general circulation sooner, with less threat to smaller veins.
- Arguments to discourage using the antecubital fossa cite restricted arm mobility when the needle is in place and increased risk for infiltration or extravasation with patient movement (eg, coughing, vomiting). An extravasation requires extensive reconstruction, which would limit use of the arm during healing and possibly decrease function and increase morbidity. Moreover, early infiltration would be difficult to see because of the subcutaneous tissue. There is the potential for venous fibrosis from chemotherapeutic agents at the site causing difficulty with drawing blood.

Needle Size

- Arguments favoring larger-gauge (eg, 19- and 21-gauge) scalp vein needles emphasize that larger needles allow potentially irritating chemotherapeutic agents to reach the general circulation quickly, without irritating peripheral veins. Larger needles decrease administration time, thereby reducing the patient's exposure to potential stress.
- Arguments favoring the use of smaller-gauge (eg, 23- and 25-gauge) scalp vein needles cite the lower likelihood of small vein wall puncture and scar formation, less pain on needle insertion, increased blood flow around the smaller-gauge needle, which increases dilution of the agent, and the belief that smaller-gauge needles minimize the risk of mechanical phlebitis. The slower rate of infusion from a small-gauge needle may decrease nausea and vomiting as well.

Drug Sequencing

- Arguments favoring administering a vesicant first cite decreases in vascular integrity over time, greater venous stability and less irritability at start of treatment, better chance for accuracy in assessing venous patency initially, and more acute patient awareness of symptomatic changes with first infusion.
- Arguments favoring administering a vesicant last cite the caustic properties of vesicants, which may increase venous fragility, potential for venous spasm at the beginning of bolus (IV push) therapy, and the benefits of receiving nonirritating drugs if an extravasation occurs.

> **Side-Arm Versus Direct Push Administration**
>
> - Arguments favoring side-arm administration cite the maximum dilution of potentially irritating drugs from freely running IV lines, ability readily to interrupt the infusion while maintaining venous access, and greater control over administration rate and amount of pressure.
> - Arguments favoring direct push administration cite the ease of assessing venous integrity and detecting signs of extravasation earlier.

■ COMPLICATIONS OF CHEMOTHERAPY

Regardless of the nurse's skills and standards, sometimes patients experience problems unique to the administration of cytotoxic agents. A common reason for the problems is the condition of the veins. Elderly, poorly nourished, and debilitated patients often have fragile veins. Unskilled nurses may unwittingly cause painful and unsightly hematomas that eliminate use of the treatment area until reabsorption is complete. Nurses should attempt to catheterize fragile veins with a loose tourniquet or with no tourniquet because distention and rapid engorgement may cause the vein wall to rupture when the tourniquet is released.

A second nurse may apply gentle hand pressure directly above the venipuncture site to distend it. Other distention techniques include application of moderate heat or asking the patient to clench or pump the fist. Gravity flow may be maximized if the patient dangles the extremity. The nurse may lightly finger-tap the site to distend the vein. Catheter gauge and length should be part of the decision process. A central line should also be a consideration. Regardless of the chosen technique, fragile veins require a cautious approach, allowing ample time to prepare for successful venipuncture on the first attempt.

Localized Acute Allergic Reactions

The nurse should be prepared for allergic reactions whenever any cytotoxic agent is administered IV. Localized allergic reactions, known as *flares*, often are associated with administration of doxorubicin hydrochloride. The first manifestation may be erythema along the venous pathways. Blotchiness, hive-like urticaria, or the rapid appearance of welts also may occur. The patient may report itchiness, stinging, or an increasing sensation of heat in the area. Some think the reaction is caused by intercellular release of histamines, which increases permeability of cell membranes. This permeability may allow drugs to leak into subcutaneous tissues. Other possibilities include drug interactions, contaminants, or molecular extravasation through vascular endothelium. Preventive measures include additional drug dilution, either by adding the drug to 100 to 200 mL solution or by administering the drug piggyback. Table 19–6 discusses some common preventive and administration tech-

text continues on page 527

T A B L E 1 9 – 6
EXTRAVASATION OF VESICANT ANTINEOPLASTIC AGENTS: PREVENTIVE STRATEGIES

Risk Factor	Preventive Strategy	Rationale
Skill of the Practitioner	Chemotherapy administration is done only by registered nurses who are specifically trained and supervised.	Procedures for management of extravasation vary according to the drug infiltrated.
		Certain drugs (streptozocin or BCNU) may cause a burning sensation during infusion, which is normal. However, it is abnormal and indicative of a problem if burning occurs during infusion of drugs such as doxorubicin and mitomycin.
	No attempts are made by practitioner to do procedures beyond his or her expertise.	
	Practitioners are skillful in venipuncture.	Procedures change rapidly. Techniques need to be learned and mastered before assuming responsibility for administration of chemotherapy.
	Practitioners are knowledgeable of the signs and symptoms of extravasation and drug therapy.	
	Practice is based on institutional policies and procedures that are routinely updated to meet the changing standards and methods of practice.	The definition of customary care in the community helps dictate standard of practice.
Condition of the Veins Small fragile veins Access limited owing to axillary surgery, vein thrombosis, prior extravasation Long-term drug therapy Multiple vein punctures	Use conventional methods for venous distention such as heat and percussion.	Risk of vesicant drug seepage exists with repeated venipuncture.
	Assess all available arm veins. Assess veins in a methodical fashion, taking time to select the most appropriate vein.	Multiple vein injections lead to thrombosis and limited availability.
	If practitioners do not feel confident in their ability to catheterize a person's veins successfully, they should seek the assistance of a colleague.	
	After attempting one or two injections without success, the practitioner should seek the assistance of a colleague before trying again.	
	A patient who consistently needs two or more attempts to secure venous access should be considered a candidate for a VAD.	Before the advent of vascular access devices (VADs), multiple venous injections to administer a drug might have been accepted as the only method of drug administration. This is no longer the case. Instead, treatment should be delayed until a VAD can be placed.
	The time to place a VAD is before an extravasation, not after.	
		Most VADs can be used immediately or within 24–48 h, so delay in drug therapy is not usually an issue.

(continued)

T A B L E   1 9 – 6 *(Continued)*

Risk Factor	Preventive Strategy	Rationale
Drug Administration Technique	Vesicant agents are never given as continuous infusions into a peripheral vein.	The risk of infiltration of a vesicant from a peripheral vein infusion is great owing to the following:
		Blood return is not assessed frequently.
		The longer the infusion, the greater the possibility of needle dislodgment.
		The patient can move the extremity, which could dislodge the IV catheter.
		Even a small amount of vesicant can cause tissue damage.
		Infiltration can be subtle and difficult to detect until a large volume has infiltrated.
		The patient may be sedated from an antiemetic and be unable to report sensations associated with extravasation.
	If peripheral line is on a controlled infusion pump, disconnect pump before injection of chemotherapy.	The pump forces drug into the tissues.
	When a vesicant is to be given as a continuous injection, the drug should be infused through an external-based central venous catheter whenever possible.	When an implanted port already exists, the patient is taught to check the needle three times a day to ensure placement during continuous infusion of a vesicant.
		The incidence of vesicant drug extravasation from ports used for continuous infusion is well documented and presents a risk to be avoided, if possible.
	Vesicant agents are most commonly administered using the two-syringe technique or through the side port of a free-flowing peripheral IV line.	The two-syringe technique allows for proper assessment of blood flow and resistance in the vein.
		A scalp vein needle causes minimal vein irritation.
	Two-Syringe Technique	
	Select an appropriate vein.	
	Begin a new IV line using scalp vein needle (25- or 23-gauge).	
	Access vein using a single approach.	A subtle leak can be caused by accidentally piercing the vein before accessing it; avoid searching for a vein with repeated approaches.
	Flush line with 8–10 mL saline. Assess for brisk, full blood return and any evidence of infiltration. Check for swelling at the site, redness or pain, and lack of blood return.	
	Once access is ensured, switch to syringe of chemotherapy.	

Risk Factor	Preventive Strategy	Rationale
	Dilute drugs according to the package insert.	Increasing the diluent increases the time it takes to administer the drug, thus increasing risk of infiltration.
	Inject drugs slowly and with minimal resistance.	The speed of the injection is determined by the resistance in the vein. Resistance varies depending on the size of the needle used.
	Assess for blood return every 1–2 mL infusion.	
	Flush with 3–5 mL of saline between each drug and 8–10 mL at the completion of the influsion of the drug or drugs.	
	Side-arm Technique	The rationale for the side-arm technique is the added dilution of the drug by the continuous drip of the IV fluid.
	Ensure proper venous access site. The IV fluid should be additive free.	
	Catheter used to access the vein should be at least a 20 gauge to ensure an adequate blood return and fluid flow.	Common pitfalls:
	Secure catheter but do not obstruct entrance site.	Not using a large enough catheter for a brisk infusion of infusate.
	Pinch off tubing and assess for blood return.	Vesicant backs up into IV line.
	Test the vein with 50–100 mL to ensure an adequate and swift drip of infusion.	IV line has to be pinched off to inject vesicant, which defeats the purpose.
	With IV fluid continuing to drip, slowly inject vesicant into IV line.	Clinician tends to take eyes off of the site of drug infusion to watch fluid drip more than with two-syringe technique.
	Do not allow vesicant to flow backward.	
	Do not pinch off tubing except to assess for blood return.	
	Assess for blood return every 1–2 mL injection.	
	Flush scalp-vein needle with saline at the completion of injection.	
Order of Vesicant Drug Administration (*Note:* Sequencing is probably unimportant. The most critical issue is adequately testing the vein with saline [8–10 mL] before administering any drug [vesicant or nonvesicant]).	Give vesicant first.	Vascular integrity decreases over time. Practitioner's assessment skills are most acute initially. Patient may be more sedated from antiemetic and less able to report changes in sensation at infusion site as time goes on.
	Give vesicant between two nonvesicants.	Chemotherapy is irritating to the veins. Nonvesicants are presumed to be less irritating than vesicants.

(*continued*)

T A B L E 1 9 – 6 (Continued)

Risk Factor	Preventive Strategy	Rationale
	Give vesicant last.	Because venous spasm occurs early during the injection, it is less likely to be confused with pain of extravasation if vesicant is given last.
		It is assumed that because the vein tolerated the nonvesticants, it will also tolerate the vesicant.
Site of Venous Access: Choosing the Best Vein	VADs, including tunneled catheters, implanted ports, and nontunneled central venous catheters, are indicated when patients have small, frail veins and are in need of long-term indefinite chemotherapy, continuous infusion of vesicant drugs, or both.	VADs are important options for patients with poor venous access. Externally based catheters are ideal for continuous infusion of vesicant chemotherapeutic agents because the risk of extravasation is very minimal.
	Although a VAD is a good way to prevent extravasation, it is not indicated just because someone is receiving a vesicant drug.	Expert technique and a knowledgeable clinician are the most cost-effective and safe means of administering vesicant drugs.
	Peripheral access is optimal in the large veins of the forearm, especially the posterior basilic vein. After these, the metacarpal veins of the dorsum of the hand are easy to access and stabilize. The veins over the wrist are risky because of potential damage to tendons and nerves should extravasation occur.	Veins in the forearm are large and adequately supporting by surrounding tissue. Adequate tissue exists around veins to provide coverage and promote healing should a problem occur.
	Note: A large, straight vein over the dorsum of the hand is preferable to a smaller vein of the forearm.	
	The antecubital fossa is to be avoided for vesicant drug administration.	The area is dense with tendons and nerves. Seepage of a vesicant can be subtle and go unnoticed. Damage here can result in loss of structure and function.
	If the antecubital fossa appears to be the only vein available for access, the patient needs an access device.	
	Hold chemotherapy—insert VAD.	Risking extravasation and subsequent tissue damage is not worth the temptation to give "just one more treatment" before considering other options.
		There is no evidence that delayed chemotherapy for 24 h in selected cases is detrimental to the overall outcome.
	Avoid administering chemotherapy in lower extremities.	Risk for thrombosis is increased when chemotherapy is given in lower extremities.

Risk Factor	Preventive Strategy	Rationale
Using a Pre-existing IV Line	Do not use a pre-existing peripheral IV line if any of the following are true: The IV catheter was placed more than 12 h earlier. The site is reddened, swollen, or sore, or there is evidence of infiltration. The site is over or around the wrist. Evidence of blood return is sluggish or absent. IV fluid runs erratically and the IV seems positional. If the IV fluid runs freely, the blood return is brisk and consistent, and the site is without redness, pain, or swelling, then there is no reason to inflict unnecessary pain by injecting the patient again.	It is unreasonable to disregard the potential for a perfectly adequate venous access line because it was not started by the person administering the vesicant drug. Our ability to assess the vein and evidence of blood return should be adequate to ensure the practitioner of an adequate and safe venous access.
	Prior dressings must be carefully removed over the catheter insertion site to fully visualize the vein during injection of the vesicant agent.	Dressings and tape can severely impede, both visually and tactilely, an assessment for an extravasation.

(From McCorkle, R., Grant, M., Frank-Stromborg, M., & Baird, S.B. [1996]. *Cancer nursing: A comprehensive textbook* (2nd ed.). Philadelphia: W.B. Saunders.)

niques. The nurse should always consult and follow the manufacturer's recommendations.

To prevent chemical cellulitis, many practitioners discontinue treatment when a localized allergic reaction occurs. Before removing the IV needle, additional drug-free fluid is infused to limit and resolve erythematous reactions. The following medications can be used to treat localized sensitivity reaction (all drugs require a physician's order before they are infused):

- Hydrocortisone sodium succinate (Solu-Cortef), slow IV push, 25 to 50 mg; anti-inflammatory agent
- Diphenhydramine (Benadryl) IV push, 25 to 50 mg; antihistamine

Venous Spasm

Some cytotoxic agents are known to produce pain or spasm along the venous pathway. Carmustine (BCNU) is diluted with absolute alcohol, which may be the offending agent. The breakdown products from the photodegradation of dacarbazine (DTIC) may be responsible for acute local burning associated with the drug's use. Mechlorethamine hydrochloride (Mustargen) also can cause pain, especially in patients who have been treated chemotherapeutically over extended times.

SAFE PRACTICE ALERT Although there are many special cautions for special drugs, it is important to remember that any agent can cause venous pain, in any patient, at any time.

Venous pain and spasm also can result from bolus (IV push) pressure too forceful for a small-gauge needle. Venous pain and spasm can be alleviated with these measures:

- Slowing the drug infusion rate
- Diluting the antineoplastic agent
- Applying warm or cool arm compresses during infusion. Some patients respond better to cool compresses, some to warm. Care must be taken to avoid second-degree burns.
- Administering lidocaine 1% (0.25 mL, 3 mL total), as needed. Patient allergy history and physician order are required before administration.

Phlebitis

The risk for chemical phlebitis exists with most IV cancer chemotherapy agents, but the risk increases when two or more antineoplastics are combined. Early phlebitis can be associated with pain, erythema, occasional limb edema, and a sensation of warmth in the affected extremity. As acute symptoms subside, venous pathways may retain dark-bluish to brown discoloration for some time, while arm use is restricted. Acute phlebitis reactions can interrupt sleep patterns and interfere with a patient's routine living activities.

Noninvestigational drugs associated with phlebitis include actinomycin, carmustine, cisplatin, dacarbazine, daunorubicin, doxorubicin hydrochloride, mechlorethamine hydrochloride, mitomycin C, streptozocin, vinblastine, and vincristine.

Nurses must exercise utmost caution to prevent phlebitis because some treatment regimens may be terminated if phlebitic reactions occur. When a time-sensitive and aggressive treatment program must be suspended until treatment sites are healed, the patient's long-term disease control may be jeopardized. Sometimes it is possible to substitute nonsclerosing agents from the same drug category as the offending agent. Occasionally a patient with history of phlebitic treatment sites manifests reactions to any IV drug administration. Evaluate the patient to determine if he or she is a candidate for a central line. To diminish the threat of phlebitis, the nurse may implement various preventive measures, including the following:

- Administering hydrocortisone sodium succinate (Solu-Cortef), 25 to 50 mg, slow IV push. After ensuring vein patency, the nurse may administer half the dose before antineoplastic administration and the other half after the final flush, immediately before the needle is removed. A physician's order is required before this drug can be administered.
- Reducing the concentration of the cytotoxic agent with further dilution.

Repetitive needle insertions for blood sampling and antineoplastic administrations increase the likelihood of both phlebitis and thrombosis. In fact, phlebitis develops in some patients despite the most meticulous clinical efforts to avoid it. Once phlebitis has occurred, elevation of the affected extremity, application of topical heat, and administration of systemic analgesics may be indicated.

A patient's venous status should be assessed carefully before chemotherapy is administered. If veins are deep and difficult to visualize and palpate with tourniquet distention, if peripheral veins are extraordinarily small, or if the proposed treatment plan is long, a central venous access device should be considered.

Generalized Anaphylactic Reaction

A nurse should be prepared for anaphylactic reaction at any time, with any drug, in any patient. Before initiating any treatment, the nurse should be aware of the institution's policies regarding emergencies arising from administration of cytotoxic agents and the location of emergency supplies and equipment. Administration of investigational drugs must be approved by the institution's pharmacy and therapeutics committees and Institutional Review Board.

To prepare for the possibility of anaphylaxis, the nurse should be vigilant for any signs of flushing, sudden agitation or anxiety, nausea, vomiting, urticaria, hypotension, generalized pruritus, respiratory distress, wheezing, coughing, shortness of breath, or asthma-type reaction. Failure to respond appropriately can result in a generalized anaphylactic reaction, seizures, or cardiopulmonary arrest.

Before therapy begins, the nurse should position the patient in a reclining position that eases management of an anaphylactic event. If the patient is seated at a table not adjacent to a bed, anaphylaxis is more difficult to handle. An emergency cart with all appropriate medications, plus stethoscope and sphygmomanometer (see Table 19–4), also should be available.

The procedures of some facilities call for a "standing order" sheet to be signed by the responsible physician before treatment. This time-saving and prudent procedure allows the nurse to begin emergency treatment even before the physician arrives. In addition, the nurse needs to record a baseline blood pressure reading before treatment. If a patient normally is hypotensive, a normal blood pressure reading is useful in case shock symptoms occur. The same is true for a baseline reference point of the patient's mental status. Particularly with metastatic brain disease or other mental alterations, early symptoms of anaphylaxis—agitation, anxiety, speech disorders, and mental confusion—can be misleading without a clear picture of the patient's pretreatment mental state.

Regardless of whether a patient displays a mild reaction (eg, generalized pruritus) or sustains complete cardiovascular collapse, the nurse should be prepared to:

- Recline the patient smoothly, safely and quickly
- Administer basic cardiopulmonary resuscitative measures
- Maintain a patent IV line for emergency drug administration
- Provide calm reassurance
- Administer appropriate drugs, as ordered
- Monitor the patient until the reaction subsides

Anaphylaxis prevention is an important goal in administration of any cancer chemotherapy. Nevertheless, the nurse must be aware of which agents are associated with anaphylaxis and prepared to administer those agents as recommended in product brochures:

- Bleomycin sulfate (Blenoxane). Package insert recommends treatment with 2 U or less, with the first two doses as test doses.
- Cisplatin (Platinol). No specific recommendations for dose attenuation or treatment duration. Product brochure lists suggestions for symptom management.
- Asparaginase (Elspar). Before the first dose of Elspar, before retreatment of any patient manifesting positive reactors, and after careful assessment of hypersensitivity risk, the nurse should consider performing desensitization.

Even though a physician may have ascertained an allergy history, the nurse should solicit and chart the same information. When the potential exists for anaphylactic reaction, these precautionary measures might be useful:

- Test dosing
- Pretreatment with antihistamines, steroids, or antiinflammatory or antipyretic agents
- Uninterrupted dosing to preclude significant reactive antibody buildup

Extravasation

Controversies surround appropriate treatment of local infiltrations of chemotherapy agents. No treatments show well-documented efficacy. Controlled clinical trials are lacking because of the low number of accruable patients treated by skilled nurses and because of ethical issues associated with a control or "no-treatment" arm. In fact, it often is difficult to ascertain that an infiltration actually has occurred. Table 19–7 outlines venous reactions compared with actual extravasations. Obviously, skilled nurses do not allow infiltration of sclerosing agents to continue to any obvious point. Therefore, there is a real ethical and moral question about involving a patient in "intentional" extravasation research. Because extravasation has a particularly morbid effect on tissue, most extravasation studies on animals use doxorubicin hydrochloride (Adriamycin). Some consequences of extensive tissue necrosis (Fig. 19–8) include the following:

- *Pain.* Extensive necrotic areas often require narcotic analgesics to relieve pain.
- *Physical defects.* Necrosis may preclude a patient from work for indefinite periods. If a patient's job requires full range of motion, permanent functional compromise may severely impinge on quality of life and activities of daily living. Moreover, the cosmetic defect may result in severe emotional impact.

T A B L E   1 9 – 7
NURSING ASSESSMENT OF EXTRAVASATION VERSUS OTHER REACTIONS

Assessment Parameter	Extravasation		Irritation of the Vein	Flare Reaction
	Intermediate Manifestations of Extravasation	Delayed Manifestations of Extravasation		
Pain	Severe pain or burning lasting minutes or hours, eventually subsiding; usually occurs while the drug is given and around needle site	48 h	Aching and tightness along the vein	No pain
Redness	Blotchy redness around needle site, not always present at time of extravasation	Later occurrence	The full length of the vein may be reddened or darkened	Immediate blotches or streaks along vein, usually subsides within 30 min with or without treatment.
Ulceration	Develops insidiously, usually 48–96 h later	Later occurrence	Not usually	Not usually
Swelling	Severe swelling usually occurs immediately	48 h	Not likely	Not likely; wheals may appear along vein line
Blood return	Inability to obtain blood return	Good blood return during drug administration	Usually	Usually
Other	Change in the quality of infusion	Local tingling, sensory deficits	—	Urticaria

- *Medical expense.* Multiple or lengthy hospitalizations or costly plastic surgeries may pose economic challenges. The effects of extravasation may require additional healing time, or secondary medical problems may occur.
- *Disease control.* Valuable time may be lost if a patient cannot sustain scheduled chemotherapy treatments to control disease. Myelosuppression from previous cancer treatments may promote secondary infection of the necrotic area, postponing treatment even further.
- *Time.* Patients with home, work, or school responsibilities may be kept from "normal life" until healing is complete. Income suspension poses additional financial hardship to the patient and family.
- *Psychological impact on nurse and patient.* The extravasation incident and its aftermath may strain trust and communication between the patient and nurse.

Prevention

Of course, years of experience in treating patients with antineoplastic drugs perfects the nurse's technique and is a good patient safeguard. It is important to keep in mind, however, that extravasation of tissue-necrosing agents can occur despite the

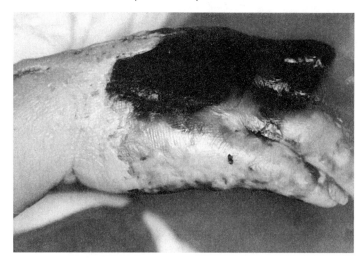

Figure 19–8. Extensive tissue necrosis following vesicant therapy. (Courtesy of Sharon Weinstein, CRNI, MS.)

nurse's skill. The nurse's focus should be on perfecting safe IV technique and implementing prudent preparation measures should an extravasation occur (Table 19–8). Although there are no guarantees, the nurse can be reasonably confident that the impact of extravasation can be minimized with early detection and treatment. Details are outlined in Procedure 19–1.

T A B L E   1 9 – 8
RECOMMENDED ANTIDOTES FOR VESICANT/IRRITANT DRUGS

Chemotherapeutic Agent	Antidote		Antidote Preparation
	Pharmacologic	Nonpharmacologic	
Mechlorethamine nitrogen mustard (Mustargen)	Isotonic sodium thiosulfate	Cold compresses	Mix 4 mL 10% Na thiosulfate with 6 mL sterile H_2O for injection. (⅙ molar solution results.) If using Na thiosulfate 25%, mix 1.6 mL with 8.4 mL sterile H_2O for ⅙ molar solution.
Vincristine (Oncovin) Vinblastine (Velban) Vindesine (Eldisine) Teniposide (VH-26) Etoposide (VP-16)	Hyaluronidase (Wydase)	Warm compresses	Mix with 1 mL NaCl (150 U/mL)
Cisplatin (Platinol) *Note:* Large extravasations of concentrated solutions produce tissue necrosis.	Isotonic sodium thiosulfate		Mix 4 mL of 10% Na thiosulfate with 6 mL sterile H_2O for injection. (⅙ molar solution results.) If using Na thiosulfate 25%, mix 1.6 mL with 8.4 mL sterile H_2O for ⅙ molar solution.

SQ, subcutaneous.
(From Oncology Nursing Society [1999]. *Cancer chemotherapy guidelines: Recommendations for the management of vesicant extravasation, hypersensitivity and anaphylaxis.* Pittsburgh: Author.)

Patient Education

The patient must be informed of possible consequences when chemotherapeutic agents are administered so that informed consent is comprehensive and legitimate. A sensitive nurse conveys the risks in such a way that the patient can react to the information appropriately and without unnecessary fear.

Constant nurse attendance is required by patients who are irrational, unconscious, or in some way unable to perceive or report early signs of extravasation. Alert and cooperative patients may report stinging, burning, and pain or an unusual sensation at the catheter insertion site. Nevertheless, extravasation can occur even without perceptible symptoms.

General Extravasation Precautions

When administering any antineoplastic drug, nurses should be prepared for potential extravasation, have antidotes available, ensure venous patency, anticipate insidious infiltration, and monitor the patient.

BEING PREPARED FOR EXTRAVASATION

Before any treatment, the nurse should be familiar with the agents known to produce tissue necrosis (see Table 19–3) and anticipate the possibility of extravasation. A chart of vesicants and their recommended antidotes and use of hot or cold compresses should be posted in a convenient place, and antidotes kept readily available for ad-

Method of Administration	Comments
• Inject 1–4 (⅙ molar) through existing IV catheter • Inject SQ if needle removed.	• Na thiosulfate neutralizes mechlorethamine. • Initiate treatment immediately. • Avoid multiple injections of antidote. Irrigate area with single injection as effectively as possible.
• Inject 1–4 mL through existing IV line catheter. • Administer 1 mL for each milliliter extravasated. • Inject SQ if needle removed.	• Enhances absorption and dispersion of the extravasated drug. • Warm compresses increase systemic absorption of the drug.
• Inject 1–4 mL (⅙ molar) through existing IV line catheter. • Administer 1 mL for each milliliter extravasated. • Inject SQ if needle removed.	• Inactivates cisplatin on contact. • Treatment not recommended unless a large amount of a highly concentrated solution is extravasated.

Procedure 19–1

Treating Extravasation Associated With Vesicants

Equipment

  Infusion apparatus

  Normal saline solution

  Appropriate antidote

  Cold packs and heat packs as appropriate

Procedure	*Rationale*
Stop the infusion.	To prevent further drug leakage into the subcutaneous tissues
Aspirate back remaining drug in the needle and tubing by drawing back on the syringe.	To remove drug from tissue if possible
Administer suggested antidotes through current device per physician's order.	To extravasate the antidote intentionally by the same route to neutralize or bind the extravasated drug
Remove the needle.	The site can no longer be used as an IV route
Administer suggested antidotes subcutaneously with multiple punctures into the suspected extravasation site, if not administered by catheter.	Direct infiltration of the antidote into the area of greatest concentration
Elevate extremity before applying cooling or heat pack and topical antidotes.	To minimize swelling and surface (skin) inflammatory and erythematous reactions
Notify physician.	To obtain further advice and direction
Obtain a plastic surgery consult.	Early plastic surgery intervention with wound débridement decreases severity
Document extravasation in official patient record.	To enhance later recall and for legal purposes
Obtain photograph of site.	To document extravasation
Maintain contact with patient.	To follow symptomatology and ensure that appropriate interventions are initiated

ministration. A delay in antidote administration increases the severity of the local tissue reaction. If standing emergency orders are available, they should be signed by the responsible physician and placed in the patient's chart.

CONFIRMING VENOUS PATENCY

A flush of at least 5 to 10 mL normal saline solution may be infused to test venous patency and needle placement before administering cytotoxic agents. Administration should be postponed until the nurse confirms that fluids are flowing unimpeded into the vein. If an immediate second venipuncture is difficult or ill advised, the nurse may choose to infuse additional normal saline solution into the original site to prove the vein competent beyond doubt. Only then should the cytotoxic agent be administered. If for any reason the nurse suspects the agent is not infusing properly, administration should be interrupted and further assessment undertaken. It is logical that the greater the extravasation volume, the more severe the local tissue destruction. When in doubt, the infusion should be stopped.

ANTICIPATING INFILTRATION

The nurse always must be alert to signs of slow leak or insidious infiltration. If the needle punctures the vein's posterior wall, chemotherapeutic agents can leak into deep subcutaneous tissues. If small-gauge needles are used, particularly when there is large volume of subcutaneous fat, infiltration is more difficult to detect. This risk underscores the need for early comparison and assessment of the venipuncture site and immediate surrounding skin.

MAINTAINING VIGILANT MONITORING

Drug and blood flow rates should be monitored frequently. When administering agents with the bolus (IV push) technique, the nurse should pull back on the syringe's plunger approximately 3 to 4 mL to check blood backflow. Although a good blood return does not always guarantee that extravasation has not occurred, any changes in blood backflow should be investigated promptly. It may be necessary to adjust and reposition the needle if the bevel is resting against the vein wall.

Because infiltration is the most frequent complication of IV therapy, it is prudent to make observations every 2 to 3 minutes, particularly when vesicants are infused. The requirements for nursing vigilance when infusing vesicants pose special problems for nurses in inpatient units because the needs of patients in other rooms often preclude adherence to the 2- to 3-minute monitoring requirement for vesicant infusion. The policies of some facilities do not permit vesicant administration with mechanical infusion devices or without constant attendance by a nurse.

COMMUNICATING EFFECTIVELY

Replacement nurses should have thorough, patient-centered orientation. If it is even remotely possible, a replacement nurse should be on the job, working alongside the predecessor nurse, ideally until he or she is entirely familiar with the medical regimen in place. To gain baseline pretreatment reference points for each patient, a successor nurse should have an opportunity to review and examine IV sites; check for venous patency; and review charts, histories, drugs, and infusion rates. This opportunity offers enormous psychological benefits for nurses and patients alike and helps ensure that a consistent quality of care will be maintained.

ENSURING SAFE TREATMENT AND CARE

During vesicant infusion, a patient should remain in the treatment area. Nurses in inpatient units should ensure that no diagnostic studies or therapies are scheduled to take a patient with cancer off the unit during infusion of vesicants. If it is essential that the patient leave the treatment area, a saline solution should be substituted while the infusion of the cytotoxic agent is temporarily discontinued. Alternatively, the nurse may accompany the patient to supervise drug infusion while diagnostic or therapeutic interventions are conducted off the treatment unit.

MANAGING EXTRAVASATION

Some extravasations are difficult to detect in early stages. It bears repeating: if vesicant extravasation is suspected, it should be treated as a presumed extravasation. Box 19–9 and Procedure 19–1 offer general guidelines for treating vesicant extravasations. Common antidotes are listed in Table 19–8. Although medical opinions and experiences differ regarding management of extravasation, most agree that ice should be applied 15 to 30 minutes four times daily for most antineoplastic extravasations; the exceptions are the vinca alkaloids, which call for local heat application.

BOX 19–9 **Warm or Cold Treatment for Extravasation?**

Desired Effect of Heat

- To increase blood supply and increase the dispersal of the enzyme hyaluronidase (Wydase) into the subcutaneous tissues.
- To promote healing after the first 24 h by increasing blood supply.
- To enhance the absorption of the vesicant agent (theoretical effect of vasodilation).

Note: Practitioners who oppose the use of heat think that vesicant agents injure the cells' metabolic mechanisms. Heat increases metabolic demands and therefore may decrease cellular destruction.

Desired Effect of Cooling

- To decrease the blood supply and decrease the absorption of drugs into the subcutaneous tissues.
- To constrict peripheral veins, which decreases blood supply to the area and thereby minimizes localized pain.
- To decrease the absorption and diffusion of the vesicant agent, thereby resulting in local tissue "pooling" (theoretic effect of vasoconstriction).

Note: Proponents think that cooling decreases many enzymatic reactions and therefore decreases the destructive effect of released white blood cell components (eg, lysozymes). Cooling also slows cellular metabolic rates and may improve survival of marginally injured tissues.

Nurses should keep in mind that detailed charting of an extravasation should be completed as soon as possible after emergency needs have been met. This is important not only for medical and legal purposes; comprehensive documentation is important for any incident review activities. Litigation rarely reaches a court until several years after an event. Because a nurse-witness is permitted to review medical documents before testimony, records should be as complete and precise as possible. Documentation should include not only the facility's nursing record and chemotherapy exposure log (Fig. 19–9A), but the extravasation record (Fig. 19–9B) and an incident report. Elements of nursing documentation include

- Date and time
- Type and size of venous access needle used
- Insertion site
- Number and location of venipuncture attempts
- Drug(s) and drug administration sequence and administration technique
- Approximate volume of drug volume extravasated or suspected of extravasation
- Patient's statements, complaints, reports
- Nursing management of extravasation
- Photographic documentation
- Description of site
- Physician notified and time
- Plastic surgery consultation/notification, if indicated
- Follow-up instructions to patient and date for return visit
- Nurse's signature

■ MANAGEMENT OF SIDE EFFECTS

Side effects of chemotherapy can be divided into two categories: temporary and permanent. Temporary toxicities are those that affect rapidly dividing cells, whereas permanent toxicities result in organ damage.

Chemotherapy has a reputation for producing potentially unpleasant side effects, which many patients fear. Fortunately, many advances have been made in methods and materials for symptom management and nurses can convey this information to reassure the patients. Nurses also have a responsibility to be an advocate for their patients, to secure appropriate orders for medications to control or relieve side effects, and to be creative within the scope of practice.

Nausea and Vomiting

Nausea and vomiting are among the most common side effects of chemotherapy. For the patient, they are very distressing symptoms that significantly interfere with quality of life. More than 70% of all patients receiving chemotherapy report nausea and vomiting, although not all chemotherapies cause nausea and vomiting. Many chemotherapeutic agents have the potential for delayed and long-lasting nausea and vom-

Chemotherapy Exposure Log

A

Date	Drug	Amount	Nature of exposure	Action Taken

B

STANFORD UNIVERSITY HOSPITAL and CLINICS
Stanford Medical Center
Stanford, California 94305

CHEMOTHERAPY DRUG EXTRAVASATION RECORD

_____ Diagnosis _____ Drug and/or Drug Regimen

Injection Site

Home Phone No. _____

DATE: _____

Route of Administration
____I.V. Push
____Piggyback
____In Dilution amt. & sol.
____I.M. (location)
____Sub. Q. (location)
____Flush only
____Other

Needle Size
____Scalp Vein Butterfly
____ #25
____ #23
____ #21
____ #19
____Other

Condition of Veins
____Soft, Pliable
____Fragile, thin-walled
____Thready
____Hard, Knotty
____Other (Specify)

Cephalic Vein — Basilic Vein
Antecubical Space
Lateral / Medial
Upper / Upper
Forearm / Forearm
Lateral / Medial
Lower / Lower
Forearm / Forearm

Dorsal Metacarpal

Sequence of Drugs
1st drug _____
Amt/Name/Method of Flus

Approx. amt. Infiltrate
_____
_____

Concentration:
_____

Doctor Notified:
____Time of extravasation.
____Time M.D. called
____Time Responded

Appearance of Infiltration Site:
Describe:

Agents and Amt. Used
____SoluCortef 25 mg. (I.V. Push)
____Xylocaine 1% (I.V. Push)
____Wydase (S.Q.)
____Decadron LA
____Na Bicarb. (I.V. Push)
____Na Bicarb. (S.Q.)
____Na Thiosulfate (I.V. push/S.Q.)
____Other

Color and Dimension of Infiltration
Site:
Describe:

Nursing Assessment/Patient Comments:

Plan and Follow-up (Use reverse side if necessary):

Signature and Date

Figure 19–9. **(A)** Example of a chemotherapy exposure log. **(B)** Example of an extravasation record.

iting with onset after the patient leaves the infusion center. As a result, the patient's distress is not seen by the health care provider, and the true magnitude of the problem may not be realized. Uncontrolled nausea and vomiting can be life threatening. It may also result in nutritional deficits, decreased energy, and fluid and electrolyte imbalances. As a general rule, it is easier to control nausea than to stop vomiting.

Predisposing factors for nausea or vomiting include a history of motion sickness or morning sickness, or prior exposure to chemotherapy (either personal or a close friend or relation, which may produce an anticipatory response). Obtaining a history and eliciting what relieved the nausea and vomiting may be helpful in implementing strategies for nausea and vomiting control.

In many instances, a slower administration of chemotherapeutic agents reduces nausea and vomiting. Ideal pharmacologic intervention for nausea and vomiting controls the symptoms without contributing additional side effects. Antiemetics alone or in combination with other drugs have demonstrated effectiveness. Because ordering practices, drug combinations, and scheduling vary depending on the physician, there is no absolute method of control. Rather, trial and error may need to be used to find what is most effective for the patient.

Nonpharmacologic interventions not only provide nurses with latitude and an opportunity for creativity but give the patient a sense of control. Regulating the environment to eliminate strong food, perfume, and other odors helps reduce nausea. Soft music, low lights, quiet atmosphere, and relaxation tapes help reduce anxiety and hence nausea. Diversional activities such as cards, movie, or crafts take the patient's mind off the chemotherapy. Other helpful strategies include hypnosis, biofeedback, and acupressure or acupuncture.

Suggestions for dietary manipulation include serving foods cold or at room temperature, and bland foods rather than spicy, fried and fatty, strong-flavored, sour, or tart foods. Clear liquids, gelatin, juice, ginger ale or other carbonated drinks, herbal teas, and sport drinks may help settle the stomach, provide hydration, and furnish electrolytes. It is advisable to avoid fried and fatty foods and foods with strong odors.

Myelosuppression

To maximize the therapeutic benefit, chemotherapy is usually escalated until myelosuppression is achieved. Myelosuppression is the most common dose-limiting factor and can affect the intensity of therapy and the quality of life. All chemotherapy affects blood counts, but certain agents or doses can cause severe myelosuppression that is potentially life threatening. Death in myelosuppressed patients usually results from infection or bleeding.

Patient education is a critical component in managing myelosuppression. The patient needs to understand clearly that infection prevention and monitoring weekly blood counts are important factors in detecting problems early so that appropriate interventions can be instituted as soon as possible (Box 19–10). Risk factors for myelosuppression include age (eg, elderly patients with aplastic marrow), malignant bone marrow involvement, prior radiation to flat bones, and prior dose-intensive chemotherapy.

Leukopenia

Leukopenia predisposes the patient to infection, and patients who are at high risk for neutropenia are sometimes placed on prophylactic broad-spectrum antibiotics. An absolute granulocyte count of $500/mm^3$ or less places the patient at severe risk of infection, and broad-spectrum antibiotics are usually started within 12 hours of a significant drop in the blood count. Bone marrow involvement from the primary tumor burden or from metastatic disease may prolong myelosuppression.

An elevated temperature may be the only sign of infection in the neutropenic patient. Because use of antipyretics may mask infection, they should be used with caution. The colony-stimulating factors have been used to manage leukopenia by shortening the nadir, which facilitates timely chemotherapy treatments with fewer reductions in dose (Box 19–11).

Thrombocytopenia

Thrombocytopenia is a potential complication of chemotherapy. The normal platelet count ranges from 150,000 to $400,000/mm^3$. Bleeding precautions are instituted when the platelet count drops below $100,000/mm^3$, and frank bleeding occurs most frequently when the count is below $20,000/mm^3$.

The nurse must be alert for thrombocytopenia, signaled by bleeding gums, petechiae, nosebleeds, multiple bruises, reports of gastrointestinal bleeding, and a change in mentation, which may indicate central nervous system bleeding. Controversy exists in the medical community over whether to transfuse platelets only in cases of active bleeding, regardless of the platelet count.

The cause of anemia should be investigated to determine if it is induced by chemotherapy, is a result of malignant bone marrow involvement, or is a consequence of bleeding. The management of anemia is controversial. A unit of packed red blood cells raises the hemoglobin value by 1 g/dL. In the absence of acute bleeding, many physicians will not order a transfusion unless the patient is symptomatic, whereas others initiate a transfusion for a hemoglobin value of 8 g/dL or lower. Erythropoietin can be effective in stimulating red blood cell production, with elevation realized in 6 to 8 weeks of therapy.

Patients with anemia frequently are fatigued and should be encouraged to have frequent rest periods to allow for activity. A significant role for nurses is teaching the patient how to conserve energy and reduce fatigue. Some teaching points are listed in Box 19–10.

Anorexia and Taste Alterations

It is well documented that both cancer and chemotherapeutic agents can cause anorexia and changes in taste. This poses a problem for maintaining adequate nutrition. Familiar foods may taste entirely different and in some circumstances may even be perceived as unpleasant. Many patients complain of a bitter or metallic taste, particularly associated with red meats. The patient may be advised to experiment with

BOX 19–10 **Patient Education: Strategies for Managing Side Effects of Chemotherapy**

Infection Prevention

- Wash hands frequently, especially after using the toilet.
- Observe good personal hygiene.
- Practice good oral hygiene.
- Avoid sources of infection, such as crowds and sick people.
- Avoid vaginal and anal intercourse.
- Wash fresh raw fruits and vegetables before eating.
- Monitor temperature.

Bleeding Precautions

- Avoid *shaving with blade razors; use an* electric razor *instead.*
- *Report* bruises *that appear for no known reason.*
- *Avoid physically* hazardous *activity* and contact sports.
- Use caution near sharp objects.
- Avoid vaginal and anal intercourse.
- Be cautious with drugs, such as aspirin, known to cause thrombocytopenia or increase bleeding; consult health care practitioner before taking any unprescribed or over-the-counter preparations.

Fatigue Reduction

- Allow for rest periods.
- Plan activities after rest periods.
- Avoid strenuous activities.
- Allow family and friends to assist with tasks.
- Choose activities that do not require high energy output.

Strategies to Reduce Constipation

- Make sure to increase fluid intake to include 2 to 3 L daily.
- Encourage fruits, vegetables, and high-fiber foods.
- Avoid constipating foods.
- Obtain order for stool softener, laxative, or cathartic.

Strategies to Relieve Stomatitis and Mucositis

- Practice good oral hygiene.
- Keep lips moist.
- Drink adequate fluids.
- Choose soft foods with smooth consistency.
- Avoid spicy foods.
- Rinse mouth with baking soda, saline solution, or stomatitis cocktail.
- Avoid alcohol-based mouthwash.

BOX 19–11 **Chemotherapy Nadir**

The nadir, which is the lowest point of the white blood cell count (WBC), usually occurs 7 to 14 days from day 1 of chemotherapy. When the marrow starts to recover, there is an increase in the bands, which are immature segmented neutrophils. The absolute neutrophil count (ANC) consists of both mature and immature neutrophils. The WBC includes all the white blood cells (eosinophils, basophils, and lymphocytes).

The following equation is used to calculate the ANC:

Segs (*segmented neutrophils*) + bands (*banded neutrophils*) × WBC = ANC

Example: (segs) 33 + (bands) 18 × (WBC) 2200 = 1122 ANC

---

different spices and flavorings to stimulate the taste buds that have been affected by the chemotherapy. Many patients report an exaggerated sensation of sweetness, which may increase. As a general rule, most patients find that cold, rather than hot, foods taste better. Eating small meals frequently may help the patient take in more total calories than eating larger but fewer meals.

Dealing with anorexia and taste alterations is an area in which patient and family education can have a positive impact on patient outcomes. Suggestions should include serving food on glass dishes rather than plastic to help control odors. The use of plastic utensils is helpful for patients who report a metallic taste sensation from silverware. Good oral hygiene and rinsing with nonirritating mouthwash is a must, especially before meals.

Xerostomia may occur in patients who are taking antiemetics or who have had radiation to the head and neck. For these patients, frequent mouth washing and chewing gum or hard candy can be helpful, and soft, moist foods are more pleasing to the palate.

When all of the usual interventions are unsuccessful, nutritional needs are usually met with supplements, such as liquid protein drinks or protein powder added to food; depending on severity of symptoms, enteral or parenteral nutrition may be added to the treatment plan (DeVita et al., 2000; Groenwald et al., 2000; Itano & Taoka, 1998; Murphy et al., 2000; Wilkes, Ingwersen, & Burk, 1997–1998).

Constipation

A patient is considered constipated when evacuation does not occur for 96 hours or when hard, dry stool causes difficulty in defecation. Because individual bowel patterns vary, it is helpful to know the patient's usual habits. Medications (including chemotherapy), anxiety, depression, hypercalcemia, immobility, dehydration, and tumor involvement resulting in intrinsic or extrinsic compression can contribute to constipation.

Intervention depends on the underlying etiology. Prophylactic laxatives, lubricants, and cathartics may help move waste through the intestinal system. Enemas should be used with caution because they can be irritating to mucous membranes and cause microscopic tears. There is a potential for bleeding in the presence of thrombocytopenia, as well as a potential for infection. Impaction is best handled with an oil retention or phosphate enema to hydrate the stool.

Teaching patients to adopt various dietary habits, such as increasing intake of fresh fruits and vegetables and fiber, may help treat and prevent constipation. Adequate fluid intake of 2 to 3 L daily is recommended. It is wise to avoid constipating foods such as cheeses, eggs, refined starches, and chocolate. Physical activity and exercise also help stimulate peristalsis. For additional strategies, see Box 19–10.

Diarrhea

It is the function of the colon to absorb fluid. When this does not happen diarrhea is the result. Diarrhea in the oncology patient can have a number of causes. Surgical procedures, such as gastric or intestinal resection, can result in a shortened tract or a malabsorption syndrome. Inflammatory bowel syndrome or *Clostridium difficile* and other intestinal infections can also cause of diarrhea, as can cancer-related chemotherapy, radiation therapy, and biologic treatments.

The nurse needs to know the degree of diarrhea so that fluid and electrolyte imbalances can be prevented or treated. Accurate intake and output measurement and the number of loose or watery stools provide valuable information for fluid replacement strategies. The major electrolyte lost with diarrhea is potassium. Therefore, potassium-rich foods should be encouraged and fluid intake should consist of at least 2 L daily. In cases of severe diarrhea, IV therapy may be initiated. Pharmacologic intervention should be started as soon as possible.

Alopecia

Not all chemotherapy causes hair loss, but most chemotherapy may cause some thinning of the hair. Many patients, especially women, have difficulty dealing with this side effect. The hair loss from chemotherapy is temporary, but for patients receiving radiation to the head, the hair loss may be permanent. Hair loss usually occurs between the second and third chemotherapy treatment. Through the years, devices involving ice caps or tourniquet have been used to reduce blood flow to the scalp, but results are mixed. Caution needs to be taken especially when the patient has disease involving the skin or metastatic lesions to the bone. Reducing the blood flow to these areas of the head gives sanctuary for cancer cells.

The patient needs to learn how to minimize trauma to the hair. Mild shampoo and gentle combing and brushing decrease breakage. Short hair is easier to manage and avoids a pulling effect present with long hair. Harsh chemicals, such as hair dyes, and devices, such as curling irons and hair dryers, should be avoided.

Once the hair falls out, lotion or moisturizer can be used on the scalp unless the patient is also receiving radiation to the area of the head. The scalp needs to be protected to avoid burns from sun and to prevent heat loss in cold weather. Wigs, scarves, and turbans can be worn.

Stomatitis and Mucositis

Other side effects of chemotherapy are stomatitis and mucositis. The mucous membranes of the gastrointestinal tract can become red, irritated, and inflamed. Chemotherapy-induced stomatitis usually begins 5 to 7 days after treatment and lasts for approximately 10 days. The patient may experience mild irritation and sensitivity to acidic or spicy foods, or painful lesions and difficulty swallowing. The specific drug, dose, and patient risk factors determine the degree of stomatitis. The nurse should be concerned about patients who have had head and neck radiation or who are receiving steroidal therapy. Patients who are nutritionally compromised and those with high oral flora due to poor dental hygiene are also at an increased risk.

Preventive measures include meticulous attention to the oral cavity with a soft toothbrush to prevent irritating delicate tissue. Commercial mouthwashes containing alcohol should be avoided because they can burn the mucous membranes. Application of balm, aloe vera, or a petroleum-based gel to lips prevents cracking and drying. Use of ice chips 5 minutes before and 30 minutes after the administration of chemotherapy reduces blood flow to the mouth and therefore limits the amount of chemotherapy agents reaching the mucous membranes. Patients with a tumor in the oral area should not use ice. Prophylactic mouthwashes containing allopurinol for patients receiving 5-FU or FUDR, or leucovorin for patients receiving methotrexate, are helpful in preventing stomatitis.

Mouthwashes containing baking soda or saline solution may soothe the irritated mucous membranes. In addition, several stomatitis cocktail formulas are available. Most contain diphenhydramine (Benadryl), antacid, and a local anesthetic with or without an antifungal agent. Soft foods with a smooth consistency and cold, wet foods are more soothing to irritated mucous membranes (see Box 19–10).

Cardiotoxicity

Cardiotoxicity can be seen with anthracycline therapy, especially Doxorubicin (Adriamycin). Paclitaxel (Taxol), mitoxantrone (Novantrone), idarubicin (Idamycin), cyclophosphamide (Cytoxan), 5-FU, and FUDR also are associated with cardiotoxicity. When doxorubicin is given before cyclophosphamide, the potential for cardiotoxicity tends to increase, particularly in bone marrow transplant recipients receiving high-dose cyclophosphamide.

Patients receiving potentially cardiotoxic drugs should have a baseline multiple-gated acquisition scan or echocardiogram and periodic follow-up testing so the ejection fraction can be tracked. Serial electrocardiograms are also helpful. Early electrocardiographic changes may show a decrease in voltage of the QRS complex or nonspecific ST segment and T-wave changes. The damage to the cardiac muscle results in decreased cardiac output with shortness of breath, nonproductive cough, and progression to congestive heart failure.

Patients at greatest risk for development of cardiotoxicity are older adults with a history of hypertension, arteriosclerotic heart disease, or other coronary artery disease. Other contributing factors include prior radiation to the mediastinum or chest wall and a lifetime cumulative dose of doxorubicin exceeding a range of 500 to 550 mg/m^2. Studies shown that cardiac damage can be decreased by administering doxorubicin by infusion rather than IV push.

Zincard (Dexrazozane) is a recently approved drug that acts as a cardioprotective agent for anthrocycline-induced cardiotoxicity. This drug was originally developed as an antiproliferative agent but was recognized for its cardioprotective properties. Zincard, an intercellular chelating agent chemically related to ethylenediamine tetra-acetic acid (EDTA), binds to iron before doxorubicin can and in turn prevents the formation of free oxygen radicals, thereby preventing cardiotoxicity. Zincard is indicated for patients who have prior doxorubicin exposure of at least 300 mg/m^2 and who need to continue with doxorubicin therapy (DeVita et al., 2000; Groenwald et al., 2000; Itano & Taoka, 1998; Murphy et al., 2000; Wilkes et al., 1997–1998).

Neurotoxicity

Many of the plant alkaloids are neurotoxic. They affect the central or peripheral nervous system, or both. Central nervous system toxicity can be manifest as acute or chronic encephalopathies. Peripheral nerve toxicity is indicated by patient complaints of numbness and tingling of hands and feet, muscle pain, weakness, and disturbances in depth perception, particularly with ambulation. Clinically, deep tendon reflexes disappear. The decreased perception and sensation that the patient experiences can result in accidents. Constipation with or without a paralytic ileus is another problem related to neurotoxicity, especially from the vinca alkaloids.

The first signs of neurotoxicity usually are seen after five or more treatments with a neurotoxic drug. Paclitaxel (Taxol), however, can produce paresthesia within 5 days of administration. When cisplatin (Platinol) is used concurrently with paclitaxel, the potential for neurotoxicity increases. It is recommended that paclitaxel be administered before cisplatin to reduce the potential of toxicity.

Amafostine (Ethyol), which was originally studied as an antidote to biologic warfare agents, was found to confer increased resistance to ionizing radiation and is considered protective against bone marrow toxicity from the alkylating agents, nephrotoxicity from cisplatin, and hemorrhagic cystitis from cyclophosphamide, without compromising the antitumor effect of any of these agents. Amafostine is labeled for platinum neurotoxicity, but has also been used with paclitaxel- and carboplatin-containing treatment plans. The major side effect of amafostine, transient hypotension, affects approximately 62% of patients. Nausea and vomiting may be severe, and premedication with antiemetics is helpful (DeVita et al., 2000; Groenwald et al., 2000; Itano & Taoka, 1998; Murphy et al., 2000; Wilkes et al., 1997–1998).

Renal Toxicity

Baseline renal function tests should be done before administering chemotherapeutic agents known for renal toxicity. The drugs most frequently associated with renal toxicity are cisplatin, methotrexate, mitomycin, and, to a lesser degree, carboplatin. When the patient demonstrates renal insufficiency (elevated blood urea nitrogen and creatinine levels), consideration needs to be given to reducing the dose to protect the kidneys from further damage and compensate for the longer half-life of the drug—a consequence of poor renal function.

Strategies used to protect the kidneys include vigorous hydration, hypertonic saline solutions, mannitol, and furosemide (Lasix). The patient needs to be monitored for renal compromise. Early intervention can avert the need for dialysis.

Tumor lysis syndrome is another factor that can cause renal damage, and the use of concurrent nephrotoxic drugs increases the patient's risk for renal toxicity (DeVita et al., 2000; Groenwald et al., 2000; Itano & Taoka, 1998; Murphy et al., 2000; Wilkes et al., 1997–1998).

Pulmonary Toxicity

Patients receiving bleomycin in doses exceeding 250 units/m^2 or 400 units/m^2 total dose, or carmustine in a total dose of 1500 mg/m^2, are at risk for development of pulmonary toxicity resulting in damage to the endothelial cells of the lung and causing pneumonitis and interstitial fibrosis. Patients at a higher risk for this complication are the elderly and those with a smoking history or a pre-existing pulmonary condition. In addition to the two previously mentioned drugs, several other drugs can cause pulmonary toxicity, including cyclophosphamide, mitomycin C, methotrexate, melphalan, procarbazine, and busulfan.

Steroids may play a role in prevention and have provided symptomatic relief of cough and dyspnea. A baseline pulmonary function test and ongoing monitoring are helpful in detecting early changes.

Gonadal Dysfunction

Chemotherapeutic agents, especially the alkylating agents, can potentially affect the function of the ovaries and testicles. There is limited information concerning fetal effects of chemotherapy, and therefore it is recommended that birth control should be practiced during chemotherapy and for 1 to 2 months postchemotherapy. The literature documents healthy live births without increased birth defects after antineoplastic therapy.

Reduction in the male sperm count can result in temporary or permanent infertility. Young men and men who wish to have children should be counseled on sperm banking.

Changes in the menstrual cycle are observed within 6 months of starting antineoplastic therapy. Women experience amenorrhea and symptoms of medical menopause (DeVita et al., 2000; Groenwald et al., 2000; Itano & Taoka, 1998; Murphy et al., 2000; Wilkes et al., 1997–1998).

References and Selected Readings

Asterisks indicate references cited in text.

Alexander, J. & Speyer, J. (1996). *Cardiotoxicity and cancer chemotherapy* (Vols. 1 & 2). Pharmacia and Upjohn.

Corrigan, A.M., Pelletier, G., & Alexander, M. (Eds.). (2000). *Intravenous Nurses Society core curriculum for intravenous nursing* (2nd ed.). Philadelphia: Lippincott Williams & Wilkins.

*DeVita, V.T., Hellman, S., & Rosenberg, S.A. (Eds.). (2000). *Cancer: Principles and practice of oncology* (6th ed.). Philadelphia: Lippincott Williams & Wilkins.

Dorr, R.T. (1980). *Cancer chemotherapy handbook.* New York: Elsevier.

Fischer, D.S. & Knobf, M.T. (1993). *The cancer chemotherapy handbook* (3rd ed.). Chicago: Year Book Medical Publishers.

*Groenwald, S.L., Frogge, M.H., Goodman, M., & Yarbro, C.H. (2000). *Cancer nursing: Principles and practice* (4th ed.). Boston: Jones and Bartlett.

*Itano, J.K. & Taoka, K.N. (1998). *Core curriculum for oncology nursing* (3rd ed.). Philadelphia: W.B. Saunders.

Intravenous Nurses Society. (1998, 2000). Intravenous Nursing Society standards of practice. *Journal of Intravenous Nursing* (Suppl.)

Lester, J. (Ed.). (1997). *Statement on the scope and standards of advanced practice in oncology nursing.*

*McCorkle, R., Grant, M., Frank-Stromborg, M., & Baird, S.B. (1996). *Cancer nursing: A comprehensive textbook* (2nd ed.). Philadelphia: W.B. Saunders.

*Murphy, G.P., Lawrence, W., Jr., & Lenhard, R.E., Jr. (Eds.). (2000). *American Cancer Society textbook of clinical oncology.* Atlanta: American Cancer Society.

Nettina, S.M. (2000). *Lippincott manual of nursing practice* (7th ed.). Philadelphia: Lippincott Williams & Wilkins.

Nursing2000 Drug Handbook. (2000). Spring House, PA: Springhouse Corp.

*Oncology Nursing Society. (1999). Fishman, M. &. Orlowski, M. (Eds.). *Cancer chemotherapy guidelines: Modules I–IV.* Pittsburgh: Author.

Oncology Nursing Society (1997). Welch J. & Silveira, J. (Eds.). *Safe handling of cytotoxic drugs: Independent study module.* Pittsburgh: Author.

Oncology Nursing Society and American Nurses Association. (1996). Brant, J. (Ed.). *Standards of oncology nursing practice.* Kansas City: American Nurses Association.

Oncology Nursing Society. (Nowatny, M., chair). (1995). *Standards of oncology nursing education: Generalist and advanced practice levels.* Pittsburgh: Author.

Oncology Nursing Society. (1989, I & II; 1990, III). (1996). *Access device guidelines, recommendations for nursing education and practice. Module I, catheters; Module II, implanted ports and reservoirs; Module III, pumps (infusion systems).* Pittsburgh: Author.

Skeel, R. (1999). *Handbook of cancer chemotherapy* (5th ed.). Philadelphia: Lippincott Williams & Wilkins.

Tenenbaum, L. (1994). *Cancer chemotherapy and biotherapy.* Philadelphia: W.B. Saunders.

Trissel, L. (1998). Drug stability and compatibility issues in drug delivery. In *Handbook on injectable drugs* (10th ed.). Bethesda, MD: American Society of Health-System Pharmacists.

U.S. Department of Health and Human Services. (1997). *NIOSH alert: Preventing allergic reaction to natural rubber latex in the workplace* (No. 97-135). Washington, DC: Author.

Wilkes, G., Ades, J., & Krahoff, I. (2000). *American Cancer Society's consumer's guide to cancer drugs.* Boston: Jones & Bartlett.

*Wilkes, G., Ingwersen, K., & Burk, M. (1997–1998). *Oncology nursing drug handbook.* Boston: Jones and Bartlett.

Review Questions

Note: Questions below may have more than one right answer.

1. If a second venipuncture site is needed, and the patient's other arm is not an option, the second site should be located:

   A. Distal to the original

   B. Proximal to the original

   C. In the lower extremity

   D. Alongside the original

2. The following drugs are classified as vesicants *except*:

   A. Dactinomycin

   B. Daunorubicin hydrochloride

   C. Doxorubicin

   D. Dacarbazine

3. All of the following elements of documentation of an extravasation are essential *except*:

   A. Mentation of the patient

   B. Date and time of the treatment

   C. Antineoplastic agents given and their sequence

   D. Approximate quantity of drug extravasated

4. Patient education and understanding of antineoplastic treatment is enhanced when:

   A. The environment is new

   B. The patient has received sedation for anxiety

   C. The patient is ready to learn

   D. The patient is bilingual

5. Precautions taken when preparing and handling antineoplastic agents include all of the following *except*:

   A. Personal protective equipment consistent with Occupational Safety and Health Administration (OSHA) guidelines

   B. Compounding under a Class II biologic safety cabinet

   C. Use of a nonaerosol needle

   D. Clipping of needle to prevent reuse

6. After chemotherapy administration, body fluids are considered to be contaminated for:

   A. 12 hours

   B. 24 hours

   C. 48 hours

   D. 72 hours

7. The glove that provides the most protection from chemotherapy is:

   A. A lightly powdered latex glove

   B. A nonpowdered latex glove

   C. A lightly powdered polyvinyl chloride (PVC) glove

   D. A nonpowdered PVC glove

8. The maximum lifetime dose of doxorubicin is usually considered to be:

   A. 150 to 75 mg/m^2

   B. 450 to 550 mg

   C. 4500 to 5500 mg

   D. 500 to 550 mg/m^2

9. The side effect most likely to affect body image is:

   A. Diarrhea

   B. Red-tinged urine

   C. Alopecia

   D. Fatigue

10. A reversible side effect of chemotherapy is:

   A. Pulmonary fibrosis

   B. Amenorrhea

   C. Myocyte damage

   D. Sterility

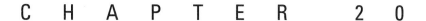

C H A P T E R   2 0

Pain Management

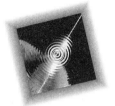

■ ROLE OF NURSES IN PAIN MANAGEMENT

Nurses and physicians are accountable for responding to and managing a patient's pain level. In 1999, the Joint Commission on Accreditation of Healthcare Organizations (JCAHO) wrote criteria for hospitals, nursing care, and long-term care facilities regarding their management of pain. Later, the JCAHO developed six standards for pain management. These standards reflect the consensus of an expert panel of physicians, nurses, pharmacists, therapists, and representatives of other health care organizations. The standards, effective January 2001, emphasize a collaborative and interdisciplinary approach, individualized pain control plans, assessment and frequent reassessment of pain, use of pharmacologic and nonpharmacologic strategies, and establishment of a formalized approach to pain management. The standards address rights and ethics, assessment of people with pain, care of people with pain, education of people with pain, continuum of care, and improvement of organization performance (Phillips, 2000). Nurses in any facility must recognize that proper pain management is a patient's right, as defined in each institution's mission statement. Documentation of protocols, educational requirements, and evaluation are significant components of the quality improvement process.

Creating institutional commitment requires administrative backing. Whatever the level of administrative support, the plan must be well thought-out and defined, and incorporate all levels of care. It should not exclude any individual or discipline.

Ideally, the institution appoints a project leader who is skilled in managing change and has knowledge of current pain management, good communication skills, and tenacity.

Initiating a Pain Management Project

The first step in developing a pain management project is to examine what is occurring in an organization in a well-defined time frame. A search of the current literature defines the basis for evidence-based practice (see Chap. 10). The literature is replete with documents that demonstrate how inadequately health care professionals have been able to control patients' pain. Many health care professionals, however, find it difficult to believe that pain management is *that bad* in their own institutions.

Data should be collected in a nonbiased, objective manner. Helpful information is gained through measuring the knowledge and attitudes about pain at all levels of nursing staff and medical staff. This information provides a baseline of comparison for measuring outcomes against educational offerings and changes in clinical intervention. Measurement tools are available through the Internet, or an institution can develop its own. An Internet site that offers measurement tools is maydaypain@smtplink.coh.org.

The institution needs to develop a time frame for completion of measures to monitor outcomes (American Pain Society, 1998). A team of data collectors can gather information about how pain is documented, what percentage of patients' charts have pain ratings documented, and what percentage of patients' charts have pain ratings within acceptable ranges (as predetermined by the lead group). The team also can gather data through interviews of care providers about what they view as barriers to effective pain management. Patient satisfaction surveys have been viewed as having little value because patients tend to rate their pain management higher than do other measurement modalities. The survey, however, may still provide insight when used in consort with other measurements. This information should be disseminated throughout the institution at multiple levels, using newsletters, magazines, staff meetings (interdisciplinary), flyers, and posters.

Motivating Change

If the results from the aforementioned measurement tools are not as desired, then change needs to occur. Three places to start are as follows:

- Staff education
- Routine pain orders
- Documentation

Staff Education

Staff education encompasses both nursing and physician education. A common mistake of institutions is that they educate only nursing staff, which leads to frustration among nurses who are unable to initiate change without challenging physicians about how they write orders. Such conflicts can become unpleasant. Education is an expensive process for institutions that have limited resources. Developing self-learning packets for nursing review and access may be necessary. Physician education usually is best done through lecture and physician-directed newsletters.

To move pain management forward in both professions, dispelling myths and misconceptions is essential. Postevaluation of the knowledge and attitudes of both disciplines should be monitored within a given time frame. Patient education could coincide with staff education; all patients should be well informed as to the options available.

Routine Pain Orders

Routine pain orders need to be rewritten. Administrative support once again is paramount for this task. Routine orders or written pain orders should be available from admission to discharge and need to continue if the patient is referred to an extended care facility or for home care. The pain orders should follow three principles:

- Decrease the use of meperidine HCl (Demerol).
- Decrease the use of intramuscular (IM) injections.
- Decrease the use of prn (as-needed) medications.

The use of Demerol has been well documented as problematic in American Pain Society publications (American Pain Society, 1999) and in the U.S. Agency for Health Care Policy and Research (AHCPR) Acute Pain Guidelines. IM injections are painful. By administering IM analgesia, the patient has to endure pain during administration of the medication before receiving relief (Ackerman, Juneja, Kaczorowski, & Colclough, 1989). When possible, the oral or IV routes should be used. A common misconception is that narcotic dosing by the IV route is equal to the IM route (American Pain Society, 1999). Routine pain orders should not reflect this mistaken belief. Analgesia delivered on an as-needed basis results in the patient experiencing hurt before receiving relief. It is preferable to administer analgesia on schedule when pain is a steady state, such as after surgery or a procedure, or for chronic cancer pain.

Routine standing orders for postoperative pain control should facilitate performance of up-to-date pain control measures. The goal of pain management is to keep the patient's pain score low enough to allow for deep breathing and coughing, early ambulation, decreased complication rates, and improved overall quality of life.

Documentation

Documentation should follow the concept that pain rating is considered the "fifth vital sign" (Pasero, 1997). If blood pressure, pulse, respirations, and temperature are documented on a graphic sheet, the pain rating also should be on the same graphic sheet. A single graphic facilitates documentation and ensures that all members of the health care team who view the graphic sheet see pain information. If the pain rating is poor (per the institution's definition) and pain medications are given, then pain evaluation needs to take place between 30 and 50 minutes after the intervention. Policies and procedures should define pain ratings and interventions as well as methods

---

BOX 20–1 **Requirements for Effective Pain Control**

- Assessment
- Intervention
- Reassessment

---

for providing patient-controlled analgesia (PCA) and epidural, intrathecal, and other forms of pain management (Box 20–1).

Conducting Follow-up and Continuing Education

A team of "pain experts" is crucial to an effective pain management plan. The properly trained and interested personnel can assist with patients who are difficult to manage or help rework systems that create barriers to effective pain management.

Evaluations need to be scheduled and completed at a predetermined time after implementation of system changes. The evaluation tool used should be identical to the first tool, so appropriate comparisons can be made. Evaluations should address knowledge and attitudes, documentation of pain, pain ratings, and patient satisfaction surveys (McNeill, Sherwood, Starck, & Thompson, 1998).

Even if the outlined goals are met, education does not stop there. Continuing education needs to be established. For example, some institutions have mandatory inservice education, similar to cardiopulmonary resuscitation training, certification, and recertification. Other institutions have yearly *Pain Fairs* in which each department, station, or floor displays how they handle pain management. Innovative ideas are shared at these fairs and may include continuous quality improvement projects.

Research Issues: PATIENT SATISFACTION AND PAIN MANAGEMENT

McNeill, J. A., Sherwood, G. D., Starck, P. L., & Thompson, C. J. (1998). Assessing clinical outcomes: Patient satisfaction with pain management. *Journal of Pain and Symptom Management, 16,* 29–40.

This study looked at patients' (N = 157) pain experience during hospitalization. It also examined the revised American Pain Society Patient Outcome Questionnaire (APS-POQ) for overall reliability and validity. A significant difference was found between dissatisfied patients and satisfied patients in their general level of pain in the last 24 hours, with both groups having high pain ratings. The mean pain score in the dissatisfied group was 9.2, and the mean pain score in the satisfied group was 8.07. The APS-POQ was compiled from several existing and widely used pain assessment instruments and has been used in three other studies. Comparison of these three studies consistently showed high patient pain rating, yet satisfaction in the physicians and nurses caring for them.

As they read forward about pain management theories, physiology, assessment, and intervention, the readers of this chapter should consider changes they want to initiate in their institutions. A methodical approach to change of this magnitude is imperative. Pain research and innovation is quite interesting, but will not succeed if it does not move toward improvement. A multitude of publications on research, theories, and clinical practice guidelines were written in the 1980s and 1990s (Bonica, 1990; Paice, 1987; Paice, Penn, & Shott, 1996; Stevens & Leon-Casasola, 1997). If improvement of the clinical practice of pain management is to take place, then nurses must (1) make it easy to do the right thing, (2) make pain management cost effective, and (3) improve patient outcome and document accordingly.

■ ACUTE PAIN

Acute pain results from an illness, injury, or surgery. This type of pain gradually improves as the body heals. Acute pain affects millions of patients worldwide. If it is not managed properly, acute pain increases the cost of health care by increasing the length of hospitalization, the time spent in intensive care settings, and patient morbidity and mortality. Effective control of acute pain is one of the most important issues in postoperative care today (Bonica, 1990). The following factors influence the incidence, intensity, and duration of postoperative pain:

- Site, nature, and duration of surgical procedure
- Type of incision
- Degree of intraoperative trauma
- Physiologic and psychological features of the patient
- Preoperative preparation
- Amount of preoperative pain
- Presence of complications
- Anesthetic management before, during, and after surgery
- Quality of postoperative care

The amount of postoperative pain varies among individuals. Nurses must pay attention to the needs of each patient to control pain effectively. They must be cognizant of individual variability and listen to what each patient says. Nurses cannot assume that, because a particular surgery is performed, the patient will experience an expected amount of pain. Having said that, nurses can assume that postoperative pain is more severe after intensive surgery such as upper abdominal, intrathoracic, renal, and lower abdominal surgery; extensive surgery of the spine; and surgery of the major joints and large bones. Based on that assumption, nurses can proactively place standing orders for postoperative pain management in these areas to cover most, but not all painful procedures.

The importance of high-quality postoperative pain control cannot be overemphasized. When a person's pain is not well controlled, the sympathetic nervous system becomes dominant, commanding the body to produce more glucocorticoids and catecholamines. This, in turn, increases the workload of the heart. Other physical stresses include a more rapid respiratory rate with shallower respirations, hyperglycemia, and decreased peristaltic action. These changes lead to postoperative complications such as hypoventilation, hypoxemia and atelectasis, cardiac arrhythmia, congestive heart failure, deep vein thrombosis, and paralytic ileus. Postoperative pain control also influences the ability to cough, breathe deeply, and ambulate after major surgery. Fortunately, much progress has been made in the field of postoperative pain management. Nurses today are fortunate to have an abundance of innovative options for postoperative pain management. Health care institutions nationwide have developed acute pain services to provide daily assessment and intervention. See Box 20–2 for available options.

■ CHRONIC PAIN

Chronic pain is defined as pain that either remains at the same level of intensity or becomes more intense over time, instead of healing or fading. It is associated with progressive cancer and long-term disability or illness. Chronic pain is complex and cannot be managed simply with one treatment. The IV nurse's technologic expertise and knowledge about infection control assists the team to provide patient care using technology-based means of pain control.

Patients who benefit from the use of pain control technology for the treatment of chronic pain include those with central nervous system or spinal cord injuries and patients with cancer pain that is refractory to conventional methods of pain control. The use of ambulatory devices facilitates the administration of pain medications (see Chap. 11). An oncology patient who in the past would have been hospitalized for pain control can be maintained safely on an outpatient basis for an extensive period (see Chaps. 19 and 23).

■ OPIOIDS

Opioid is another term for *narcotic;* the terms can be used interchangeably. Opioids are effective when they bind with particular opioid receptors in the body. This chap-

---

BOX 20–2 **Options for Pain Control**

- Systemic analgesics and adjuvant drugs (administered orally, rectally, transdermally, intramuscularly, IV, subcutaneously, by continuous infusion, or by patient-controlled analgesia
- Intraspinal opioids, including epidural and intrathecal
- Regional analgesia using local anesthetic agents
- Topical anesthetic agents
- Nonsteroidal anti-inflammatory drugs
- Electrical analgesia through transcutaneous electrical stimulation or electroacupuncture
- Psychological analgesia in the form of hypnosis, relaxation techniques

ter addresses only the mu and kappa receptors. The mu is the most powerful opioid receptor and requires stimulation when serious pain control is necessary. Particular opioids combine with the mu receptor, such as morphine sulfate, meperidine HCl, hydromorphone, and fentanyl citrate. Other opioids combine with the kappa receptor; nalbuphine and buprenorphine HCl (Buprenex) are examples. An opioid that combines with the mu receptor used with an opioid that combines with the kappa receptor will compete with each other for the mu receptor. Clinically, when a patient is receiving a morphine sulfate infusion of 3 mg/hour and the nurse administers a high dose of nalbuphine, the morphine sulfate becomes ineffective and pain intensifies. If the patient is physically dependent on an opioid, he or she may experience physical withdrawal. Opioids that combine with the kappa receptor are weaker analgesics (Box 20–3).

For lengthy procedures in which it is uncomfortable for the patient to maintain a certain position, an opioid often is given to provide analgesia. Opioids are also given during conscious sedation to provide analgesia for the injection of the local anesthetic and for tourniquet pain (Yaney, 1998). Practice criteria for IV conscious sedation have been developed by the INS (INS, 2000).

Side Effects

Side effects and complications associated with opioids include:

- Respiratory depression
- Mental status changes (euphoria)
- Urinary retention
- Nausea, vomiting
- Pruritus
- Constipation
- Orthostatic hypotension
- Bradycardia

Respiratory depression (6 to 8 respirations/minute) is caused by an accumulation of carbon dioxide in the blood, which communicates with the brain (medulla oblongata) to slow respirations until the carbon dioxide level returns to normal. A person may normally experience respiratory depression and simultaneous apnea during regular sleep patterns. Institutional protocol should address assessment of

---

BOX 20–3 **Opioid Receptors**

1. Mu
2. Kappa
3. Sigma
4. Delta
5. Epsilon

respiratory depression during sleep. Protocol also should address patients with a history of sleep apnea. Precautions must be observed for patients who use continuous positive airway pressure (CPAP) machines while in the hospital, especially when opioids are administered. All opioids directly depress brain stem–regulated ventilation, producing a dose-dependent reduction in respiratory rate (Yaney, 1998).

Oxygen saturation monitors are reliable indicators of the patient's oxygen level in the blood; however, the monitors do not measure the level of carbon dioxide. The oxygen saturation may remain normal for 2 to 4 minutes of apnea. More sophisticated continuous carbon dioxide monitors are needed. No machine, however, replaces thorough bedside nursing assessment of respiratory rate, depth, and quality.

Mental status changes are indicative of significant levels of narcotic in the blood and impending respiratory depression. Mental status change may reflect hyponatremia or infection, especially in the elderly. Good nursing assessment differentiates symptoms by considering the complete picture, such as the patient's baseline mental status, respiratory rate, blood chemistries, amount and type of narcotic, and other clinical diagnoses or potential diagnoses.

Urinary retention may be related to narcotic administration, and is caused by relaxation of the detrusor muscle located in the floor of the bladder. The patient may or may not feel the urge to void. Administration of bethanechol contracts the bladder, allowing it to empty. Catheterization is another option for immediate relief of urinary retention; however, risk of nosocomial infection increases.

Nausea may be reversed by either narcotic antagonists, such as nalbuphine HCl (Nubain) or naloxone HCl (Narcan), or by antiemetics. If narcotic antagonists are used, the doses should be kept low to prevent reversal of analgesia. If antiemetics are used, a synergistic effect with the narcotic can result in sedation. When reversal of nausea is not accomplished with antiemetics or low-dose narcotic antagonism, the physician should be notified and further evaluation performed.

Systemic narcotics may cause histamine release and *pruritus*, which may be relieved with antihistamines and by changing the medication. When narcotics are administered intraspinally (epidural or intrathecal), pruritus is related to the action of the narcotic at the spinal cord and may be reversed with low-dose narcotic antagonists.

Narcotics slow the peristaltic action of the bowel, as does pain. Adequate pain control with close bowel monitoring and possible administration of both a stool softener and a peristaltic agent alleviates *constipation*.

Methods of Opioid Administration

Routes of administration include IV PCA, subcutaneous analgesia, and intraspinal analgesia. Each of these routes requires specific nursing assessment, planning, implementation, and evaluation.

Intravenous Patient-Controlled Analgesia

Patient-controlled analgesia allows the patient to control IV delivery of an analgesic and to maintain therapeutic serum drug levels. The physician's order for PCA should include:

1. Loading dose, given IV push at initiation of therapy
2. Lock-out interval, during which the PCA device cannot be activated
3. Maintenance dose
4. Bolus dose
5. Maximum amount the patient may receive within a given time

The loading dose of opioid is achieved through a technique called **titration to effect.** This technique calls for administering small doses of narcotic frequently to obtain a level of analgesia. Titration to effect usually occurs within 40 minutes. The patient is monitored during this time through observation of mental status, level of pain relief, respiratory rate, and amount of narcotic. The nurse should be qualified to manage this technique; an anesthesiologist often provides training. For IV PCA to be effective, the loading dose must be given. Once the loading dose is given and analgesia is increasing, the IV PCA can be piggybacked into the proximal port on the IV tubing.

The *lock-out* interval is a safety system that prohibits the patient from frequently administering narcotic without giving it adequate time to achieve analgesia. The usual amount of time between patient-controlled boluses is 5 to 10 minutes.

The maintenance dose is the amount of narcotic that is infusing continuously. For example, an average, middle-aged, 70-kg adult would receive morphine sulfate at a rate of 1 mg/hour. This maintenance dose usually is administered for the first 12 to 24 hours, after which the rate is reduced or the infusion is stopped and analgesia is maintained through self-administered boluses. This dosage is determined by the patient's age, weight, renal function, history of chemical use or abuse, and level of pain rating (Snell, Fothergill-Bourbonnais, & Durocher-Hendriks, 1997).

The anesthesiologist, surgeon, or primary care physician determines the maximum amount of narcotic the patient may self-administer in a given time. This amount is programmed into the infusion pump and offers another safety system to protect the patient from an overdose of narcotic.

 SAFE PRACTICE ALERT Family members or friends of the patient must not administer boluses to the patient. Accidental overdose may occur if assessment is incorrect or the narcotic starts to accumulate in the bloodstream.

The PCA device has an integral system to activate the bolus. Various devices are available. Factors to consider in device selection include the following:

- Compatibility with currently used IV systems, poles, or conversion to ambulatory system
- Battery life
- Memory retention
- Display features
- Security and safety features
- Cost effectiveness
- Delivery mode (bolus vs. continuous infusion)
- Durability
- Ease of use

A discussion of ambulatory infusion systems is found in Chapter 11. These devices have greatly enhanced the ability to manage acute, postoperative, and chronic pain in the hospital or alternative care setting. Devices such as the CADD PCA (Fig. 20–1) are flexible; programmable in milligrams or milliliters for use with a diversity of drugs and concentrations, appropriate for subcutaneous, IV, and epidural delivery; safe to use; and comfortable; they provide a total system of pain management and comprehensive support.

Subcutaneous Narcotic Infusions

The subcutaneous infusion of narcotics provides analgesia to patients when IV access is unacceptable or unavailable. The level of analgesia obtained through subcutaneous infusions of narcotics is similar to that obtained through IV infusions. The selection of narcotic is important to the success of subcutaneous infusions. Morphine sulfate and hydromorphone HCl are the drugs of choice. The goal of a subcutaneous infusion is to offer a reduced volume of more concentrated solution with minimal chemical irritation. The quality of analgesia is limited to the amount of absorption of narcotic at the subcutaneous site. The conversion from oral narcotic to subcutaneous is equivalent to the conversion from oral narcotic to IM. Table 20–1 shows the appropriate conversions (Watanabe, Pereira, Hanson, & Bruera, 1998).

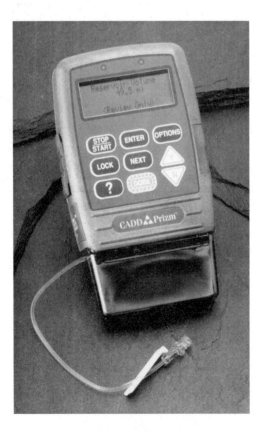

Figure 20–1. Prizm ambulatory infusion pump (Courtesy of Sims-Deltec, St. Paul, MN).

T A B L E   2 0 – 1
CONVERSION TO SUBCUTANEOUS NARCOTIC

	Equianalgesic Dose (mg)	
Analgesic	Oral	IM or SC
Morphine sulfate	30.0	10.0
Hydromorphone HCl	7.5	1.5

IM, intramuscular; SC, subcutaneous

The technique for subcutaneous access is simple; however, the use of proper equipment and stabilizing methods enhances patient comfort and compliance. Supplies needed for subcutaneous access include a small-gauge scalp vein needle or catheter, transparent dressing, povidone–iodine swab stick, and an adhesive bandage. The site of choice is commonly the subclavicular area, abdomen, or anterior chest wall. The site is prepared with povidone–iodine, and the needle is inserted either at an angle or perpendicular to the skin, depending on the needle used. The needle is then stabilized using the manufacturer's recommended methods.

The most common problems with subcutaneous infusion of narcotics are local irritation at the needle insertion site and subcutaneous scarring. Frequent site changes (every other day) and reducing the infusion volume can minimize these complications.

The development of transdermal fentanyl has enabled a subcutaneous deposit of narcotic through diffusion from a rate-controlling membrane in the Duragesic (Janssen Pharmaceuticals, Titusville, NJ) patch. Doses of fentanyl are 25, 50, 75, and 100 μg/hour. When applied to the patient's torso, the patch takes 12 to 15 hours to reach its peak effect. The patch provides analgesia for 72 hours, with subsequent changes providing steady-state analgesia without the initial 12-hour delay to peak. If the patient's pain level increases after 48 hours, the physician should be consulted. The patient may require a fast-acting narcotic through another route until the dose is adjusted to provide steady-state analgesia. The character of the skin is important with transdermal fentanyl; the skin surface must be dry and body hair clipped, not shaved. The patch does not adhere to oily skin. The skin surface should be free of abrasions to avoid bolus administration of fentanyl (INS, 1998, 2000).

Intraspinal Administration

Epidural catheter placement to deliver pain medication offers analgesia, low narcotic dosages, and decreased sedation; it also facilitates earlier ambulation and enhances patient comfort. A working knowledge of relevant anatomy and physiology ensures a high level of care.

Epi refers to "outside," and *dura* refers to the covering of the spinal cord that encloses the cerebrospinal fluid (CSF). The epidural space is a potential space that is part of the spinal canal outside the dura mater, enclosed by protective ligaments. Extending from the base of the skull to the coccyx, the epidural space ends at approximately S1 in many patients (the spinal cord ends at approximately L1; Fig. 20–2).

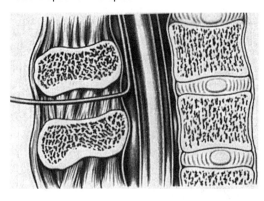

Figure 20–2. Close-up of L1 epidural catheter placement.

The epidural space contains a network of large-bore, thin-walled veins. It also contains fat (directly proportional in amount to a person's body fat) and extensions for nerves that travel out from the spinal cord. The epidural space is also called the peridural and extradural space.

The **intrathecal** space, containing the CSF that bathes the spinal cord, runs parallel to the epidural space. The dura and arachnoid mater separate the intrathecal and epidural spaces. Other terms used to identify the intrathecal space are subarachnoid space and spinal space. The term *intraspinal* is used to describe both the epidural and intrathecal spaces.

When the epidural space is accessed, the anesthesiologist must insert the needle between the spinous processes and through the ligaments, and enter the epidural space with a technique called *loss of resistance*. Loss of resistance occurs when the needle enters the epidural space, and the pressure placed on the plunger of the syringe allows the contents to empty into the space. When an anesthesiologist accesses the intrathecal space, the needle penetrates through the same route into the epidural space and continues through the epidural space until it punctures the dura mater. The intrathecal space contains CSF, which can be aspirated by the syringe attached to the accessing needle.

Elimination of narcotics from the intraspinal space occurs through two mechanisms: diffusion up the neuraxis in the CSF and vascular uptake in the epidural space. The analgesic action occurs in the spinal cord at the location of the substantia gelatinosa of the dorsal horn. Opiate receptors are located at the substantia gelatinosa and bind with the intraspinal narcotic, blocking the pain pathway through the dorsal horn to the brain. The lipid-solubility of the narcotic determines the amount of narcotic used, the volume needed, the placement of the epidural catheter tip, the time to produce analgesia, and the elimination time.

Extremely lipid-soluble narcotics have a more rapid action than water-soluble narcotics. Lipid-soluble narcotics create analgesia in a narrow segment, following the **dermatomes** that surround the level of narcotic injection. Water-soluble narcotics create a wider spread of analgesia and take longer to achieve analgesia, which in turn is longer lasting because of the increased elimination time. An example of a water-soluble narcotic is morphine sulfate; fentanyl citrate is an example of a lipid-soluble narcotic.

Local anesthetics are often used to create analgesia in the epidural space. Pain transmission is blocked at the sympathetic chain ganglion, which lies on either side of and runs parallel to the spinal cord. Local anesthetic agents result in a sympathetic blockade and reduce the amount of narcotic required to create analgesia. They increase the peristaltic action of the bowel, reduce workload on the heart, increase tidal volume of the lung, and increase vascular graft flow, reducing the incidence of deep vein thrombosis. Potential side effects are a significant reduction of blood pressure and numbness along the dermatomal distribution of the catheter tip placement.

 SAFE PRACTICE ALERT   If local anesthetics are used in the epidural infusion, caution must be used in raising the patient from a lying to sitting position and a sitting to a standing position. When position elevation occurs, the blood pressure may decrease, making the patient dizzy or even syncopal.

 SAFE PRACTICE ALERT   *Determine safety before ambulation.* When the patient has an epidural catheter placed in the lumbar region during infusion of local anesthetics, use caution when assisting the patient to a standing position. First, determine the strength in the patient's legs by asking him or her to lift the legs off the bed one at a time (testing for quadriceps strength). Second, determine sensation by touching the patient's thigh. If he or she can feel touch and has the ability to lift the leg off the bed, then proceed. Third, have the patient stand by the side of the bed, and ask him or her to bend the knees slightly and straighten them (again to determine quadriceps strength). If the patient is able to do this, proceed with ambulation. If not, check with the physician because adjustments can be made in the epidural solution or rate to facilitate ambulation.

Research Issues: PATIENT-CONTROLLED ANALGESIA AND INTRAMUSCULAR INJECTIONS

 Snell, C. C., Fothergill-Bourbonnais, F., & Durocher-Hendriks, S. (1997). Patient controlled analgesia and intramuscular injections: A comparison of patient pain experiences and postoperative outcomes. *Journal of Advanced Nursing, 25,* 681–690.

Outcomes of patients receiving intramuscular (IM) injections versus patient-controlled analgesia (PCA) for postoperative pain showed a slight difference in improved pain scores with PCA. No statistical difference in pain score was found. The authors state that a meta-analysis, however, showed that patient satisfaction was greater with PCA than with IM injections. Therefore, the choice of PCA should be made on the basis of patient satisfaction or financial considerations, rather than on improved analgesia.

Epidural access may be achieved through the placement of a percutaneous epidural catheter, a fully **implanted** epidural access portal system, or a fully implantable drug infusion pump. The epidural space is accessed by using a special needle (ie, the Touhy needle), which is placed between the spinous processes and penetrates through the ligaments entering the epidural space through loss of resistance. When the needle is properly placed, the catheter is threaded through the needle. When the epidural catheter is used for temporary analgesia, the catheter is taped to the back and connected to the external infusion pump. When the epidural catheter is used for long-term analgesia, the catheter is connected to the implantable pump, port, or external catheter for connection to an external infusion pump (Caballero, Ausman, & Himes, 1986; DuPen, 1987; Krames, 1996; Paice, 1987; Paice et al., 1996; Samuelsson, Malmberg, Eriksson, & Hedner, 1995).

Before the epidural catheter is placed, the patient should be informed of the potential risks involved and informed consent should be obtained. Bleeding can occur in the epidural space and exit out the insertion site of the catheter. Patients who receive anticoagulant therapy or who have liver damage should have a bleeding time determined before catheter placement. If the bleeding time is less than 10 minutes, the catheter may be safely placed.

▲ Legal Issues: LOW-MOLECULAR-WEIGHT HEPARIN

In 1997, the U.S. Food and Drug Administration issued a warning regarding the use of low–molecular-weight heparin in conjunction with an epidural catheter. The nurse must be aware of the risk of an epidural hematoma.

Sterile technique consistent with established standards of practice is used during catheter placement. The physician should be notified if a patient is febrile before placement or has a known infection. Patients may express concerns related to placement, care, and potential problems. They should be told the catheter is placed into the tissue around the spinal cord, not into the spinal cord itself. They need to know that their blood pressure may decrease because of muscle relaxation and sympathetic blockade when local anesthetic is injected. Administration of IV fluids usually remedies this problem (Box 20–4).

BOX 20–4 Points to Cover in Obtaining Informed Consent for Epidural or Intrathecal Administration

- Bleeding may occur.
- Infection is a possibility.
- An allergic reaction to the local anesthetic agents may occur.
- Injection is not into the spinal cord but into the tissue around the spinal cord.
- During the procedure, the patient may feel a "tickle" down the leg, which is the catheter coming into contact with the nerve. The patient needs to tell the anesthesiologist about this feeling.
- Blood pressure may decrease because the medication relaxes the muscle.
- A headache may occur if the needle enters the cerebral spinal fluid or intrathecal space.

A spinal headache may occur if the needle enters the CSF or intrathecal space and discharges CSF into the epidural space. This leak decreases the fluid padding around the brain. Classic spinal headaches are "positional," that is, the patient experiences a headache when upright but not when lying down. The location of the headache varies. Spinal headache may be relieved with a blood patch, a procedure in which the anesthesiologist realigns the needle in the epidural space close to the dural puncture site. The anesthesiologist then withdraws 10 to 15 mL of blood from the patient's arm and injects the blood into the epidural needle. He or she then removes the epidural needle and instructs the patient to avoid the Valsalva maneuver, either through lifting or bearing down, for 24 hours. The blood patch plugs the leaking dural membrane and increases pressure in the epidural space, forcing the CSF in the intrathecal space toward the brain to relieve the headache soon after the patch is performed.

EPIDURAL CATHETERS

A small-lumen, temporary catheter made of nylon or Teflon is placed initially. Long-term delivery is possible through the use of a long-term epidural catheter or an epidural portal system.

According to the literature (Hassenbusch et al., 1990; Patt, 1989; Waldman, 1990; Yablonski-Peretz et al., 1985), potential candidates for epidural pain management should be evaluated for:

- Confirmed patient response to epidural analgesia
- Normal bleeding parameters
- Absence of active, untreated bacterial infection
- Acceptance of the therapy and understanding of potential side effects
- Adequate support systems to meet the patient's needs

Care and Management. Consistent with Intravenous Nurses Society (INS) Standards of Practice (INS, 2000), the delivery of medications and maintenance of epidural catheters should be established in IV policies and procedures specific to the Nurse Practice Act. Policies and procedures for obtaining, delivering, administering, documenting, and discarding medication should be in accordance with state and federal regulations (INS, 2000).

All medications administered by epidural catheter should be preservative free. Alcohol is contraindicated for preparing the site or accessing the catheter because of the potential for migration of alcohol into the epidural space and possible resultant nerve destruction. Povidone–iodine may be used; however, it can irritate the nerves if it migrates into the epidural space. A 0.2-μm filter without surfactant should be used for medication administration. Before use, the catheter should be aspirated to determine the absence of CSF. Epidural catheters may be placed for short- or long-term use.

Mechanical problems may occur with the epidural catheter system, including leaking catheter hub, disconnected catheter, occluded catheter, or leaking at the skin site. Leakage at the catheter hub is common with temporary epidural catheter systems. The patient experiences breakthrough pain from leakage of medications, and bedding or clothing is wet. The nurse must tighten the hub or replace the hub if it is

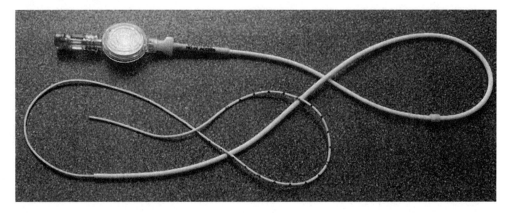

Figure 20–3. DuPen Eupucath. (Courtesy of Davol, Inc., Subsidiary CR Bard Inc., Salt Lake City, UT.)

cracked. Clean technique is appropriate for manipulating the catheter hub (Figs. 20–3 and 20–4).

When the catheter is disconnected from the medication infusion, it may be in the patient's bed or on the floor. If the catheter is not grossly contaminated, a sterile scissors can be used to clip the catheter 1/2-inch from the distal end. The new end may then be reconnected to the hub of the catheter and tightened. If the catheter is found on the floor, the epidural catheter must be removed and another form of analgesia used. No alcohol or povidone–iodine is necessary for removal of the catheter.

When the epidural catheter is occluded, the electronic infusion device should stop and the alarm should sound. Nursing interventions include ensuring that all clamps are open and checking the tubing for kinking. The hub is loosened and then retightened to secure it to the catheter, and the infusion restarted. If this is unsuccessful, the anesthesiologist or pain management team should be called. Supplemental pain medication may be given by an alternative route.

The dressing over the catheter exit site may be damp from leaking at the skin site. The nurse needs to assess whether the patient is experiencing pain. If the patient is comfortable, no treatment is necessary other than to replace the wet dressing. If the patient is uncomfortable, the dressing should be removed to see if the catheter has pulled out of the epidural space. The physician should be notified that there is leaking and the patient is uncomfortable. Supplemental analgesia should be initiated.

Aspiration. Aspiration of the epidural catheter is required to determine if the catheter is displaced, either in an epidural vein or in the CSF. Positive aspiration of

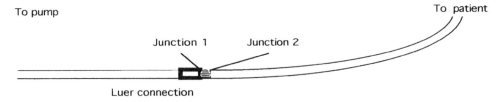

Figure 20–4. Epidural catheter and points at which damage may occur. 1 = tighten catheter; 2 = Leak may occur.

the catheter, however, does not guarantee either condition, and should not be considered conclusive. The physician should be notified. If the patient is oversedated, the epidural catheter may have migrated into the intrathecal space. If the patient is receiving epidural local anesthetic and feels numbness in the toes only, the catheter may be intrathecal. Aspiration of a small amount of blood (1 to 2 mL) is also inconclusive because the pool of medication in the epidural space may have mixed with a pool of blood in the epidural space that resulted from the trauma of insertion. If the syringe fills with greater than 3 mL blood and the patient is receiving inadequate analgesia, however, the nurse can conclude that the epidural catheter is in an epidural vein. If so, the epidural catheter needs to be pulled back out of the vein and into the epidural space. Only an anesthesiologist or trained member of a pain management team should do this. If there is more than 5 mL clear fluid, the nurse can assume it is CSF unless there is a high-volume infusion of medication and poor diffusion through the dura, resulting in higher pools of medications in the epidural space. The clear fluid can be tested to determine glucose level. A higher level of glucose indicates CSF, and the physician should be consulted.

▲ Legal Issues: DISLODGING THE CATHETER

> There is always the risk of pulling the catheter out of the epidural space. The patient needs to be advised of this risk. The nurse must not allow the patient to suffer while the epidural system is being managed. An alternative form of analgesia is necessary.

Flushing with Preservative-Free Saline. Flushing is performed to determine patency of the catheter; 3 mL preservative-free saline is instilled. If resistance is met, the connector to the epidural catheter should be loosened and a second attempt to flush made. If leaking occurs, the epidural catheter connector should be tightened.

Breakthrough Pain. Breakthrough pain may indicate that the pump is programmed incorrectly, the epidural catheter is disconnected and leaking, the epidural catheter is no longer epidural, the catheter has migrated into an epidural vein, or the patient is receiving too low a dose. Regardless of the reason for breakthrough pain, intervention must be initiated to provide pain control.

Breakthrough pain when an epidural catheter is not functioning adequately can be remedied by administration of 2 to 4 mg IV morphine sulfate, every 20 minutes as needed. If the patient is sensitive to morphine sulfate, 0.2 to 0.3 mg IV hydromorphone may be substituted, every 20 minutes as needed.

EPIDURAL PORT

The epidural port consists of the portal and catheter and contains a filter to remove large particulate matter. The catheter portion of the port system is positioned in the epidural space using the technique discussed earlier, and the catheter is then threaded through a percutaneous tunnel. A subcutaneous pocket is prepared for the port. The system is intended for repeated injection or infusion of preservative-free morphine sulfate into the epidural space (Fig. 20–5).

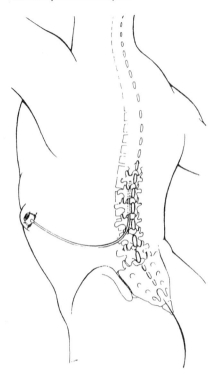

Figure 20–5. Epidural port (Courtesy of Sims-Deltec, St. Paul, MN.)

Research Issues: EPIDURAL MORPHINE TREATMENT

Samuelsson, H., Malmberg, F., Eriksson, M., & Hedner, T. (1995). Outcomes of epidural morphine treatment in cancer pain: Nine years of clinical experience. *Journal of Pain and Symptom Management, 10,* 105–112.

After 9 years of clinical experience, Samuelsson, Malmberg, Eriksson, and Hedner published their outcome study of 146 cancer patients in a community hospital–based pain service. One hundred twenty-one patients stayed on lifelong or chronic epidural opioids. Mean time was 92 days, with a range of 2 to 2040 days. Forty-nine percent of patients were managed on an outpatient basis. The authors concluded that long-term epidural morphine therapy was a beneficial alternative in the treatment of intractable cancer pain.

IMPLANTED PUMPS

In the 1980s and 1990s, advancements in medical technology facilitated convenient alternatives to conventional methods of long-term drug delivery. Systems such as the implanted pump (including pump, catheter, and optional access port) are implanted surgically and require periodic refilling. The pump weighs approximately 6 oz and stores and releases prescribed amounts of medication into the body. A physician or nurse may use a computer during refill and check-up sessions to communicate by telemetry with the pump and to set the prescription as ordered. The pump delivers a controlled amount of medication through a catheter to the area in the body where it will be most effective. These pumps are battery operated and usually last 3 to 4 years. Potential risks include infection at the implant site, catheter plug or kinking, dislodgment, and leaking.

Patients should be cautioned to report redness, swelling, and pain near the incision and to avoid such activities as scuba diving, which results in pump underinfusion and diminished drug effect. The pump site should be avoided during diathermy and ultrasound treatments. Atmospheric pressure, body temperature, blood pressure, and concentration and viscosity of the medication may affect flow rates.

Possible complications include cessation of therapy due to battery depletion, migration of the catheter access port, pocket seroma, complete or partial catheter occlusion, CSF leak, and drug toxicity. The use of needles larger than 22 gauge may compromise the self-sealing properties of the septum. Noncoring needles are recommended to minimize septal damage. The IV nurse is cautioned to follow procedures for the use of implanted pumps, consistent with the manufacturer's guidelines and institutional policy (Fig. 20–6).

Patient Identification Card. When the pump is implanted, the surgeon should complete the patient registration and implantation record. The manufacturer issues the patient a wallet-sized identification card containing information pertinent to the implanted pump. The physician should fill in the space provided for any medical emergency instructions. This patient should carry this card at all times.

Postimplantation Care. After the implantation is complete, the pump can be filled with the medication. The 10-mL pump is filled with 6 mL, and the 18-mL pump is

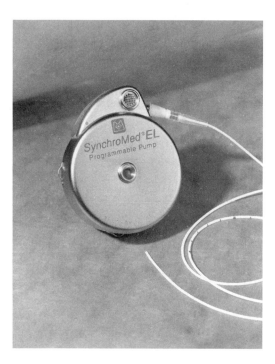

Figure 20–6. SynchroMed Pump (Courtesy of Medtronic, Minneapolis, MN).

BOX 20–5 **Instructions for Patients After Implantation**

Action

1. Avoid traumatic physical activity.
2. Avoid long, hot baths, saunas, and other activities that increase body temperature.
3. Consult physician during febrile illness.
4. Consult the physician before air travel or change of residence.
5. Avoid deep sea or scuba diving.
6. Report any unusual symptoms or complications relating to the specific drug therapy or the device.
7. Return at the prescribed time for pump refill.

Result

1. Prevent tissue damage around the implant site.
2. Increased drug flow.
3. Assess the effects of increased drug flow.
4. Adjustments in drug dosage may be required to compensate for anticipated change in drug flow.
5. Dosage may require modification.
6. Ensure safety.
7. Ensure compliance.

---

filled with 10 mL. The reduction is necessary only for the first infusion. Thereafter, the refills can completely fill the chamber. Patients should be monitored carefully after implantation to confirm proper pump performance, wound healing, and favorable response to therapy. Instructions for patients with implanted pumps are listed in Box 20–5.

Pump Refill Procedure. The pump requires refills at specific intervals, depending on the volume of the reservoir and rate of administration. The technique used to refill the pump should be sterile.

KEY INTERVENTIONS: Refilling the Pump

---

1. Obtain the following equipment: sterile fenestrated drape (1), sterile extension tubing with clamp (1), sterile towel (1), sterile gloves (1 pair), 20-mL syringe with drug solution, sterile 2 x 2-inch sponge (1), sterile empty 20-mL syringe (1), povidone–iodine swabs (3), sterile 22-gauge noncoring needle (2), 0.22-μg filter, pressure monitor, template.
2. Warm 20-mL syringe with drug solution to room temperature.
3. Identify the outer perimeter of the pump by palpating the pump pocket. Locate pump septum.
4. Wash hands thoroughly and dry.
5. Using sterile technique, place all sterile items on opened sterile towel. Put on sterile gloves.

6. Disinfect pump site with povidone–iodine. Use three separate preps. Start at the center of the pump and work outward beyond the periphery of the pump.
7. Place fenestrated drape over prepared pump site. Sterile template may be aligned over septum.
8. Securely connect barrel of empty 20-mL syringe and extension tubing to the non-coring needle. Close clamp.
9. Using a perpendicular angle, insert needle into center of septum.
10. Open clamp, allowing pump to empty.
11. Close clamp. Record returned volume, adding 1 mL for amount of drug remaining in extension tubing. Disconnect and discard syringe barrel.
12. Securely attach air-purged syringe with drug solution to extension tubing. Open clamp.
13. To instill the solution into the pump, release extension tubing clamp and allow drug to return to syringe. This test confirms proper needle placement. Continue to inject and check needle placement at 5-mL increments until syringe is emptied.
14. Pull needle out quickly and apply digital pressure with sterile sponge. If necessary, apply a sterile adhesive bandage.

STATIONARY INFUSION DEVICES

Abbott Laboratories' (North Chicago, IL) LifeCare PCA Classic and PCA Plus II meet the needs of the sedentary patient receiving pain management. The Classic is a single-mode PCA device for low-cost PCA procedures. The Plus II has the ability to dose in micrograms or milligrams (Fig. 20–7).

■ STAFF EDUCATION

Although information on the safe administration of epidural medication and monitoring of potential side effects is available, little has been written about preparing the

text continues on page 576

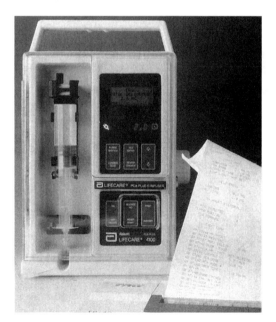

Figure 20–7. LifeCare PCA Plus II Infuser (Courtesy of Abbott Laboratories, Inc., North Chicago, IL.)

CURRICULUM FOR NURSE INVOLVEMENT WITH EPIDURAL/INTRATHECAL INFUSIONS

Criteria	Rationale
If epidural analgesia is already being used without proper staff education, the analgesia should be maintained by trained personnel (MDA, CRNA) until staff nurse(s) are proficient, meet preapproved criteria, and are RNs.	Ensure patient safety during learning period.
Instructions include:	
Epidural/intrathecal medications, including morphine, hydromorphone, fentanyl, and local anesthetics	• Nurse understands action of medication in intraspinal space.
Epidural/intrathecal equipment	• Nurse is familiar with equipment and can differentiate epidural infusion and IV infusion.
Monitoring of mental status and respiratory rate, depth, and quality	• Nurse appropriately monitors effects of narcotic and local anesthetics given in the intraspinal spaces.
Dressing changes	• Temporary epidural catheters can easily fall out during dressing changes; precautions are needed during dressing changes. Nurse avoids alcohol at epidural site.
Medication changes	• Nurse verifies only preservative-free narcotics or local anesthetics are used.
Pump programming	• Nurse trouble-shoots pump to minimize delays in pain control.
Trouble-shooting catheter	• Nurse understands occlusion management and leaking of the epidural catheter when it occurs.
Managing side effects	• Nurse understands interventions for nausea, vomiting, constipation, pruritus, and other side effects.
Epidural/intrathecal administration of medications in patients with:	Nurse understands the patient selection criteria.
Postsurgery pain	
Post-trauma pain	
Intractable cancer pain	
Refractory nonmalignant pain with appropriate psychological/physical evaluation	
The nurse notifies the anesthesiologist when there is:	These problems require assessment by an anesthesiologist or personnel from the pain management team.
Pain at insertion site	
Inadequate analgesia	
Pain with administration of infusion or injection	
Drainage from catheter exit site that requires multiple dressing changes, especially when accompanied by inadequate analgesia	
Clear drainage greater than 8–10 mL when catheter is aspirated	
Before injection	
An unresolveable occlusion	
Intrathecal infusions are not connected to an external pump.	The intrathecal space contains cerebrospinal fluid and is a good medium for bacterial growth, increasing the risk of infection.
The nurse removes the epidural catheter when ordered.	Nurse with special training in the technique of epidural catheter removal and documentation of this removal ensures safe patient care.

In. date / Initials	NURSING DIAGNOSIS/PATIENT PROBLEM / DESIRED OUTCOME	ACTIONS/INTERVENTIONS SET & REVIEWED W/PATIENT/FAMILY [ ] YES [ ] NO	TARGET DATE	DATE OF DAILY REVIEW/INITIALS	RESOLUTION DATE / EVALUATION
	1. Knowledge deficit related to the use of epidural analgesia for post-operative pain control	1. Describe the placement of the catheter, its use, who will administer pain medication and the use of an apnea monitor for immediate post-op period			
	:. Patient demonstrates knowledge related to epidural catheter use for post-operative pain control and verbalizes understanding of need to report pain as soon as perceived				
	2. Potential for injury due to catheter displacement (i e intrathecal space).	1. RN will monitor: a The patency of the catheter b The condition of the dressing c Observe catheter site of intactness and hash marks indicating length d Negative aspiration before each medication administration			
	:. Catheter will remain in epidural space or will be removed immediately if dislodged				
	3. Potential for ineffective breathing pattern related to respiratory depression secondary to epidural analgesia	1. Maintain apnea monitor for first 24 hours or until a baseline dose is established to maintain patient comfort			
	:. Patient will exhibit effective breathing pattern: • respirations of six or greater, regular and non-labored				

Initials	RN Signatures	Initials	RN Signatures

Primary Nurse

Social Worker:

Other

Figure 20-8. Patient care plan for postoperative pain control using epidural analgesia. Reprinted from *Oncology Nursing Forum* with permission from Oncology Nursing Press, Inc. (Camp-Sorrel, D., Fernandez, K., & Reardon, M.B. [1990]. Teaching oncology nurses about epidural catheters. *Oncology Nursing Forum, 17*[5], 683–689.)

Init date / Initials	NURSING DIAGNOSIS/PATIENT PROBLEM DESIRED OUTCOME	ACTIONS/INTERVENTIONS SET & REVIEWED W/PATIENT/FAMILY [ ] YES [ ] NO	TARGET DATE	DATE OF DAILY REVIEW/INITIALS	RESOLUTION DATE	EVALUATION
	3 Potential for ineffective breathing (Continued)	2 Have Naloxone (Narcan) 4mg available at all times while epidural narcotics are being used				
		3 Maintain IV access at all times while epidural catheter is in place				
		4 Monitor for signs of restlessness, miosis				
	4 Potential urinary retention related to atonic bladder from sacral analgesia	1 If urinary catheter not in place, measure intake and output every four hours for first 24 hours and every eight hours thereafter				
	: Patient will demonstrate adequate urinary elimination.					
	5 Potential for alteration in comfort related to displacement or dysfunction of the catheter	1 Use visual analog scale and Pain Flow Sheet to monitor patient comfort level every four hours				
	: Patient will report adequate pain control	2 Administer medication as ordered or notify anesthesiologist of inadequate pain control. * Note: No other narcotics, tranquilizers or sedatives may be given unless ordered by anesthesiologist				

Initials	RN Signatures	Initials	RN Signatures

Primary Nurse

Social Worker:

Other

Figure 20-8. (*continued*)

Initials / In. date	NURSING DIAGNOSIS/PATIENT PROBLEM, DESIRED OUTCOME	ACTIONS/INTERVENTIONS SET & REVIEWED W/PATIENT/FAMILY [ ] YES [ ] NO	TARGET DATE	DATE OF DAILY REVIEW/INITIALS	RESOLUTION DATE / EVALUATION
	6. Potential for discomfort related to pruritis secondary to release of histamine from the morphine effect. :Patient will inform caregiver when itching begins. Patient will report relief of itching.	1 Administer antipruritic as ordered by anesthesiologist PRN			
	7. Potential for hypotension related to vasomotor disturbance :Blood pressure will be maintained at adequate level	1 Monitor vital signs every four hours while epidural is in use			
		2 Maintain adequate intravenous or oral fluid intake			
		3 Elevate lower extremities			
		4 When getting OOB, allow patient to dangle at bedside first			
	8. Potential for injury related to infection secondary to epidural catheter. :Patient will remain infection-free as evidenced by absence of purulent drainage, redness or tenderness at catheter insertion site	1 Monitor catheter insertion site every shift for redness, edema, drainage			
		2 Maintain strict sterile technique during preparation and administration of medications			
		3. Monitor temperature and WBC to detect possible infection.			

Initials	RN Signatures	Initials	RN Signatures

Primary Nurse

Social Worker:

Other

Figure 20-8. *(continued)*

573

PAIN ASSESSMENT FLOW SHEET

DATE: _____
MEDICATION ORDERED: _____
CONTINUOUS RATE: _____
PCA DOSE: _____
LOCKOUT: _____

CHECK ONE:

EPIDURAL: _____
INTRATHECAL: _____
IV-PCA: _____

(Addressograph Plate)

Checks Made Here - See Nurse's Notes:

1 Hour Assessment

Date	Time	Sed. Scale	Respir. Rate	Mod. Inf. As Ordr'd. Tubing Secure

4-HOUR ASSESSMENT

Local Anesthetic

Pain Scale	B.P./ Pulse Lying	B.P./ Pulse Sitting	No Loss Of Sens. Lower Extrem.	Drsg. Dry Intact. No Edema S/S of Inf.	Urinary Ret.	Pruritus	Break Through Pain	Catheter Checked For Placement	Drsg. Chg. (Kit Utlzd.)	Catheter Flushed 3cc NS.	Nausea Vomiting	Pulse Ox.	R.N.'s Initials

RN SIGNATURE / INITIALS: _____

N/V ECOG SCALE:
0 - No Nausea or Vomiting
1 - Nausea/Vomiting X 1/day
2 - Nausea/Vomiting Less Than X 6/day
3 - Vomiting X 6/day
4 - Dehydration - IV Therapy

PAIN SCALE:
0 - No Pain
1 - 2 - Discomfort
3 - 4 - Mild Pain
5 - 6 - Distress
7 - 8 - Severe Pain
9 - 10 - Excruciating Pain

SEDATION SCALE:
0 - No Sedation-Pt. Found Awake.
S - Normal Sleep-Easy To Awake.
1 - Mild Drowsy, Easy To Arouse.
2 - Moderate, Frequently Drowsy, Still Able To Arouse.
3 - Severely Somnolent, Unable To Arouse.

Figure 20–9. Pain assessment form. (Courtesy of Midwestern Regional Medical Center, Zion, IL.)

PAIN ASSESSMENT ORDERS:

_____

_____

_____

_____

_____

_____

_____

_____

NURSE'S NOTES:

_____

_____

_____

_____

_____

_____

_____

_____

_____

_____

_____

_____

_____

_____

_____

_____

_____

_____

_____

_____

_____

_____

_____

Figure 20–9. (_continued_)

PATIENT-CONTROLLED ANALGESIA

Sample Flow Sheet

HOSPITAL I.D.	PATIENT I.D.

DATE_____

MEDICATION_____

LOADING DOSE_____
(IF APPLICABLE)

TIME	12MN	2A	4A	6A	8A	10A	12N	2P	4P	6P	8P	10P
DOSE VOLUME (ML)												
LOCK-OUT												
4 HR LIMIT (ML)												
# DOSE DEL.												
TOTAL VOL. DEL.												
SEDATION (1-5)												
PAIN (1-5)												
RESP. RATE												
NURSE'S SIG.												

ADMIN. SET CHANGE	
NEW PCA UNIT	
CONDITION I.V. SITE	

SCALES

SEDATION

1 = WIDE AWAKE
2 = DROWSY
3 = DOZING INTERMITTENTLY
4 = MOSTLY SLEEPING
5 = ONLY AWAKENS WHEN AROUSED

PAIN

1 = COMFORTABLE
2 = IN MILD DISCOMFORT
3 = IN PAIN
4 = IN BAD PAIN
5 = IN VERY BAD PAIN

Figure 20–10. Sample flow sheet for patient-controlled analgesia.

registered professional nurse for administering and monitoring epidural analgesia. The initial step is to establish the rationale and criteria on which the policy and procedure for administration of epidural analgesia will be based, as outlined in Table 20–2.

Development of a care plan illustrating potential side effects and appropriate nursing interventions is an essential component of the process. A sample care plan is detailed in Figure 20–8. The clinical program should be intensive and, ideally, skills checklists used to identify criteria for assessing appropriate techniques.

BOX 20-6 **American Pain Society Quality Assurance Pain Relief Standards**

- Recognize and treat pain promptly.
  - Chart and display pain and relief. (Process)
  - Define pain and relief levels to initiate review. (Process)
  - Survey patient satisfaction. (Outcome)
- Make information about analgesics readily available. (Process)
- Promise patients attentive analgesic care. (Process)
- Define explicit policies for use of advanced analgesic technologies. (Process)
- Monitor adherence to standards. (Process)

■ INTRAVENOUS CONSCIOUS SEDATION

Intravenous conscious sedation (IVCS) requires a physician's order and should be provided in a controlled clinical setting. Practice criteria for IVCS has been defined by the INS. Consistent with the criteria, only a qualified anesthesia provider or attending physician selects and orders the medication. The patient's infusion nurse should be competent, and the institution should have an educational and competency verification system. Informed patient consent should be obtained, and the patient should be monitored and IV access should be continuously maintained (INS, 2000).

■ CONTINUOUS LOCAL ANESTHETICS

Local anesthetics block nerve conduction and may offer excellent postoperative pain control by achieving uninterrupted pain relief, minimizing opioid requirements, and avoiding the adverse effects of opioids. Continuous local anesthetic is given through a 16-gauge introducer needle placed under the subcutaneous tissue and above the fascia or muscle adjacent to or in the wound site after surgery. After placing the introducer, the surgeon threads a 20-gauge epidural catheter through the needle. The surgeon removes the introducer and secures the site with a semipermeable transparent dressing. The patient receives a loading dose of local anesthetic before beginning the continuous infusion, via disposable infusion pump or electronic infusion device. Pain intensity is monitored and documented. Breakthrough pain may be managed with oral analgesics, such as oxycodone. Toxic effects of continuous local anesthesia include dizziness, ringing in the ears, a metallic taste, perioral anesthesia, and slowed speech. If signs of toxicity are recognized early, decreasing the infusion rate may alleviate the problem. Elderly patients may be at a higher risk for toxicity due to a decreased ability to clear local anesthetics. The nurse should instruct the patient and family about what to do and whom to call about unrelieved pain, symptoms of infection, determining when the infusion is complete, removing the catheter, and dressing the site (Pasero, 2000).

■ DOCUMENTATION

Documentation should include the type of pain management provided, route of administration, methods used, IV or other access route, site care and maintenance, assessment of pain and degree of pain relief, and problems encountered in dealing with the particular type of access used. Flow sheets facilitate accuracy of documentation and provide a guideline for all areas of concern, including pain rating (intensity) and level of consciousness (Figs. 20–9 and 20–10).

When PCA systems are implemented, the nurse records the date, time, medication, patient's name and room number, physician's name, and his or her name on an appropriate flow sheet. The continuous nature of the injection does not permit the nurse to record the exact dosage administered on the standard control sheets found in many health care institutions. Many such facilities have developed individualized flow sheets specifically for PCA control. The American Pain Society has developed quality assurance standards for pain relief (Box 20–6).

References and Selected Readings

Asterisks indicate references cited in text.

*Ackerman, W.E., Juneja, M.M., Kaczorowski, D.M., & Colclough, G.W. (1989). A comparison of the incidence of pruritus following epidural opioid administration in the parturient. *Canadian Journal of Anaesthesia, 36*(4), 388–391.

*American Pain Society. (1999). *Principles of analgesic use in the treatment of acute pain and cancer pain* (4th ed.). Skokie, IL: Author.

American Pain Society Quality of Care Committee. (1995). Quality improvement guidelines for the treatment of acute pain and cancer pain. *Journal of the American Medical Association, 274*(23), 1874–1880.

Barnason, S., Merboth, M., Pozehl, B., & Tietjen, M.J. (1998). Utilizing an outcomes approach to improve pain management by nurses: A pilot study. *Clinical Nurse Specialist, 12*(1), 28–36.

*Bonica, J.J. (1990). Management of post-operative pain. In J.J. Bonica (Ed.), *The management of pain* (2nd ed., pp. 461–480). Philadelphia: Lea & Febiger.

*Caballero, G.A., Ausman, R.K., & Himes, J. (1986). Epidural morphine by continuous infusion with an external pump for pain management in oncology patients. *American Surgeon, 8*, 402–405.

Clarke, E.B., French, B., Bilodeau, M.L., Capasso, V.C., Edwards, A., & Empoliti, J. (1996). Pain management knowledge, attitudes and clinical practice: The impact of nurses' characteristics and education. *Journal of Pain and Symptom Management, 11*, 18–31.

Davidson, J. (1997). The nurse's role in monitoring a patient who is consciously sedated. *Critical Care Nurse, 17*, 102–104, 106.

Davol, Inc. Subsidiary of C.R. Bard, Inc., P.O. Box 8500, Cranston, RI ONC 60290-88810M.

Dufault, M.A. & Sullivan, M.C. (1999). Generating and testing pain management standards through collaborative research utilization. *Journal of Nursing Scholarship, 31*, 355–356.

*DuPen, S.L. (1987). A new permanent exteriorized epidural catheter for narcotic self-administration to control cancer pain. *Cancer, 59*, 986–993.

Edwards, A.D. (1999) The role of systemic lidocaine in neuropathic pain management. *Journal of Intravenous Nursing, 22*(5), 273–279.

*Hassenbusch, S.J., Pillay, P.K., Magdinec, M., Currie, K., Bay, J.W., Covington, E.C., & Tomaszewski, M.Z. (1990). Constant infusion of morphine for intractable cancer pain using an implanted pump. *Journal of Neurosurgery, 73*, 405–409.

*Intravenous Nurses Society. (2000). *Core curriculum for intravenous nursing* (pp. 16–18, 196). Philadelphia: Lippincott Williams & Wilkins.

*Intravenous Nurses Society. (1998). Revised intravenous nursing standards of practice. *Journal of Intravenous Nursing, 23* (Suppl.).

Intravenous Nurses Society. (2000). Revised standards of practice.

Janssen Pharmaceuticals. (1999). Product literature: Duragesic™. Titusville, NJ: Author.

Joint Commission on Accreditation of Healthcare Organizations. (1998). *Anesthesia care: Comprehensive manual for ambulatory care.* Oakbrook Terrace, IL: Author.

*Krames, E.S. (1996). Intraspinal opioid therapy for chronic nonmalignant pain: Current practice and clinical guidelines. *Journal of Pain and Symptom Management, 11*, 333–352.

Max, M. (1990). American Pain Society quality assurance standards for relief of acute pain and cancer pain. In M.R. Bond, J.E. Charlton, & C.J. Woolf (Eds.), *Proceedings of the VI World Congress on Pain* (pp. 196–189). Amsterdam: Elsevier.

McCaffery, M. & Pasero C. (1999) Pain control: Teaching patients to use a numerical pain-rating scale. *American Journal of Nursing, 99*(12), 22.

*McNeill, J.A., Sherwood, G.D., Starck, P.L., & Thompson, C.J. (1998). Assessing clinical outcomes: Patient satisfaction with pain management. *Journal of Pain and Symptom Management, 16,* 29–40.

Messinger, J.A., Hoffman, L.A., O'Donnell, J.M., & Dunworth, B.A. (1999). Getting conscious sedation right. *American Journal of Nursing, 99*(12), 44–50.

*Paice, J.A. (1987). New delivery systems in pain management. *Nursing Clinics of North America, 22,* 715–726.

*Paice, J.A., Penn, R.D., & Shott, S. (1996). Intraspinal morphine for chronic pain: A retrospective, multicenter study. *Journal of Pain and Symptom Management, 11,* 71–80.

*Pasero, C.L. (1997). Pain ratings: The fifth vital sign. *American Journal of Nursing, 97,* 15–16.

Pasero, C. (2000). Pain control: Continuous local anesthetics. *American Journal of Nursing, 100*(8), 22.

*Patt, R.B. (1989). Interventional analgesia: Epidural and subarachnoid therapy. *American Journal of Hospice Care, 11*–14.

Phillips, D.M. (2000). JCAHO pain management standards unveiled. *Journal of the American Medical Association, 284*(4), 428.

*Samuelsson, H., Malmberg, F., Eriksson, M., & Hedner, T. (1995). Outcomes of epidural morphine treatment in cancer pain: Nine years of clinical experience. *Journal of Pain and Symptom Management, 10,* 105–112.

*Snell, C.C., Fothergill-Bourbonnais, F., & Durocher-Hendriks, S. (1997). Patient controlled analgesia and intramuscular injections: A comparison of patient pain experiences and postoperative outcomes. *Journal of Advanced Nursing, 25,* 681–690.

Stevens, R.A. & de Leon-Casasola, O. (1997). What have we learned about acute postoperative epidural pain management since 1988? *Techniques in Regional Anesthesia and Pain Management, 1,* 59–63.

*Waldman, S.D. (1990). The role of spinal opioids in the management of cancer pain. *Journal of Pain and Symptom Management, 5,* 163–168.

*Watanabe, S., Pereira, J., Hanson, J., & Bruera, E. (1998). Fentanyl by continuous subcutaneous infusion for the management of cancer pain: A retrospective study. *Journal of Pain and Symptom Management, 16,* 323–326.

*Yablonski-Peretz, T., et al. (1985). Continuous epidural narcotic analgesia for intractable pain due to malignancy. *Journal of Surgical Oncology, 29,* 8–10.

*Yaney, L.L. (1998). Intravenous conscious sedation: physiologic, pharmacologic, and legal implications for nurses. *Journal of Intravenous Nursing, 21,* 9–19.

Review Questions

Note: Questions below may have more than one right answer.

1. Which pain management modality is to be avoided if at all possible?

   A. IV administration

   B. Continuous infusion of narcotic

   C. Intraspinal infusion of narcotic

   D. Intramuscular administration

2. When a patient experiences breakthrough pain, the first nursing intervention should be to:

   A. Believe the patient and record the level of pain

   B. Increase medication dose consistent with nursing judgment

   C. Contact the physician

   D. Verify the physician's order in the clinical record

3. Which of the following narcotic antagonists may be administered to reverse nausea?

   A. Nubain

   B. Nortriptyline

   C. Neupogen

   D. Naloxone

4. Epidural morphine has been associated with a high incidence of pruritus thought to be related to:

   A. An allergic reaction causing histamine release

   B. Opiate receptors binding with the opiate at the substantia gelatinosa

   C. Activity of the narcotic at the chemoreceptor sites

   D. Rostral spread of the narcotic in the CSF

5. Alcohol is contraindicated for site preparation or when accessing the catheter because of the potential for:

   A. Migration into the epidural space

   B. Possible nerve damage

   C. Obliterating the catheter

   D. Damage to the Silastic

6. Temporary epidural catheters are typically used for:

   A. Postoperative pain management

   B. Trial of epidural analgesia for patients with intractable cancer pain

   C. Long-term use for patients with intractable cancer pain

   D. A and B only

7. Aspiration of 3 mL of clear fluid from an epidural catheter could mean which of the following?

   A. The aspirant is medication.

   B. The aspirant is CSF.

   C. The epidural catheter is in a vein.

   D. All the above

8. Presence of up to 10 mL of clear fluid in the syringe after aspiration of an epidural catheter is evidence of which of the following?

   A. Catheter patency

   B. Catheter kinking

   C. Catheter migration into the intrathecal space

   D. Catheter damage

9. Nursing standards of practice for pain management have been established by which of the following organizations?

   A. American Pain Society

   B. American Epidural Society

   C. American Association for Pain

   D. American Society of Pain Management Nurses

10. Factors to be considered in pain assessment include:

   A. Patient's self-report of pain rating

   B. Nurses' report of patient's pain rating

   C. Physicians' report of patient's pain rating

   D. All of the above

U N I T 5

SPECIAL APPLICATIONS OF INTRAVENOUS THERAPY

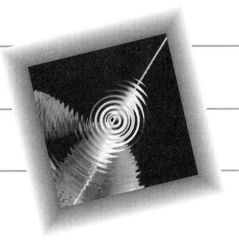

581

Pediatric Intravenous

Therapy

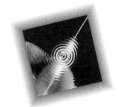

K E Y   T E R M S

Intraosseous Infusion
Play Therapy

■ INTRAVENOUS THERAPY IN INFANTS AND CHILDREN

This chapter focuses on features of IV therapy that are unique to pediatric patients. It highlights developmental considerations, IV therapies commonly used in children and adolescents, and necessary adaptations and adjustments to vascular access techniques and devices for pediatric patients. Two ongoing considerations in the administration of pediatric IV therapy are emotional preparation of the child and initiation of IV access. This chapter examines these topics in detail, along with special nursing considerations and specific IV therapeutic modalities.

■ PHYSICAL AND EMOTIONAL CONSIDERATIONS IN PEDIATRIC PATIENTS

Human beings change both physically and emotionally throughout childhood, whereas parameters remain relatively constant after adulthood. For example, body circumference increases more than 3-fold in length and approximately 20-fold in weight from birth through adolescence (Batton, Maisels, & Applebaum, 1982). The body circumference of the adult, however, changes relatively little throughout the remainder of life. Thus, the stress levels and basal metabolic rates of the child are much higher than those of the adult.

A more subtle area of concern is the child's emotional needs, which require patience, education, and understanding from IV nurses. Psychological age and ability as well as each child's particular developmental stage exert major influences on emotional needs. For example, when hospitalized, some children regress and exhibit behaviors more common in a younger age group (eg, a child who is toilet trained may regress to the diaper stage). These children resume developmental landmarks once treatment ends or the child's condition stabilizes. Thus, even though children of varied ages and intellectual capacities receive similar IV therapies, they require education before, during, and after IV therapy that considers their particular emotional and developmental variables.

Developmental Stages

A full understanding of each developmental stage enables the health care team to provide appropriate, nonthreatening care. It enhances the ability of staff to recognize that children's needs vary markedly, not only according to stress levels but by growth and developmental levels.

The pediatric population can be divided by age into the following stages: infant (0 to 12 months), toddler (1 to 3 years), preschool (4 to 5 years), school age (6 to 12 years), and adolescent (12 to 18 years) (Whaley & Wong, 1993). A subdivision of the infant group is neonates or newborns (0 to 28 days); the unique IV therapy needs of premature infants also are considered within the infant stage (Sater, 1998). The health care team should gear pre-IV and post-IV care according to these stages, including preparation for the procedure, IV site protection, and mobility and safety needs. For example, most children are not able to understand the significance of IV therapy, including the importance of not manipulating the IV site, until they reach age $3\frac{1}{2}$ to 5 years, depending on the individual child. Thus, younger children and their families require appropriate adjustments. A review of growth, development, and useful approaches when working with children of different developmental stages is highlighted in Table 21–1.

Although developmental stages are important, nurses must remember to explain all procedures to the child or parent and to assess each child individually, not just according to age or physiologic maturity. In some cases, children have disease processes, such as renal disease, that can result in growth delays, causing staff to mistake the child's actual age.

Play Therapy and Coping Mechanisms

Play therapy, consisting of practicing IV therapy on a doll, is an ideal teaching strategy that enhances emotional preparation through acting out. It may not, however, always be practical because of the urgency of IV therapy or the availability of dolls. When it is pragmatic, nurses certainly can use play therapy for teaching purposes, or they may seek such assistance from child-life workers, ancillary members of the health care team who specialize in child development.

A "coping" or "comfort basket," filled with items for various age groups, is easy and inexpensive to put together. The basket can include a Slinky, a clear, sealed acrylic "magic wand" with floating sparkles, a kaleidoscope, and a bottle of bubbles for blowing. Such items are easy to clean and small enough to keep in a hospital treatment room, pediatric care office, or equipment bag. An adolescent may find a portable stereo with headphones a useful distraction during IV insertion (Frederick, 1991; Heiney, 1991).

Establishing Rapport

Another important aspect of IV therapy is establishing rapport with the family and child through good communication. Communication differs for all age groups and according to the child's intellectual level.

Usually it is best to tell the child that the venipuncture will hurt but only for a short time. Define the term *time* not by minutes (young children will not understand) but by comparison with other procedures. For example, say, "The actual IV puncture takes about the same time it takes me to take your temperature, get you a glass of orange juice, or for you to finish your dinner." Inform the child that even though this therapy may be painful initially, it should make him or her feel better, like before the illness. Always be honest with a child. Specifically, do not promise a certain number of IV attempts or "only one stick" because a child will lose trust if several attempts turn out to be necessary. Give the child the opportunity to cry, providing as much privacy as possible. Allow children who are old enough to participate in the therapy. Tearing tape, opening alcohol swabs, or holding tubing may provide distraction and a sense of involvement, particularly if the child is of school age. Nurses may be able to assuage a child's fear of needles by telling the child that once the IV is in place, the needle is no longer there, and only a small "straw" is in the vein.

An IV therapy teaching tool with pictures and large-print words in simple language can help preschoolers understand the procedure. The learning tool can be used as a hospital coloring book (Thompson, 1994). Adolescents, in particular, require a great deal of individual attention and allowance for their independent nature versus their dependent situation. Adolescents believe they are mature and desire the chance to assess their disease status; they deserve the opportunity to participate in the decision-making aspects of their care. They feel grown up but lack the adult's experience and knowledge. Therefore, educational techniques practiced with adolescents should encompass a common-sense approach that provides adolescents with the opportunity to deal with IV therapy to the best of their ability.

The presence of parents during a painful or invasive procedure is controversial and needs to be evaluated on a case-by-case basis. One study concluded that patients aged 1 to 7 years are likely to experience less distress during venipuncture if parents are present, and that parental presence is unlikely to affect experienced health care providers (Wolfram, Turner, & Philput, 1997). Parents may provide emotional support and represent security during an actual procedure, but they should not be used to restrain a child unless no other assistance is available (eg, in home care).

If a parent chooses not to accompany a child into the treatment room for IV insertion, the IV nurse should honor this decision and not make parents feel guilty. Provision of comfort and praise after an IV insert is an ideal means of parental involvement after the procedure is completed.

text continues on page 588

T A B L E   2 1 – 1

GROWTH, DEVELOPMENT, AND INTRAVENOUS INSERTION TIPS
FOR VARIOUS PEDIATRIC DEVELOPMENTAL STAGES

Stage (Age)	Growth	Development	IV Insertion Tips
Infancy (birth to 12 mo) (includes neonatal period from birth to 28 d)	• Physical and developmental changes are rapid. • Head and body grow very rapidly. • Major body systems undergo progressive maturation. • Birth weight usually doubles by age 6 mo and triples by age 1 y.	• Trust vs. mistrust • Child displays social affective play. • Attachment to caregivers is paramount. • Separation anxiety begins approximately age 6 mo.	• Infants require caregivers to meet their needs consistently. • Do not feed the baby before IV placement or aspiration may occur. • Provide comfort during and after the procedure, using a pacifier and distraction, such as a mobile.
Toddler (12 to 36 mo)	• Growth slows down. • Birth weight quadruples by 30 mo. • Height at age 3 y is usually approximately half adult height. • Head circumference growth slows, and chest circumference is larger than the head or abdomen.	• Autonomy vs. shame • Child displays cause and effect thinking. • Exploration is prominent. • Child shows imaginative play and may be reckless at times. • New gross motor skills develop.	• Toddlers require short, concrete explanations immediately before the IV is started. • Do not give a toddler a choice, such as "Can we start your IV now?" or the answer will be "No!" • The nurse will need an assistant to position and restrain the toddler.
Preschool/early childhood (36 mo to 6 y)	• Growth stabilizes. • Average annual weight gain is approximately 2.2 kg (5 lbs). • Average height increase ranges from 6.4 to 7.6 cm (2.5 to 3 in.). • Most height growth is in legs, resulting in a more slender physical appearance.	• Fantasy vs. reality • Child follows simple commands. • Child fears blood loss and invasive procedures. • Play is solitary and interactive. • Child is fascinated with superheroes/monsters. • Child may fantasize about procedures based on understanding.	• Preschoolers require preparation immediately before the procedure and may be distracted with age-appropriate toys. • Play therapy using medical toys works well with this age group. • Nurse may still need help to hold the child still.

School age (6–12 y)	• Growth and development is gradual. • Average annual weight gain is 2–3 kg (4.5–6.5 lbs). • Average height increase is approximately 5 cm (2 in.).	• Industry vs. inferiority • Logic, reasoning, and concept of permanence develop. • Child develops skills and can dramatize. • Self-esteem and values emerge. • Child finds role models.	• School-age children can be told about the IV a short time in advance and can assist with small tasks, such as ripping pieces of tape and helping to keep a record of intake and output. • Allow for privacy. • Allow the child to cry; don't force him or her to "be brave."
Adolescence Divided into three substages: early adolescence (11–13 y), middle adolescence (13 to 15 y), and late adolescence (15 y and older)	• Early, little size difference between boys and girls. • Toward the end of early adolescence, a growth spurt occurs. • Girls first surpass boys in height and weight, then boys surpass girls. • Body proportions approach adult parameters by the end of adolescence.	• Identity vs. role confusion • Abstract and deductive reasoning emerge. • Child needs independence, yet wants to be cared for at times. Early • Teen seeks independence from parents/guardians. • Peers are very important. Middle • Sexual identity and body image are very important. • Teen grapples with mortality. Late • Career plans take shape. • Teen shows high idealism and favors close, intimate relationships. • Teen looks for a significant other.	• Adolescents vacillate between dependence and independence; approach a teen using adult language • Prepare teens for procedures in advance, allowing them a part in their care.

(Data From Guhlow, L. & Kolb, J. [1979]. Pediatric IVs: Special measures you must take. *RN, 42*, 40–52; and Whaley, L. F. & Wong, D. I. [Eds.]. [1995]. *Nursing care of infants and children* (5th ed., p. 107) St. Louis: Mosby.)

Pain Reduction

Studies indicate that infants and children respond to noxious stimuli and experience pain. In one study, infants and children showed significant behavioral changes and toddlers demonstrated measurable increases in heart rate during venipuncture and IV insertion (Van Cleve, Johnson, & Pothier, 1996). By using pain reduction techniques, such as imagery and the coping basket, nurses can reduce the anxiety associated with IV insertion. In addition, local anesthetics, such as topically applied eutectic mixture of local anesthetics (EMLA) cream or intradermal saline at the IV site, may decrease pain sensation in children. A summary of some medications for pain reduction is provided in Table 21–2. In some cases, IV conscious sedation may be necessary to provide a more generalized sedation for invasive procedures such as insertion of a peripherally inserted central catheter (PICC), and noninvasive procedures, such as diagnostic studies (Deady & Gorman, 1997).

■ COMMON PEDIATRIC INTRAVENOUS THERAPIES

Primary indications for pediatric IV therapy include fluid therapy, medication administration, antineoplastic therapy, nutritional support, and transfusion therapy. Although these topics are covered fully in other chapters, features unique to pediatric patients are highlighted in the following sections.

Fluid Therapy

Fluids are delivered through a peripheral or central IV device by gravity using a volume control chamber or, for more accuracy, through an electronic infusion device. For fluid therapy that is short-lived and can be advanced quickly to oral rehydration therapy, a peripheral catheter is usually the device of choice. If hypertonic solution or chronic fluid therapy is indicated, a central access device may be recommended. Accurate intake requires precision in IV administration. Delivery of a constant flow of IV fluids is paramount. Even the smallest error can cause serious problems, especially in the compromised child. If the child's fluid requirements are not met, a number of physiologic and metabolic problems may ensue, including weight loss associated with hyperosmolality, hypernatremia, and increased hematocrit, as well as evidence of metabolic acidosis, dehydration, and, frequently in infants, multiple apnea spells and increased bilirubin.

Assessing Fluid Needs

At what rate should IV fluids be administered to a child? The child's stature and metabolic rate determine the answer. The amount of fluid required for maintenance levels depends on insensible water losses from the lungs, skin, urine, and stools and from metabolic expenditures based on both internal and external stress levels. The younger the child, the greater his or her fluid requirements because he or she has a higher percentage of total body water. For example, the water content of a 28-week-gestational-age infant comprises 85% of total body weight, compared with the term

T A B L E 2 1 – 2
LOCAL NUMBING METHODS FOR PEDIATRIC INTRAVENOUS ACCESS PROCEDURES

Method	Administration	Advantages	Disadvantages
EMLA cream (topical)	Cream is placed on potential venipuncture sites and covered with transparent dressing 1 or more hours before procedure.	• Topical • Noninvasive • Easy to use • May be applied at home	• Takes a relatively long time to work • May cause vasoconstriction • Precautions necessary in neonates
NUMBY Stuff (topical), Iomed, Inc., Salt Lake City, UT	Iontophoresis—a liquid solution containing anesthetics is placed on an electrode, and the electrode is pasted to the skin and stimulated with a mild current of electricity.	• Works quickly • More depth of penetration than EMLA	• Electrical stimulation may be uncomfortable for some patients • Takes 10 min to work
Ethyl chloride (chloroethane; topical)	Spray bottle directs pressurized liquid to cool the skin and produce instant local anesthesia.	• Easy to use • Works quickly • Lasts only a few seconds to 1 min	• May obscure site or constrict vein • May cause frostbite, skin ulceration, muscle damage • Very flammable
Lidocaine hydrochloride 0.5%, 1% without epinephrine (intradermal)	An intradermal wheal of approximately 0.05 to 0.1 mL is made near the IV insertion site by using a very tiny needle (26- or 29-gauge insulin needle).	• Works immediately and provides good level of local anesthesia • Useful for such procedures as peripherally inserted central catheter placement	• Two sticks needed • May sting if acidity not neutralized • Can inadvertently be injected IV • May cause allergic reaction
Normal saline with preservative (intradermal)	An intradermal wheal of approximately 0.05 to 0.1 mL is made near the IV insertion site by using a very tiny needle (26- or 29-gauge insulin needle).	• Works immediately and provides equivalent level of local anesthesia to lidocaine • Does not have the potential side effects of lidocaine (stinging, allergic reaction, possible IV injection)	• Two sticks needed • Limited duration of local numbing (2 min) • Cannot be used in preterm and low–birth-weight neonates

EMLA, eutectic mixture of local anesthetics (Astra Zeneca International, Wilmington, DE).
(Data From Fein et al., 1998; Lewis & Stephen, 1997; Milliam, 1995; Robieux et al., 1991.)

infant, whose water content is only 70% of total body weight (Klaus & Fanaroff, 1979). In general, rates for pediatric patients vary from 5 to 80 mL/hour, depending on the child's size. Requirements vary among term, low–birth-weight, and premature, high-risk infants. Adolescent fluid requirements are similar to those for adults, ranging from 100 to 175 mL/hour.

A precise record of intake and output is the most valuable assessment tool for determining fluid requirements. To ensure accuracy in judging fluid needs, intake and output, including diaper weights, are monitored strictly for children receiving IV therapy. Infants have a greater urine volume per kilogram of body weight and a smaller bladder volume capacity than older children. Expected urine output with adequate intake should be 2 to 3 mL/kg/hour for infants, 2 mL/kg/hour for toddlers, 1 to 2 mL/kg/hour for school-age children, and 0.5 to 1 mL/kg/hour for adolescents (Whaley & Wong, 1995). Expected urine output for children and adolescents is 1.0 mL/kg/hour.

MAINTENANCE REQUIREMENTS

Maintenance fluid requirements for neonates and children differ in terms of the volume allowed over 24 hours, but all fluid needs are calculated in milliliters per kilogram of weight (Holiday & Segar, 1957) (Table 21–3). Familiarity with three different methods of assessing 24-hour maintenance fluids is crucial: namely, the meters-squared, caloric, and weight methods (Graef & Cone, 1977). These methods address only maintenance requirements for normal metabolism; they do not address insensible losses or additional metabolic expenditures that require further replacement therapy.

1. In the meters-squared method, the child's height and weight are plotted on a nomogram to obtain a surface area in meters squared (m^2). This method uses an arbitrary estimated requirement of 1500 to 1800 mL of fluid per square meter. The advantage of this method is its simplicity; its disadvantage is the need for an accessible visual nomogram.
2. In the weight method, fluid needs are estimated based on the child's weight in kilograms. The advantage of this method also is its simplicity; its disadvantage is its decreased accuracy in patients who weigh more than 10 kg.
3. In the caloric method, usual fluid expenditure is calculated at approximately 150 mL for every 100 calories metabolized. This method, too, is simple, but not totally accurate unless actual calorie requirements and energy intake are assessed continuously. This method is the most frequently used to calculate fluid requirements.

T A B L E 2 1 – 3
FORMULA FOR CALCULATING MAINTENANCE FLUID REQUIREMENTS FOR CHILDREN

Newborn:	60–100 mL/kg/24 h (used up to 72 h of age)
0–10 kg:	100 mL/kg/24 h for the first 10 kg
11–20 kg:	100 mL/kg/24 h for the first 10 kg, PLUS 50 mL/kg/24 h for each kilogram over 10 kg
21–30 kg:	100 mL/kg/24 h for the first 10 kg, PLUS 50 mL/kg/24 h for each kilogram over 10 kg, PLUS 20 mL/kg/24 h for each kilogram over 20 kg

Examples:

A 6-kg infant would receive 600 mL divided by 24 h: 6 kg × 100 mL/kg = 600 mL

A 32-kg child would receive 1740 mL divided by 24 h:

```
10 kg ×  100 mL/kg  =  1000 mL, PLUS
10 kg ×   50 mL/kg  =   500 mL, PLUS
12 kg ×   20 mL/kg  =  +240 mL
32 kg                  1740 mL divided by 24 h
```

CAUSES OF ALTERATIONS IN FLUID NEEDS

The most common cause of altered fluid and caloric needs is changes in temperature. An increase in temperature by 1°C raises the child's caloric needs by 12%, thereby increasing fluid needs as well. In the neonate, use of radiant warmers and single-walled incubators may effectively maintain the newborn's temperature, but this temperature elevation in turn increases the infant's insensible fluid losses. Phototherapy, although effectively used to treat newborn hyperbilirubinemia, increases insensible fluid losses and water requirements (Klaus & Fanaroff, 1979). These various losses must be included when determining fluid replacement needs. Conversely, a child who is hypothermic experiences a 12% decrease in caloric needs for every 1°C lost, which in turn decreases fluid requirements. Other conditions that affect fluid requirements include diarrhea and presence of nasogastric tubes.

Managing Fluid and Electrolyte Imbalances

Infants and children are especially prone to fluid and electrolyte imbalances because their bodies are made up of more water in proportion to surface area than those of adults. Moreover, their immature body organs compromise their ability to handle imbalances.

DEHYDRATION

Dehydration can occur rapidly in children who lose more water than they receive. Being alert for signs of dehydration is an important aspect of caring for pediatric patients. Physical assessment parameters for dehydration are outlined in Table 21–4.

T A B L E   2 1 – 4
ASSESSMENT PARAMETERS USED TO DETERMINE DEGREE OF DEHYDRATION

Parameter	Degree of Dehydration		
	Mild	Moderate	Severe
Weight loss	3%–5%	6%–9%	≥10%
Skin turgor	Normal	Decreased	Decreased
Mucous membranes	Slightly dry	Dry	Dry
Eyes	Normal	Sunken orbits	Deeply sunken orbits
Extremities	Warm, normal capillary refill	Delayed capillary refill	Cool, mottled
Fontanelle	Normal	Sunken	Sunken
Blood pressure	Normal	Normal	Normal to reduced
Pulse quality	Normal	Normal or slightly decreased	Moderately decreased
Heart rate	Normal	Increased	Increased; bradycardia in severe cases
Mental status	Normal	Normal to listless	Normal to lethargic or comatose
Urine output	Slightly decreased	<1 mL/kg/h	<0.5–1 mL/kg/h

(From Fann, B. D. [1998]. Fluid and electrolyte balance in the pediatric patient. *Journal of Intravenous Nursing, 21,* 153–159.)

Dehydration is characterized by type, depending on level of serum sodium, and by degree, depending on weight loss, patient history, and physical assessment. The three types of dehydration are as follows:

- Isotonic—Sodium is within normal limits and electrolyte and water deficits are equal (eg, mild vomiting and diarrhea)
- Hypertonic—Sodium is elevated and water losses are greater than electrolyte losses (eg, too concentrated formula intake)
- Hypotonic—Sodium is low and electrolyte losses are greater than water losses or water intake is large (eg, diabetes insipidus, drowning in fresh water)

To determine the degree of dehydration, nurses must calculate the percentage of weight lost. For each 1% of weight loss, the patient also has lost 10 mL/kg of fluid, which must be made up in addition to maintenance and ongoing losses. If a child presents with severe dehydration, a fluid bolus of normal saline or lactated Ringer's at a dosage of 20 to 40 mL/kg should be initiated and repeated if necessary. Oral rehydration should be initiated at a rate of 50 to 100 mL/kg if the child is mild to moderately dehydrated. IV therapy continues if the child does not tolerate oral rehydration therapy or the type of dehydration warrants IV correction (American Academy of Pediatrics, 1996).

FLUID OVERLOAD

Fluid overload and intoxication are less common than dehydration, but can occur more readily in infants, whose immature kidneys are unable to excrete excess fluid. A serum sodium less than 130 mEq/L in an infant that is not associated with dehydration is a sign of water intoxication (Fann, 1998). Causes of water intoxication include too rapid dialysis, too rapid reduction of glucose levels in diabetic ketoacidosis, and administration of overly diluted formula (Wong, 1995). Treatment includes reducing fluid delivery and administering IV furosemide.

ELECTROLYTE IMBALANCES

Laboratory values to monitor in children include sodium, potassium, chloride, calcium, and glucose. Gastrointestinal disturbances, such as diarrhea, most often alter potassium levels. Children usually do not experience cardiac symptoms until the serum potassium falls below 3 mEq/L. Hyperkalemia is more common, especially in premature infants. For children with renal failure, hyperkalemia does not decrease as expected during rehydration (Barnard & Hazinski, 1992). The hallmarks of hyperkalemia in children are similar to those in in adults—tented T waves and prolonged P-R intervals on the electrocardiogram. Other common electrolyte imbalances in children include hypocalcemia, hyponatremia or hypernatremia (as seen with dehydration), and chloride disturbances. Infants are especially prone to hypocalcemia because more calcium is deposited in the bones when the infant is stressed and growth hormone is secreted. Other causes of hypocalcemia include transfusion of citrated blood, pancreatitis, newborn intake of cow's milk, hyperphosphatemia, hypomagnesemia, vitamin D deficiency, and malabsorption. Conversely, lower calcium can result from excessive use of diuretics, tumor breakdown when initiating chemotherapy, and immobilization (Fann, 1998).

ACID–BASE IMBALANCES

Acid–base balance is part of the overall picture of fluid balance. When a child has diarrhea, he or she loses bicarbonate in the stool. Metabolic acidosis results. Conversely, when a child is vomiting or has a nasogastric tube, metabolic alkalosis can result from the large amount of acid lost in gastric secretions. When replacing electrolytes, frequent (at least hourly) monitoring of laboratory values and fluid balance is necessary to prevent acid–base imbalances.

Antibiotic and Medication Therapy

Multiple-drug therapy is routine for today's highly acute pediatric patient. Drugs administered through IV therapy include antibiotics, antivirals, and antifungals for such conditions as cystic fibrosis, meningitis, osteomyelitis, Lyme disease, joint infections, prophylaxis before and after abdominal surgery, bacterial and fungal central line infections, and systemic herpes infection. The most common pediatric disorder requiring antibiotic therapy is sepsis. Length of antibiotic therapy differs according to diagnosis, so choice of IV device is based on those factors as well as the child's vein availability. For short-term therapy (1 to 2 weeks), a peripheral IV may suffice, whereas for longer than 2 weeks, a midline catheter or PICC may be indicated (Frey, 1995; Schuman, 1990).

In addition, many IV medications used in adults are used in children. These medication categories include but are not limited to the following:

- Analgesics, such as morphine sulfate
- Antiarrhythmic agents, such as adenosine (Adenocard)
- Anticoagulants, such as heparin sodium (Liquaemin)
- Anticonvulsants, such as phenytoin (Dilantin)
- Antiemetics, such as ondansetron (Zophran)
- Chelating agents, such as deferoxamine mesylate (Desferal Mesylate)
- Corticosteroids, such as dexamethasone (Decadron, Hexadrol)
- Gastric acid inhibitors, such as ranitidine hydrochloride (Zantac)
- Vasoactive drugs, such as dopamine (Intropin) and isoproterenol (Isuprel)
- Bronchodilators, such as aminophylline
- Immunosuppressant agents, such as cyclosporine (Sandimmune)

In many cases, drugs have not yet been approved for pediatric IV administration but are used based on ongoing and published research studies, experience with adults, and the emergency status of the child. For this reason, children often are referred to as *therapeutic orphans,* indicating the lack of information about interactions between medications and children's body processes (Berner-Howry, McGillis-Bindler, & Tso, 1981; Jew, 1997–1999).

Pharmacokinetics

Pharmacokinetic parameters must be considered when administering IV medications to a child. These parameters include absorption, distribution, metabolism, and excretion. Each of these is affected by the patient's level of maturity and the disease process itself (Matyskiela-Frey, 1985).

Absorption depends on adequacy of IV access and length of delivery; it usually is immediate with IV medications. Distribution occurs when a drug enters the circulatory system (it takes approximately 1 minute for blood to circulate through a child's body) and is delivered to the tissues (Holiday & Segar, 1957). Most drugs are distributed by the extracellular fluid; others are distributed by binding with protein or fat molecules.

Because neonates have a higher level of total body water than adults, water-soluble drugs, such as theophylline, must be given at higher doses (Matyskiela-Frey, 1985). Neonates and malnourished children have decreased levels of plasma proteins, and drugs that bind to protein may be given in lower doses to these children. Some drugs also may compete with binding sites on the albumin molecule, displacing bilirubin from these sites in neonates and increasing the risk of hyperbilirubinemia. Such drugs include salicylates, sulfonamides, phenytoin (Dilantin), furosemide (Lasix), and sodium benzoate (Guyon, 1989). Many commercially available medications and drug diluents contain sodium benzoate in the form of the preservative benzyl alcohol, which has been linked with toxicity and death in premature infants. Thus, care should be taken to stock only preservative-free diluents in the nursery and neonatal intensive care unit (Meyer, 1982).

Because neonates have less subcutaneous fat, lipid-soluble medications such as diazepam (Valium) should be given in smaller doses. The liver plays a large part in drug metabolism. In neonates with immature hepatic systems or children with liver disease, decreased liver function may alter the metabolism of such drugs as phenobarbital, phenytoin, and carbamazepine (Guyon, 1989).

Many drugs are excreted by the renal system. Again, less efficient renal function due to immaturity in the neonate or disease process in the older child may decrease excretion of drugs, causing longer half-life and possible toxicity. In these patients, penicillins and aminoglycosides are given with longer intervals between doses (every 12 or 18 hours vs. every 6 or 8 hours). In children with cystic fibrosis, whose extrarenal clearance pathways eliminate drugs more quickly, IV aminoglycosides such as tobramycin (Nebcin) must be given at two to three times the normal dose (Matyskiela-Frey, 1985).

Pediatric Dosages

Dosages for pediatric patients are individualized, based on the patient's weight and metabolism. Dose and volume of medications for children can differ from those used in adults, depending on the child's age and size. Drug dosages are calculated in grams, milligrams, micrograms, units, and milliequivalents. However, a full dose of a drug may amount only to tenths of 1 mL in volume. A rule of thumb is that most drugs are packaged in single adult-sized doses, so a portion of a vial is usually needed for a child's dose. If more than two vials of a drug are needed for a single pediatric dose, calculations should be rechecked.

Before and after IV administration of certain drugs, levels of medication in the blood are tested to determine the safe dosage range for therapeutic effectiveness. These levels are known as trough level, or the lowest drug level drawn just before giving a scheduled dose, and peak level, or the highest drug level, drawn 30 minutes after the drug and postflush have infused (Korth-Bradley, 1991). Monitoring these levels and the patient's clinical status, coupled with an awareness of pharmacokinetic parameters, provides a good picture of the effects of IV medication administration in the child.

Techniques for Medication Administration

One of the most frequently encountered problems with administration of medications to pediatric patients is limiting the amount of fluid used to administer and flush the drug through the IV tubing. When a child receives multiple-drug therapies, the potential to exceed fluid requirements exists. Volumes can be limited by using microbore tubing and minimal dilution volumes. Sample minimal dilution guidelines are provided in Table 21–5.

Each method of drug administration is applicable to specific drugs and desired therapeutic outcomes. Methods of IV medication administration in children include direct IV push or bolus, continuous infusion, and intermittent infusion (Gura, 1993).

Direct IV push or bolus is usually defined as an IV injection given over 5 minutes or less. Examples of IV push or bolus medications include antibiotics (eg, ampicillin), anticonvulsants (eg, phenytoin), sedatives (eg, midazolam), and antineoplastic drugs (eg, vincristine). The IV push or bolus method is used when therapeutic serum levels are needed quickly to achieve the desired effect, whether it be a high serum level of an antibiotic, cessation of seizure activity, or sedation for a procedure. Not all medications can be given in this manner because of local and systemic effects, such as phlebitis, cardiac dysrhythmias, hypotension, or anaphylaxis. The nurse administering an IV push or bolus dose must administer the drug at a certain rate and dilution, which usually is specified in drug references, and monitor the child closely to avoid adverse effects.

Continuous infusions are used primarily for administration of drugs that require maintenance of a steady blood level, or of potent drugs that must be highly titrated to individual needs. Intermittent infusions are used mainly for antimicrobials. They can be administered by several different methods:

- Calibrated chamber
- Retrograde
- Syringe pump
- Individual pump

CALIBRATED CHAMBER
The in-line calibrated chamber is used commonly in general pediatric settings. Medication is injected into the in-line calibrated chamber and infused at a prescribed rate. Once the infusion is complete, the usual practice is to flush the chamber and tubing with 10 to 20 mL (depending on tubing volume) of IV solution compatible with the medication, such as 5% dextrose in water or 0.9% sodium chloride. The advantage of this method is its simplicity; however, in neonates, the tubing volume may be too large for the child's fluid needs.

RETROGRADE INFUSION
Retrograde infusion is practiced mainly in the neonatal intensive care units. A specific retrograde administration set, with a volume of less than 1 mL, is required for

text continues on page 598

TABLE 21–5
MAXIMUM RECOMMENDED CONCENTRATIONS AND MINIMUM RECOMMENDED ADMINISTRATION TIMES FOR THE ADMINISTRATION OF ANTIBIOTICS TO THE FLUID-RESTRICTED PATIENT

Antibiotics	Recommended Final Concentration for Administration	Recommended Duration of Infusion	Antibiotics	Recommended Final Concentration for Administration	Recommended Duration of Infusion
Acyclovir	7 mg/mL	1–3 h	Miconazole	6 mg/mL	30–60 min
Amikacin	6 mg/mL	15–30 min	Nafcillin*	50 mg/mL	10–30 min
Ampicillin*	50 mg/mL	10–30 min	Penicillin G	Infants: 50,000 U/mL	10–30 min
Amphotericin B†‡	0.1 mg/mL	2–4 h		Large child: 100,000 U/mL	
Azlocillin*	50 mg/mL	15–30 min	Pentamidine	2.5 mg/mL	1 h
Aztreonam	20 mg/mL	20–60 min	Pipiricillin*	50 mg/mL	10–30 min
Carbenicillin*	50 mg/mL	10–30 min	Ticarcillin	50 mg/mL	10–30 min
Cefazolin*	50 mg/mL	10–30 min	Tobramycin	2 mg/mL	15–30 min
Cefotaxime*	50 mg/mL	10–30 min	Trimethoprim–sulfamethoxazole	1 mL in 15–25 mL (5 mL = 80 mg TMP, 400 mg SMX)	60 min
Cefoxitin*	50 mg/mL	15–30 min	Vancomycin§	5 mg/mL	60 min
Ceftazidime*	50 mg/mL	15–30 min	Vidarabine	0.45 mg/mL	12–24 h
Ceftriaxone*	50 mg/mL	10–30 min			
Cefuroxime*	50 mg/mL	15–30 min			
Cephalothin*	50 mg/mL	15–30 min			
Chloramphenicol	50–100 mg/mL	10–30 min			

Clindamycin	6–12 mg/mL	15–30 min
Erythromycin	5 mg/mL	20–30 min
Gentamicin	2 mg/mL	15–30 min
Imipenem–cilastatin	5 mg/mL	30–60 min
Methicillin*	50 mg/mL	15–30 min
Metronidazole	5–8 mg/mL	60 min
Mezlocillin*	50 mg/mL	10–30 min
Experimental		
Flucytosine (do not dilute)	10 mg/mL	30 min–1 h
Ganciclovir (DHPG)	10 mg/mL	1 hour
Rifampin	6 mg/mL	<3 h
Trimetrexate	4 mg/mL	30 min

The main determinant of the maximum recommended concentration of antibiotics for IV administration is the development of phlebitis. The table lists the maximum recommended concentration for infusion of antimicrobial agents. Infusions exceeding these guidelines may cause the development of severe phlebitis and loss of the IV site. Administration of medication faster than the infusion times listed above may lead to an increase in adverse drug reactions.

* The concentration of beta-lactam drugs (penicillins and cephalosporins) may be increased from 50 to 100 mg/mL when administered to large children in whom excessive volumes of fluid would be required with the 50 mg/mL concentration.

† Amphotericin B is incompatible with saline.

‡ Amphotericin B (Fungizone IV) must be given by *slow* IV infusion (see package insert). Side effects may be reduced, however, by using a shorter infusion time.

§ Vancomycin should not be infused over <60 min because of the association of a characteristic rash over the head and neck with more rapid infusion rate.

‖ May infuse over a longer period of time if the fluid volume necessitates.

(From Farrington, E. [1990]. Pediatric drug information. *Pediatric Nursing, 16*, 310.)

Section Editor's Note:

- If an antibiotic has been noted to be irritating to the veins, the concentration may be decreased to no more than half of what is recommended.
- When infusing antibiotics a central line, a concentration of twice that listed above may be used to reduce the fluid volume administered to a patient.

this purpose. A three-way stopcock or access port is at each end of the tubing. To administer medications through the system, a medication-filled syringe is attached to the port most proximal to the patient, and an empty syringe is connected to the port most distal from the patient. The clamp between the port and the child is closed, and the medication is injected distally up the tubing (away from the child). The fluid in the retrograde tubing is displaced upward in the tubing into the empty syringe. Both syringes are removed, the lower clamp is opened, and the medication is then infused into the patient at the prescribed rate. The medication volume is then automatically incorporated into the regulated amount of fluid to be infused. This method is often used in infants or children who cannot tolerate a rapid infusion rate or additional fluid volume.

SYRINGE PUMP

An increasingly popular and accurate method of IV medication administration in children is the syringe pump. The syringe pump can be connected by an extension set directly onto a heparin lock or in a piggyback fashion into the primary line. A syringe of diluted medication, prefilled by the pharmacy or by the nurse caring for the patient, is attached to microbore tubing, and the medication can then be infused at a prescribed rate.

INDIVIDUAL PUMP

This system of IV medication infusion is very popular in home care. Individual patient doses may be premixed by the home care pharmacy in an elastomeric infusion pump or other single-use device. After administration of the dose, the disposable pumps are either returned to the home care pharmacy or discarded. Individual dosing systems provide premixed diluted drug doses that are easy for the caregiver or patient to administer.

Emergency Intravenous Medication Administration

Of great concern to many practitioners is correct administration of IV medications given to a child during advanced life support. These medications are administered by weight, age, or both; patient length also has been used to determine weight with a high degree of accuracy (Luten, 1997). Some institutions, particularly in pediatric critical care areas, use bedside charts that list the individual doses of emergency drugs for the weight of that particular child. In addition, large multidose charts listing doses of drugs and sizes of equipment used in a pediatric code may be posted in the emergency or treatment room areas. This information is extremely helpful to nursing and medical personnel who work with adult patients and are not familiar with these dosages from experience. Tables 21–6 and 21–7 list pediatric life support medications, dosages, and infusions.

Although most medications are administered by peripheral or central IV, emergency medications and fluids to treat respiratory and cardiac arrest may be administered by the intraosseous (IO) route (discussed later in this chapter) if IV access cannot be obtained.

TABLE 21-6
INFUSIONS FOR PEDIATRIC AND NEONATAL RESUSCITATION

Medication	Preparation (add amounts calculated to D$_5$W to = 100 mL)	Dosage	Range
Dopamine (μg/kg/min)	(6 × kg) mg	1 mL/h = 1 μg/kg/min	2.0–15.0
Dobutamine (μg/kg/min)			2.0–15.0
Epinephrine	(0.6 × kg) mg	1 mL/h = 0.1 μg/kg/min	0.1–1.0 μg/kg/min
Norepinephrine	(60 × kg) mg	1 mL/h = 10 μg/kg/min	10.0–50.0 μg/kgmin
Lidocaine	≤ 20 kg: (0.6 × kg) mg	1 mL/h = 0.1 μg/kg/min	0.1–1.0 μg/kg/min
Isoproterenol	20–40 kg: (0.3 × kg) mg	1 mL/h = 0.05 μg/kg/min	
	≥ 40 kg: (0.12 × kg) mg	1 mL/h = 0.02 μg/kg/min	

Antineoplastic Therapy

Because of research, new drug combinations, and aggressive therapy, the mortality rate for children with cancer has decreased greatly since the 1960s. Still, cancer remains the primary cause of death from disease in children between the ages of 1 and 14 years (Bertolone, 1997). Common cancers in children include neuroblastoma,

TABLE 21-7
INTRAVENOUS DRUGS FOR PEDIATRIC AND NEONATAL RESUSCITATION

Drug	Dosage
Sodium bicarbonate (8.4%) (dilute to half strength in neonates/infants)	1.0–2.0 mEq/kg
Epinephrine (1:10,000)	0.1 mL/kg
	0.01 mg/kg
Atropine (0.4 mg/mL)	0.02 mg/kg
	Min dose = 0.15 mg
	Max dose = 2.0 mg
Naloxone (Narcan) (0.4 mg/mL)	0.1 mg/kg
	Min dose = 0.5 mg
	Max dose = 2.0 mg
Dextrose 10% by peripheral IV	5.0 mL/kg
Dextrose 25% by central IV	2.0 mL/kg

(Adapted from *Emergency pediatric and neonatal resuscitation reference,* courtesy of Robert Brown, RN, MSN, PNP, Nurse Manager, Emergency Department and Transport Team; and nursing staff of Pediatric/Neonatal Transport Team, St. Christopher's Hospital for Children, Philadelphia, 1991.)

leukemia, Wilms' tumor, rhabdomyosarcoma, lymphoma, retinoblastoma, Hodgkin's disease, and brain tumors. Many of these cancers are now curable (Bertolone, 1997).

The health care team that works with children who have cancer includes physicians, clinical nurse specialists, staff nurses, social workers, child-life therapists, pharmacists, surgeons, and home IV and hospice to supportive care or palliative care nurses. Childhood cancer is treated with a combination of surgery, radiation, chemotherapy, and biotherapy. Children are usually randomized to be treated according to certain protocols, which are the subject of widespread, ongoing, multicenter research studies in one of two large study groups: the children's cancer group (CCG), established in 1955, or the pediatric oncology group (POG), established in 1979. Treatment in a center belonging to one of these groups ensures access to state-of-the-art treatment protocols based on ongoing cooperative data collection.

Because of efficacious absorption, the IV route is used to administer most antineoplastic or anticancer chemotherapy drugs required for treating childhood cancers. Many more IV protocols are designed for the child with cancer compared with the adult, primarily because many types of cancer are unique to children (eg, Wilms' tumor, neuroblastoma, retinoblastoma). Precision in regulating the specific IV chemotherapy along with monitoring IV clearance is crucial because of the incremental risk of fluid overload, electrolyte imbalances, and chemotherapy side effects. The aggressive therapy usually requires adequate long-term IV access because attempts to administer a vesicant drug by peripheral IV in an agitated child can result in extravasation injury to the child and occupational exposure to a toxic drug for the nurse. Many children with cancer benefit from the flexibility of single- or double-lumen, nontunneled, tunneled, or implanted central access devices. The function of various antineoplastic agents and administration guidelines is discussed in Chapter 19; a listing of antineoplastic agents is provided in Table 21–8.

Nutrition Therapy

Parenteral nutrition (PN) is the IV administration of a balanced solution that contains all the components of a balanced diet (Bilodeau, Poon, & Mascarenhas, 1998). PN has become one of the most important therapeutic parameters in the successful management of certain pediatric diseases. PN may be administered through a peripheral or central IV catheter. Indications for PN in pediatric patients include congenital or acquired gastrointestinal disorders, such as gastroschisis and Crohn's disease; respiratory diseases, such as cystic fibrosis and bronchopulmonary dysplasia; hypermetabolic states, such as major trauma and burns; and miscellaneous disorders, such as liver disease, inborn errors of metabolism, cancer, and prematurity. Although it has saved the lives of many pediatric patients, PN is not without risks. Close monitoring is necessary.

Supplemental PN, which is usually peripheral PN but may be central, does not provide all calories and nutrients. It is used as a boost to oral intake for short-term benefit. Total PN (TPN) is used for the child whose gut is not functional for congenital or acquired reasons, such as prematurity, short bowel syndrome, Crohn's disease, acquired immunodeficiency syndrome (AIDS), or cancer. TPN is administered through some type of central access device (described later in this chapter).

T A B L E   2 1 – 8
ANTINEOPLASTIC AGENTS USED FOR PEDIATRIC PATIENTS

Category	Drugs
Alkylating agent	Busulfan
	Carboplatin
	Cisplatin
	Ifosfamide
Nitrogen mustard	Chlorambucil
	Cyclophosphamide
	Mechlorethamine hydrochloride
	Melphalan
Nitrosourea	Carmustine
	Lomustine
Antibiotic	Bleomycin sulfate
	Dactinomycin
	Daunorubicin hydrochloride
	Doxorubicin hydrochloride
	Idarubicin hydrochloride
	Mithramycin
	Mitomycin
	Streptozocin
Antimetabolite	Cytarabine hydrochloride
	Fluorouracil
	Mercaptopurine
	Methotrexate
	Thioguanine
Hormone	Leuprolide acetate
Mitotic Inhibitor	Etoposide phosphate
	Vinblastine sulfate
	Vincristine sulfate
Purine	Mercaptopurine
Miscellaneous	Asparaginase
	Dacarbazine
	Hydroxyurea
	Pegaspargase
	Procarbazine hydrochloride

(From Jew, R. [Ed.] [1997–1999]. *Pharmacy handbook and formulary, the Children's Hospital of Philadelphia*. Hudson, OH: Lexi-Comp, Inc.)

Peripheral PN usually is reserved for patients who have normal nutritional status but need short-term supplemental nutrition until they can resume oral intake. Peripheral PN therapy should be limited to less than 2 weeks because of limitations in the amount of calories that can be delivered while still maintaining fluid balance, and difficulty in maintaining peripheral IV access (Heird, 1993). If PN is required for a longer period, central venous PN (TPN) should be prescribed.

With the addition of TPN to their therapy, affected children can be expected to gain weight normally with only parenteral nutrients. In addition, TPN supplies enough calories to maintain the positive nitrogen balance required for normal growth and development. The parameters used to determine caloric needs are age, resting energy requirements, level of physical activity, and severity of illness.

Constituents of Parenteral Nutrition

Usually, hospital or home IV agency pharmacy staff formulate PN solutions and perform admixture of solutions under a laminar-airflow hood. The general constituents for PN are protein, carbohydrates, fat, electrolytes, minerals, trace elements, and vitamins. Pediatric requirements for IV nutrition follow general guidelines and are based on protein, calorie, and fluid needs per kilogram of body weight.

Protein is provided in the form of crystalline amino acids; in infants younger than 6 months, a special formulation of protein, based on serum aminograms of healthy 1-month-old, breast-fed, term infants, is administered (Bilodeau et al., 1998). This solution differs from adult formulations in content of amino acids. PN protein is limited in critically ill patients who have renal, liver, and protein metabolism disorders. One gram of protein should deliver at least 30 calories (Testerman, 1989).

Carbohydrates are provided as dextrose, which provides energy for body tissue function. If carbohydrate supply is inadequate, the body breaks down protein or fat to provide metabolic needs. Dextrose, administered in milligram per kilogram per minute increments, provides the main calorie source; because the dextrose in PN is in monohydrated form, it provides not 4 but 3.4 kcal/g. For example, 100 mL 5% dextrose in water solution contains 5 g dextrose, or 17 kcal; 100 mL 10% dextrose in water solution contains 10 g dextrose, or 34 kcal. The strength of dextrose that can be administered peripherally in a child is 10% to 12.5% (Bilodeau et al., 1998; Heird, 1993; Jew, 1997–1999; Testerman, 1989). Greater concentrations given through a peripheral IV can cause sclerosis, phlebitis, and extravasation injury if infiltration occurs. Although concentrated dextrose is needed to provide calories, the volume of fluid needed to dilute very concentrated dextrose is often deleterious to fluid balance in children, especially neonates. Higher concentrations of dextrose (up to 25%) in less volume of fluid may be delivered by central catheter. Excessive carbohydrate use can result in fatty infiltration of the liver (Bilodeau et al., 1998).

The other source of nonprotein calories is lipids, delivered as a fat emulsion used to supply essential fatty acids that are needed for brain and somatic growth, immune system function, skin integrity, and wound healing. Originally, fat infusion was kept to a minimum (only 2% to 10% of daily calorie intake) because it was thought that a higher fat intake resulted in pulmonary changes. This hyperlipidemia is now thought to have been brought on by rapid infusion rates, so a slower infusion rate over a longer period is now the rule. Fat intake now comprises 30% to 40%, to a maximum of 60% of total calories required daily (Bilodeau et al., 1998; Testerman, 1989). Fat emulsions come in strengths of 10%, with 1.1 kcal/mL, and 20%, with 2 kcal/mL. Both may be infused peripherally or centrally, but the 20% solution is used most often. Fats are essential for neurologic development in the infant; however, fatty acids may displace bilirubin from albumin, causing a rise in bilirubin level and an increased risk of kernicterus. In infants with hyperbilirubinemia, the lipid intake is initially 0.5 g/kg/day, increased gradually as tolerance is demonstrated (Heird, 1993).

Electrolytes usually are added to the PN solution in amounts established for IV maintenance requirements, based on recommended dietary allowances. Because calcium, magnesium, phosphorus, and magnesium are incompletely absorbed from the gastrointestinal tract, IV dosages may exceed the recommendations for oral intake. Calcium and phosphorous may precipitate in PN solution when higher levels are prescribed; adjustment of the protein and pH level of the solution may assist in solubility. Minerals and trace elements also are included in a balanced PN solution. Vitamins are added according to children's recommended daily allowances; IV preparations are designed to meet the needs of preterm and term infants and children. The yellow color of the TPN solution results from the addition of multivitamins. Because multivitamins limit the shelf life of TPN, patients on home TPN are taught to add vitamins and other medication additives such as heparin.

In some cases, total nutrient admixtures (TNA), in which all the nutrients are added to one bag, have been used in children. The more common practice is to infuse the dextrose/amino acid solution separately in one bag, using a 0.22-μm filter into one arm of a "Y" set, and to infuse the fat, unfiltered, into the other arm of the "Y." If a TNA solution is used, use of a 1.5- to 5-μm in-line filter decreases the chance that an unseen precipitate will be infused. Two deaths have been reported from pulmonary emboli when TNA solutions were used (Hill, Heldman, Goo et al., 1996).

Nursing Assessment and Management

Once the child has been deemed a candidate for PN, a complete physical assessment, including height, weight, head circumference, and nutrition and laboratory evaluations, is completed. Duration and route of PN are determined, and the appropriate catheter is placed. The patient then is started on 75% to 80% of goal calories, which gradually is increased by 10% to 20% daily until the goal of the PN regimen is reached (Bilodeau et al., 1998). Infusions may run over 24 hours for the very sick hospitalized child, or may be cycled down gradually by 4-hour increments daily, maintaining the same volume of infusion over less time. Cycling down to between 8 to 18 hours of daily infusion TPN allows the child far more freedom. This is particularly true for children on home TPN, who may infuse at night while asleep and still follow a fairly normal lifestyle of school and activities. Cycling the PN also may mobilize hepatic fat stores, decreasing hepatic steatosis (Bilodeau et al., 1998). Although common in adults, cycling has been shown to be safe even in infants younger than 6 months (Collier, Crouch, Hendricks, & Cacallero, 1994). Initially, when patients were cycled on and off their PN solution, it was thought that glucose would rise once the infusion began and fall once the infusion was finished. Evidence now shows that in children younger than 3 years of age receiving more than 10% dextrose solutions, PN does not need to be tapered when starting; however, when completing the cycle, the PN rate should be decreased by 50% for the last hour to prevent rebound hypoglycemia (Bendorf, Friesen, & Roberts, 1996).

The nurse frequently monitors the patient's physical status and screens, intervenes for, and reports abnormal findings: temperature spikes, inappropriate glucose spills, chills, rashes, irritability, decreased level of consciousness, and any changes in growth or clinical picture. The nurse immediately reports any observable abnormality to the nutrition team. Results of various serum chemistry and hematology tests are assessed daily for the first week and then weekly for the stable patient in the hospital or at home. Table 21–9 provides a sample schedule for assessing these parameters.

Another major area of nursing intervention in a child receiving TPN is psychological support. Most such patients are acutely ill infants. Even though a child on central TPN may be NPO, cuddling and holding the child should assist in meeting maternal needs. Also, allowing parents and caregivers every opportunity to participate in their child's care is extremely important. First, the nurse should assess the family's level of comprehension about TPN and intervene by offering support to decrease parental anxiety. As soon as the decision is made to place a child on TPN, it is best to use the preoperative teaching methodology of explaining purpose, procedures, and potential complications. Of course, all further questions can be handled daily. Permitting this open channel of communication not only supplies parents with the knowledge they need to become involved but assists them in comprehending the purpose of TPN and why adherence to protocols is so important.

T A B L E   2 1 – 9
PARENTERAL NUTRITION MONITORING RECOMMENDATIONS

Parameter	Initially	Daily	Weekly	Monthly
Weight	✓	✓ <2 y; every other day for >2 y		
Height/length	✓			✓
Head circumference (<3 y)	✓			✓
Arm anthropometrics	✓			✓
Complete blood count without differential	✓			✓
Total parenteral nutrition panel*	✓		✓	
Prealbumin	✓		✓	
Iron studies: serum iron, total iron-binding capacity, ferritin and percentage saturation (in children >2 mo)	✓			✓

* Sodium, potassium, chloride, bicarbonate, glucose, creatinine, blood urea nitrogen, calcium, phosphorus, magnesium, total protein, albumin, triglycerides, cholesterol, alkaline phosphatase, alanine aminotransferase, gamma-glutamyltranspeptidase, and total bilirubin, plus unconjugated bilirubin if total is >1.5 mg/dL.
(Data from Bilodeau et al., 1998; Heird, 1993; Jew, 1997–1999; and Testerman, 1989.)

Complications

Disadvantages of TPN are its potential complications. Every nurse must fully understand the possible complications of TPN, including the specific symptoms of each. Complications are subdivided into two categories: catheter related and metabolic. Catheter-related complications have been previously addressed. Metabolic complications include the following:

- Glucose disturbances
- Electrolyte imbalances
- Mineral disturbances
- Acid–base imbalance
- Hepatic disorders
- Metabolic bone disease
- Refeeding syndrome

Close attention to detail during the initial assessment and ongoing monitoring can treat or even prevent most of these complications. Some predisposing metabolic abnormalities, however, may require immediate medical intervention. With the incremental advances in technology and the formation of nutrition support teams, the incidences of even the more common complications have decreased to acceptable rates. See Chapter 16 for more information on nutrition support.

Transfusion Therapy

Although transfusion therapy is covered fully in Chapter 17, an overview of the therapeutics unique to pediatric patients is presented here. Transfusions of blood and blood components may be administered to a child through a peripheral IV for one-time or infrequent transfusion or through a central device for chronic transfusions. Because transfusion carries the risk of iron buildup, IV chelating agents are often prescribed in addition to transfusion therapy.

The major differences related to transfusion therapy from neonate to adult include a gradual decrease in blood volume, maturation of the immune system with regard to blood typing, changes in blood counts, and changes in requirements. Table 21–10 lists blood volumes for various ages. The red blood cell of the infant is nucleated at birth and has a reduced half-life (23.3 days) compared with the adult (26 to 35 days) (Luban & Keating, 1983). Synthesis of fetal hemoglobin (HbF) declines rapidly after birth, whereas that of adult hemoglobin (HbA) rises concomitantly. The higher affinity for oxygen of HbF facilitates transfer of oxygen from mother to fetus in utero, but persistence of HbF after birth may result in neonatal respiratory distress and tissue hypoxia because of the inability of HbF to release oxygen to the tissues (Cahill-Alsip & McDermott, 1996). Manipulations of the infant, such as suctioning and IV starts, as well as crying, can increase peripheral leukocyte counts. In the newborn, neutropenia rather than neutrophilia is a more common indicator of sepsis. Platelet counts do not differ greatly from neonate to adult, but thrombocytopenia may easily develop in neonates from extrinsic sources. The immune system matures during infancy. Circulating antibodies are derived from the mother during the last several prenatal weeks; therefore, premature infants have a less efficient humoral immunity. As an infant is exposed to outside antigens, antibody production begins.

T A B L E   2 1 – 1 0
AVERAGE TOTAL BLOOD VOLUMES
AT VARIOUS AGES

Premature infant	95 mL/kg
Term infant	80 mL/kg
1–12 mo	75 mL/kg
1–6 y	70 mL/kg
7–18 y	80 mL/kg
Adult	80 mL/kg

(From Luban, N., & Keating, L. [Eds.] [1983]. *Hemo-therapy of the infant and premature.* Arlington, VA: American Association of Blood Banks; Nathan, D.G. & Orkin, S.H. [Eds.] [1998]. *Nathan & Oski's Hematology of infancy and childhood* (5th Ed.) Philadelphia: W.B. Saunders.)

Indications for Transfusion Therapy

Indications for transfusing blood and blood products to children are similar to those described for adults in Chapter 17. In general, indications for transfusion therapy in children include acute hemorrhage, anemia, abnormal component function or component deficiency, and removal of harmful substances, such as bilirubin, during exchange transfusion. Reduction in the blood volume of a child by 30% to 40% produces clinical evidence of shock. When 20% of blood volume is lost and loss may recur, transfusion also is indicated (Nathan & Orkin, 1998). Decreased production or altered function of platelets usually results from a maternal problem or disorder (ie, prenatal aspirin intake), congenital disorder, acquired disorder (ie, idiopathic thrombocytopenic purpura [ITP]), or chemotherapy-induced thrombocytopenia.

The most common blood components given to children are packed red blood cells, platelets, and fresh frozen plasma, as well as plasma derivatives given for congenital or acquired lack or dysfunction of that component. These products are administered in milliliters per kilogram; dosages are based on the volume limits of the child and the desired therapeutic outcome. Blood products may be modified before transfusion through several methods to reduce the risk of complications in at-risk children. These modifications include irradiation, leukocyte depletion, and warming.

Irradiation reduces the ability of leukocytes to engraft in the patient and cause graft-versus-host disease (Cahill-Alsip & McDermott, 1996; Roth, 1997). Recipients of irradiated blood include transplant recipients, children with lymphoma or leukemia, and neonates. Leukocyte depletion, by one of several methods, reduces the risk of febrile, nonhemolytic reactions, especially in patients who have had multiple prior transfusions. Leukocyte-depleted red cells and platelets also are given to prevent alloimmunization in children who receive platelets frequently or transmission of cytomegalovirus (CMV) when CMV-negative blood products are not available. They also are given to prospective renal allograft recipients (Cahill-Alsip & McDermott, 1996). Warmed blood products, heated in a controlled system, are used in exchange transfusions, patients with cold agglutinin disease, hypothermic patients, and in those receiving large amounts of blood quickly (more than 1 unit every 10 minutes) (Cahill-Alsip & McDermott, 1996). Although not indicated for routine transfusion therapy, warming reduces the chance of hypothermia, dysrhythmias, and cardiac arrest in these situations.

Indications for transfusion of platelets, plasma, and plasma components are similar to those in adults. Table 21–11 lists some parameters for blood component therapy in children.

Infusion of IV gamma globulin or IV IgG warrants specific mention because the use of this plasma derivative in children has grown substantially since the 1980s, when safe, effective IV preparations became licensed in the United States. Before that time, children with humoral immunodeficiencies were treated with intramuscular injections or infusions of plasma. The large volume of intramuscular IgG required adequate muscle mass, the procedure was uncomfortable because the injected volume was large, and IgG levels rose slowly and were maintained only for a short time before another injection was needed to help bolster infection-fighting capabilities. Larger doses of IgG can be given by the IV route, thus maintaining adequate serum levels with more convenient administration. Approved indications for IV IgG include deficiencies of the humoral immune system and ITP, and this product is being

TABLE 21–11
BLOOD COMPONENT THERAPY FOR PEDIATRIC PATIENTS

Blood Product	Indication	Dosage/Rate
Red blood cells (packed)	Treatment of anemia without volume expansion	10 mL/kg, not to exceed 15 mL/kg at 2–5 mL/kg/h
		IV drip by gravity or transfusion approved pump
Platelets	To control bleeding associated with deficiency in platelet number or function (platelet count <20,000 or <50,000 with active bleeding)	1 unit (50–70 mL)/7–10 kg body weight
		Run over 30 min to maximum of 4 h; IV push or drip
Fresh frozen plasma	Occasionally volume expansion in acute blood loss; to increase levels of plasma coagulation factors in children with demonstrated deficiency	Acute hemorrhage: 15–30 mL/kg as indicated
		Clotting deficiency: 10–15 mL/kg at 1–2 mL/min
		IV push or drip
Cryoprecipitate	To replace factors not present or present in inadequate amounts due to congenital disease	1 U/5 kg not faster than 1 mL/kg/min
		IV push or drip
Albumin	Hypovolemia	5%: 10–20 mL/kg as fast as tolerated, usually IV push or gravity
		25%: 2–4 mL/kg over 30–60 min regulated by pump

(Adapted from Cahill-Alsip, C. & McDermott, B. [1996]. Hematologic critical care problems. In M.Q. Curley, J.B. Smith, & P.A. Moloney-Harmon [Eds.], *Critical care nursing of infants and children* [pp. 793–817]. Philadelphia: W.B. Saunders; and National Institutes of Health. [1990]. *Transfusion therapy guidelines for nurses.* National Blood Resource Education Program, Public Health Service. Washington, DC: U.S. Department of Health and Human Services.)

studied as a means of heightening the immune response in many other adult and pediatric disorders, such as AIDS, neonatal sepsis, and cystic fibrosis (Frey, 1991). Antibodies against specific organisms also have been developed, allowing a more specific plan of treatment, such as anti-CMV immune globulin used in transplant recipients (Stiehm, 1991).

Techniques for Pediatric Transfusion Therapy

For the first several days of life, the mother's serum is used for compatibility testing. In infants older than 1 week and those previously transfused, compatibility testing is done on the child's blood. Group O red blood cells that are Rh negative or the same Rh as the infant are used frequently. In addition, red blood cells are tested for CMV and are given to neonates only if CMV negative. The freshest cells possible are used to avoid potassium loading in infants.

Blood and blood products in children may be administered by a 24-gauge peripheral catheter in neonates and by a 24- or 22-gauge catheter in older children. As stated by Keller (1995), "A review of the literature revealed that red blood cells could safely be transfused through needles smaller than 18–20 gauge at relatively high infusion rates without increasing the risk of hemolysis." A pump capable of infusing blood is recommended for transfusion therapy in children; in neonates, blood may be prefiltered by the blood bank and then infused from a syringe on a syringe pump. Pediatricians request blood and blood products in milliliter per kilogram increments, instead of units, because a single unit of packed red blood cells may equal the entire blood volume of several infants. In children, volume and fluid balance considerations negate the simultaneous infusion of saline, particularly in neonates; instead, the peripheral or central IV device must be flushed with 1 to 3 mL saline before and after the transfusion. Rate of blood transfusion may be very slow or even staggered with boluses of dextrose in neonates. Five to 10% of red cell volume should be infused slowly over the first 15 minutes, then the rate increased to an hourly IV rate tolerated by the child (Landier, Barrell, & Styffe, 1987).

Nursing Assessment and Management

Central venous pressure is the best indicator for restoration of blood volume to normal; pulse rate is less reliable, and 24 to 36 hours may pass before hemoglobin reflects the true extent of blood loss. A red blood cell mass deficit occurs with chronic anemia; transfusion with packed cells is not indicated until the hemoglobin level drops below 6 g/dL (Nathan & Orkin, 1998). The patient's cardiopulmonary status, activity level, and hemoglobin should be assessed before transfusion because an unstressed child can tolerate hemoglobin values of 3 to 6 g/dL without showing signs of heart failure. Also, because the most common form of anemia seen in children is iron-deficiency anemia (which rarely is treated with transfusion), other treatments may be indicated, including iron therapy, folic acid, or vitamin B_{12}.

Specific physical assessment areas indicative of hematologic function in children include color changes in skin, lips, conjunctivae, mucous membranes, and nails, such as blue for cyanosis, pale for anemia, or yellow for jaundice. The fingernails and toenails should be examined for clubbing, the skin for petechiae, and the mucous membranes for bleeding. Blood oozing from old venipuncture sites often is a precursor to the onset of disseminated intravascular coagulation. When a tourniquet is placed on an extremity, evidence of petechiae distal to the tourniquet may indicate ITP or other platelet disorders. Laboratory values as simple as the commonly done complete blood count, which includes hemoglobin, hematocrit, white cell count, platelet levels, and cell differential, can provide a very good picture of the child's hematologic status. These values vary among age groups. Clotting studies and levels of specific factors may be analyzed if a bleeding disorder is suspected.

In addition to physical assessment, history should include previous exposure to toxins (which may cause aplastic anemia) and any previous transfusions, including the reason and the patient's reaction. Psychological support of the family is indicated, as is education about transfusion therapy and available alternatives. Institutional policy is necessary regarding refusal of transfusion by a parent or guardian, and state laws differ on this topic; in most cases, parents must sign a waiver if they refuse transfusion.

Possible Complications

As with other therapies, transfusion therapy is not without risks. Potential complications include acute hemolytic reactions, nonhemolytic reactions (eg, febrile and allergic reactions), alloimmunization, circulatory overload, citrate toxicity, infectious disease transmission, and coagulopathy (Cahill-Alsip & McDermott, 1996). The type of reaction may be difficult to ascertain initially. These reactions are discussed in more detail in Chapter 17.

Exchange Transfusion

A procedure unique to the neonatal population is exchange transfusion, in which most or all of the infant's blood volume is replaced with compatible red blood cells and plasma from one or several donors. Exchange transfusion was first used in the early 1950s for management of hemolytic disease of the newborn [HDN]. With the introduction of anti-D immune globulin (Rhogam) in the 1960s, the number of infants with HDN greatly declined; however, HDN is still the most common indication for exchange transfusion. Other indications include disseminated intravascular coagulation, sepsis, respiratory distress syndrome, and polycythemia. Exchange transfusions optimally are undertaken using two IV sites or an IV and an intra-arterial site. A combination of peripheral, central, or umbilical access devices can be used.

CONSIDERATIONS RELATED TO HEMOLYTIC DISEASE OF THE NEWBORN

Two causes of HDN include Rh incompatibility and ABO incompatibility. In Rh incompatibility, the anti-D antibodies that an Rh^- mother developed during her first pregnancy with an Rh^+ fetus cross the placenta and destroy the red blood cells of subsequent Rh^+ fetuses. At birth, subsequent infants are anemic and have increased levels of unconjugated (indirect) bilirubin. Deposition of excess bilirubin in the brain can cause kernicterus, a type of encephalopathy. Exchange transfusion is considered when bilirubin levels increase more than 1 mg/dL each hour or reach 15 to 16 mg/dL in the premature neonate and 20 mg/dL in the full-term infant (Kasprisin, 1985). ABO incompatibility occurs most frequently when a type O mother carries a type A or B fetus (Nathan & Orkin, 1998). Although HDN from ABO incompatibility is more common than HDN from Rh incompatibility, it usually is mild enough to be treated with phototherapy or a single blood transfusion, until the infant's liver matures enough to clear bilirubin from the blood. For either type of HDN, red blood cells alone or with fresh frozen plasma may be used for exchange transfusion. To treat Rh HDN, type O Rh blood crossmatched with the mother should be used; for ABO HDN, Rh-compatible, type O blood should be used.

TECHNIQUES AND SPECIAL CONSIDERATIONS

A double-volume or two-volume exchange usually is performed when exchange transfusion equals twice the patient's blood volume. This replaces approximately 85% of the newborn's blood and lowers the bilirubin level approximately 50%, but has no effect on extravascular bilirubin. Albumin may be administered before the exchange to bind bilirubin, allowing a greater amount to be removed during the procedure. Ideally, two vascular access sites are used to allow simultaneous withdrawal and infusion. Common sites include the umbilical vessels and peripheral or central veins. If only one access is available, the push-pull method is used. Calcium and dextrose levels are monitored closely during the exchange because blood preservatives may cause levels to decrease. Complications can include those related to the catheter as well as those related to transfusion therapy.

■ PERIPHERAL INTRAVENOUS ACCESS

This section focuses on peripheral sites and devices appropriate for IV therapy. Depending on the child's age, finding a site for administering IV therapy typically is more difficult than in the adult. Both hydration status and previous IV therapy may be used as predictors of difficulties in obtaining an intact venous access. In the child, the site selected for IV therapy should involve minimal risk and allow maximum efficacy and safety.

Peripheral IVs are used to administer fluids, medications, and PN and even to draw frequent blood samples. Although the standards of the Intravenous Nurses Society (INS) (INS, 1998, 2000) state that indwelling peripheral IV catheters should not be used routinely to acquire blood samples in children, the frequency of venous sampling for certain diagnostic tests necessitates the use of peripheral IV devices (INS, 1998, 2000). Examples include short-duration blood tests that require blood sampling every 15 minutes (eg, growth hormone) to every 4 to 6 hours (eg, clotting studies or blood glucose levels) (Roulston-Betts, 1998). In such cases, the IV would be used only for that purpose to avoid skewing results of the laboratory tests.

Peripheral Intravenous Sites

When selecting the optimal site for IV therapy, nurses should follow certain basic strategies. These include using veins distally to proximally and inserting the IV device in line with venous flow—for example, facing down or toward the heart in a scalp vein or facing up in an arm or leg vein. A vein in the nondominant extremity should be chosen when possible. The thumb should be left untaped or another extremity used if the child sucks his or her thumb (Frey, 1998b). In addition, the nurse always closely monitors an infusing IV, at least every 1 to 2 hours, depending on the type of infusate, size of the patient, and location of the IV access device.

Traditionally, the head was frequently used in the neonate and young infant because the scalp has an abundant supply of superficial veins (Fig. 21–1). The bilateral superficial temporal veins just in front of the pinna of the ear and the frontal vein, which runs down the middle of the forehead, are usually easy to find and involve minimal risk to the patient. Scalp veins are readily available until approximately 12 to 18 months of age, when hair follicles mature and superficial layers of skin thicken, making venous access difficult. The scalp as an IV site, however, can be distressing to parents, who may believe that the IV is in the brain. Moreover, a scalp IV can restrict mobility and be easily dislodged. With the advent of small IV catheters for peripheral access, scalp veins are no longer the first choice for IV access in infants.

If the scalp is chosen as the IV site and the head must be shaved, the smallest area possible should be shaved or clipped, saving the hair for the parents as the child's first haircut, which should help alleviate some distress at the use of this site. When inserting an IV in the scalp, the nurse should be aware of artery location, because distinguishing veins from arteries in this area is difficult. Use of an "arterial" IV could damage the artery and the area to which oxygenated blood is delivered. In-

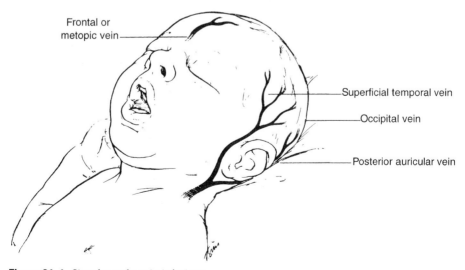

Frontal or metopic vein

Superficial temporal vein

Occipital vein

Posterior auricular vein

Figure 21–1. Sites for scalp vein infusions.

advertent arterial puncture reveals bright red blood, pulsation, and blanching of the skin caused by arteriospasm when the IV device is flushed (Fay, 1983). Should arterial puncture occur, the IV device should be removed and pressure held on the site until bleeding stops.

Other favorable peripheral IV sites, moving from distal to proximal locations, include the hand, forearm, upper arm, foot, and antecubital fossa (Fig. 21–2). Some unusual sites such as the axilla, abdomen, and popliteal area also have been used when chronically ill infants and children exhibit greatly diminished peripheral venous access from long use (Table 21–12).

Foot veins are used up to walking age and occasionally in older children when other usual sites are not available, such as in patients with burns or multiple trauma. Depending on the regulations of the state's Board of Nursing and institutional policy, external jugular and femoral veins may be used for IV access and blood samples, although these last two sites usually are accessed by a physician, nurse practitioner, or emergency personnel.

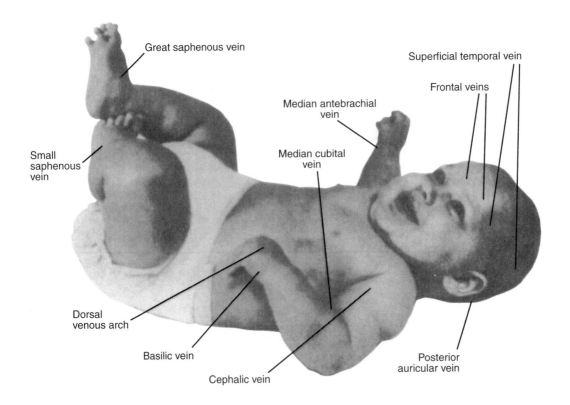

Figure 21–2. Pediatric venipuncture sites. (Used with permission from Fay, M.J. [1983]. The special challenges of pediatric IVs. *Dimensions of Critical Care Nursing, 2,* 24. Hall-Johnson Communications. Photo by Randi Boyette.)

TABLE 21-12
PERIPHERAL INTRAVENOUS ACCESS SITES FOR PEDIATRIC PATIENTS[*]

Sites	Veins
Preferred Sites	
Hand	Metacarpal, digital
Forearm	Accessory cephalic, basilic, median antebrachial
Antecubital fossa	Median basilic, median cephalic, median cubital
Upper arm (below axilla)	Basilic, cephalic
Foot	Greater saphenous, lesser saphenous, median marginal
Scalp	Frontal, temporal, posterior auricular, occipital
Lower leg	Greater saphenous, lesser saphenous
Secondary Sites[†]	
Wrist	Superficial veins on the ventral surface: infiltration in this area may result in pressure on the radial nerve
Knee	Popliteal vein: usually limited to neonates because of decreased mobility
Axilla	Axillary vein: usually limited to neonates; infiltration may cause pressure on structures in chest cavity
Abdomen	Superficial veins: rarely used, usually limited to chronically hospitalized patients; infiltration may result in damage to abdominal wall

[*] Sites listed in order of preference.
[†] Secondary sites should be considered only when preferred sites are not available.

Peripheral Intravenous Devices

Until the late 1970s, the winged infusion needle was the device of choice for short-term IV therapy and withdrawal of blood samples for laboratory analysis in pediatric patients. Then, 22-gauge catheter-over-needle devices made of plastic, then Teflon, became available and could be used for longer-lasting IV access in pediatric patients (Batton et al., 1982). Many pediatric institutions still use winged infusion needles for blood sampling because the vacuum withdrawal method used in adults is often too aggressive for tiny pediatric veins.

Catheter-over-needle device design has advanced to include thin-wall catheters (Fig. 21–3) for greater flow rates, smaller gauge (24 and 22), shorter length, and nonkinking material. Although several companies now manufacture devices intended to prevent needlestick injuries from the stylet of the IV catheter, these protective devices were deemed to be of "unwieldy design" for placing IVs in children (Friedland & Brown, 1992).

Small-gauge catheters such as the 24 for neonates and the 24 and 22 for children and adolescents are the choice when up to 2 weeks of IV therapy is prescribed (Wickham, 1990). After 2 weeks, peripheral access sites become increasingly unavailable, and use of a longer-lasting or central device may be warranted.

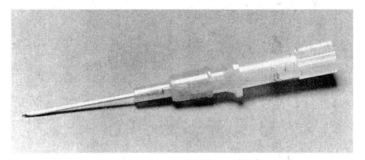

Figure 21–3. Small-gauge thin-walled Teflon peripheral IV catheter, suitable for use with children. (Courtesy of Johnson & Johnson, Inc., Tampa, FL.)

Peripheral Intravenous Insertion

General IV insertion techniques have been described previously and are not discussed in this chapter; however, some special techniques for achieving venous access in children are highlighted. To dilate veins in children, a smaller tourniquet may be necessary. In neonates, a rubber band with a tape tab provides an easily removable tourniquet for scalp IVs (Fig. 21–4). In some cases, especially when placing an IV in a premature neonate, no tourniquet is used. Additional aids to locate and dilate veins may include warm soaks or transillumination (Mattson & O'Connor, 1986).

Insertion of IVs in children requires stabilization of the extremity before venipuncture so that movement of the child does not dislodge the newly inserted device, necessitating subsequent sticks (Frey, 1998b). An arm board usually is an adequate restraint (Fig. 21–5) and can be taped to the treatment room table to provide passive restraint during IV insertion. Box 21-1 refers to core competencies associated with peripherally inserted central catheters. Many of those same competencies apply to standard peripheral insertion as well.

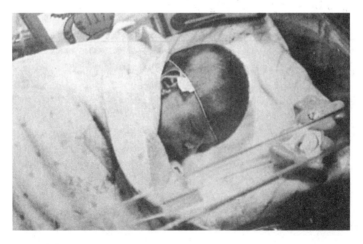

Figure 21–4. Rubber band used as a tourniquet on infant's scalp. (Courtesy of A.M. Frey.)

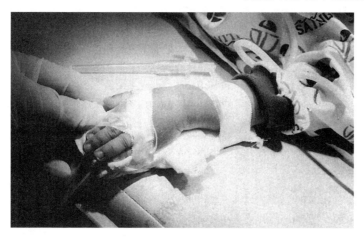

Figure 21–5. An arm board is used to support the area of the IV site and provide light restraint during IV insertion. (Courtesy of A.M. Frey)

Equipment

Equipment and supplies are set up before venipuncture, usually in a treatment room, if possible, thus preserving the child's room and bed as a "safe" place where invasive procedures are not performed (Piercy, 1981). In an intensive care environment, supplies may be prepared away from the bedside so as not to cause undue anxiety before the actual venipuncture. In the home, supplies usually are set up in an area where lighting is maximized and a flat surface, such as a kitchen table, can be used as a work area. The nurse will need:

- Peripheral IV catheter in 24- or 22-gauge size
- Luer-locking microbore connector tubing
- Needleless cap
- 1 to 2 mL of flush solution in a syringe
- Padded arm board
- 1/2- and 1-inch tape
- Semipermeable transparent dressing
- Gauze pads
- Alcohol solution to clean the site
- Nonsterile gloves
- Latex-free tourniquet or rubber band
- Site protector (optional)
- Warm packs (optional)

Technique

Intravenous insertion in children requires patience and practice until the learning curve is diminished and skill level increases. No more than two or three attempts at IV access should be made. If unsuccessful, the nurse should consult a more experienced person or consider alternate access. Limiting the number of venipuncture at-

text continues on page 618

PICC Insertion Skills Checklist for: _____ **Date:** _____
Preceptor: _____ *(Complete one checklist for each insertion)*

Original PICC course completed: Date _____

Initial clinical competency verification: **Circle age group:**

Date: _____ PICC Precepted by: _____   neonatal   pediatric

Date: _____ PICC Precepted by: _____   neonatal   pediatric

Date: _____ PICC Precepted by: _____   neonatal   pediatric

Date: _____ PICC Precepted by: _____   neonatal   pediatric

Date: _____ PICC Precepted by: _____   neonatal   pediatric

Periodic competency verification: (Concentrate on items noted from CQI report of individual's PICC insertion/outcomes.)

Date: _____ PICC Precepted by: _____ satisfactory   unsatisfactory
Review specific aspects of PICC insertion/care listed below based on CQI data:
_____

Date: _____ PICC Precepted by: _____ satisfactory   unsatisfactory
Review specific aspects of PICC insertion/care listed below based on CQI data:
_____

Date: _____ Continuing Education [describe]: _____

Date: _____ Continuing Education [describe]: _____

Date: _____ Continuing Education [describe]: _____
Individual maintains competency according to CQI review and agency policy. Use additional forms if needed.
_____

Insertion Method: Break-away-needle / Peel-away-sheath / Modified Seldinger/ Other _____

COMPETENCY CRITERIA (Place a check in the column[s] to the right)	MET	NOT MET	N/A
Consults with MD/NP as needed to plan correct catheter type for therapy ordered and for patient specific needs/activities.			
Checks MD/NP order for placement, number of lumens, local anesthetic or conscious sedation protocol, and tip location verification.			
Applies tourniquet briefly to select appropriate vein and measures for correct catheter length (double-checking this measurement).			

continued

Uses barrier precautions according to procedure, including: hand washing, masks, gloves, goggles, sterile drapes, and powder-free sterile gloves (gown if indicated).			
Maintains sterility when setting up equipment and throughout procedure. Places all needed supplies on sterile field.			

COMPETENCY CRITERIA (Place a check in the column[s] to the right)	MET	NOT MET	N/A
Wearing sterile gloves, prepares equipment in kit for use. (Draws up flush solutions, assembles and preflushes extension set and needle-free cap, and so forth.			
Correctly measures catheter and cuts to premeasured length appropriate for brand used.			
Positions patient appropriately to facilitate threading catheter.			
Prepares skin according to procedure guidelines.			
Positions sterile drapes to maintain sterility of site and equipment during procedure.			
Follows standard precautions to avoid contact with blood and body fluids throughout procedure.			
Injects local anesthetic if ordered.			
Applies tourniquet and positions it for ease of removal after venipuncture. Changes sterile gloves.			
Performs venipuncture using technique appropriate for brand.			
Releases tourniquet once venous access is achieved.			

COMPETENCY CRITERIA (Place a check in the column[s] to the right)	MET	NOT MET	N/A
Follow steps specific to insertion method, using instruments/technique appropriate for brand of device.			
Instructs patient to turn head toward insertion site with chin on chest if using upper extremity.			

continued

Threads catheter to premeasured length.			
Removes introducer using technique appropriate for brand.			
Removes guidewire (if applicable) using technique appropriate for brand.			
Attaches connector tubing and needleless cap (if applicable to brand) and verifies catheter patency with saline flush.			
Applies skin protectant solution around periphery of dressing area.			
Secures catheter to skin using appropriate technique for procedure (sterile tape strips, hub-lock device, or sutures).			

COMPETENCY CRITERIA (Place a check in the column[s] to the right)	MET	NOT MET	N/A
Applies dressing. Places small pressure dressing over site using folded gauze covered with transparent dressing for first 24–48 hours.			
Labels dressing appropriately.			
Flushes catheter with heparinized saline if indicated by brand.			
Arranges for radiographic or fluoroscopic verification of catheter tip placement.			
Charts procedure, including patient teaching, catheter brand, gauge, length, local anesthetic, type of dressing, and patient's response/tolerance of procedure.			

tempts decreases physical and emotional trauma to the child and can preserve venous integrity (Frey, 1998b). Consideration should be given to using an IV specialty nursing team for IV procedures in children because such teams have a higher rate of success when placing IVs and can be quite cost effective. One study demonstrated that using staff nurses and physicians who were not IV specialists to place IVs in children resulted in a low rate of success for IV placement and increased cost to the hospital (Frey, 1998a).

A firm but gentle insertion technique is necessary for a successful venipuncture in a child because blood return in the flashback chamber may not appear as readily

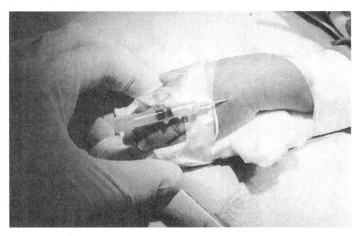

Figure 21–6. Blood enters the flashback chamber of the IV catheter, then the 24-gauge catheter is advanced slightly. (Courtesy of A.M. Frey.)

as in the adult, and the nurse may not feel the characteristic "pop" of entering a vein (Frey, 1997). Threading the IV catheter occasionally can be difficult in children. After initial flashback of blood, but before threading the catheter into the vein, the nurse verifies that the catheter tip and the stylet have entered the vein lumen by advancing the IV device slightly. Other measures include attaching a small connector tubing with flush solution and flushing gently as the catheter is advanced. Sometimes, just waiting a few seconds until the child has calmed down can decrease the incidence of venous spasm and facilitate catheter threading. Figures 21–6 through 21-8 demonstrate IV insertion in a 5-month-old infant with meningitis who is receiving IV antibiotics intermittently through a heparin lock.

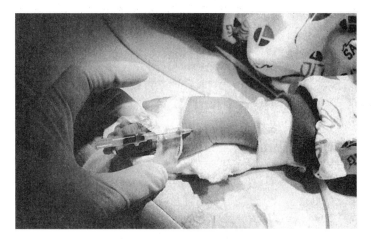

Figure 21–7. The catheter is advanced fully, stylet is pulled back, and tourniquet is removed. (Courtesy of A.M. Frey.)

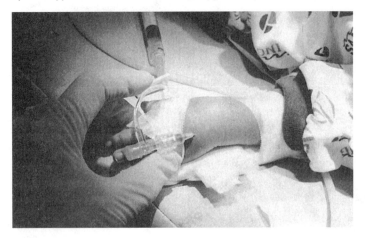

Figure 21–8. The stylet is removed and T-connector is attached to hub of IV catheter. Catheter is flushed gently to assess patency. (Courtesy of A.M. Frey.)

Postinsertion Care of the Peripheral Intravenous Site

Frequent assessment of the site must be done, range of motion maintained, and usage of restraints documented. Dressing changes usually are done only when the IV site is changed, as recommended by infection control research (Pearson, 1996). Peripheral and central catheter care is summarized in Table 21–13.

Stabilization of the Intravenous Site

Stabilization is essential, primarily in the younger child whose comprehension of the importance of not manipulating the IV site is minimal. The nurse should tape IVs in a "U"-shaped chevron or "H" pattern and loop the extension tube so that if the child pulls on the IV, the tension affects the loop, not the IV site (Hutchinson, 1991). Sites requiring stabilization include those over joints, such as the dorsum of the hand near the wrist. The advantage of using a padded arm board for stabilization is that it restricts the child's range of movement, thereby decreasing the risk of dislodging the IV needle. The foot also demands stabilization, primarily when using the large saphenous vein (Fig. 21–9). An important aspect of IV access in the foot involves maintaining normal joint configuration by placing padding under the foot, thus preserving the natural bend at the ankle and preventing foot drop or contracture injuries. See "Legal Issues: Site Monitoring" for a comprehensive review of legalities associated with monitoring pediatric infusion patients.

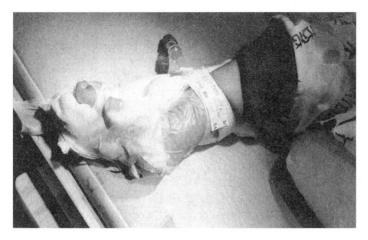

Figure 21–9. Foot IV site. Note that joint configuration is maintained and toes and IV site are visible. (Courtesy of A.M. Frey.)

Use of Restraints

In younger children, especially toddlers, great care must be taken to protect the IV site. Coverings such as a clear plastic IV protector, an easily removable wrap secured with Velcro, or stretch netting may keep little fingers away from the IV site, while providing easy visualization (Vallino, 1998). The top "ribbed" portion of a sweat sock slipped over the IV can serve the same function for home IV access. A roller bandage should not be used to cover an IV site because it is time consuming to unravel and makes site assessments difficult (INS, 1998, 2000). In general, children's medical centers rarely use restraints because restraints not only are confining but foster a sense of frustration and mistrust in the child. Restraints should be used only with an extremely uncooperative child or a child who may injure himself or remove the IV. In those cases, alternate resources, such as parental monitoring, should be considered.

Site Rotation

Although 48 to 72 hours is the recommended interval for site rotation, a survey indicated that most (71.9%) children's hospitals changed peripheral IV sites only when necessary (Bossert & Beecroft, 1994). One large study done in a pediatric critical care unit demonstrated that peripheral IV sites could remain in place safely for up to 144 hours (6 days), after which the incidence of bacterial colonization increased threefold. In fact, this same study demonstrated that newer sites had an increased chance of complications over those sites left in place (Garland, Dunne, Havens et al., 1992). Removal of the IV should be done carefully, without using scissors near the site.

text continues on page 624

TABLE 21–13

ROUTINE CARE AND MAINTENANCE OF PEDIATRIC INTRAVENOUS ACCESS DEVICES

Device	Patency	Dressing	Connector Tubing/ Cap Change	Comments
Peripheral IV	• 1 mL of 10 U/mL heparinized saline every 8 h or after each medication infusion • Consider saline flushes for catheters 22 gauge and larger or for intervals of every 4 h or more often • Use benzyl alcohol–free flushes for neonates	• Transparent • Changed only with site change	• Connector tubing changed when site is changed or if compromised • Cap changed if removed or compromised	• Inexpensive • Maximum dwell: 6 days, according to latest research • May be placed for frequent blood samples (for tests requiring samples be taken every 15 min to every 4–6 h)
Peripherally inserted central catheter (PICC)	• 2 mL of 10–100 U/mL heparinized saline every 12–24 h • For any age child with one or more medication doses daily, use 10 U/mL • If more than one lumen, flush each lumen as needed	• Initially: transparent dressing over gauze, changed in 48 h to transparent only • Second dressing is not changed on PICCs unless loose, soiled, wet, compromised • Steri-Strips not changed unless very soiled	• T-connector tubing considered part of catheter if placed aseptically during insertion procedure • Not changed unless compromised • Cap changed weekly, if removed, or if compromised	• Moderately inexpensive • Used for intermediate-term therapies, but no dwell limit set • Can clot, dislodge, or break if care not taken • 3-French or larger may be used for blood sampling; discard volume = 3× device and attached tubings or ~2 mL.

Device	Flushing	Dressing	Tubing/Cap	Comments
Non tunneled catheter Jugular Subclavian Femoral	• 2 mL of 10–100 U/mL heparinized saline every 12–24 h • For child of any age with one or more medication doses daily, use 10 U/mL • If more than one lumen, flush each lumen as needed	• Initially: transparent dressing over gauze, changed in 48 h to transparent only, then weekly dressing change, or if loose, soiled, wet, compromised	• T-connector tubing not used • Cap changed weekly, if removed, or if compromised	• Short-term catheter placed in emergencies, traumas, intensive care unit • High infection rate, especially with femoral site • May have one, two, or three lumens
Tunneled catheter (Broviac)	• 2 mL of 10–100 U/mL heparinized saline every 12–24 h • For child of any age with one or more medication doses daily, use 10 U/mL	• Initially: transparent dressing over gauze, changed in 48 h to transparent only, then weekly dressing change, or if loose, soiled, wet, compromised	• Connector tubing not usually used • Cap changed weekly, if removed, or if compromised	• Long-term catheter placed for months to years of therapy • Expensive to place and maintain, prone to infection, breakage, clotting • May be used for blood sampling; discard volume = 3× device or ~1–4 mL
Implanted port	• 2 mL of 10 U/mL heparinized saline for child of any age with one or more medication doses daily • At discharge and monthly: use 5 mL of 100 U/mL heparinized saline flush	• Use noncoring needle in 22 to 20 gauge, ½" to 1½" • Initial septum access while child sedated during insertion of port if port is being used after • Pad under needle wings with gauze • Dressing change with needle change weekly	• Connector tubing already attached to noncoring needle set • Cap change with weekly needle change, or if removed or compromised	• Long-term device placed for years of therapy, especially in larger children and adolescents needing intermittent treatments • May be used for blood sampling; discard volume = 3× device or ~3 mL for small arm port, or 5–7 mL for larger chest port

Research Issues: WHAT ARE CORRECT FLUSHING TECHNIQUES FOR PERIPHERAL IV DEVICES?

Source: Bossert & Beecroft, 1994; Crews et al., 1997; Danek & Noris, 1992; Gyr et al., 1995; Hanrahan et al., 1994; Heilskov et al., 1998; Kotter, 1996; Krueger-Paisely et al., 1997; LeDuc, 1997; McMullen et al., 1993

Flushing techniques for peripheral and central devices are a topic of controversy. Studies done in the early 1990s indicate that saline alone may be efficacious in maintaining the patency of 22-gauge catheters in children; however, the numbers of 24-gauge catheters reported was small, and one study demonstrated increased patency in 24-gauge catheters when a dilute heparin flush was used. More recently published research revealed increased patency and decreased tenderness when IVs were flushed with heparinized saline (10 U/mL), whereas several studies in neonates demonstrated no significant difference between normal and heparinized saline flush. In all the neonatal studies, 24-gauge catheters were used, and the IVs were flushed at least every 4 hours. One study evaluated flushes used for short-term IVs in patients in the emergency department, noting that saline was equivalent to heparin flush for patency. Another recent study examined intervals between heparin flushes, noting that 8 hours was optimal for flushing 22-gauge catheters in pediatric patients. Several studies also noted that positive-pressure flush technique, where the connector tubing was clamped before syringe removal, helped to maintain patency of IV catheters. The most common practice reported in a survey of children's hospitals was irrigation of peripheral IVs with 1 mL of a solution of 10 units of heparin per milliliter of saline every 8 hours. Clearly, more research, especially with 24-gauge catheters, and flush intervals longer than 4 hours, is needed to come to a scientific conclusion regarding flush solution and technique for flushing peripheral IVs in children.

Managing Complications

Complications of IV therapy in children are similar to those of adults and are de-scribed earlier in this textbook. The most common peripheral IV complication is in-filtration, which can lead to an extravasation injury, depending on the infusate IV site (dorsal metacarpal veins of the foot are a high-risk site), skill of the inserter, and the child's activity. Current pediatric treatment modalities include application of cold, el-evation of the extremity, and local pharmaceutical intervention with such agents as hyaluronidase (Wydase), nitroglycerin ointment, and glyceryl trinitrate (Brown, Hoelzer, & Piercy, 1979; Denkler & Cohen, 1989; Flemmer & Chan, 1993).

Young children very rarely exhibit a phlebitic response to peripheral IV access, which differs from the much higher rates of phlebitis found in adults. Phlebitis rates reported in children hospitalized in intensive care units were 13%, whereas for those children on general units, phlebitis rates were 10%. In children older than 10 years, phlebitis rates reported (21%) approached those of adults (Nelson & Garland, 1987; Tully, Friedland, Baldini, & Goldman, 1981). Risk factors for development of phlebitis include catheter location, infusion of hyperalimentation fluids with continuous IV lipid emulsions, and length of intensive care stay before catheter insertion (Garland et al., 1992).

 SAFE PRACTICE ALERT   Decreased rates of phlebitis are reported in the following instances:

- Use of 24- and 22-gauge catheters
- Catheters placed in the operating room
- Catheters in surgical patients
- Catheters through which blood products were transfused

Intermediate-Term Midline Intravenous Access

A midline catheter, longer than the peripheral IV of 5/8 to 2 inches, reaches the larger vessels of the upper arm, and in neonates and children the upper thigh (Lesser, Chhabra, Brion, & Suresh, 1996). These larger blood vessels provide greater blood flow and better hemodilution of infusions. Midline catheters are available in 24- and 22-gauge sizes, with lengths of 3 to 6 inches for children. Midline catheters are still considered peripheral IV access devices and are most commonly used for 2 to 4 weeks. Their use is associated with a lower rate of complications than use of central lines (Kupensky, 1998).

Because the tip of a midline catheter does not extend beyond the extremity in which it is placed, radiographic confirmation of tip placement is optional and recommended only when there is difficulty in catheter insertion or flushing (INS, 1998). As with most medical equipment, adult-sized versions of these devices are tested initially, and then studies in children are undertaken. Although very few research studies or outcome data have been published regarding midlines in neonates and children, these catheters have been used to administer IV fluids, medications, and blood products. Complications reported in children include phlebitis, pain, erythema at the insertion site, occlusion, and dislodgment (BeVier & Rice, 1994). Varying degrees of success have been reported with use of these devices in children; more research, particularly in the pediatric population, is certainly a mission for the IV nurse. When using such catheters, manufacturers' recommendations should be followed.

■ CENTRAL INTRAVENOUS ACCESS

When long-term or emergency IV access is desired because of unavailability of peripheral sites, or extended or even lifelong therapy is needed, central venous access is indicated. Pettit & Hughes (1999) most aptly state, "Most authors suggest that placement of a central venous catheter should be considered if parenteral therapy is needed for more than a few weeks or long-term, if PN requiring 12.5% dextrose or greater becomes necessary, if an infant requires more than two IV starts a day, or if vesicants are being infused." Many types of central IV access devices exist, including nontunneled catheters, PICCs, surgically placed cuffed tunneled catheters, totally implanted devices, and, in the neonate, umbilical venous catheters, which are considered a central access device. Umbilical venous and arterial catheters are discussed in the section on Umbilical Catheterization, later. Choice of device depends on the duration and type of therapy prescribed, input from the patient and family, and disease process. Although these devices are described in detail in earlier chapters, features unique to the pediatric population are outlined in the following sections.

Of concern to children and parents is catheter care, safety, cost, and body image. For instance, in toddlers, catheter dislodgment may occur easily; an infant may bite through the catheter during the teething period. A child who is extremely afraid of needles may not do well with an implanted port, which has to be accessed with a needle periodically. Conversely, an older child or adolescent may choose an implanted port over a tunneled catheter to avoid disturbance of body image. If the central device is to be used for continuous infusions or cycled daily therapies, such as TPN, a tunneled catheter, such as a Broviac, may be the best choice; if intermittent treatments are prescribed, a port might be best. Pediatric hospitals often use clinical nurse specialists who can demonstrate pros and cons of each device, assist families in their choice of venous access, introduce children with similar devices, and help decrease anxiety about insertion and care.

Nontunneled Central Venous Catheters

For the purposes of this chapter, nontunneled catheters include percutaneously placed femoral, jugular, and subclavian catheters. These catheters are referred to as *nontunneled* to distinguish them from longer-dwelling cuffed Silastic catheters that are surgically tunneled under the skin. In children and adults, nontunneled catheters often are used for IV access in critical situations, such as in a patient with multiple trauma or in children in the pediatric intensive care unit who need several weeks of IV access and possibly PN.

Size and Insertion

Nontunneled percutaneously placed catheters usually are short and may have from one to four lumens (Fig. 21–10). They usually are made of a stiffer material such as polyurethane for easier insertion by percutaneous skin puncture. Catheter sizes range from 3 to 5 French. In children, these catheters may be inserted nonsurgically, usually by a physician, using local anesthetic and mild sedation.

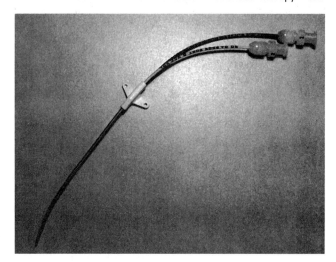

Figure 21–10. Nontunneled double-lumen catheter. (Courtesy of A.M. Frey.)

Site Selection

Although venous anatomy is similar in all age groups, some differences in children necessitate choosing specific sites over others. The preferred sites for percutaneous placement of nontunneled central lines in children are femoral veins, internal and external jugular veins, and subclavian veins, in that order (Lavelle & Costerino, 1997). For anatomic reasons, the right side is preferred when catheterizing the internal jugular or subclavian veins.

The femoral site is the first choice in children because it has easily identifiable landmarks for catheter placement, it is easy to apply pressure to the site if needed, and its location will not hinder any cardiopulmonary resuscitation efforts (Stenzel, Green, Fuhrman et al., 1989) (Fig. 21–11). The internal and external jugular veins are

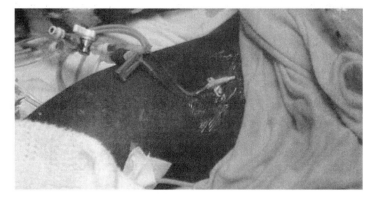

Figure 21–11. Double-lumen nontunneled right femoral catheter in multiple-trauma patient in pediatric intensive care unit. (Courtesy of A.M. Frey.)

chosen next. Their advantages include ease of identification of landmarks and accessibility. They also have a larger diameter, present fewer technical difficulties with catheterization, and carry fewer risks of complications than subclavian veins. The right internal jugular vein runs an almost straight course to the superior vena cava, whereas the left is more angled (Cobb, Vinocur, Wagner, & Weintraub, 1987). Use of the internal jugular vein carries a risk of carotid artery puncture; thus, it should not be used in a child with a clotting disorder. Even though it is located superficially, valves and angles in the external jugular vein make threading a catheter difficult (McGee & Mallory, 1988).

The subclavian vein is the least common site because of anatomic considerations. In infants younger than 1 year of age, higher arching of the subclavian vein causes acute angles that can obstruct placement. After 1 year of age, the subclavian arch assumes the horizontal position similar to that of the adult (Cobb et al., 1987). Curvature and softness of the chest and clavicles make landmarks difficult to identify, and the apices of the lungs are higher in children. Subclavian catheter insertion in neonates is technically difficult and can result in life-threatening complications such as pneumothorax, hydrothorax, hemothorax, and massive hemorrhage (Dolcourt & Bose, 1982).

Maintenance

Maintenance includes daily flushing. Dressing changes should be done weekly or more often, as needed (see Table 21-13).

Problems and Contraindications

Catheter stiffness, high incidence of thrombus, and easy dislodgment limit use of these catheters to a relatively short period, ranging from a few days to 4 weeks (Viall, 1990). Catheters placed in jugular and femoral locations may be occluded because infants tend to have a shortened neck and frequently adduct their legs, causing kinking in the catheter placed in the neck or groin. Femoral location is also the diaper area, and the dressing may become soiled frequently and exposed to infective organisms prevalent in this region. These factors, in addition to potential for air embolism, also limit use of this device for home infusion, particularly in younger children. Contraindications to percutaneous insertion of a nontunneled central line include vascular abnormality or disease in the involved extremity, skin compromise or injury at the proposed entry site, presence of a clotting disorder, or a treatment plan requiring a different type of device.

Peripherally Inserted Central Catheters

A PICC is defined as a catheter inserted into a peripheral vein, usually of the arm or leg, with the tip residing in the superior or inferior vena cava (INS, 1988; Tip location of peripherally inserted central catheters, 1998). Published reports from the 1970s and 1980s mainly described two purposes for the use of PICCs in neonates and children: provision of PN in neonates (Dolcourt & Bose, 1982; Filston & Johnson, 1971; Loeff et al., 1982; Shaw, 1973; Sherman et al., 1982) and provision of several weeks of IV antibiotics in children with cystic fibrosis (Dietrich & Lobas, 1988; Williams et al., 1988; Zanni, Shutack, Schuler, et al., 1985). Before reports of PICC use in neonates and children, central venous access was accomplished using a medical or surgical procedure to place a nontunneled, tunneled, or implanted device or an umbilical catheter in neonates. The development of smaller, easier to insert, more biocompatible catheters resulted in renewed interest in the PICC as a central access device in neonates and children ensued (Frey, 1995; Weeks-Lozano, 1991).

Sizes and Insertion

Pediatric-sized PICCs are manufactured of polyurethane, or softer Silastic material shown to have low incidence of irritation and thrombus formation, allowing PICCs to remain in place for months to years (Markels, 1990). Catheter size should be chosen according to vein size and availability and prescribed treatment plan. Appropriate PICC sizes for children, from the smallest to largest, include:

- Single-lumen devices
- 28-gauge neonatal size
- 2 French (23 gauge)
- 3 French (20 gauge)
- 4 French (18 gauge)
- Double-lumen PICCs
- 3.5 French (18 gauge) to 5 French (16 gauge) (Fig. 21–12).

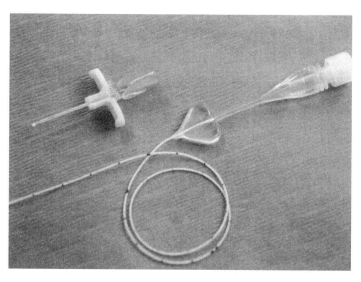

Figure 21–12. 2-French NeoPICC. (Courtesy of Klein-Baker Medical, Inc., San Antonio, TX.)

Insertion can be done without general anesthesia. PICCs may be inserted in children in the hospital, outpatient, or home setting. Restraint and use of local anesthetic or conscious sedation may provide for easier insertion.

Insertion of PICCs is similar in adults and children, although a child may be more anxious and less likely to cooperate. The PICC may be inserted in neonates and children by one of four methods:

1. Winged steel needle—used as prototype for later PICCs and in neonates (Dolcourt & Bose, 1982; Loeff et al., 1982; Sherman et al., 1982).
2. Winged breakaway metal introducer needle—less popular than methods 3 and 4 below because of the potential for catheter shear (Chathas, Paton, & Fisher, 1986; Frey, 1995)
3. Peel-away IV catheter—very popular method because of the ease of use, and most similar to insertion of a peripheral IV catheter, with which many nurses are familiar (BeVier & Rice, 1994; Frey, 1995; Thiagarajan, Ramamoorthy, Gettemann, & Bratton, 1997).
4. Modified or unmodified Seldinger technique—the latter method is becoming increasingly popular because the inserter is able to place a larger-gauge catheter using a small-gauge introducer needle or catheter (Cardella et al., 1993, 1996; Chait et al., 1995; Crowley et al., 1997; Donaldson et al., 1995; Dubois et al., 1997; Goodwin, 1989; Valk, Liem, & Gevin, 1995). Both nurses and physicians use the modified Seldinger technique, whereas physicians only tend to use the unmodified Seldinger technique.

Site Selection

In neonates, PICCs are inserted into the veins of the antecubital fossa, as well as the axillary, saphenous, popliteal, and external jugular veins (Chathas, 1986) (Fig. 21–13).

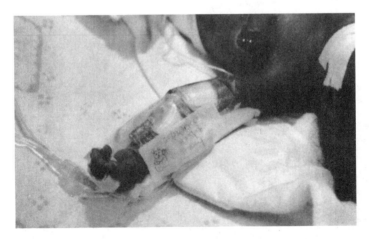

Figure 21–13. 2-French (23 gauge) PICC in place, with dressing on site, in left basilic vein of neonate with hypoplastic ventricle. Patient is receiving prostaglandin infusion through the PICC. (Courtesy of A.M. Frey.)

In older children, the median cubital basilic, basilic, and cephalic veins in the ante-cubital fossa, or slightly above or below this site, are ideal (Fig. 21–14).

Maintenance

Maintenance of PICC catheters in pediatric patients includes dressing care, mainte-nance of patency, changing of end caps, site protection, and avoidance of complica-tions (see Table 21–13). Care must be taken to avoid undue pressures when flushing these small catheters, and flush never should be forced if resistance is felt (Hadaway, 1998b). In addition, rapid injectors used in radiology are avoided with PICCs because the catheter may rupture (Kaste & Young, 1996; Rivitz & Drucker, 1997; Ruess, Bulas, Rivera, & Markle, 1997).

Problems and Contraindications

Although PICCs are associated with fewer complications than surgically placed catheters, PICC use in neonates and children is not without complications, some of which can be severe or fatal (Clarke & Reddy, 1979). Major complications in neonates with PICCs include mechanical complications (10% to 40%), especially catheter oc-clusion. Catheter-related bloodstream infection (Bryant, 1990; Flemmer & Chan, 1993; Frederick, 1991) was the next most frequent reported complication in neonates (0% to 19.1%) (Chathas et al., 1990; Oellrich, Murphy, Goldberg, & Aggarwal, 1991; Trot-ter, 1996). In reports of mixed neonatal/pediatric and pediatric/adult PICC pro-grams, complications, noted from most commonly reported to least, were occlusion, pain/phlebitis, dislodgment, and catheter fracture. The rate of catheter-related bloodstream infection in older children is low (0.8% to 8%) compared with neonates (Frey, 1999). Research is still lacking on the best type of PICC materials, best methods of care, duration of dwell, securement, and other practices, although more studies are being published about PICCs in children.

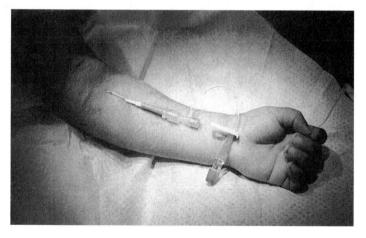

Figure 21–14. 3-French [20 gauge] Silastic PICC in place prior to dressing application, in left median cubital basilic vein of a 3-year-old for TPN af-ter repeat surgery for Hirschsprung's disease. (Courtesy of A.M. Frey.)

Tunneled Central Venous Catheters

Tunneled catheters are most often chosen for long-term venous access, as are implanted ports, which are discussed in the next section. In the early 1970s, Broviac developed the first tunneled catheter for patients who required long-term TPN (Broviac, Cole, & Schribner, 1973). Broviac catheters have since become a popular choice when long-term central IV access is needed, such as with children who have cancer. The Groshong catheter with a valved internal tip, developed in the 1980s, also is tunneled, but is made of thinner-walled silicone than the Broviac (Wickham, 1990).

Sizes and Insertion

Single- and double-lumen Broviacs and single- and double-lumen Groshongs are used in children; the triple-lumen devices tend to be somewhat large for pediatric use. Both catheters contain a Dacron polyester cuff that anchors the catheter in place subcutaneously several weeks after insertion (Camp-Sorrell, 1990) (Fig. 21–15). Both catheters have a Luer-locking proximal hub or hubs outside the patient; the Broviac has an open distal tip on the internal portion, whereas the distal tip of the Groshong is closed with a two-way slit valve. Other companies also manufacture pediatric-sized tunneled catheters.

If no contraindications to general anesthesia exist, tunneled catheters are often inserted in the operating room or radiology suite by a surgeon or interventional radiologist. Often, several procedures are coordinated with catheter insertion to avoid unnecessary trauma while the child is awake; for example, a patient newly diagnosed with leukemia may have one visit to the operating room for Broviac insertion, bone marrow biopsy, and lumbar puncture.

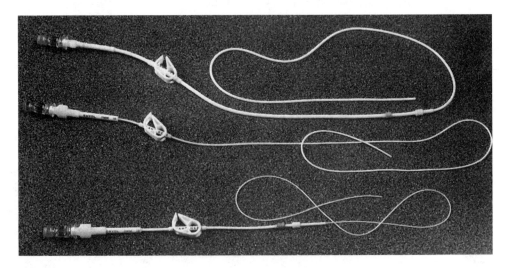

Figure 21–15. Neonatal- and pediatric-sized Broviac catheters with and without Dacron cuff and Vitacuff. (Courtesy of Bard Access Systems, Cranston, RI.)

Site Selection

In older children, the catheter usually is inserted percutaneously into the subclavian vein. In infants and neonates, because of the small size of the subclavian vein and proximity of other structures, this approach can be extremely dangerous. Therefore, in children younger than 5 years, the catheter usually is inserted through the facial vein or the external or internal jugular vein to the superior vena cava (Fig. 21–16).

After proper placement is verified by chest radiography, subcutaneous tunneling of the catheter is done either up the parietal occipital area or down the chest wall to the fourth or fifth intercostal space, depending on the catheter type. This distal exit site from the original phlebotomy site provides a barrier against infection (Meyenfeldt, Stapert, Deong et al., 1980), facilitates catheter maintenance, and provides the child with full-range neck mobility.

In some children, chest access sites are not available because of many previous central lines, vein thromboses, or other surgery or complications. An alternate site for catheter placement is the femoral vein to the inferior vena cava, particularly in children younger than walking age. The proximal portion of the catheter is then tunneled under the skin of the abdomen or out onto the thigh.

Maintenance

Care of tunneled catheters, detailed in Table 21–13, includes dressing changes, flushing to maintain patency, and prevention of infection, occlusion, and dislodgment. Care of tunneled catheters is continually researched, and procedures for children are based on manufacturers' guidelines, catheter volume, experience with adults, and ongoing and previously published research studies. These protocols vary among in-

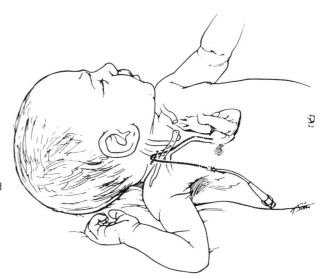

Figure 21–16. Example of inserted pediatric infant-sized Broviac catheter. Note that the catheter is threaded into the external jugular to the right atrium and tunneled subcutaneously down the chest wall.

stitutions and should be reviewed regularly, based on research studies and the needs of the child.

Problems and Contraindications

The complications most frequently reported for tunneled catheters in children include infection, with the highest risk in the first 100 days of use, and mechanical complications, such as occlusion and dislodgment. Toddlers exhibit the highest rate of complications (Wiener & Albanese, 1998).

Tunneled catheter infection rates can range from 5% to 31.6% and should be reported in terms of rate per 1000 catheter days to maintain consistency of data (Decker & Edwards, 1988). The most common infectious organisms reported include coagulase-negative *Staphylococcus,* coagulase-positive *Staphylococcus, Pseudomonas, Escherichia coli, Candida,* and *Enterococcus* (Wiener & Albanese, 1998). In the past, tunneled catheters were removed when catheter-related bloodstream infection was suspected. However, more recent studies have shown promising results in treating infected tunneled catheters and implanted ports in children with a combination of antibiotics and urokinase. In a 1998 publication, Jones concluded that "catheter-related infections, including bacteremia and exit site, tunnel, and pocket infections, can be treated in many cases without removal of the device."

Occlusion may be mechanical, thrombotic, or nonthrombotic. Mechanical occlusions may be evaluated by assessing the catheter for kinking or clamping, repositioning the child, and further assessing as needed using dye studies. Thrombotic occlusions may be corrected with tissue plasminogen activator (TPA); nonthrombotic occlusions are treated with hydrochloric acid, ethanol, or sodium bicarbonate, depending on the cause and pH of the occlusion (Bagnall-Reeb, 1998; Hadaway, 1998a; Ruble, Long, & Connor, 1994). Dislodgment may be prevented by carefully looping the external "tail" of the catheter under the dressing or taping it to the chest. Children of all age groups who have tunneled catheters should wear T-shirts to prevent inadvertent catheter trauma. If breakage occurs, a permanent splicing procedure can be accomplished using a manufacturer's repair kit that matches the broken segment of the tunneled catheter (Viall, 1990).

Because of the complications possible with tunneled catheters, activities such as swimming and contact sports, where exposure to organisms or catheter damage can occur, may be prohibited. Alternate activities should be planned carefully (Marcoux, Fisher, & Wong, 1990). Tunneled catheter removal is a surgical procedure, and because of adherence of the Dacron cuff to tissue in the subcutaneous tunnel, it usually is done using local anesthesia and conscious sedation.

Implanted Ports

Low-profile pediatric ports have been available for several years and are made of stainless steel, titanium, plastic, or a combination of these materials (Fig. 21–17). Ports are ideal for children who require intermittent therapy, can tolerate the needle access, and do not like the inconvenience of an external catheter, such as patients

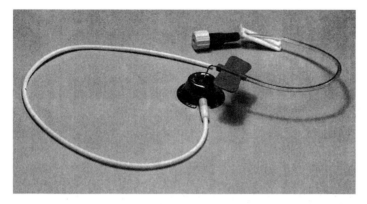

Figure 21–17. Low-profile pediatric implanted port accessed with 22-gauge, 3/4-inch, 90-degree angle, noncoring needle. (Courtesy of A.M. Frey.)

with cancer, short bowel syndrome, or cystic fibrosis (Marcoux et al., 1990). Ports are a good long-term choice for children older than 1 year. Before that age, lack of subcutaneous tissue may cause the port to erode through the skin. In children with cancer, one author reports ports being used the least frequently in children younger than 3 years and most frequently in children older than 15 years of age. When advising patients and family about venous access devices, an important consideration is that the port requires access with a needle at least monthly. Ports are accessed from the top or side, depending on the design, with a noncoring needle or, in some brands, an IV catheter.

Sizes and Insertion

Venous access ports are implanted in the chest, upper abdomen, or forearm, with the catheter threaded into a central vein. A 22- to 20-gauge, 1/2-inch needle for a forearm port and a 22- to 20-gauge, 3/4- to 1-inch needle for a chest port are usually adequate for the viscosity and flow of pediatric infusions.

A hospital or home IV nurse, parents, or patients themselves in some cases may access the port after return demonstration of correct technique. Of concern in patients with cystic fibrosis is use of the arm port versus the chest port. Chest physiotherapy, involving chest percussion, is a large part of the treatment plan for cystic fibrosis. A chest port may obstruct this therapy.

Maintenance

Needles are changed every 7 days while the port is being used; dressings over the accessed port can be changed with the needle or more frequently. When the port is not being used for infusion of medications, PN, transfusion therapy, or blood sample withdrawal, patency is maintained by flushing the port with heparinized saline (Marcoux et al., 1990). Care of implanted ports is detailed in Table 21–13. More on port description and care may be found in Chapter 14.

Problems and Contraindications

Complications reported with ports are similar to those identified for tunneled catheters, including infection and occlusion; in most studies, implanted ports had longer survival times and fewer complications than tunneled catheters (Pearson, 1996). Although risk of port dislodgment is minimal, the noncoring needle may be dislodged and cause infiltration and possible tissue injury if vesicant drugs are being administered. Slight discomfort has been reported with needle access of the port, but this diminishes in time, and a high level of satisfaction also has been reported (Poole, Ross, Haas, & Odom, 1991).

▲ Legal Issues: SITE MONITORING

Site monitoring is of the utmost importance in pediatric patients because infiltration can occur quickly, and effects can be devastating if the infiltrated infusate has caustic properties. Risk factors for an infiltration injury include age younger than 1 year, catheter dwell time less than 72 hours, administration of anticonvulsant medications, and use of steel butterfly needles instead of catheters. IV sites in those areas with very little superficial tissue, particularly the dorsum of the foot in infants, are more prone to extravasation injury. Patients who are unable to communicate because of age, sedation, or physical condition also can be at higher risk for IV injury. Infiltration injuries can be a reason for litigation if the injury is extensive or limits function. Recommended frequency for peripheral IV site assessment, while therapies are infusing, ranges from every 1 to 2 hours, or more often if the infusate is known to be an irritant or vesicant. Peripheral IV sites used as heparin or saline locks, without an infusate running, should be assessed at least once per shift (every 8 to 12 hours). In home care as well, patients and caregivers are taught how to recognize signs of IV complications and to take corrective actions. Peripheral IV access should not be used for continuous infusions in alternative settings, such as the home, unless the site can be monitored. For this reason, central venous access is often used in the home and alternative setting.

(From Brown et al., 1979; Denkler & Cohen, 1989; Garland et al., 1992; Guhlow & Kolb, 1979; INS, 1998, 2000.)

■ OTHER ROUTES OF VASCULAR ACCESS IN CHILDREN

Umbilical Catheterization

Most sites for neonatal IV therapy are similar to those discussed earlier in this chapter. A site unique to the newborn population is the umbilicus, which contains two arteries and one vein. Umbilical catheterization is common practice in many neonatal and intensive care units for treatment of acutely ill infants. This mode of therapy provides an easy route for vascular administration of transfusions, medications, fluids, PN, and blood withdrawal, although it is not without complications. Risks include thrombosis, embolism, vasospasm, vascular perforation, infection, and hemorrhage

(Bryant, 1990). To prevent these complications, a specially designed umbilical catheter with the following features should be selected:

- Flexibility
- Relatively rigid walls for accurate pressure monitoring
- Smoothness of the tip to prevent perforation of the vessel wall during catheter insertion
- Radiopacity to visualize the location of the catheter tip by radiography
- Small-volume capacity so that only a small amount of blood need be withdrawn to clear the catheter for blood sampling
- Size from 3.5 to 5 French, single- or double-lumen (Figs. 21–18 and 21–19)

Procedure

Within minutes of birth, the umbilical arteries normally constrict; delays in the process, however, occur in states of hypoxia and acidosis. Most infants are catheterized in the first day of life because umbilical catheterization is more difficult or impossible past the fourth day of life. The procedure for umbilical catheterization begins with aseptic technique, including hand washing, gloving, masking, and gowning. Equipment is set up using a cutdown tray and recommended catheter size. All IV tubing must be purged of air. The infant is restrained temporarily using leg/arm restraints and an assistant. The umbilical stump is cleaned with a povidone–iodine solution; excess should not be allowed to pool at the infant's side or skin irritation or blistering may occur (Lipton & Schafermeyer, 1997). The sterile field is set up around the umbilicus, using a fenestrated drape that exposes the umbilical area. Dissection

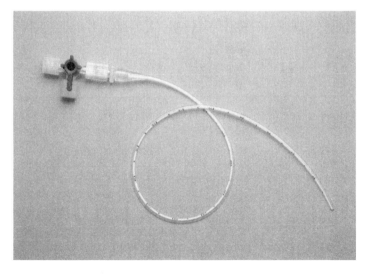

Figure 21–18. Neo-Care photo of single-lumen umbilical vessel catheter. (Courtesy of Klein-Baker Medical, Inc., San Antonio, TX.)

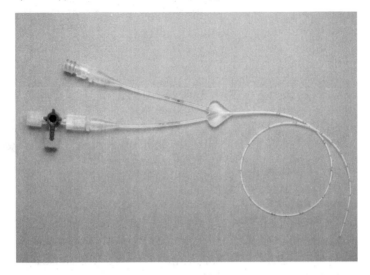

Figure 21–19. Neo-Care photo of dual-lumen umbilical vessel catheter. (Courtesy of Klein-Baker Medical, Inc., San Antonio, Texas.)

begins at the umbilical cord approximately 1.5 cm from the skin until the umbilical vessels are identified. Two thick-walled, pinpoint-sized arteries are easily distinguishable from a large, thin-walled vein. The heparinized catheter is passed through either the umbilical artery or vein, depending on the type of therapy desired.

There are important differences between arterial and venous umbilical catheterization (Table 21–14). Arterial catheterization accomplishes five goals: blood sampling; measurements of arterial pressures; parenteral or antibiotic therapy in the vascularly compromised child; exchange transfusions; and measurements of arterial pH and blood gases. Venous umbilical catheterization accomplishes four goals: blood sampling; parenteral or antibiotic therapy in the vascularly compromised child; direct measurement of central venous pressure; and infusion of TPN (Klaus & Fanaroff, 1979). Placements differ between the umbilical arterial and venous routes. Ideally, the umbilical arterial catheter (UAC) is positioned above the level of aortic bifurcation in good position for arterial measurements and exchange transfusions. Comparatively, the tip of the umbilical venous catheter (UVC) should be positioned in the inferior vena cava near the right atrium in good position for central venous pressure and TPN administration.

Once the catheter is placed correctly and position is confirmed radiographically, a suture may be placed superficially through the stump and tied firmly to the catheter for anchorage. The umbilical catheter is taped to the infant's abdomen using goalpost taping, often referred to as a tape "bridge." The UAC usually is connected to a three-way stopcock for pressure monitoring, blood drawing, and fluid administration. In the UVC, when fluid administration is not necessary, the line may be heparinized. It is of the utmost importance to maintain patency of the indwelling catheter because blood clots can otherwise form. Flushing with heparin (1 to 10 U/mL preservative-free normal saline) should be done frequently.

T A B L E 2 1 – 1 4
DIFFERENCES BETWEEN UMBILICAL VESSELS

	Umbilical Arteries	**Umbilical Vein**
Anatomy	Two thicker-walled vessels	One larger, thinner-walled vessel
Number of days vessel can be catheterized	• Constrict within minutes of birth • Arteries close before umbilical vein • Can occasionally be used up to 7 days after birth	Usually used within the first 4 days of life; may be able to be catheterized for up to 14 days after cord is clamped and cut
Indications for catheterization	Respiratory compromise requiring mechanically assisted ventilation in neonates	Central venous access immediately after birth, especially when long-term care and venous access needs are anticipated.
Contraindications	• Omphalitis • Impetiginous skin lesions • Suspected necrotizing enterocolitis or intestinal hypoperfusion • Should not be inserted for routine fluids/medications/blood sampling	
Catheter size/type	<2 kg: 3.5–4-French catheter >2 kg: up to 5-French catheter	Larger catheter can be used because of larger vessel size: 5–8 French
Depth of catheter tip	• Above diaphragm: spinal level T6–T9 (at the level of the thoracic aorta between the ductus arteriosus and the origin of the celiac axis) • Below diaphragm: spinal level L3–L5 (between the inferior mesenteric artery and the bifurcation of the aorta)	Above the diaphragm, at the junction of the inferior vena cava and the right atrium
Use of catheter	• Blood gas sampling • D_5W or $D_{10}W$ with heparin Reported use varies by neonatal intensive care unit and includes: • Fluids • Blood products • Blood sampling • Furosemide [Lasix] • Bicarbonate • Cimetidine [Tagamet] • Access for cardiac catheterization • Angiocardiography • Antibiotics • Diazepam • Phenobarbital	• Central venous pressure monitoring • Medications • Parenteral nutrition solutions • Infusions given by central line

(Adapted from Bryant, B.G. [1990]. Drug, fluid, and blood products administered through the umbilical artery catheter: Complication experiences from one NICU. *Neonatal Network, 9,* 27–46; and Lipton, J.D. & Schafermeyer, R.W. [1997]. Umbilical vessel catheterization. In F.M. Henretig & C. King [Eds.], *Textbook of pediatric emergency procedures* [pp. 515–22]. Philadelphia: Lippincott–Raven.)

Nursing Assessment and Management

Nursing care and assessment (Lipton & Schafermeyer, 1997; Stanford, 1990; Wheeler & Frey, 1995) should include the following:

• Examine buttocks and extremities hourly to detect blanching or color changes caused by arterial spasms or catheter malposition. If color changes are noted,

apply warm soaks to opposite extremity for 15 minutes to trigger reflex vasodilation in the affected limb.
- Use Luer-lock connections to prevent disconnection of the tubing with resultant hemorrhage.
- Closely monitor peripheral edema, unequal femoral pulses, and respiratory distress, which could indicate emboli formation.
- Observe and document the quality of the arterial waveform on the monitor; change in quality or dampening of the waveform may indicate a problem with the umbilical arterial line.
- Monitor the umbilicus daily for signs of infection during treatment and for 12 hours after catheter removal; provide routine cord care daily.

Risks and Complications

Reported risks and complications associated with UACs include aortic, mesenteric, or renal artery thrombus formation resulting in visceral infarction and subsequent necrotizing enterocolitis; renal insufficiency; hypertension; congestive heart failure; lower limb ischemia; sepsis; aortoiliac aneurysms; and hypoglycemia from glucose infusion into the pancreatic circulation. Risks and complications associated with UVCs include those complications associated with other central venous lines in infants, such as sepsis, arrhythmias, and vessel or heart perforation, and cardiac tamponade (Sigda, Speights, & Thigpen, 1992).

Studies of infectious complications associated with umbilical catheters indicate that incidences for catheter colonization are similar, ranging from 40% to 55% for UACs and 22% to 59% for UVCs. The documented bloodstream infection rates reported were 5% for UACs and 3% to 8% for UVCs (Pearson, 1996). Neonates with very low birth weight receiving prolonged antimicrobials were at increased risk for UAC bloodstream infection; neonates with higher birth weight receiving PN were at increased risk for UVC related infection (Landers, Moise, Fraley et al., 1991).

Mechanical complications include hemorrhage, occlusion, and air embolism (Lipton & Schafermeyer, 1997; Stanford, 1990). If complications arise, report them immediately to the appropriate physician/practitioner so immediate assessment and treatment can be provided. Early intervention can reduce the risk of morbidity and mortality when using umbilical access for IV therapy. Because of the risk of complications and the short dwell time when using the umbilical vessel for IV therapy, many physicians now prefer to use an alternate peripheral or central site as soon as possible.

Surgical Cutdown

Although alternative choices of access, such as the IO and central venous routes, have diminished the need for venous cutdown, this method remains a viable option for emergency vascular access in resuscitation of the pediatric patient. When acute hypovolemia and acidosis cause severe enough peripheral vasoconstriction that percutaneous placement of venous access is impossible, and if IO access cannot be achieved, venous cutdown may be warranted (Gauderer, 1992).

The most common cutdown sites are the distal saphenous vein at the ankle, the proximal saphenous vein at the groin, the basilic vein at the antecubital, and the axillary vein, which is used in newborns (Winci, 1997). Because this procedure requires venous laceration or minor surgery, a physician or surgeon usually performs it. Meticulous sterile technique is required. The size of the IV catheter placed can range from 22 to 16 gauge, depending on the size of the vessel. Complications reported with venous cutdown include local injury of contiguous structures, such as an artery or nerve, hemorrhage, hematoma, extravasation, phlebitis with prolonged use, localized cellulitis, suppurative phlebitis, and catheter-related bloodstream infection (Winci, 1997).

Obtaining successful IV access is essential to provide efficacious pediatric advanced life support. In many cases, during a "code" situation, peripheral veins have collapsed because of cardiac arrest and poor perfusion. Time for performance of a surgical cutdown can range from 2 to 40 minutes, with a median time of 8 minutes (Kanter, Zimmerman, Straus, & Stoeckel, 1986).

Intraosseous Access

Intravenous access should be obtained within 5 minutes from the start of a resuscitation effort. After traditional routes have been attempted or often simultaneously, IO access is a realistic goal. **Intraosseous infusion** is defined as infusion of blood, fluids, or drugs through a rigid needle directly into the bone marrow cavity (Manley, Haley, & Dick, 1988). This technique was widely used from 1922, when first described by Drinker, Drinker, and Lund (1922), through the 1960s. As IV device technology improved, facilitating peripheral venous access, IO technique lost popularity. Since 1983, however, interest in IO therapy has increased because of a letter to the editor of *American Journal of Diseases of Children* that questioned the abandonment of this route (Turkel, 1983).

The IO technique is based on the fact that the extensive network of venous sinusoids quickly takes up fluid injected into the medullary cavity of the bone, and drugs given by the IO and central venous routes are equally effective, working faster than those administered by peripheral IV (Manley et al., 1988). The tibia and femur are the preferred sites for IO administration because the limbs are readily accessible during resuscitation efforts and the marrow cavity is well developed, even in neonates (Tocantins & O'Neil, 1945).

The preferred site for IO infusion in children up to 5 or 6 years of age is the anterior medial aspect of the tibia, 1 to 3 cm below the tibial tuberosity, thus avoiding the growth plate at the end of the bone (Kanter et al., 1986; Manley et al., 1988; Miccolo, 1990) (Fig. 21–20). The tibial sites are preferred because less subcutaneous tissue over the bone enhances ease of access, as opposed to the femur, where subcutaneous tissue may make IO access difficult. Other sites include distal medial tibia, mid-anterior distal femur, iliac crest, and humerus, and the sternum in children older than 3 years of age, before which the sternum is too thin to support the IO needle (Miccolo, 1990). Contraindications to IO access include site infections, fractures, burns, and bone disorders, such as osteogenesis imperfecta (brittle bone disease) and osteopetrosis (marble bone disease), where bones may fracture easily (Manley et al.,

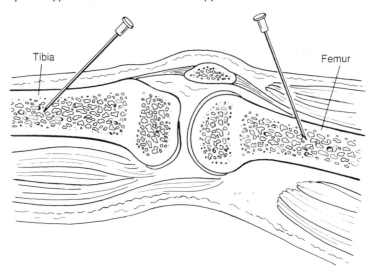

Figure 21–20. The anterior medial aspect of the tibia (lateral view) is the best site for intraosseous access in the child younger than 6 years of age.

1988; Miccolo, 1990). IO access is indicated during emergencies, such as respiratory or cardiac resuscitation efforts or when two attempts at peripheral IV access are unsuccessful (Manley et al., 1988).

A short, rigid needle with a stylet is used to obtain IO access (Fig. 21–21); alternatively, a lumbar puncture needle may be used for infants, although this needle can bend easily and is awkward to insert. Disposable bone marrow aspiration needles are now manufactured for IO access; 16, 18, or 20 is the recommended gauge because a small-lumen needle can become blocked with bone fragments or bend on insertion.

After antimicrobial cleansing of the desired site, the IO needle is inserted perpendicular to the bone surface at a slight angle away from the epiphyseal plate. A

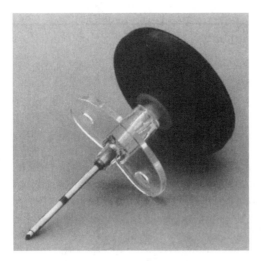

Figure 21–21. Intraosseous needle with Diekmann modification (two laterally opposed side ports, positioned near distal tip to ensure flow if tip is obstructed by fragment). (Courtesy of Cook Critical Care, Bloomington, IN.)

screwing motion is used to insert the needle into the bone until decreased resistance is noted and the needle stands without support, usually at a depth of 1 cm in an infant or child (Hodge, 1997). Further advancement may cause penetration of the opposite wall of the bone and result in extravasation of infusates. Some IO needles are now manufactured with a premarked shaft to indicate depth. After insertion, the stylet is removed and bone marrow content, similar to blood, is aspirated; this sample may be used for readings of Pa_{CO_2} and pH, important parameters indicating success of resuscitative efforts (Manley et al., 1988).

A short connector tubing and flush solution, similar to that used with IV catheters, is connected to the hub of the IO needle, and a split sterile gauze dressing and tape are placed to secure the site. If the child is awake, intradermal anesthesia before IO needle placement is advised. The site should be observed for infiltration of infusates into surrounding tissues; the same bone should not be used for repeated access if infiltration occurs. Types of infusions given by the IO route are listed in Table 21–15. Infusates may be administered by gravity, manual pressure, or infusion pump.

Complications are relatively rare. A 0.6% incidence of osteomyelitis, the most common complication (Rosetti, Thompson, Miller et al., 1985), has been reported in the literature and is related to long-term use and infusion of hypertonic solutions. Other complications can include the following (Hodge, 1997; Manley et al., 1988; Simmons et al., 1994):

- Cellulitis
- Compartment syndrome
- Abscess
- Local necrosis
- Fat embolism (although a possibility, this has not been reported in children, probably because of the low fat content of bone marrow in children, especially those younger than 4 years of age)
- Bilateral tibial fractures

TABLE 21–15
INTRAOSSEOUS INFUSIONS

Fluids	Medications	Blood Products
• 5%, 10%, and 50% dextrose	• Analgesics	• Albumin
• Saline	• Anesthetics	• Dextran
• Lactated ringer's solution	• Antibiotics	• Packed red blood cells
• Parenteral nutrition	• Anticonvulsants	• Plasma
	• Antisera	• Whole blood
	• Catecholamines	
	• Contrast media	
	• Miscellaneous (eg, atropine, calcium, dopamine, dobutamine, epinephrine, heparin, insulin, lidocaine, levarterenol, phenytoin, sodium bicarbonate)	

(Adapted from Arbeiter & Greengard, 1944; Chameides, 1994; Dieckmann et al., 1997; Glaesser & Losek, 1986; Miccolo, 1990; and Mofenson, 1988.)

To prevent complications, the site should be monitored closely, especially during infusion of potential vesicants. Success rates with IO therapy have been reported as high as 97% (Roth, 1997). Replacement of the IO needle with IV access is recommended as soon as conventional IV access is feasible.

■ INTRAVENOUS ADMINISTRATION EQUIPMENT

Options for volume control, delivery of small doses of medication, and assurance of safety in pediatric patients include microdrip administration sets, microbore tubing, Luer-lock connections, volume control chambers, and infusion pumps (Jackson & Saunders, 1993). None of these devices, however, can replace close surveillance of the patient by the health care provider.

Tubing and Administration Sets

Large-bore tubing holds a great deal of volume. Attempts to deliver a small amount of medication through this type of tubing could result in delivery of too much volume to a small child. Microbore tubing is incorporated into IV administration sets and connection devices for pediatric patients.

Minimal flow rates in neonates, infants, and children necessitate proper choice of intravascular administration set. Special sets are required to avoid the possibility of medication overdose or fluid volume overload.

Microdrip administration sets for gravity infusion (60 gtt/minute) are specific for infants and children. IV tubing with an in-line calibrated volume control chamber (50-, 100-, and 150-mL sizes are available) should be used on all children whose prescribed fluid rate is less than the volume of the chamber. The calibrated chamber also is used to administer intermittent doses of medications.

Because acutely ill patients often need multiple therapies, extension sets with a three-way stopcock are used frequently in critical care units. However, such stopcocks can present concerns about infection and safety. In place of stopcocks, some institutions use multiple-arm connectors with two or more arms, each with its own clamp. These connectors provide a closed system for administration of multiple infusates into one IV site. In this case, consultation with pharmacy experts regarding compatibility issues is advisable.

Containers

Plastic rather than glass solution containers should be used whenever possible to avoid breakage in case the container falls off its pole. To avoid the risk of fluid volume overload, the volume of the solution container should be based on the age and size of the child and should not contain greater than 500 mL of fluid, unless rates exceed that limit. In premature infants and neonates, smaller solution containers should be considered.

Electronic and Pressurized Infusion Devices

Devices that electronically control volume, rate, and, sometimes, dose, have become the norm rather than the exception in pediatric IV therapy. Electronic infusion devices with a high degree of accuracy, no free-flow capacity, ability to infuse rates from tenths of a milliliter to hundreds of milliliters, controlled pressure settings, and microbore tubing sets are available for use in neonatal and pediatric patients. Syringe pumps are often used in intensive care and medical surgical units to deliver small-volume medications accurately.

There is debate over whether the chambered IV set is required when an electronic infusion device is used. Manufacturers of electronic infusion devices claim that their product is guarded against free-flow fluid, and products that are safety tested in proven clinical trials should be chosen for neonatal and pediatric patients. In one such trial, an intensive care nursery eliminated the use of volume control chambers with electronic infusion pumps after assessing the need for this redundant volume control (Reiser, 1999).

In the home setting, single-use pressurized pumps are convenient for individual doses. Small electronic pumps that can be hidden in a backpack are often used for intermittent and continuous doses, and large-volume pumps can be used for such therapies as cycled TPN. When choosing a pump for a pediatric patient, accuracy and safety are of utmost importance. Independent consumer groups for medical devices provide excellent, unbiased reviews of these devices for the agency to consult before purchasing a pump for use in children.

■ ALTERNATIVE-SITE PEDIATRIC INTRAVENOUS THERAPY

Much routine and some high-acuity stable neonatal and pediatric IV therapy has moved out of the hospital and into the home or subacute care facility or outpatient infusion center. Home infusion is estimated at one-third the costs of hospitalization (Ringel, 1995). Disorders treated at home or other locations with IV modalities include but are not limited to cystic fibrosis; hemophilia; bone, soft tissue, and joint infections; neonatal sepsis; gastrointestinal disorders; immunologic dysfunction; and oncologic disorders and treatment sequelae (Ferris, 1990; Schuman, 1990). IV therapies administered in the home or at alternate sites include fluids, antibiotics or antifungals, PN, chemotherapy, analgesics, chelating agents, chemotherapy, pain control medications, and blood components. Even neonates and infants are sent home safely under the care and supervision of agencies skilled in neonatal and pediatric care (Cady & Yoshioka, 1991).

Pediatric patients usually receive one or more doses in a controlled environment to verify that there is no adverse reaction. With TPN, the therapy is usually cycled to infuse over several hours before discharge home or transfer to alternative site care. Intermediate- to long-term catheters are often used for IV therapy at home to avoid the trauma and possible omitted therapy for frequent peripheral IV site changes. Occasionally peripheral IVs, but more often, midline, PICC, and tunneled or implanted central devices are chosen for pediatric home or alternate site care.

Readiness, willingness, and ability of the patient and family and extensive teaching with demonstrated feedback should be documented before patient discharge, and be ongoing during the patient's course of treatment until service is discontinued. School-age and older children can participate in their own care. Outcome data on pediatric home care, lacking in the published literature, is another opportunity for nursing research. The pediatric home infusion nurse must be an experienced IV practitioner, as might be indicated by CRNI status, as well as an expert in recognition and treatment of pediatric abnormal states. In 1995, Ringel summarized this concept, "Pediatric infusion has to be done by a company dedicated to pediatrics or that has a pediatrics division . . . . If children are given to a provider that does not have the expertise for high-acuity patients, they (children) can end up back in the hospital" (Ringel, 1995). Pediatric home care is now the fastest growing portion of the home care market (see Chap. 23) (Ferris, 1990; Schuman, 1990).

References and Selected Readings

Asterisks indicate references cited in text.

*American Academy of Pediatrics. (1996). The management of acute gastroenteritis in young children. *Practice Guideline, 97*(3), 1–24.

*Arbeiter, H.I. & Greengard, J. (1944). Tibial bone marrow infusions in infancy. *Journal of Pediatrics, 25,* 1.

*Bagnall-Reeb, H. (1998). Diagnosis of central venous access device occlusion. *Journal of Intravenous Nursing, 21* (Suppl. 5), S115–S121.

*Barnard, J. & Hazinski, M.F. (1992). Pediatric gastrointestinal disorders. In M. F. Hazinski (Ed.), *Nursing care of the critically ill child* (pp. 715–803). St. Louis: Mosby.

*Batton, D.G., Maisels, J., & Applebaum, P. (1982). Use of peripheral intravenous cannulas in premature infants: A controlled study. *Pediatrics, 70,* 488.

*Bendorf, K., Friesen, C.A., & Roberts, C.C. (1996). Glucose response to discontinuation of parenteral nutrition in pediatrics less than 3 years of age. *JPEN Journal of Parenteral and Enteral Nutrition, 20*(2), 10–22.

*Berner-Howry, L.B., McGillis-Bindler, R., & Tso, Y. (1981). *Pediatric medications.* Philadelphia: J.B. Lippincott.

*Bertolone, K. (1997). Pediatric oncology: Past, present, and new modalities of treatment. *Journal of Intravenous Nursing, 20,* 136–140.

*BeVier, P.A. & Rice, C.E. (1994). Initiating a pediatric peripherally inserted central catheter and midline catheter program. *Journal of Intravenous Nursing, 17,* 201–205.

*Bilodeau, J.A., Poon, C., & Mascarenhas, M.R. (1998). Parenteral nutrition and care of central venous lines. In S.M. Altschuler & C.A. Liacouras (Eds.), *Clinical pediatric gastroenterology* (pp. 637–652). Philadelphia: Churchill Livingstone.

*Bossert, E. & Beecroft, P.C. (1994). Peripheral intravenous lock irrigation in children: Current practice. *Pediatric Nursing, 20,* 346–355.

*Broviac, W., Cole, B., & Schribner, B.H. (1973). A silicone rubber atrial catheter for prolonged parenteral alimentation. *Surgery, Gynecology and Obstetrics, 136,* 602.

*Brown, A.S., Hoelzer, D., & Piercy, S.A. (1979). Skin necrosis from extravasation of intravenous fluids in children. *Plastic and Reconstructive Surgery, 64,* 145–150.

*Bryant, B.G. (1990). Drug, fluid, and blood products administered through the umbilical artery catheter: Complication experiences from one NICU. *Neonatal Network, 9,* 27–46.

*Cady, C. & Yoshioka, R.S. (1991). Using a learning contract to successfully discharge and infant on home total parenteral nutrition. *Pediatric Nursing, 17,* 67–74.

*Cahill-Alsip, C. & McDermott, B. (1996). Hematologic critical care problems. In M.Q. Curley, J.B. Smith, & P.A. Moloney-Harmon (Eds.), *Critical care nursing of infants and children* (pp. 793–817). Philadelphia: W.B. Saunders.

*Camp-Sorrell, D. (1990). Advanced central venous access, selection, catheters, devices, and nursing management. *Journal of Intravenous Nursing, 13,* 361–370.

*Cardella, J.F., et al. (1993). Interventional radiologic placement of peripherally inserted central catheters. *Journal of Vascular Interventional Radiology, 4,* 649–656.

*Cardella, J.F., et al. (1996). Cumulative experience with 1,273 peripherally inserted central catheters at a single institution. *Journal of Vascular Interventional Radiology, 7,* 5–13.

*Chait, P.G., et al. (1995). Peripherally inserted central catheters in children. *Radiology, 197,* 775–778.

Chameides, L. (1994). *Textbook of pediatric advanced life support.* Dallas, TX: American Heart Association.

*Chathas, M.K. (1986). Percutaneous central venous catheters in neonates. *Journal of Obstetric, Gynecologic, and Neonatal Nursing, 141,* 324–332.

*Chathas, M.K., Paton, J.B., & Fisher, D.E. (1990). Percutaneous central venous catheterization: Three years' experience in a neonatal intensive care unit. *American Journal of Diseases of Children, 41,* 1243–1250.

*Clarke, T.A. & Reddy, P.G. (1979). Intravenous infusion technique in the newborn. *Clinical Pediatrics, 18,* 550–554.

*Cobb, L.M., Vinocur, C.D., Wagner, C.W., & Weintraub, W.H. (1987). The central venous anatomy in infants. *Surgery, Gynecology and Obstetrics, 165,* 230–234.

*Collier, S., Crouch, J., Hendricks, K., & Cacallero, B. (1994). Use of cyclic parenteral nutrition in infants less than 6 months of age. *Nutrition in Clinical Practice, 9,* 65–68.

*Crews, B.E., Gnann, K.K., Rice, M.H., & Kee, C.C. (1997). Effects of varying intervals between heparin flushes on pediatric catheter longevity. *Pediatric Nursing, 23,* 87–91.

*Crowley, J.J., et al. (1997). Peripherally inserted central catheters: experience in 483 children. *Radiology, 204,* 577–521.

*Danek, G.D. & Noris, E.M. (1992). Pediatric IV catheters: Efficacy of saline flush. *Pediatric Nursing, 18,* 111–113.

*Deady, A. & Gorman, D. (1997). Intravenous conscious sedation in children. *Journal of Intravenous Nursing, 20,* 245–252.

*Decker, M.D. & Edwards, K.M. (1988). Central venous catheter infections. *Pediatric Clinics of North America, 35,* 579–612.

*Denkler, K.A. & Cohen, B.E. (1989). Reversal of dopamine extravasation injury with topical nitroglycerin ointment. *Plastic and Reconstructive Surgery, 84,* 811–813.

*Dieckmann, R., et al. (1997). *Pediatric emergency and critical care procedures.* St. Louis: Mosby–Year Book.

*Dietrich, K.A. & Lobas, J.G. (1988). Use of a single silastic IV catheter for cystic fibrosis pulmonary exacerbations. *Pediatric Pulmonology, 4,* 181–184.

*Dolcourt, J.L. & Bose, C.L. (1982). Percutaneous insertion of silastic central venous catheters in neonates. *Journal of Obstetric, Gynecologic, and Neonatal Nursing, 15,* 324–332.

*Donaldson, J.S., et al. (1995). Peripherally inserted central venous catheters: US-guided vascular access in pediatric patients. *Radiology, 197,* 499–504.

*Drinker, C.K., Drinker, K.R., & Lund, C.C. (1922). The circulation in the mammalian bone marrow. *American Journal of Physiology, 62,* 1–92.

*Dubois, J., et al. (1997). Peripherally inserted central catheters in infants and children. *Radiology, 204,* 582–586.

*Fann, B. D. (1998). Fluid and electrolyte balance in the pediatric patient. *Journal of Intravenous Nursing, 21,* 153–159.

*Farrington, E. (1990). Pediatric drug information. *Pediatric Nursing, 16,* 310.

*Fay, M. (1983). The special challenges of pediatric IVs. *Dimensions of Critical Care Nursing, 2,* 24.

*Fein, J.A., Boardman, C.R., Stevenson, S., & Selbst, S.M. (1998). Saline with benzyl alcohol as intradermal anesthesia for intravenous line placement in children. *Pediatric Emergency Care, 14,* 119–122.

*Ferris, E.W. (1990). A neonatal home intravenous therapy program. *Journal of Intravenous Nursing, 13,* 383–387.

*Filston, H.C. & Johnson, D.G. (1971). Percutaneous venous cannulation in neonates and infants: A method for catheter insertion without "cutdown." *Pediatrics, 48,* 896–901.

*Flemmer, L. & Chan, S.L. (1993). A pediatric protocol for management of extravasation injuries. *Pediatric Nursing, 19,* 355–358.

*Frederick, V. (1991). Pediatric IV therapy: Soothing the patient. *RN, 54*(12), 40–42.

*Frey, A.M. (1991). The immune system: Part II. Intravenous administration of immune globulin. *Journal of Intravenous Nursing, 14,* 397–405.

*Frey, A.M. (1995). Pediatric peripherally inserted central catheter program report: A summary of 4,536 catheter days. *Journal of Intravenous Nursing, 18,* 280–291.

*Frey, A.M. (1997). Tips for pediatric IV insertion. *Nursing 97, 27*(9), 32.

*Frey, A.M. (1998a). Success rates for peripheral IV insertion in a children's hospital: Financial implications. *Journal of Intravenous Nursing, 21,* 160–165.

*Frey, A.M. (1998b). When a child needs peripheral IV therapy: Use these suggestions to choose the right site. *Nursing 98, 38*(4), 18.

*Frey, A.M. (1999). Pediatric and neonatal PICC complications. *Journal of Vascular Access Devices, 4* (Suppl. 2), 4.

*Friedland, L.R. & Brown, R. (1992). Introduction of a "safety" intravenous catheter for use in an emergency department: A pediatric hospital's experience. *Infection Control and Hospital Epidemiology, 13,* 114–115.

*Garland, S., Dunne, M., Havens, P., et al. (1992). Peripheral intravenous catheter complications in critically ill children: A prospective study. *Pediatrics, 89,* 1145–1150.

*Gauderer, M.W.L. (1992). Vascular access techniques and devices in the pediatric patient. *Surgical Clinics of North America, 72,* 1267–1284.

Glaesser, P.N. & Losek, D. (1986). Emergency intraosseous infusions in children. *American Journal of Emergency Medicine, 4,* 35.

*Goodwin, M.L. (1989). The Seldinger method for PICC insertion. *Journal of Intravenous Nursing, 12,* 238–240.

*Graef, J. & Cone, T. (1977). *Manual of pediatric therapeutics.* Boston: Little, Brown.

*Guhlow, L. & Kolb, J. (1979). Pediatric IVs: Special measures you must take. *RN, 42,* 40–52.

*Gura, K.M. (1993). Parenteral drug administration guidelines for the pediatric patient: One hospital's recommendations. *Hospital Pharmacy, 28,* 221–242.

*Guyon, G. (1992). Pharmacokinetic considerations in neonatal drug therapy. *Neonatal Network, 7,* 9–12.

*Gyr, P., Burroughs, T., Smith, K., Mahl, C., Pontious, S., & Swerczek, L. (1995). Double blind comparison of heparin and saline flush solutions in maintenance of peripheral infusion devices. *Pediatric Nursing, 21,* 383–389, 366.

Hadaway, L. (1990). A midline alternative to central and peripheral venous access. *Caring, 9,* 45–50.

*Hadaway, L. (1998a). Major thrombotic and nonthrombotic complications. *Journal of Intravenous Nursing, 21*(Suppl. 5), S143–S160.

*Hadaway, L. (1998b). Catheter connection. *Journal of Vascular Access Devices, 3*(3), 40.

*Hanrahan, K.S., Kleiber, C., & Fagan, C.L. (1994). Evaluation of saline for IV locks in children. *Pediatric Nursing, 20,* 549–552.

*Heilskov, J., Kleiber, C., Johnson, K., & Miller, J. (1998). A randomized trial of heparin and saline for maintaining intravenous locks in neonates. *Journal of the Society for Pediatric Nursing, 3,* 111–116.

*Heiney, S.P. (1991). Helping children through painful procedures. *American Journal of Nursing, 91,* 24.

*Heird, W.C. (1993). Parenteral support of the hospitalized child. In R.M. Suskind & L. Lewinter-Suskind (Eds.), *Textbook of pediatric nutrition* (2nd ed., pp. 225–238). New York: Raven Press.

*Hill, S.E., Heldman, L.S., Goo, E.D.H., et al. (1996). Fatal microvascular pulmonary emboli from precipitation of total nutrient admixture solution. *Journal of Parenteral and Enteral Nutrition, 20,* 81–87.

*Hodge, D. (1997). Intraosseous infusion. In F. Henretig, & C. King (Eds.), *Textbook of pediatric emergency procedures* (pp. 289–298). Baltimore: Williams & Wilkins.

*Holiday, M.A. & Segar, W.E. (1957). The maintenance need for water in parenteral fluid therapy. *Pediatrics, 14,* 698–704.

*Hutchinson, D.B. (1991). Pediatric IV therapy: Starting the line. *RN, 54*(12), 43–48.

*Intravenous Nurses Society. (1988). *Peripherally inserted central catheters* (Position Paper #8). Cambridge, MA: Author.

*Intravenous Nurses Society. (1998). Intravenous nursing standards of practice. *Journal of Intravenous Nursing, 23*(Suppl.).

*Intravenous Nurses Society. (2000). Revised intravenous nursing standards of practice (publication pending).

*Jackson, D. & Saunders, R. (Eds.). (1993). *Child health nursing.* Philadelphia: J.B. Lippincott.

*Jew, R. (Ed.). (1997–1999). *Pharmacy handbook and formulary, the Children's Hospital of Philadelphia.* Hudson, OH: Lexi-Comp, Inc.

*Jones, G.R. (1998). A practical guide to evaluation and treatment of infections in patients with central venous catheters. *Journal of Intravenous Nursing, 21(Suppl. 5),* 134–142.

*Kanter, R.K., Zimmerman, J.J., Straus, R.H., & Stoeckel, K. (1986). Pediatric emergency intravenous access: Evaluation of a protocol. *American Journal of Diseases of Children, 140,* 133.

*Kasprisin, C.A. (1985). Transfusion therapy for the pediatric patient. In R. Rutman & W. Miller (Eds.), *Transfusion therapy* (pp. 179–185). Rockville, MD: Aspen.

*Kaste, S.C. & Young, C.W. (1996). Safe use of power injectors with central and peripheral venous access devices for pediatric CT. *Pediatric Radiology, 26,* 469–501.

*Keller, S. (1995). Small gauge needles promote safe blood transfusions. *Oncology Nursing Forum, 22,* 718.

*Klaus, M.H. & Fanaroff, A. (1979). *Care of the high risk neonate* (2nd ed.). London: W.B. Saunders.

*Korth-Bradley, M. (1991). A pharmacokinetic primer for intravenous nurses. *Journal of Intravenous Nursing, 14,* 124.

*Kotter, R., (1996). Heparin vs. saline for intermittent intravenous device maintenance in neonates. *Neonatal Network, 15*(6), 43–47.

*Krueger-Paisely, M., Stamper, M., Brown, J., Brovan, N., & Ganong, L. (1997). The use of heparin and normal saline flushes in neonatal intravenous catheters. *Pediatric Nursing, 23,* 521–527.

*Kupensky, D.T. (1998). Applying current research to influence clinical practice: Utilization of midline catheters. *Journal of Intravenous Nursing, 21,* 271–274.

*Landers, S., Moise, A.A., Fraley, J.K., et al. (1991). Factors associated with umbilical catheter-related sepsis in neonates. *American Journal of Diseases of Children, 145,* 675–680.

*Landier, W.C., Barrell, M.L., & Styffe, D.J. (1987). How to administer blood components to children. *Maternal and Child Nursing, 12,* 178–184.

*Lavelle, J. & Costarino, A. (1997). Central venous access and central venous pressure monitoring. In F.M. Henretig & C. King (Eds.), *Textbook of pediatric emergency procedures* (pp. 251–278). Baltimore: Williams & Wilkins.

*LeDuc, K. (1997). Efficacy of normal saline solution versus heparin solution for maintaining patency of peripheral intravenous catheters in children. *Journal of Emergency Nursing, 23,* 306–309.

*Lesser, E., Chhabra, R., Brion, L.P., & Suresh, B.R. (1996). Use of midline catheters in low birth weight infants. *Journal of Perinatology, 16,* 205–207.

*Lewis, L. & Stephan, M. (1997). Local and regional anesthesia. In F.M. Henretig & C. King (Eds.), *Textbook of pediatric emergency procedures* (pp. 465–475). Baltimore: Williams & Wilkins.

*Lipton, J.D., & Schafermeyer, R.W. (1997). Umbilical vessel catheterization. In F.M. Henretig & C. King (Eds.), *Textbook of pediatric emergency procedures* (pp. 515–522). Baltimore: Williams & Wilkins.

*Loeff, D.S., et al. (1982). Insertion of a small central venous catheter in neonates and young infants. *Journal of Pediatric Surgery, 17,* 941–948.

*Luban, N. & Keating, L. (Eds.) (1983). *Hemotherapy of the infant and premature.* Arlington, VA: American Association of Blood Banks.

*Luten, R.C. (1997). Emergent drug dosing and equipment selection. In F.M. Henretig & C. King (Eds.), *Textbook of pediatric emergency procedures* (pp. 39–42). Baltimore: Williams & Wilkins.

*Manley, L., Haley, K., & Dick, M. (1988). Intraosseous infusion: Rapid vascular access for critically ill or inured infants and children. *Journal of Emergency Nursing, 14,* 63.

*Marcoux, C., Fisher, S., & Wong, D. (1990). Central venous access devices in children. *Pediatric Nursing, 16,* 123–133.

*Markels, S. (1990). Impact on patient care: 2652 PIC catheter days in the alternative setting. *Journal of Intravenous Nursing, 13,* 347.

*Mattson, D. & O'Connor, M. (1986). Transilluminator assistance in neonatal venipuncture. *Neonatal Network, 4,* 43.

*Matyskiela-Frey, A.M. (1985). Pediatric dosage calculations. *Journal of the National Intravenous Therapy Association, 8,* 373–379.

*McGee, W.T. & Mallory, D.L. (1988). Cannulation of the internal and external jugular veins. *Problems in Critical Care, 2,* 217–241.

*McMullen, A., Fioravanti, I.D., Pollack, V., Rideout, K., & Sciera, M. (1993). Heparinized saline or normal saline as a flush solution in intermittent intravenous lines in infants and children. *Maternal Child Nursing, 18,* 78–85.

*Meyenfeldt, M., Stapert, J., Deong, P., et al. (1980). TPN catheter sepsis: Lack of effect of subcutaneous tunneling of PVC catheters on sepsis rate. *Journal of Parenteral and Enteral Nutrition, 4,* 514–517.

*Meyer, H.M. (1982, May). *Letter to hospital pharmacists.* Rockville, MD: U.S. Department of Health and Human Services, Federal Drug Administration.

*Miccolo, M.A. (1990). Intraosseous infusion. *Critical Care Nurse, 10,* 35–47.

*Milliam, D. (1995). The use of anesthesia in IV therapy. *Journal of Vascular Access Devices, 1,* 22–29.

*Mofenseon, H.C. (1988). Guidelines for intraosseous infusions (Letter). *Journal of Emergency Medicine, 6,* 145–146

*Nathan, D.G. & Orkin, S.H. (Eds.). (1998). *Nathan and Oski's hematology of infancy and childhood* (5th Ed.). Philadelphia: W.B. Saunders.

*Nelson, D.B. & Garland, J.S. (1987). The natural history of catheter associated phlebitis in children. *American Journal of Diseases of Children, 141,* 1090–1092.

*Oellrich, R.G., Murphy, M.R., Goldberg, L.A., & Aggarwal, R. (1991). The percutaneous central venous catheter for small or ill infants. *Maternal Child Nursing, 16,* 92–96.

*Pearson, M.L. (1996). Guideline for prevention of intravascular-device-related infections. *Infection Control and Hospital Epidemiology, 17,* 438–473.

*Pettit, J. & Hughes, K. (1999). Neonatal intravenous therapy practices. *Journal of Vascular Access Devices, 4*(1), 7–15.

*Piercy, S. (1981). Children on long term IV therapy. *Nursing 81,* 11, 66–69.

*Poole, M.A., Ross, M.N., Haase, G.M., & Odom, L.F. (1991). Right atrial catheters in pediatric oncology: A patient/parent questionnaire study. *American Journal of Pediatric Hematology/Oncology, 13,* 152–155.

*Reiser, D.J. (1999). Intensive care nursery eliminates solusets. *Infusion Management Update, 8*(2), 6–8.

*Ringel, M. (1995a). For pediatric infusion, there's no place like home. *Infusion, 2*(1), 10–16.

*Ringel, M. (1995b). Providing pediatric infusion therapies: Putting the pieces together. *Infusion, 2*(2), 20–25.

*Rivitz, S.M. & Drucker, E.A. (1997). Power injection of peripherally inserted central catheters. *Journal of Intravenous Radiology, 8*(5), 853–863.

*Robieux, I., Kumar, R., Radhakrishnan, S., & Koren, G. (1991). Assessing pain and analgesia with a lidocaine-prilocaine emulsion in infants and toddlers during venipuncture. *Journal of Pediatrics, 118,* 971–973.

*Rosetti, V.A., Thompson, B.M., Miller, J., et al. (1985). An alternative route of pediatric intravascular access. *Annals of Emergency Medicine, 14,* 885–888.

*Roth, D. (1997). A comprehensive review of blood transfusion therapy: Part 2. *Journal of Vascular Access Devices, 2*(4), 13–21.

*Roulston-Betts, K. (1998). Pediatric growth hormone deficiency. *Journal of Intravenous Nursing, 21,* 143–147.

*Ruble, K., Long, C., & Connor, K. (1994) Pharmacologic treatment of catheter-related thrombus in pediatrics. *Pediatric Nursing, 20,* 553–557.

*Ruess, L., Bulas, D.I., Rivera, O., & Markle, B.M. (1997). In-line pressures generated in small-bore central venous catheters during power injection of CT contrast media. *Radiology, 203,* 625–629.

*Sater, K.J. (1998). Treatment of sepsis in the neonate. *Journal of Intravenous Therapy, 21,* 275–281.

*Schuman, A. (1990). Homeward bound: The explosion of pediatric home care. *Contemporary Pediatrics, 7,* 26–29, 32–47, 50–54.

*Shaw, J.C. (1973). Parenteral nutrition in the management of sick low birthweight neonates. *Pediatric Clinics of North America, 20,* 333–354.

*Sherman, M.P., et al. (1982). Percutaneous and surgical placement of fine silicone elastomer central catheters in high-risk newborns. *Journal of Pediatric Surgery, 7,* 75–78.

*Sigda, M., Speights, J.T., & Thigpen, J. (1992). Pericardial tamponade due to umbilical venous catheterization. *Neonatal Network, 11*(2), 7–9.

*Simmons, C., et al. (1994). Intraosseous extravasation complication reports. *Annals of Emergency Medicine, 23,* 363–366.

*Stanford, A. (1990). Umbilical artery and venous catheters. In J.L. Blumer (Ed.), *A practical guide to pediatric intensive care* (pp. 846–849). Philadelphia: Mosby–Year Book.

*Stenzel, J.P., Green, T.P., Fuhrman, B.P., et al. (1989). Percutaneous femoral venous catheterizations: A prospective study of complications. *Journal of Pediatrics, 114,* 411–415.

*Stiehm, E.R. (1991). New pediatric indications for IVIG. *Contemporary Pediatrics, 8,* 29–52.

*Testerman, E. (1989). Current trends in pediatric total parenteral nutrition. *Journal of Intravenous Nursing, 12,* 152–162.

*Thiagarajan, R., Ramamoorthy, C., Gettemann, T., & Bratton, S. (1997). Survey of the use of peripherally inserted central venous catheters in children. *Pediatrics, 99,* 1–8.

*Thompson, V. (1994). An IV therapy teaching tool for children. *Pediatric Nursing, 20,* 351–355.

*Tocantins, L.M. & O'Neil, J.F. (1945). Complications of intraosseous therapy. *Annals of Surgery, 122,* 266–277.

*Trotter, C.W. (1996). Percutaneous central venous catheter related sepsis in the neonate: An analysis of the literature from 1990 to 1994. *Neonatal Network, 15*(3), 15–28.

*Tully, J.L., Friedland, G.H., Baldini, L.M., & Goldman, D.A. (1981). Complications of intravenous therapy with steel needles and Teflon catheters: A comparative study. *American Journal of Medicine, 70,* 702–706.

*Turkel, H. (1983). Intraosseous infusions (Letter to the editor). *American Journal of Diseases of Children, 137,* 706.

*Valk, W.J., Liem, K.D., & Geven, W.B. (1995). Seldinger technique as an alternative approach for percutaneous insertion of hydrophilic polyurethane central venous catheters in newborns. *JPEN Journal of Parenteral and Enteral Nutrition, 19*(2), 151–155.

*Vallino, L. (1998). IV house: Pediatric nurses contribute to refinement of IV protector. *Journal of Pediatric Nursing, 13,* 196–198.

*Van Cleve, L., Johnson, L., & Pothier, P. (1996). Pain responses of hospitalized infants and children to venipuncture and intravenous cannulation. *Journal of Pediatric Nursing, 11,* 161–168.

*Viall, C.D. (1990). Your complete guide to central venous catheters. *Nursing 90,* 20, 34.

*Weeks-Lozano, H. (1991). Clinical evaluation of Per-Q-Cath for both pediatric and adult home infusion therapy. *Journal of Intravenous Nursing, 14,* 246–252.

*Whaley, L.F. & Wong, D.I. (Eds.). (1993). *Nursing care of infants and children.* St. Louis: Mosby.

*Wheeler, C. & Frey, A.M. (1995). Intravenous therapy in children. In J. Terry, L. Baranowski, R.A. Lonsway, & C. Hedrick (Eds.), *Intravenous therapy: Clinical principles and practice* (pp. 467–494). Philadelphia: W.B. Saunders.

*Wickham, R.S. (1990). Advances in venous access devices and nursing management strategies. *Nursing Clinics of North America, 25,* 345–364.

*Wiener, E.S. & Albanese, C.T. (1998). Venous access in pediatric patients. *Journal of Intravenous Nursing, 21*(Suppl. 5), S122–S133.

*Williams, J., et al. (1988). Silastic catheters for antibiotics in cystic fibrosis. *Archives of Diseases in Children, 63,* 654–655.

Willmore, D.W. & Dudrick, S.J. (1968). Growth and development of an infant receiving all nutrients exclusively by vein. *Journal of the American Medical Association, 203,* 860.

*Winci, R.J. (1997). Venous cutdown catheterization. In F.M. Henretig & C. King (Eds.), *Textbook of pediatric emergency procedures* (pp. 279–287). Baltimore: Williams & Wilkins.

*Wolfram, W., Turner, E.D., & Philput, C. (1997). Effects of parental presence during young children's venipuncture. *Pediatric Emergency Care, 13,* 325–328.

Wong, D.L. (Ed.). (1995). *Nursing care of infants and children* (5th ed., pp. 107, 1136, 1219, 1233–1281). St. Louis: Mosby.

*Zanni, R.L., Shutack, J.G., Schuler, P.M., et al. (1985). Peripherally inserted central venous catheters for treatment of cystic fibrosis. *Pediatric Pulmonology, 1,* 328–332.

Review Questions

Note: Questions below may have more than one right answer.

1. When starting an IV in a toddler, the best approach would be:

   A. "Let's go and start your IV now."

   B. "You were bad, so we're going to give you a needle."

   C. "Where do you want your IV?"

   D. "Can we start your IV now?"

2. An IV in the frontal vein might be the site of choice in which of the following children?

   A. 2-month-old with hydrocephalus

   B. Neonate with sepsis on 3 days of antibiotic therapy

   C. 20-month-old with leukemia

   D. 16-month-old in respiratory arrest

3. What size peripheral IV catheters are recommended for use in children?

   A. 18 and 20 gauge

   B. 14 and 16 gauge

   C. 5 and 7 French

   D. 24 and 22 gauge

4. The ideal location to place an IV in a child is:

   A. At the bedside

   B. In the treatment room

   C. On the mother's lap

   D. In the home of the patient

5. After two attempts at IV access during resuscitative efforts, the following site should be used:

   A. Intracardiac

   B. Intra-arterial

   C. Intrathecal

   D. Intraosseous

6. A vascular access site unique to the newborn population is:

   A. The umbilicus

   B. The anterior fontanel

   C. The subclavian area

   D. The antecubital fossa

7. What type of vascular access device would you recommend to an adolescent with cystic fibrosis, who receives intermittent IV antibiotics several times annually?

   A. Broviac catheter

   B. Subclavian catheter

   C. Implanted port

   D. Hickman catheter

8. The best method for calculating maintenance fluid requirements for a child is:

   A. Caloric method

   B. Weight method

   C. Age method

   D. Meters-squared method

9. In parenteral nutrition solutions, which component provides energy for body tissue function?

   A. Amino acids

   B. Selenium

   C. Carbohydrates

   D. Fatty acids

10. The purpose of neonatal exchange transfusion is to:

    A. Elevate neutrophil count

    B. Prevent congestive heart failure

    C. Change blood type

    D. Lower bilirubin level

Intravenous Therapy in an

Older Adult Patient

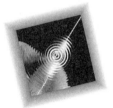

K E Y   T E R M S

Cellular
Homeostasis
Older Adult
Organic
Systemic

■ DEMOGRAPHICS: AN AGING POPULATION

Advances in medical science and technology have resulted in an increased life span; older patients today represent 13% of the U.S. population. According to the U.S. Census Bureau (1998), 61,000 centenarians lived in this country in 1998, making this group the fastest-growing segment of the population. The Census Bureau predicts 834,000 centenarians in the year 2050. The burgeoning elderly population will continue to place great strains on the health care resources of the United States, which will need to expand its services to those older adults who have chronic diseases. In the 1990s, the number of nursing homes and nursing home beds has risen by approximately 20%. Acute care facilities are licensing their excess beds as transitional care units to retain patients under a separate reimbursement program (Hoechst, 1999). Nursing professionals now require an increased awareness of the changes associated with the aging process and the special needs of this patient population (American Association of Retired Persons, 1998). These older citizens have age-related health problems requiring medications and treatment, many of which are given IV.

This chapter addresses the important considerations in initiating, delivering, and maintaining IV therapy in the older adult patient. The term **older adult** describes a broad category that ranges from 50 to 80 years of age because many physiologic changes associated with the older adult begin in the sixth decade of life. Variations do exist among individuals. Principles of fluid volume assessment, patient teaching, and available resources are provided.

■ THE OLDER PATIENT AS A HEALTH CARE CONSUMER

The older adult patient may require administration of complex IV therapies to treat a multitude of clinical conditions that may occur simultaneously. The older patient may be more acutely ill for a longer time than a younger patient, and he or she may need additional resources to regain strength and health status. As a health care consumer, the older adult patient has special needs associated with the aging process that challenge the health care system and health care providers.

For example, an 82-year-old patient with chronic pulmonary disease and congestive heart failure is in need of complicated inpatient treatment. Her children live out of state and must travel frequently to her Florida home to deal with one medical crisis after another. During each hospitalization, a phalanx of case managers besieges the patient and confers about her care. These professionals represent the hospital, the insurer, and the skilled care facility where she has been residing. A new level of case manager may be added to the picture: one representing the patient and her long-distance family. Professionals with an understanding of the economics and medical aspects of providing care for the elderly are entering this field (Greene, 1999). The National Association of Professional Geriatric Care Managers offers a directory of advocates.

Although to the health care system, the patient may be a product, such as a covered life, a patient day, or an encounter, patients see it differently. They view health care as the product and themselves as the consumer (Haugh, 1999). Estimates are that caregivers spend an average 50% more time on health care Web sites than do other types of Internet health users (Haugh, 1999). Caregivers (for the elderly) largely comprise women in their 40s with children (Haugh, 1999). Caregiver Zone.com is a site specifically aimed at seniors (Katzman, 2000).

■ PHYSIOLOGY OF AGING

Aging occurs at the cellular, organic, and systemic levels. **Cellular** refers to the changes in cell structure that affect the cells' ability to respond to illness. **Organic** changes are those that affect specific organs, such as the liver's ability to detoxify medications or the kidney's propensity to slow down with aging. Major **systemic** changes affecting IV therapy practice and delivery to the older patient include those related to homeostasis, the immune and cardiovascular systems, and skin and connective tissue. Implications related to nursing care are featured in Table 22–1.

Homeostasis

Homeostasis is the ability of the body to maintain balance of volume and composition of body fluids within normal ranges (see Chap. 7). The kidneys, heart and blood ves-

T A B L E 2 2 – 1
NORMAL CHANGES ASSOCIATED WITH THE AGING PROCESS

Physiologic Component	Normal Aging Changes	Nursing Implications
Total body water	Reduction of 6%; decreased ratio of intracellular to extracellular fluid	Patient is at increased risk of fluid volume deficit.
Renal function	Reduced body weight; loss of 30%–50% of glomeruli by age 70; thickening of glomerular and tubular basement membranes; decreased ability to concentrate urine	Patient has greater difficulty in eliminating heavy solute loads (eg, drugs, glucose, proteins); slower conservation of fluids occurs in response to fluid restriction; drug excretion slows.
Regulatory functions	Decrease in secretion of aldosterone from adrenal cortex, response of distal tubule to vasopression, ability to form and excrete ammonia, glucose tolerance, and sensation of thirst	Ability to conserve sodium and excrete potassium is diminished. Ability to correct an acid–base imbalance is reduced. Patient is at increased risk for hyperglycemia and osmotic diuresis. Ability to recognize fluid volume deficit is decreased.
Skin changes	Decreased elasticity; atrophy of sweat glands; diminished capillary bed	Skin turgor is a poor indicator of hydration; skin is less effective in cooling body temperature.
Cardiovascular function	Decrease in cardiac output, stroke volume, renal plasma flow, elasticity of arteries; increase in vascular rigidity	Diminished ability to manage hypotension associated with shock; increased incidence of peripheral edema; risk of orthostatic hypotension, dizziness, falls
Respiratory function	Decrease in compliance of chest wall, elasticity of lung tissue, numer of alveoli, strength of expiratory muscles, normal partial pressure of oxygen	Increased difficulty in regulating pH during episode of illness, surgery, burns, trauma
Gastrointestinal function	Decrease in volume of saliva and gastric juice, calcium absorption	Dry mouth; increased risk for hyponatremia and hypokalemia during vomiting and gastric suction

(Adapted from Metheny, N. M. [2000]. *Fluid and electrolyte balance* [4th ed., p. 352] Philadelphia: Lippincott Williams & Wilkins.)

sels, lungs, skin, adrenal glands, hypothalamus, pituitary gland, parathyroid gland, and gastrointestinal tract are the regulatory organs associated with maintaining the body's homeostasis. Recall from Chapter 7 that the kidneys are a primary force in homeostasis because they work to adjust the amount of water and electrolytes that exit the body in an amount equal to the quantity of solution entering the body, either through IV or oral feedings. Circulating blood reaches the kidneys in sufficient volume to regulate water and electrolytes, and the pumping action of the heart provides circulation through the kidneys, which produce and excrete urine. The lungs are involved in homeostasis through ventilation. Antidiuretic hormone (ADH), which causes fluid retention, is manufactured in the hypothalamus and stored in the pituitary gland. ADH also is involved in controlling blood volume. When blood volume is increased, ADH secretion is decreased and water is excreted through the kidneys. Parathyroid hormone affects calcium and phosphate concentrations and influences reabsorption of calcium, a key factor in maintaining fluid and electrolyte monitoring and replacement. The gastrointestinal tract also plays a major role in homeostasis by absorption and reabsorption through the small intestine, or "great absorbing organ." For the body to maintain homeostasis, all these organs must work in synchronicity.

Normal homeostatic mechanisms in aging become less efficient in the face of external trauma, surgical intervention, disease process, or infection. The older patient is vulnerable to complications associated with routine IV therapy.

The Immune System

In aging, the normal immune system becomes hyporesponsive to foreign antigens and hyper-responsive to self (Metheny, 2000). These changes may contribute to decreased resistance to infection, increased autoimmunity, and development of other immune disorders. The immunocompromised patient is at increased risk for IV-associated infection.

The Cardiovascular System

Cardiovascular changes are profound, contributing to a slower response to the stress of blood loss, fluid depletion, shock, and acid–base imbalances. Changes in renal and cardiac status have the potential to place the patient at great risk for development of infusion-related complications (see Table 22–1).

Skin and Connective Tissue

The skin, the body's first defense against disease, changes in texture, depth, and integrity as the person ages. After age 60 years, epidermal cell replacement decreases, resulting in a marked thinning of the epidermis and an increased fragility of the skin's surface. The result is dry, transparent, paper-thin tissue that tears easily and heals slowly. Changes in the dermis create a loose, wrinkling effect. The skin becomes pale, and nerve endings are less sensitive. The patient is at risk for thermal injuries. Subcutaneous fat cells decrease, resulting in changes to the superficial fascia, including decreased production of sebum and sweat (Metheny, 2000). Loss of subcutaneous tissue and resultant thinning of the skin present a venous access challenge. Purpura and ecchymoses may appear because of dermal fragility; minor trauma may inflict bruising (Hankins, 1995).

Fluid Balance

Physiologic changes of aging affect the older adult's fluid balance. Fluid reserves are limited, and total body water is reduced by 6%, creating a potential for fluid volume deficit. Gastrointestinal changes such as decreased volume of saliva and gastric juice and decreased calcium absorption cause the mouth to be drier and increase potential for sodium and potassium deficit during episodes of vomiting and gastric suction. Assessment guidelines may be found in Box 22–1.

BOX 22–1 **Fluid Volume Assessment Parameters in the Older Adult Patient**

Skin turgor of forehead/sternum
Temperature <98.6°F
Decreased rate/filling of hand veins
Intake and output
Daily weight
Tongue—center should remain moist
Blood pressure—possibility of orthostatic hypotension
Swallowing function
Functional assessment of patient's ability to obtain fluids

(Adapted from Metheny, N.M. [2000]. *Fluid and electrolyte balance* [4th ed., p. 352]. Philadelphia: Lippincott Williams & Wilkins.)

The usual assessment measures to determine fluid balance should be adjusted when providing care to the older adult. For example, testing skin turgor on the forearm is no longer a valid measure because skin loses elasticity with age. Skin turgor is best assessed in the older patient by tenting the tissue on the forehead or over the sternum. Alterations in skin elasticity are less marked in those sites (Metheny, 2000).

Senses

Changes in sensation affect the patient's response to treatment; changes in vision, hearing, and tactile sensation may alter communication. After age 50 years, subtle changes in the hearing process result in difficulty in differentiating sounds. For example, the older patient often cannot hear someone speaking within an otherwise normal range because of the outside influence of loud music or traffic (Metheny, 2000; S. Weinstein, personal communication, March, 1998). Older patients may need assistive devices, such as hearing aids, eyeglasses, and visual aids, to learn the skills associated with infusion therapy. Because of decreased tactile sensation, infiltration might go unnoticed, contributing to the potential for development of tissue necrosis, infection, or compartment syndrome (Metheny, 2000) (see Chapter 9).

Vascular System

Chronic disease, such as asthma, chronic obstructive pulmonary disease, hypertension, and the changes associated with atherosclerosis and arteriosclerosis affect the blood vessels in the older patient. Vessels are fragile, with small, thin-walled surface capillaries easily observed across the extremities and chest of the older patient. Vascular fragility is a potential problem for IV access; a tourniquet sometimes is not used to decrease the potential for bruising.

Psychological Changes

A confused patient or one experiencing the ill effects of senile dementia will respond differently to treatment. Teaching may become complicated because the patient has difficulty in differentiating between recent and remote memory. For example, the patient forgets what he or she learned the previous day, but remembers all the details of early childhood.

■ ACCESS AND EQUIPMENT

When providing IV therapy to older adult patients, careful consideration should be given to the type of treatment ordered, the duration of therapy, and availability of IV access. A biocompatible catheter material is preferred, including products manufactured from silicone, elastomeric hydrogels, and others (see Chap. 11); these products are nonthrombogenic. The smallest gauge possible for the therapy being delivered should be used. Consideration must be given to the type of catheter–tubing connection used; some products are more irritating to frail skin and usually must be padded to prevent injury to the skin surface and underlying tissue.

When a central venous access device is needed for long-term therapy, the type of device should be determined carefully. Consideration should be given to the patient's living circumstances, availability of family or other support systems, and ability to manipulate the equipment involved and to maintain a secure, intact dressing (Intravenous Nurses Society [INS], 1998, 2000).

Flow Control

Electronic flow control devices (electronic infusion devices) should be used liberally in the older adult to prevent overhydration and resultant fluid imbalances. Pump infusion pressures should be monitored carefully. As with all patients, the device used should be biomedically safe and meet and exceed standards developed by ECRI, formerly the Emergency Care Research Institute, and internal safety committees (see Chap. 11). ECRI publishes a diversity of information helpful in the selection of products for all patient populations, but especially those significant for older adults.

An electronic flow control device should be an accessory to quality patient care and not a substitute for ongoing monitoring. The nurse should refer to technical information provided by the manufacturer of equipment and institutional guidelines for use. The alarm on a pump with a fixed pressure of 4 psi activates when the peripheral venous pressure reaches 200 mm Hg (1 psi = 50 mm Hg). This setting can seriously harm the patient when infiltration occurs; the alarm will sound only after the damage has been noted. An infiltrated site exerts a mean pressure gradient at 100 mm Hg or 2 psi. Pumps that continue to infuse or that do not have a free-flow alarm system pose potential risks to the older patient (ECRI, 1999).

Site Selection

Principles of site selection applied to the younger patient (see Chap. 21) also may be used to determine appropriate venous access in the older patient. Assessment of available peripheral venous access is necessary. Avoiding bruised, fragile veins and conserving veins for future use are major considerations. The nurse should secure adequate lighting and ensure patient comfort.

Technique

Although a tourniquet may be used, it also may not be necessary. Excessive distention of the veins may contribute to bruising and subsequent tearing of the venous wall and hematoma. The veins should be palpated carefully to determine state of health and condition. Corded veins may indicate thickening, occluded vein walls, and valve blockage. Threading a catheter into such vessels may be difficult; venous stasis and dependent edema may result (Metheny, 2000).

Table 22–2 lists the special techniques required in an older adult. Skin tension is determined by assessing the direction or axis of the vessel. Traction is ensured by placing the thumb directly along the vein axis 2 to 3 inches below the intended venipuncture site. The palm and fingers of the hand used to apply traction hold and stabilize the patient's extremity. Traction is maintained throughout the procedure (INS, 1998, 2000).

T A B L E   2 2 – 2
SPECIAL TECHNIQUES IN THE OLDER ADULT PATIENT

Intervention	Rationale
Avoid tourniquet in patients with fragile veins or who are taking anticoagulants or steroids.	Tourniquet may not be needed; use of tourniquet may contribute to hematoma formation.
If tourniquet is used, release it quickly.	Quick release decreases backflow of blood.
Multiple-tourniquet technique may be an option to facilitate venous distention.	
Grasp the patient's mid-upper arm and stroke the arm downward toward the hand. Place a tourniquet on the extremity.	Stroking promotes venous filling.
Wait 1–2 min and then place a second tourniquet below the antecubital fossa and continue to stroke the lower forearm.	Placement of the second tourniquet stimulates venous pressure and forces venous distention to small veins that otherwise would not be visible.
A third tourniquet may be placed after an additional 1–2 min at a point just above the wrist.	The third tourniquet promotes additional venous distention, particularly in the very small veins of the digits and lower wrist. Although not *ideal* for infusion purposes, the veins in this area will fill due to venous pressure and provide adequate hemodilution for infusion purposes.
Release the first tourniquet and evaluate inner wrist, thumb, knuckle, and fingers for distention.	
In edematous patient, use anatomic landmarks.	Facilitates location of appropriate veins
Gently tap the vein to distend; do not slap.	Avoids hematoma formation and bruising
Use transillumination.	Assists in visualizing veins
Insert catheter with steady, firm motion	Prevents bruising associated with difficult venipuncture
Consider preflushing catheter in patients with spidery, capillary-type veins.	Avoids trauma associated with sudden flushing
Use a one-handed approach.	Facilitates proper skin tension

The directional line of the vessel is determined. If the vein is very small, venous distention may be inadequate, and imaging techniques may be used. Imaging uses magnetic light to visualize hard-to-find veins.

A small-gauge IV catheter should be selected and positioned with the bevel up. The catheter should be aligned parallel to the vein track and brought close to the skin directly above the insertion site. A lower angle decreases vein trauma on insertion (INS, 1998, 2000; Metheny, 2000).

The direct or indirect technique may be applied (see Chap. 12); however, for patients with small, fragile veins, the clinician may find the two-step technique more beneficial. If the veins are extremely fragile and if a tourniquet has been used, it may be helpful to release the tourniquet as soon as blood return is evident. Doing so prevents damage from high-pressure backflow of blood from the catheter insertion point. The "hooded" technique also may help reduce vein damage. In this approach, the clinician advances the catheter forward over the bevel tip into the vein. This action retracts the stylet tip inside the catheter. Then, the clinician threads the catheter into the vein by grasping the hub of the catheter and advancing the catheter and stylet as a unit up the vein. This procedure minimizes the possibility of perforating the vein during threading. The clinician must maintain stabilization and skin tension throughout the process.

Maintenance and Monitoring

Securing, dressing, and stabilizing the IV catheter are unique challenges when providing infusion care to the elderly patient. Although the catheter should be secure, use of excessive tape is discouraged because of the fragility of the patient's skin. Adaptations to taping technique should be used as needed. The use of additional protection such as a skin polymer solution should be considered. The polymer solution is best applied in a concentric circle from the center to the periphery and allowed to air dry before the dressing is applied (INS, 1998, 2000). The elderly patient may be confused owing to physiologic reasons or medications, and the nurse should make every effort to ensure safety with the infusion device. Patient education is essential to ensure compliance with the plan of care. See Box 22–2 for principles of patient teaching.

BOX 22–2 Principles of Patient Teaching for the Older Adult Patient Receiving Intravenous Therapy

- Speak slowly, clearly, and directly to the patient.
- Hearing impairment and sensitivity to outside sounds require patience.
- Address the patient by his or her proper name.
- Explain steps in logical order.
- Take steps to decrease anxiety.
- Use familiar terminology.

Care should be taken when securement devices or restraints are used. The IV tubing should be long enough to provide adequate range of motion, but not so long as to dangle on the floor or get caught on the bedside or IV pole. A Luer-locking device provides added protection. Surgical stretch mesh gauze also may be used to cover the IV site, providing stability and protecting the catheter from snagging bed garments. Roll-type gauze should be avoided, consistent with institutional guidelines and established practice standards (INS, 1998, 2000).

The IV site should be evaluated at regularly established intervals and as needed to ensure patency. Site rotation is recommended every 72 hours; however, deviations may be acceptable (see Chaps. 4, 9, and 12). If a routine site change is not performed because of limited access or the patient's clinical condition, a full description of the site, dressing change, and reasons for not completing the site rotation should be documented in the clinical records.

References and Selected Readings

Asterisks indicate references cited in text.

*American Association of Retired Persons. (1998). *A profile of older Americans*. Washington, DC: U.S. Department of Health and Human Services.

Bulger, R. (1999). What will health care look like in the future? In E. Sullivan (Ed.), *Creating nursing's future* (pp. 16–17). St. Louis: Mosby.

Chyna, J.T. (2000). The consumer revolution: An age of changing expectations. *Healthcare Executive, 15*(1), 7–9.

*ECRI. (1999). *Continuing care risk management system* (pp. 28–30). Plymouth Meeting, PA: Author, Health Devices.

Elsner, R.J., Quinn, M.E., & Fanning, S.D. (1999). Ethical and policy considerations for centenarians—the oldest old. *Image: Journal of Nursing Scholarship, 31*, 263–267.

Gordon, S. (1997). *Life support: Three nurses on the front lines*. Boston: Little, Brown.

*Greene, J. (1999). Case management: Consumer consultant. *Hospitals and Health Networks, 73*(12), 24–25.

*Hankins, J., in Intravenous Nurses Society. (1995). *Core curriculum for intravenous nursing*. (pp. 165–166). Philadelphia: J.B. Lippincott.

*Haugh, R. (1999; December). The new consumer. *Hospitals and Health Networks*, 30–32.

*Hoechst, M.R. (1999). *Managed care digest series*[TM] *nursing home industry summary/institutional digest* (pp. 24–27).

*Intravenous Nurses Society. (1998). *Revised standards of practice*. Philadelphia: Lippincott Williams & Wilkins.

*Intravenous Nurses Society. (2000). *Standards of practice draft*. Philadelphia: Lippincott Williams & Wilkins. In press.

*Katzman, C.N. (2000). Catching the eldercare wave. *Healthcare Business, 3*(4), 22.

*Metheny, N.M. (2000). *Fluid and electrolyte balance* (4th ed.). Philadelphia: Lippincott Williams & Wilkins.

Sansivero, G.E. (1998). Venous anatomy and physiology. *Journal of Intravenous Nursing 21*(Suppl. 5), S207–S209.

*U.S. Census Bureau. (1998). Resident population of the United States: Middle series projections, by age and sex. [On-line]. Available: http://www.census.gov/population/estimates/nation/nas/npas.3550.txt

Review Questions

Note: Questions below may have more than one right answer.

1. Principles of education in the older adult patient include which of the following?

   A. Speak slowly, clearly, and directly.

   B. Address the patient by name.

   C. Use familiar terminology.

   D. All of the above

2. Which of the following skin layers is associated with development of dry, transparent surfaces?

   A. Deep fascia

   B. Dermis

   C. Epidermis

   D. Superficial fascia

3. Skin turgor in the adult patient should be measured at what location?

A. Forehead

B. Sternum

C. Abdomen

D. Inner aspect of forearm

4. All the following are true when determining skin tension *except:*

A. Assess direction of vessel

B. Assess axis of vessel

C. Eliminate traction

D. Determine direction line of vessel

5. The alarm on an electronic infusion device with fixed pressure of 4 psi activates when peripheral venous pressure reaches how many mm Hg?

A. 100

B. 150

C. 200

D. 250

6. The name of the technique used to reduce vein damage is known as:

A. Retraction

B. Hooded

C. Threaded

D. Advanced

7. Total body water in the older patient is reduced by what percentage?

A. 2%

B. 5%

C. 6%

D. 8%

8. Respiratory function in the adult patient is associated with which of the following?

A. Decreased elasticity of lung tissue

B. Increased number of alveoli

C. Decreased compliance of chest wall

D. All of the above

9. Which of the following statements is true concerning skin turgor in the adult patient?

A. It is a poor indicator of hydration.

B. It is a good indicator of hydration.

C. It diminishes ability to conserve sodium.

D. It is more effective at cooling body temperature.

10. Communication skills in the elderly patient may be compromised by changes in which of the following?

A. Vision

B. Hearing

C. Tactile sensation

D. All of the above

Intravenous Therapy in

Alternate Clinical Settings:

Cost Factors and

Treatment Modalities

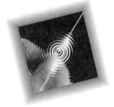

K E Y   T E R M S

Ambulatory Infusion Centers   Long-term Care
Home Care   Medicare
Hospice   Subacute Care
ICD9 Code

■ THE CHANGING HEALTH CARE ENVIRONMENT

In today's complex health care industry, hospitals have strong financial incentives to discharge patients as soon as possible. Hospitals and other health care providers face an increasingly complex dilemma: how to provide the highest quality care at the lowest price. Because of advances in medical science and technology and the influence of managed care insurance contracts, patients discharged from hospitals now can receive complex, high-level services, once available only in hospitals, in alternate care settings. The patient populations who receive treatment outside the hospital range from critically ill newborns to chronically ill older adults. The nurse needs an array of clinical and critical thinking skills to care for these patients, often while working within an autonomous practice setting.

Cost-cutting measures have enhanced the growth of new ways to provide IV therapy services. The growth of home infusion therapy and alternate clinical settings has created countless opportunities for IV nurses nationwide. Infusion nurse specialists must assess the level of skills and services currently being provided and determine venues where they can best use their skills, including, but not limited to settings such as:

- Hospitals
- Physicians' offices
- Home care
- Long-term care facilities
- Subacute settings
- Teaching for other professionals
- Ambulatory infusion centers
- Insertion of peripherally inserted central catheters (PICCs) and midline catheters
- Hospice

This chapter examines alternate settings for the delivery of IV therapy. It discusses the influence of managed care and cost-containment efforts. It thoroughly explores home care infusion therapy, along with the parameters mandated by Medicare, patient selection, the role of various health care team members, and typical IV therapies conducted in the home. It also explores other sites for IV care delivery, including hospice, subacute care, ambulatory infusion centers, and long-term care.

■ INFLUENCE OF MANAGED CARE

Managed care is a system of controls to manage access, costs, and quality of health care services. The controls may include any or all of the following:

- Preferred provider contracts
- Prior approval/authorization
- Patient education/incentives
- Utilization review/quality assurance

Two other controls used in managed care include case management and capitation. Case management is a program to manage high-cost health care cases by exploring alternative care options to achieve the same patient outcomes while better controlling costs. Case management requires the insurance company and the provider of services (eg, home care) to discuss the necessary IV therapy orders for the patient before the initiation of services. Usually, the parties determine and agree on a number of nurse visits for the IV therapy. Periodic updates and communication continue throughout the duration of the therapy. Patients and caregivers are encouraged to learn self-care with limited nursing monitoring, which results in decreased nursing visits and costs.

Capitation is a system of prepayment for health care in which a provider receives a flat monthly fee for agreeing to provide specified services to members of health maintenance organizations (HMOs) assigned to the provider for a contracted time (usually a year). Unlike traditional fee-for-service (FFS) systems, capitated systems pay providers, either individually or collectively, the same amount per member each month, in advance, regardless of how many times the members use their services. Usually, risk sharing is involved, meaning that the HMO and contracted provider share the financial risks and rewards to provide cost-effective care.

Under the auspices of the "managed care umbrella":

- Payers are changing.
- New delivery systems are designed around risk sharing.
- Payers/providers are competing for managed care savings (profits).
- Competition is increasing.
- Risk is shifting (in both directions).
- Attitudes of providers, payers, and employers are changing.

Under the old system, providers were paid on a fee-for-service basis; they are now paid discounted fee-for-service or by capitation. Under the old system, the patient base was the local community; now it is covered members/patients. Under the old system, the philosophy of care was to "treat the disease and restore wellness"; now it is to maintain health. When providers are reimbursed under bundling or capitated contracts, the incentive is to keep members healthy, provide care in the least costly setting, and decrease total costs. The members are scheduled to have IV therapy care and procedures performed in alternative clinical settings such as home care, outpatient clinics, or ambulatory infusion centers, rather than in the hospital, to avoid the higher costs.

■ HOME CARE

Home care originally was conceived as a stage in the continuum of care after hospitalization, during which recovery and rehabilitation could continue effectively in the patient's home at a lower cost than if furnished in a hospital. Today, home care services often are used as low-cost substitutes for hospital care. Provision of services in the home decreases Medicare dollars spent and improves access to health care for many older adults.

Reimbursement for Home Care Services

Third-party payers for home care therapies include Medicare, Medicaid, commercial insurance, HMOs, preferred provider organizations, and managed care companies. Managed care payers, HMOs, and preferred provider organizations determine payments on a case-by-case basis and usually do not go "out of contract." Medicaid, third-party payers, and managed care programs have various payment methods along with specific criteria. An overview of various payment plans for therapies may be found in Table 23–1.

TABLE 23-1
HOME INTRAVENOUS INFUSION COVERAGE

Payer	Antibiotic	Chemotherapy	Hydration	Pain	Total Parenteral Nutrition
Medicare A	—	Yes	Yes	No	—
Medicare B	No	Yes	No	Yes	No
Medicaid	Yes	Yes	Yes	Yes	Yes
HMO/PPO	Yes	Yes	Yes	Yes	Yes
Commercial	Yes	Yes	Yes	Yes	Yes
Champus	Yes	Yes	Yes	Yes	Yes

HMO, health maintenance organization; PPO, preferred provider organization; Champus, Civilian Health and Medical Programs for Uniformed Services.

Combined with a working knowledge of precisely what types of therapy that various payer sources cover, it is essential that the written record of care, including the diagnosis, be consistent with the type of therapy provided. As in the tertiary care setting, a series of codes has been developed to reflect procedures (current procedural terminology [CPT]) and diagnoses (International Category of Disease [ICD9]). In the physician's office, application of the appropriate CPT code combined with a *correct* diagnosis ensures third-party payment. In home care, the ICD9 descriptors are applied. The **ICD9 code** filed by the third-party payer should match the diagnosis and the type of therapy provided. For example, blood transfusion is appropriate for a diagnosis of anemia; the ICD code is 285.9. Antibiotics are appropriate for a diagnosis of osteomyelitis; the ICD code is 730.2. Refer to Table 23–2 for more information.

Specific Considerations Related to Medicare

Home care is one of the fastest growing benefits in the **Medicare** program, which is the largest purchaser of home health services in the United States (Disbrow, 1999). The number of Medicare beneficiaries has been expanding by approximately 2% each year (Disbrow, 1999) and is expected to accelerate even more rapidly with the enrollment of the baby-boomer generation. Eligibility for the home care benefit within the Medicare program requires that the following conditions be met (Disbrow, 1999):

- The patient must be at least 65 years of age and have received acceptance for Medicare coverage.
- The patient must be confined to the home in such a way that leaving requires considerable effort and the assistance of another person or an adaptive device such as a cane, walker, or wheelchair. Absences from the home must be infrequent, of short duration, and for the purposes of receiving additional medical care.
- Home care services must be provided under a Plan of Care established and reviewed by a licensed physician directly involved in the patient's care. Written physician orders are required for home care.

text continues on page 669

T A B L E   2 3 – 2
POTENTIAL HOME INFUSION DIAGNOSIS AND SUGGESTED THERAPIES

Diagnosis	ICD9 Description Code	Suggested Therapy
Abscess, general	682.9	Antibiotic
Abscess, brain	324.0	Antibiotic
Abscess, pelvic	614.4	Antibiotic
Achalasia, digestive organs, congenital	751.8	TPN
Achalasia, esophagus	530.0	TPN
Acquired immunodeficiency syndrome	279.3/D43	Anti-infective/TPN
Actinomycosis	039.9	Anti-infective
Adhesions, intestinal with obstruction	560.81	TPN
Amyotonia	728.2	Antibiotic/TPN
Anemia	285.9	Blood
Aphagia	783.0	TEN
Arthritis, bacterial	040.89	Antibiotic
Arthritis, infective	711.9	Antibiotic
Asthma	493.9	Aminophylline
Atresia, alimentary organ or tract	751.8	TPN
Bacteremia	790.7	Antibiotic
Bacteremia caused by organism	038.8	Antibiotic
Blastomycosis	116.0	Anti-infective
Blood transfusion	V58.2	Blood
Bronchiectasis	494.0	Antibiotic
Bronchitis	491.0	Antibiotic
Cachexia caused by cancer	199.1	TEN/TPN
Cachexia caused by malnutrition	261.0	TEN/TPN
Candidiasis	112.9	Anti-infective
Carcinoma	194.3	Chemotherapy
Celiac disease	579.0	TEN/TPN
Cellulitis	682.9	Antibiotic
Chemotherapy	V58.1	Chemotherapy
Coccidioidomycosis	114.9	Anti-infective
Colitis	558.9	TEN/TPN
Colitis, ulcerative	556.0	TEN/TPN
Congestive heart failure	428.9	Dobutamine
Cooley's disease	282.4	Deferoxamine mesylate
Crohn's disease	555.9	TEN/TPN
Crush injury with infection	929.9	Antibiotic
Cryptococcoses	117.5	Antibiotic
Cytomegalovirus	363.2	Antibiotic
Deficiency, α_1-antitrypsin	277.6	Prolastin
Deficiency, antihemophilic factor	286.0	Blood product
Deficiency, growth hormone	253.3	Growth hormone

T A B L E   2 3 - 2 (Continued)

Diagnosis	ICD9 Description Code	Suggested Therapy
Deficiency, immunoglobulin	279.0	Gamma globulin
Decubitus ulcer	707.0	Antibiotic
Degenerative heart disease	429.1	Dobutamine
Dehydration	276.5	Hydration
Diabetes	250.0	Antibiotic
Diabetes with gangrene	250.7	Antibiotic
Diabetic ulcer	250.8	Antibiotic
Diarrhea, chronic	558.9	TEN/TPN
Diarrhea, infectious	009.2	TEN/TPN
Disease, pelvic inflammatory, chronic	614.4	Antibiotic
Embolism, pulmonary	415.1	Antithrombolytic
Encephalitis, viral	049.9	Anti-infective
Encephalitis, viral, arthropod-borne	064.0	Anti-infective
Endocarditis, infectious	421.0	Antibiotic
Enteritis, viral	008.6	Anti-infective
Enteritis, bacterial	008.5	Antibiotic
Fibrosis, cystic	277.0	Antibiotic/TEN/TPN
Fistula, abdomen	569.8	TEN/TPN
Fracture, open	829.1	Antibiotic
Fungal disease	117.9	Anti-infective
Gangrene	785.4	Antibiotic
Gonococcal joint infection	098.5	Antibiotic
Gonococcal pelvic infection, chronic	098.39	Antibiotic
Hemophilia	286.0	Blood products
Herpes simplex, complicated	054.8	Anti-infective
Histoplasmosis	115.9	Anti-infective
Hodgkin's disease	201.9	Chemotherapy
Human immunodeficiency virus	044.9	Anti-infective/TEN/TPN
Hyperalimentation	783.6	TPN
Hyperemesis gravidarum	643.0	TPN/hydration
Hypogammaglobulinemia	279.0	Gamma globulin
Ileus	560.1	TPN
Infarct, bowel	557.0	TPN
Infection	136.9	Antibiotic
Infection, atypical mycobacteria	031.9	Antibiotic
Infection, bacterial	041.9	Antibiotic
Infection, brain	323.9	Antibiotic
Infection, cytomegalovirus	771.1	Anti-infective
Infection, skin	686.9	Antibiotic
Ischemic, bowel	557.1	TPN

(continued)

T A B L E   2 3 - 2 (*Continued*)

Diagnosis	ICD9 Description Code	Suggested Therapy
Ixodiasis	134.8	Antibiotic
Kaposi's sarcoma	173.9	Chemotherapy
Labor, premature	644.2	Tocolytics
Leukemia	208.9	Chemotherapy
Leukemia, acute myelogenous	205.9	Chemotherapy
Lymph node removal	088.8	Chemotherapy
Lymphoma	202.8	Chemotherapy
Malabsorption	579.9	TEN/TPN
Malnutrition	263.9	TEN/TPN
Melanoma	172.9	Chemotherapy
Meningitis	322.9	Antibiotic
Metaplasia, agnogenic myeloid	289.8	Antibiotic/TEN
Mycobacterium avium-intracellulare	031.0	Antibiotic
Mycosis	117.9	Anti-infective
Myeloma	203.0	Chemotherapy
Myocarditis	429.0	Antibiotic
Neoplasm	199.1	Chemotherapy
Neoplasm, alimentary tract	159.9/197.8	Chemotherapy
Neoplasm, bone	170.9/198.5	Chemotherapy
Neoplasm, breast	174.9/198.81	Chemotherapy
Neoplasm, digestive organs	159.9/197.8	Chemotherapy
Neoplasm, esophagus	150.9/197.8	Chemotherapy
Neoplasm, intestine	159.0/197.8	Chemotherapy
Neoplasm, large intestine	153.9/197.5	Chemotherapy
Neoplasm, larynx	161.9	Chemotherapy
Neoplasm, lung	162.9/197.0	Chemotherapy
Neoplasm, metastatic	275.4	Chemotherapy
Neoplasm, neck	195.0/198.89	Chemotherapy
Neoplasm, prostate	185.0	Chemotherapy
Obstruction, intestine	560.9	TPN
Osteomyelitis	730.2	Antibiotic
Otitis, external malignant	380.14	Antibiotic
Pain, bone	733.9	Pain
Parkinson's disease	332.0	TEN/TPN
Pneumonia	486.0	Antibiotic
Pneumonia, *Pneumocystis carinii*	136.3	Anti-infective
Prematurity	765.1	PEN
Prostatis	601.9	Antibiotic
Pseudomonas	250.8/682.6	Antibiotic
Pseudo-obstruction, intestinal	564.8	TPN

T A B L E   2 3 – 2 (*Continued*)

Diagnosis	ICD9 Description Code	Suggested Therapy
Pulmonary disease, chronic obstructive	416.9	α_1-Proteinase inhibitor
Purpura, idiopathic thrombocytopenic	287.3	Biologics
Pyelonephritis	590.8	Antibiotic
Septicemia	038.9	Antibiotic
Short bowel syndrome	579.2	TPN
Sinusitis, chronic	473.9	Antibiotic
Stomatitis	528.0	Partial enteral nutrition
Thalassemia	282.4	Deferoxamine mesylate
Thrombophlebitis	451.9	Anticoagulants
Wound, complicated	879.8	Antibiotic

TEN, total enteral nutrition; TPN, total parenteral nutrition.

- The home care services the patient needs must be skilled intermittent nursing, physical therapy, occupational therapy, or speech therapy.
- A certified Medicare program provider who agrees to adhere to the extensive Medicare Conditions of Participation regulations and requirements and accepts Medicare's reimbursement for the provision of those services must provide home care (Health Care Finance Administration Medicare [HCFA], 1999).

The following are the requirements of Medicare Conditions of Participation (HCFA, 1999):

1. Nursing services must require the skills of a registered nurse.
2. Intermittent care is defined as consisting of up to 35 hours total per week by all professional disciplines combined.
3. No more than 8 hours of combined services may be provided per 24-hour day. Daily visits are not to last longer than a specified number of days per month.

Services eligible for Medicare reimbursement fall under Part A or B (see Table 23–1). Congress decided in the 1980s to eliminate cost-based reimbursement to hospitals to reduce health care costs. Medicare introduced its prospective payment system (PPS) in the form of diagnosis-related groups (DRGs) (Disbrow, 1999). Implementation of PPS reduced the costs of hospitalization by shifting the end point of care to the home, thereby contributing to the growth of the alternative care delivery system. Before January 1, 1998, Medicare-certified home health agencies were reimbursed retrospectively for the costs they incurred in providing services to patients. On January 1, 1998, reimbursement provisions for Medicare home health services underwent significant changes in legislation and regulations. Prospective payment for home care is now making the transition to an interim payment system that was planned to be implemented in October, 1999 but was postponed until October, 2000.

This form of prospective payment will result in lump-sum payments for services provided to home care patients, a system similar to the DRG system used for hospital care. The transition from retrospective and cost-based payment to prospective payment is expected to affect this market dramatically. Medicare has begun to redefine benefits it previously covered by limiting access to services, tightening eligibility requirements, and re-examining homebound status. As the government continues to struggle with rising costs, further changes are anticipated.

Reimbursement for Home Infusion Therapy

Reimbursement for home infusion therapies is very complex and depends on the nature of the home infusion business itself. For example, a Medicare-certified home health agency may bill for supplies associated with a Medicare Part A visit, but the same agency may not bill under Part A for home total parenteral nutrition (TPN). When a managed care company is involved, services are provided on a per diem basis.

Patient Criteria for Home Care Infusion Therapy

In addition to meeting Medicare criteria for home care, patients must meet other criteria to qualify as candidates for home infusion therapy. Patients will be responsible for specific aspects of IV therapy, including monitoring, catheter line management, operation of electronic infusion equipment, and other duties. The patient, caregiver, or both must be able to learn signs and symptoms of complications to report to the nurse, and be able to identify any other situations that require immediate attention. An emergency phone number should be available for patients and families to call for help (Box 23–1).

Appropriate Diagnosis

Often the type of drug therapy ordered determines a candidate's appropriateness for home infusion therapy. Many drugs given in the inpatient setting are acceptable for

---

BOX 23–1 Criteria for Patient Selection for Home Infusion

1. Appropriate diagnosis
2. Medical stability
3. Venous access
4. Evaluation of drug therapy
5. Laboratory profile
6. Presence of a support system
7. Technical criteria, including desire and willingness to receive therapy at home, educability, manual dexterity, appropriate home environment
8. Financial resources

home infusion programs. Table 23–2 lists potential home infusion diagnoses and suggested therapies.

The home infusion therapy ordered must be consistent with the patient's diagnosis and ability to receive therapy in the home. Common diagnoses for antibiotic therapy include osteomyelitis, otitis media, sinusitis, cryptococcal meningitis, pneumonia, subacute bacterial endocarditis, primary bacteremia, cellulitis, urinary tract infections, pyelonephritis, septic arthritis, histoplasmosis, peritonitis, toxic shock syndrome, Lyme disease, rickettsial infection, opportunistic infections related to acquired immunodeficiency syndrome, and others. All types of patients with cancer are appropriate candidates for home infusion of antineoplastic agents, especially combination protocols. Many third-party payers restrict reimbursement for antineoplastic agents to alternate clinical care settings and have set limits on inpatient treatments. Related infusion therapies for the oncology patient may include nutritional support, IV pain management, antiemetics, and leucovorin rescue regimens.

Medical Stability

Medical stability is essential if patients are to perform all required procedures themselves. If a patient is not medically stable but has medical approval for home care, then a family member or other caregiver may assume full responsibility for performing all techniques. Another person may be needed as a backup, depending on the home situation. The patient should have a comprehensive assessment before discharge from the hospital.

Venous Access

Vascular access appropriate to the planned type of therapy is essential. Some patients may be discharged with an IV device in place that was used in the hospital, including a jugular vein catheter, subclavian vein catheter (triple lumens), tunneled catheters (Hickman/Broviac, Groshong), implanted ports (chest or arm), PICCs, midline catheters, or peripheral catheters. Other times, the home care nurse initiates the vascular access device placement in the home, such as a peripheral catheter for short-term therapy or a midline catheter for long-term therapy, after she has demonstrated competency. Teaching protocols for catheter care management and flush procedures for the type of access are required and must be patient-specific to address all areas of maintenance for self-care.

Evaluation of Drug Therapy

Each drug ordered is evaluated for all aspects of the administration: length of time required for the administration; the dosing frequency; duration of time for therapy; whether the insurer will approve an electronic device; and patient risks. For example, antibiotics may be administered over 30 minutes to 2 hours, depending on the drug and volume of solution. Dosing may be every 4, 6, 8, 12, or 24 hours. Duration may be 4 to 8 weeks. Other drugs must be administered with an electronic pump or device. Some drugs require close monitoring and the presence of a nurse in the event of an anaphylactic reaction. Some drugs require the availability of emergency medical services.

Laboratory Profile

Procedures must be established for routine laboratory studies and transmission of reports to the physician, home infusion pharmacist, and home care agency. The nurse should report changes in laboratory values, high or low, immediately to the physician so that adjustments can be made in the treatment plan consistent with the patient's clinical condition. Laboratory testing of blood levels and white blood cell counts may be weekly or biweekly for patients receiving TPN, antineoplastic therapy, and antibiotics or antifungal agents that may require routine peak and trough levels to avoid toxicity.

Presence of a Support System

Even if the patient meets the criteria for home care as discussed earlier, many adjustments need to be made in the home. The patient often is very ill and still recovering from whatever condition necessitated the hospitalization. The IV therapy orders usually are a continuation of IV therapy the patient received as an inpatient. Planning is necessary to provide 24-hour support from a family member or other caregiver until the patient can assume some of the procedures and self-care. The home care nurse visits as frequently as required to perform some of the procedures and begin teaching the patient and caregiver, and is on call for assistance. A home health aide may be available to help the patient with personal care.

Technical Criteria

The compliant patient or caregiver administers drugs and treatments as ordered, follows aseptic technique, reports signs and symptoms of complications, and monitors and records intake and output, weights, temperature, blood glucose, and other parameters as indicated. The elderly patient must be evaluated for manual dexterity to perform the required procedures. Many patients have arthritis in their fingers and hands and are unable to assemble and manipulate the IV equipment to participate in their care. Some patients have a limited educational background and are unable to learn the procedures they are taught. Some patients experience dementia, depression, or mental illness and are incapable of assuming responsibility for their care. The home environment must be evaluated for basic needs (eg, telephone, electricity, hot and cold water, refrigeration). When these basic needs are unmet, the physician must be notified so that another plan of care that is safe for the patient can be considered.

Financial Resources

Before acceptance to home care, the patient's insurance benefits are assessed. Although many patients may have outstanding health care benefits for inpatient care, they may have limited or no benefits for home care. Some patients may have insurance coverage for home care services, but no prescription coverage. Some patients may be able to pay out of pocket for the cost of the drugs and supplies needed to receive IV therapy in the home. If the patient is unable to pay, the physician is notified, who must consider alternate plans or place the patient in a subacute facility paid for by insurance.

Role of Health Care Professionals in Home-Based Intravenous Therapy

The home care infusion program must be full service, available 24 hours a day, and able to meet the patient's total needs for nursing, supplies, delivery, inventory, and storage. Qualified professional personnel must be responsible for the direction, coordination, and supervision of all professional services. Care should be consistent with the highest standards of the two accrediting organizations that provide guidelines: the Joint Commission on Accreditation of Healthcare Organizations (JCAHO) and the Community Health Accreditation Program (CHAP) of the National League for Nursing (NLN). Table 23–3 compares JCAHO and CHAP.

Policies and procedures for the provision of home infusion services must be consistent with published practice standards. The Intravenous Nurses Society (INS) has published IV Standards for all patients regardless of their clinical setting (INS, 1998, 2000). The procedures must be comprehensive and address all the infusion therapies provided. The home infusion therapy program must be consistent with the organization's philosophy and purpose.

Positive outcomes should be the treatment goal for restoring the patient to a functional capacity and enabling the patient and family to return to a level consistent with the stage of disease and its process. Outcome measurements, based on those developed by JCAHO and CHAP, enhance the level of care provided and ensure excellence.

TABLE 23–3
COMPARISON OF JCAHO AND CHAP

	JCAHO	CHAP
Number of accredited providers:		
Home care organizations	3500	100
Infusion providers	1500	0
Cost of accreditation	$3000–$10,000	$1300–$24,000
Accredits networks	Yes	Yes
Accredits ambulatory centers	Yes	Yes
Year accrediting for home care facilities began	1988	1965

CHAP, Community Health Accreditation Program; JCAHO, Joint Commission Accreditation of Healthcare Organizations.
(Adapted with permission from Epstein, D. [1995]. Struggling for recognition. *Infusion, 1*(7), 36–37.)

The Discharge Planner/Home Care Coordinator

Discharge planning begins during hospitalization. The home care coordinator may be involved in identifying appropriate candidates for home infusion therapies. The discharge orders must be consistent with the type of IV therapy, medication, dose, route, duration, frequency interval, and method of administration. The discharge planner arranges final coordination with the supplier before the patient is discharged from the hospital to ensure the safe and timely arrival of IV pump, solutions, medications, and related equipment. Open lines of communication enable the infusion provider to meet the patient's current and ongoing needs for care and ensure a high degree of confidence.

The Physician

The physician orders the referral to the appropriate alternate care setting. He or she writes the plan of treatment for the patient in need of home infusion therapy. In addition to routine infusion orders and other treatments, the individualized plan also should define functional limitations, goals, and duration of treatment. For some modalities, a letter of medical necessity is required. The physician also maintains the role of "gatekeeper," providing recertification for ongoing care, reviewing progress notes, and coordinating the home care plan.

The Nurse as Home Care Infusion Provider

The home care nurse maintains ongoing communication with the physician regarding the patient's status and changes in orders. The nurse continues to assess the patient, and whenever the patient's condition deteriorates, he or she notifies the physician and may send the patient to the physician's office or to the hospital.

The home care nurse must demonstrate competency in drawing blood samples by peripheral venipuncture or by central venous access devices. Once the referral to home care has been completed and insurance coverage or other reimbursement is verified, the nurse should complete a referral checklist (Fig. 23–1). The nurse should review the Patient's Bill of Rights, Responsibilities for Participation in the Home Infusion Program, and the assignment of benefits document. Then the nurse performs an initial patient assessment that includes review of body systems, review of current and past medical history, psychosocial assessment, evaluation of available support systems, and assessment of functional limitations, environment, and cognitive and technical skills. He or she clarifies IV orders if needed; develops the patient's plan of care; coordinates interdisciplinary communication for physical therapy, occupational therapy, speech therapy, social worker, or nurse aide as needed; and orients the patient to the services being provided.

A designated nurse case manager must coordinate services for each patient. The infusion therapy nurse case manager is selected for his or her expertise and experience, and preferably is a Certified Registered Nurse in Intravenous Therapy (CRNI). A list of case manager responsibilities is provided in Box 23–2. This nurse is the home

Home Infusion Referral Checklist

Home Care Provider:

[   ] _____

[   ] _____

	DATE/INITIAL
INFORMATION TO:	
A. DISCHARGE PLANNER INFORMED	_____
B. IV TEAM INFORMED	_____
C. HOME AGENCY INFORMED:	_____

Name of agency _____

Address _____

Phone # _____ FAX # _____

Local contact _____

D.   LOCAL PHYSICIAN IDENTIFIED (if applicable)   _____

Name _____

Address _____

Phone # _____ FAX # _____

TYPE OF REFERRAL:

A.   Parenteral nutrition   _____

B.   Enteral nutrition   _____

C.   IV antibiotics   _____

D.   Pain management   _____

E.   Nupogen   _____

F.   Chemotherapy   _____

G.   Catheter care   _____

H.   Other _____   _____

TEACHING COMPLETED:

A.   HOME INFUSION _____   _____

B.   SUBCLAVIAN/CATHETER CARE   _____

[   ] Port   Type _____

[   ] Hickman/Groshong   [   ] Subclavian   [   ] Other _____

Lumens _____

SUPPLIES NEEDED FROM HOSPITAL UPON DISCHARGE:

_____

_____

_____

_____

DELIVERY DATE _____   START OF INFUSION _____

DATE OF REFERRAL FROM PHYSICIAN _____   DATE OF DISCHARGE _____

SIGNATURE/INITIAL _____ _____   TITLE _____

_____ _____   _____

_____ _____   _____

Figure 23–1. Home infusion referral checklist.

BOX 23–2 **Responsibility of the Case Manager**

- Initial assessment of the patient, family, and home environment
- Development of a plan of care
- Appropriate referral and follow-up
- Coordination of services
- Implementation of the plan of care
- Ongoing evaluation
- Plan for termination of home care

---

care nurse who is assigned as a case manager to the patient and is responsible for coordinating care among all disciplines: nursing, physical therapy, occupational therapy, speech therapy, social work, and home health aides. Also, the nurse case manager monitors the patient's progress toward goals, independence, and discharge from home care.

The plan of care should include patient teaching for the ordered IV therapy, including managing the catheter, using aseptic technique, changing dressings, flushing the IV line and heparin-locking the catheter, hooking up and disconnecting continuous or intermittent administration, changing tubings and other devices, handling IV equipment, performing emergency interventions, noting signs and symptoms of possible complications, handling inventory, and managing the pump.

 SAFE PRACTICE ALERT   The nurse should provide teaching with return demonstrations until the patient or caregiver is confident and independent. Even then, the nurse provides ongoing support and monitoring.

The nurse should provide specific teaching packets with pictures and individualize the teaching plan to the patient's specific needs. Once therapy is initiated in the home, the nurse must take adequate time to ensure the patient's compliance with the therapeutic regimen. Language barriers often inhibit a successful teaching program. Every effort should be made to address the patient in the language he or she best understands. Figure 23–2 provides an example of IV teaching in Spanish.

The nurse should develop, review, and sign the teaching plan for the patient. A copy should become part of the patient's clinical record, with a second copy given to the patient and kept in the place of residence.

Home care providers should offer infusion classes for nurses before patient assignment to enhance skills and learning with verification and documentation of IV competencies. Ongoing education is necessary to keep abreast of the latest technologies, equipment, and infusion therapy procedures. Competency of infusion skills for nurses should be documented and validated on an annual basis. The resources of professional societies and the role that such organizations play in development of the nurse's knowledge base cannot be overlooked. These societies provide the collegiality and professional camaraderie that enable nurses to grow in this rapidly changing field. IV nursing professionals should be encouraged to publish case studies about

¿Cómo está? Soy la enfermera encargada de administrarle el suero intravenoso.
▲ HELLO, I AM YOUR I.V. NURSE. (FEMALE)

Como esta? Soy el enfermero encargado de administrarle el suero intravenoso.
▲ HELLO, I AM YOUR I.V. NURSE. (MALE)

Vengo a revisarle la aguja del suero intravenoso.
▲ I AM HERE TO CHECK YOUR I.V.

Voy a aplicarle el suero intravenoso.
▲ I AM HERE TO START YOUR I.V.

Le cambiaremos la aguja intravenoso de lugar cada (2) - (3) dias.
▲ WE CHANGE THE I.V. SITE EVERY (2) - (3) DAYS.

Le duele en donde tiene inyectada la aguja intravenosa?   Si   No
▲ DO YOU HAVE PAIN AT YOUR I.V. SITE?   YES   NO

Tengo que cambiarle el lugar de la aguja intravenosa debido a que:
▲ I NEED TO   CHANGE YOUR I.V. TODAY BECAUSE OF:

(a) le duele,	(b) tiene inflamacion,	(c) tiene la piel roja,	(d) es un procedimiento de rutina.
▲ (A) PAIN	(B) SWELLING	(C) REDNESS	(D) ROUTINE

Si le duele o si se le inflama el lugar donde tiene la aguja del suero intravenoso, hagaselo saber a la enfermera.
▲ IF PAIN OR SWELLING BEGINS, TELL YOUR NURSE.

SPANISH

Figure 23–2. Language for IV patient teaching: Spanish. (Courtesy of Jaclyn Tropp, CRNI, Evanston, IL.)

their success stories in home infusion care and to share their knowledge and expertise with others. Box 23–3 lists available resources.

The Pharmacist

The roles and responsibilities of the pharmacist vary in different parts of the country. In general, the pharmacist is responsible for reviewing medical records for current and past medical history and nutritional and medication history; obtaining and correlating physician orders; checking allergies and drug compatibilities; and facilitating delivery of medications, solutions, supplies, and equipment to the patient's place of residence. The pharmacist also reviews laboratory data and monitors pharmacokinetic dosing with the physician for certain drugs and therapies.

Types of Home Infusion Therapy

Home infusion therapies are diverse and encompass many modalities. Such modalities include antibiotics and anti-infectives, hydration, antiemetics, antineoplastics,

---

BOX 23–3 **Available Resources**

American Association of Blood Banks (AABB)
American Hospital Association (AHA)
American Society of Health-System Pharmacists (ASHP)
American Society for Parenteral and Enteral Nutrition (A.S.P.E.N.)
Association for Practitioners in Infection Control (APIC)
Case Management Society of America (CMSA)
Centers for Disease Control and Prevention (CDC)
Community Health Accreditation Program (CHAP)
Intravenous Nurses Society (INS)
Joint Commission on Accreditation of Healthcare Organizations (JCAHO)
National Association of Vascular Access Networks (NAVAN)
National Association for Home Care (NAHC)
National Home Infusion Association (NHIA)
National Hospice Organization (NHO)
National Subacute Care Association (NSCA)
Oncology Nursing Society (ONS)

---

nutritional support, pain management, blood and component therapy, cardiovascular drugs, drugs to prevent transplant rejection, and venous sampling.

Some health care providers prefer that the first dose of some drugs be administered in a monitored clinical setting, but many first doses are now administered in the patient's residence in the presence of a nurse. This change may be attributed to changes in technology and pharmaceuticals as well as to the increased availability of professional nurses with appropriate IV therapy credentials.

▲ Legal Issues: FIRST DOSING

> The patient who is scheduled to receive the first dose in the home should have a thorough allergy profile and history, including a risk assessment for first dosing.

An appropriate order for emergency anaphylaxis should be provided. The medication should be available immediately and sent to the home before the first administration of the medication. Components of the anaphylactic kit may include epinephrine, diphenhydramine, hydrocortisone, acetaminophen, sodium chloride solution, IV administration set, needles, and syringes. Allergic reactions may occur with subsequent doses of medication as well. The home care IV clinician must be able to identify and differentiate allergic responses from anaphylactic reactions and teach the patient and caregiver.

In the home care program, provision must be made for handling infectious patient waste. The U.S. Environmental Protection Agency (EPA), a federal regulatory board, has developed many advisories regarding infectious waste. With the passage of the Medical Waste Tracking Act of 1988, Congress mandated to the EPA the investigation and development, if needed, of guidelines for handling home-generated waste. Prepackaged kits are available from various manufacturers and include sharps disposal systems and several types of spill kits. Today's emphasis on safety in the workplace has enhanced these efforts (see Chaps. 11 and 19).

Antibiotics and Anti-infectives

The delivery of antibiotics and anti-infective agents in the home is a rapidly growing home care service. To qualify, the patient should be medically stable and compliant, the infection should be treatable in the home, and a reliable venous access should be available. Disease conditions amenable to home care IV antibiotic therapy include long-lasting and deep-seated infections. Awareness of a patient's medication history and allergic reactions allows guided monitoring before, during, and after IV antibiotic administration. Recognition of potential adverse drug reactions associated with each class of anti-infectives is an important part of safe and effective IV antibiotic infusions (Barrio, 1998).

Nutritional Support

The advent of TPN in the 1960s enabled physicians to support intestinally compromised patients indefinitely. Technical barriers have diminished over time. Advanced products, catheters, and technologies have enabled advanced nutritional support to be provided to patients with appropriate diagnoses. If the patient is under the Medicare program, he or she must require TPN for 90 days or more to qualify. For diagnoses associated with TPN, see Box 23–4.

In the home setting, the patient usually receives TPN as a cyclic administration rather than a continuous 24-hour infusion. With the cyclic infusion, the patient receives a full day's prescribed requirement of fluid, glucose, protein (amino acids), lipids, and other additives over 12 to 18 hours. The pharmacist prepares the TPN solution, but the nurse, patient, or caregiver must add some drugs to the solution just before administration. Home monitoring must be done, including daily weights, temperature, blood glucose monitoring, intake and output, and weekly blood sampling.

Many patients begin their TPN solution in the evening, to be administered while they are sleeping, and disconnect in the morning. The patient, caregiver, or both learn to flush the IV catheter and perform catheter maintenance to keep the line patent. This allows the patient to be free from using the IV pump during the day. When it is necessary to visit the physician's office, the patient does not have to deal with TPN administration and equipment, especially when nonambulatory equipment is supplied (see Chap. 16).

Hydration

Elderly patients often become dehydrated, especially during very hot weather, the influenza season, or periods of inadequate fluid intake. The goal for home hydration

---

BOX 23–4 **Applicable Diagnoses for Total Parenteral Nutrition**

Kwashiorkor
Cystic fibrosis
Nutritional marasmus
Disorders involving the immune mechanism
Severe protein-calorie malnutrition
Anorexia nervosa
Malnutrition
Nutritional and metabolic cardiomyopathy
Unspecified vitamin deficiency or other nutritional deficiency
Obstruction of duodenum
Disorders of amino acid transport and metabolism
Regional enteritis
Intestinal disaccharidase deficiencies
Idiopathic proctocolitis
Malabsorption
Disorders of lipid metabolism
Chronic liver disease and cirrhosis
Disorders of fluid, electrolyte, and acid–base balance
Postsurgical nonabsorption
Cancer cachexia

---

is to maintain the patient's fluid balance by providing multiple electrolytes, supplemental vitamins, or plain IV solutions (without additives) and also to avoid hospitalization for those people who resist admission for this therapy.

Pain Management

Continuous or intermittent self-administration of IV analgesics in the home allows those in need of pain relief to remain with their families while experiencing a degree of comfort not previously available. Manufacturers have developed sophisticated equipment to ensure safe administration of these drugs in an unmonitored environment. Pain medications may be administered by a patient-controlled analgesia pump through IV, epidural, intrathecal, subcutaneous, or other routes of administration. The most frequently ordered medications are morphine sulfate, meperidine, and hydromorphone. A common concern among patients and families is addiction. Health care providers should assure patients and caregivers that addiction is a minimal concern and that doses should be administered as needed (see Chap. 20).

Antiemetics

Antiemetic protocols aimed at intermittent infusion facilitate the care of the patient receiving antineoplastic therapy and ensure patient comfort. Protocols may call for antiemetic infusions as a single-agent treatment or combined with TPN therapies. Patients with a diagnosis of hyperemesis gravidarum may benefit from home IV antiemetic therapy.

Antineoplastics

Chemotherapeutic agents are administered by various IV systems to patients in their homes. Vesicant and nonvesicant agents are administered through centrally placed IV catheters, PICCs, implanted chest or arm ports, tunneled catheters, and implanted pumps. In some patients, the chemotherapeutic agents may be initiated in a chemotherapy clinic or physician office. The infusate is connected to an ambulatory infusion pump and sent home. The home care nurse monitors the patient, changes tubings and dressings, and disconnects the equipment at the end of therapy (see Chap. 19).

Blood and Component Therapy

Transfusion of blood and blood components may be performed in the home whenever the policies and procedures required by the American Association of Blood Banks can be followed and the procedure itself is cost effective. See Chapter 17 for more information.

▲ Legal Issues: TRANSFUSION PARAMETERS

The availability of the physician *as well as paramedic services* should be determined before the transfusion. Policies should be written for safe administration and compatibility checks, identification checks and verification, transportation of the blood unit or component, emergency measures, registered nurse monitoring (including remaining with the patient for the duration of the procedure and for approximately 90 minutes after the completion of the transfusion), and signs and symptoms of various types of blood reactions.

Venous Sampling

Venous sampling for all types of laboratory testing is available in home infusion programs. Peak and trough levels, chemistry panels for patients on TPN, white cell counts for patients receiving antineoplastic therapy, and other tests may be performed. Venous samples may be drawn through peripheral venipuncture or central line sampling. Procedures should be established for blood draws from central line catheters, including the amount of blood to discard before the sampling, the volume at which to flush the catheter after the draw, and change of any equipment.

■ HOSPICE

Hospice is a specialized program of care for any person with a limited life expectancy. Available through a national network (1-800-658-8898;www.nho.org), hospice seeks to enhance, preserve, and encourage the dignity of life for patients and families by providing medical care, supportive care, and grief educational services. Hospice emphasizes the management of pain and other symptoms, so the patient is comfortable, alert, and able to maintain the highest quality of life possible. One of the major fears of the seriously ill is pain (Flores, 1998). In a hospice program, medications are prepared for any patient with pain to achieve constant pain control without impairing alertness. A team of physicians, nurses, pharmacists, psychologists, dietitians, social workers, clergy, and volunteers provides 24-hour care. The hospice team develops an individualized plan of care for each patient. Hospice care may be provided in the home with a primary caregiver, or in a hospice center when no primary caregiver is available or for short-term acute symptom management that cannot be given at home. Each eligible Medicare patient must decide whether to choose the hospice benefit, which means that the hospice will provide all care related to the terminal illness. Regular Medicare coverage can be used for any services provided by a personal physician or for illnesses or accidents unrelated to the terminal illness. Hospice care also is provided under other insurances, HMOs, and Medicaid.

■ SUBACUTE CARE FACILITIES

Subacute programs are a new level of care for patients in various stages of an acute illness or injury, usually after, but sometimes instead of, hospitalization for an acute episode (Levenson, 1998). **Subacute care** is sometimes called *transitional care*. Two organizations developed the definition: the National Subacute Care Association (NSCA) and JCAHO (Griffin, 1998). Subacute care facilities respond to the need for the treatment of patients with complex medical conditions and rehabilitation needs and provide for a more cost-effective approach.

Beginning in the 1980s, the earliest subacute care units were located in skilled nursing facilities. Later, hospitals began to add subacute units and called them *extended acute care* or *specialty hospitals*. These specialty hospitals typically have 40 beds or more and usually are located in a separate wing or floor of the host hospital. They have an independent admission and discharge function, are licensed separately as a long-term acute care hospital, and are accredited by JCAHO. Their costs are 30% to 60% lower than general acute care hospitals.

The extended acute care hospital provides high-quality, cost-effective, long-term care for high-acuity patients. These specialty hospitals manage patients with medically complex conditions who require extended stay, and whose medical condition will resolve sufficiently for transfer to lower levels of care within a few days with an achievable positive outcome for the patient. The types of patients admitted are those who have multiple body system complications with difficult medical and therapeutic needs: patients with challenges of pulmonary care, ventilator dependency, cardiovascular complications, complicated wounds, major multiple trauma, disease management problems, burns, or other special needs. Infusion therapy treatments include antibiotic or anti-infective therapy, pain management, nutritional support, hydration, and various other infusions, including PICC/midline insertions and central venous catheter care management.

■ AMBULATORY INFUSION CENTERS

Ambulatory infusion centers (AICs) are another alternative site for delivering IV therapies. Ideally, the physical layout of an AIC is in a medical office building, either adjacent to or near an inpatient hospital. The standard components are a small laboratory, IV admixture room, education and training area, medical record station, nourishment area, and individualized patient rooms. The patient is seated in a recliner-type chair, with access to IV teaching videotapes or other movies during treatment. Laboratory parameters are reviewed, along with the physician's orders. If needed, additional laboratory studies are obtained and processed. The patient is offered juices and appropriate snacks during the visit. A nurse assigned to and familiar with the patient performs a complete assessment (including vital signs) and initiates treatment, which may take from 30 minutes to more than 4 hours.

Ambulatory infusion centers may be physician practice based or hospital based. Some organizations provide a stand-alone infusion center, but this model has faced many reimbursement constraints, limiting its viability and growth. With the introduction of PPS in long-term care and home care, the need for AICs will be even greater as the pressure to lower costs continues, and the AIC may help patients to avoid rehospitalization.

Under Medicare Part B reimbursement, physician practice–based infusion centers are reimbursed for medications and clinical nursing time spent on medication administration. Hospital-based infusion centers are able to bill Medicare through the outpatient billing modality. Traditionally, Medicare has reimbursed hospitals for outpatient services based on their costs. The Balanced Budget Act of 1997, however, required Medicare to begin paying for hospital outpatient services on a prospective basis. The program began in 2000. (Hallam, 2000). Stand-alone (independent) infusion centers are not covered. When Medicare is not the main payer source and reimbursement billing is through private insurers, stand-alone infusion centers may be the most effective model (Flores, 1998).

Patient selection for the AICs depends on reimbursement. The types of patients appropriate for AICs are those who do not have a caregiver in the home or who are unable to learn or perform self-administration. Another appropriate referral is a patient who is not homebound, does not qualify for home care, or does not have insurance coverage for home health care services. Patients can still recover at home and schedule visits for their infusions as prescribed by the physician.

Other benefits of AICs include improved documentation, teaching, monitoring, follow-up, quality assurance, patient satisfaction, and outcomes (Liebert & Bryant-Wimp, 1997). Types of IV therapy provided at AICs are addressed in Box 23–5. Because this model focuses on positive patient outcomes, other therapies provided may include allergy desensitization injections, diabetes education, hormone therapy, immunizations, protease inhibitors, rabies vaccination, respiratory therapy (aerosolized pentamidine), and wound care (Liebert & Bryant-Wimp, 1997). Patient care, education, continuity of care, and positive patient outcomes are the keys to patient satisfaction, physician satisfaction, and the success of AICs.

BOX 23–5 **Types of Intravenous Therapy Provided at Ambulatory Infusion Centers**

Antibiotics/anti-infectives and first dosing
Anticoagulants–heparin therapy
Biologics
Blood transfusion and component therapy
Catheter placement and maintenance (peripheral, peripherally inserted central catheter/midline insertion)
Chemotherapy
Drug monitoring (peak and trough)
Hydration
Intravenous immune globulin
Parenteral nutrition
Pain management
Steroids
Venous sampling

■ LONG-TERM CARE

Long-term care, often provided in skilled nursing facilities or nursing homes, is part of the continuum of care and an ongoing element of integrated health care. Long-term care services are intended for people of all ages with chronic disabilities and functional deficits to maintain their physical, social, and psychological functioning. The initiation of long-term care services may be preceded by an acute medical illness or the inability to perform activities of daily living independently for 90 days or more (Nazarko, 1998). The care ranges from skilled nursing care, to supportive services provided in the home, to informed assistance given by family and friends.

Many residents of long-term care facilities have complex medical problems and receive skilled care for tracheostomies, gastric feeding tubes, ventilators, mobility disabilities, impaired nutrition, IV medications, and deficits in activities of daily living associated with Alzheimer's disease. Other than acute care and subacute care hospitals, nursing homes are the only places that offer 24-hour nursing services (Nazarko, 1998). Professional nurses are essential to care for the residents by assessing and coordinating patients' needs for care, focusing on rehabilitation and convalescence, providing high-quality care, reducing complications and mortality, and being cost effective.

Infusion therapy is frequently required for the long-term patient. Commonly used modalities include antibiotic/anti-infective therapy, TPN, pain management, blood products, immune globulin, central venous catheter care and management, and PICC and midline catheter insertion. Several credentialed infusion nurse consultants offer educational in-service sessions for the staff to enhance patient care and reduce complications.

As the population ages, chronic illness and disability also will increase, thus creating a growing need for long-term care. The greatest surge in the aging population will occur as the baby boomers reach old age. Estimates are that 20% of the U.S. population will be 65 years or older by 2020 (Nazarko, 1998). Demographic increases also are expected in the segment of the population aged 85 years and older. Based on such projections, the number of people needing long-term care services will triple within the next 30 years (Beck & Chumbler, 1997) (see Chap. 22).

■ FUTURE INFUSION TECHNOLOGY FOR ALTERNATE CARE PROGRAMS

Technology is one of the most important factors affecting infusion therapy for alternate care programs. In the future, patient care will change to accommodate new technologies, new drug therapies, and new equipment. The greatest obstacle will be reimbursement. Many professionals recognize that patients have multiple, medically complex needs that will necessitate more intensive clinical monitoring of the therapy, requiring improvements in staff and caregiver education.

Health care providers are being challenged to become more efficient and cost conscious about what they do and how they do it. The delivery of antibiotics and anti-infectives is one of the fastest-growing therapies in alternative care programs. Over the years, tremendous changes have occurred in how these therapies are administered. Both high- and low-technology devices and methods are available for these therapies: gravity infusion, stationary infusion pumps, ambulatory electronic pumps, IV push, syringe delivery, and elastomeric devices with rate-restricted IV systems (Saladow, 1999).

As pressure builds to contain costs, studies are being done to evaluate techniques and procedures. Providers are looking at IV push administration for selected therapies as a safer and more efficient means of delivery than the traditional piggyback method (Poole & Nowobilski-Vasilios, 1999). Positive patient outcome monitoring is essential. Concerns related to IV push administration are increased phlebitis and vein irritation, increased infiltration, safety, therapeutic benefit for specific patients, and difficulties in patient/caregiver training. Manufacturers' warnings of side effects must be acknowledged and followed, especially for some medications. Some drugs are not appropriate for IV push administration, and the IV push method should not become the universal procedure of choice when attempting to control costs and reduce reimbursement rates.

References and Selected Readings

Asterisks indicate references cited in text.

Barrio, D. (1998). Antibiotic and anti-infective agent use and administration in home care. *Journal of Intravenous Nursing, 21,* 50–58.

*Beck, C. & Chumbler, N. (1997). Planning for the future of long-term care: Consumers, providers, and purchasers. *Journal of Gerontological Nursing, 23*(8) 6–13.

Benco, L.B. (2000). The exodus escalates: Medicare market pullouts to double in 2001. *Modern Healthcare, 30*(27), 14.

*Bowers, M. (1999). The JCAHO home health mock survey made simple. New York: Opus Communications.

*Disbrow, R. (1999). *The impact of prospective payment implementation on Medicare beneficiary access to home health services.* Unpublished master's thesis. Flint, MI: University of Michigan.

*Epstein, D. (1995). Struggling for recognition: Meet CHAP—the "other" accrediting body. *Infusion, 1*(7), 36–37.

*Flores, K. (1998). AIC—What's your role in the most talked about Delivery Model? *Infusion, 4*(11) 35–38.

*Griffin, K. (1998). Evolution of transitional care settings: Past, present, future. *AACN Clinical Issues, 9,* 398–408.

*Health Care Financing Administration. (1999). *Medicare health insurance manual (HIM)*. U.S. Department of Health and Human Services Washington, DC: Author.

*Intravenous Nurses Society. (1998). Revised intravenous nursing standards of practice. *Journal of Intravenous Nursing, 21*(Suppl. 1) 51–59.

*Intravenous Nurses Society. (2000). Revised intravenous nursing standards of practice. *Journal of Intravenous Nursing,* (in press).

*Levenson, S. (1998). Subacute settings: Making the most of a new model of care. *Geriatrics, 53,* 69–74.

*Liebert, L. & Bryant-Wimp, J. (1997). Ambulatory infusion centers: Hospitals survival in an outpatient world. *Infusion, 4*(3), 25–29.

Malone-Rising, D. (1994). The changing face of long-term care. *Nursing Clinics of North America, 29,* 417–426.

*Nazarko, L. (1998). Continuing to care. *Nursing Management, 5*(5), 29–33.

*Poole, S.M. & Nowobilski-Vasilios, A. (1999). To push or not to push. *Infusion, 5*(9), 53–55.

*Saladow, J. (1999). History in the making: Health care delivery and pump technology continue to evolve. *Infusion, 5*(9), 15–48.

Review Questions

Note: Questions below may have more than one right answer.

1. The fastest-growing alternate clinical setting for infusion is:

   A. Home care

   B. Hospice

   C. Ambulatory infusion center

   D. Long-term care

2. The plan of treatment in a home care program is written by the:

   A. Pharmacist

   B. Nurse

   C. Physician

   D. Branch manager

3. A case manager is responsible for which of the following activities?

   A. Initial assessment

   B. Development of a care plan

   C. Appropriate referral and follow-up

   D. All of the above

4. The most frequently prescribed home infusion therapy is:

   A. Antibiotics

   B. Parenteral nutrition

   C. Hydration

   D. All of the above

5. The most limiting control of the managed care system is:

   A. Preferred provider contracts

   B. Prior approval/authorization

   C. Utilization review

   D. All of the above

6. Capitation is a system of prepayment in which providers receive:

   A. Prepayment on a monthly basis

   B. Prepayment on a quarterly basis

   C. Payment based on utilization

   D. Increased payment on utilization

7. Types of patients admitted to subacute care facilities are:

   A. Patients with multiple body system complications

   B. Patients who are ventilator dependent

   C. Patients with complicated wounds

   D. Patients with endocarditis

8. One type of patient appropriate for services at an ambulatory infusion center is:

   A. A patient with inadequate insurance coverage

   B. A patient who is homebound

   C. A patient who is not homebound

   D. A patient who is totally independent

9. One type of infusion therapy administered for the long-term patient is:
   A. Enteral food supplements
   B. TPN
   C. Pain drug patches
   D. Antibiotic intramuscular injections

10. The need for infusion nurses in alternate clinical settings will increase because of their credentialing and high skill level in:
    A. Subacute hospitals
    B. Ambulatory infusion centers
    C. Long-term care
    D. All of the above

APPENDIX A

Licensed Practical/Vocational Nurse Role in Infusion Therapy

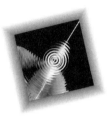

Many IV teams nationwide recognize the valuable contribution that a licensed practical/vocational nurse (LPN/LVN) may make as a member of an IV team. Other institutions have a career ladder and development for the LPN/LVN articulating to the professional registered nurse (RN) role.[2]

More than 20 states have identified that the LPN/LVN has a designated role in IV therapy; however, the scope of practice is left up to each individual state agency. States with these expanded role guidelines are identified in Box A–1.[1]

The states that identify the role of the LPN/LVN to include IV therapy, but who delegate the responsibility of education, competency, and role delineation to each agency, are found in Box A–2.[1]

Four states indicate that the role of the LPN/LVN is not in the maintenance or initiation of IV therapy. These are identified in Box A–3.[1]

The health care system in the United States is consistently challenged to deliver the highest level of care to the greatest number of people at the lowest cost. Nurse managers are now more than ever involved in managing the fiscal responsibility for their areas in addition to patient care. With an emphasis on re-engineering and restructuring the workload, many hospitals have added LPN/LVN and nurse extender positions at a lower cost than that of the professional RN. Given the acute nature of IV therapy, and the need for a highly trained professional to deliver this intense level of care, the workload for IV nurses has expanded dramatically, both within and outside the hospital setting. The RN may be responsible for mentoring an LPN/LVN in the IV nursing practice, consistent with the guidelines of the scope of practice for that level of caregiver.

The Intravenous Nurses Certification Corporation (INCC) has in the past provided an entry-level credential to those LPN/LVNs who achieve success in a standardized curriculum and who possess the body of knowledge and clinical skills to pass an examination administered by the INCC.

Currently, LPN/LVN responsibilities are limited by the guidelines of individual state nursing boards and institutional policy. LPN/LVN responsibilities usually do not include administration of IV medications, blood products, and antineoplastic agents. Routine duties include monitoring, dressing and tubing changes, and site maintenance.

BOX A–1 **States With Expanded Role Guidelines**

Alabama	Maryland
Alaska	Mississippi
Arizona	Missouri
California	Nevada
Colorado	New Hampshire
Connecticut	New York
Delaware	North Carolina
District of Columbia	Ohio
Florida	Oregon
Idaho	Pennsylvania
Kansas	South Carolina
Kentucky	South Dakota (adults only)
Louisiana	Wyoming
Maine	

BOX A–2 **States That Identify the Role of the LPN/LVN in IV Therapy***

Arkansas	Rhode Island
Georgia	Tennessee
Illinois	Texas
Indiana	Utah
Massachusetts	Vermont
Michigan	Virginia
Minnesota	Washington
Montana	West Virginia
New Mexico	Wisconsin
Oklahoma	

*All delegate the responsibility of education, competency, and role delineation to each agency.

BOX A–3 **States That Do Not Include IV Therapy in the Role of the LPN/LVN**

Hawaii
Iowa
Nebraska
New Jersey

References

1. Phillips, L. D. (1997). *Manual of IV therapeutics,* 2nd ed. Philadelphia: F. A. Davis.
2. Intravenous Nurses Society. (1998, 2000). Revised intravenous nursing standards of practice. *Journal of Intravenous Nursing (Supplement),* November 2000. Philadelphia: Lippincott Williams & Wilkins.

A P P E N D I X   B

Certification and Recertification

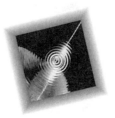

The Intravenous Nurses Certification Corporation (INCC) was created to develop and administer a credentialing program that meets judicial, regulatory, and professional testing standards (Box B–1). Although specialty nursing certification is voluntary, programs must exist for public protection and cannot violate antitrust legislation by restraining trade or restricting competition. Eligibility criteria for participants in credentialing programs should not be overly restrictive (Box B–2). Certification examinations must be flexible and open to innovation evidenced by empirical data, and they must reflect the skills and knowledge in the content area being assessed.

The benefits of certification are many. Registered nurses who become CRNIs demonstrate their commitment to their practice, improve their skills and knowledge about the specialty, enhance their professional image as IV therapy nurses, and provide better patient care. National certification ensures competency! National nursing certification provides the public with competent practitioners by validating the competency of practicing nurses.

In addition to inpatient programs, an increasing number of home infusion providers are acknowledging the value of having certified nursing professionals on their staffs. To promote nursing certification, the American Nurses Credentialing Center (ANCC) and several specialty nursing organizations established the National Credentialing Research Coalition (NCRC). The purpose of the coalition is to conduct quantitative and qualitative research on the impact, role, and benefits associated with the credentialing process. INCC is a member of the coalition. INCC also has also recently expanded the opportunities for recertification (Table B-1).

BOX B-1 **Intravenous Nurses Certification Corporation**

✔ Assesses, validates, and documents the clinical eligibility and continued clinical competency of nurses delivering IV therapy in all practice settings
✔ Validates reliability of credentialing mechanisms and their relationship to clinical practice
✔ Promotes recognition of credentialed nurses to the public, other health care organizations, and to the nursing profession

---

BOX B-2 **INCC Eligibility Criteria**

Eligibility Criteria

- Current RN license in U.S. or Canada
- Minimum 1600 hours of experience within the last two consecutive years prior to the date of application

Recertification by

- Continuing education
- Examination

T A B L E   B - 1
REVISED RECERTIFICATION OPPORTUNITIES

Education Program	Recertification Units
INS National Meetings	30 (minimum)
• Annual Meeting and Industrial Exhibition	
• National Academy of Intravenous Therapy	
• Other programs approved by INCC for recertification units	
Item Writers Workshops	10 (maximum)
INS Chapter education (accredited by the state nursing regulatory agency for continuing education)	5 (maximum)
Educator for clinical IV educational programs (accredited by the state nursing regulatory agency for continuing education	5 (maximum)
Continuing education through Journal of Intravenous Nursing	

Continuing Education Opportunities

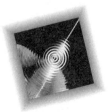

The nurse with an interest in infusion therapy has a multitude of educational opportunities available. Programs provided by the Intravenous Nurses Society also award recertification units for the credentialed intravenous nursing specialist. Providers of continuing education include:

- The Intravenous Nurses Society
  Annual meeting
  National Academy
  Continuing medical education programs
  Item writing workshops
  Core curriculum
  Journal of Intravenous Nursing
  Videotapes
  Audiotapes
  PICC educational series
- Local chapters of the Intravenous Nurses Society
- The Association for Parenteral and Enteral Nutrition
- The Association of Practitioners in Infection Control
- National Association of Vascular Access Nurses
- The Oncology Nursing Society
- Hospitals and home care agencies
- Internet resources

A P P E N D I X   D

Drug Enforcement Agency Schedules of Controlled Substances

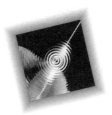

The Controlled Substances Act of 1970 regulates the manufacturing, distribution, and dispensing of drugs that are known to have abuse potential. The Drug Enforcement Agency (DEA) is responsible for the enforcement of these regulations. The controlled drugs are divided into five DEA schedules based on their potential for abuse and physical and psychological dependence.

Schedule I *(C-I):* High abuse potential and no accepted medical use (heroin, marijuana, LSD)

Schedule II *(C-II):* High abuse potential with severe dependence liability (narcotics, amphetamines, and barbiturates)

Schedule III *(C-III):* Less abuse potential than Schedule II drugs and moderate dependence liability (nonbarbiturate sedatives, nonamphetamine stimulants, limited amounts of certain narcotics)

Schedule IV *(C-IV):* Less abuse potential than Schedule III and limited dependence liability (some sedatives, antianxiety agents, and nonnarcotic analgesics)

Schedule V *(C-V):* Limited abuse potential. Primarily small amounts of narcotics (codeine) used as antitussives or antidiarrheals. Under federal law, limited quantities of certain Schedule V drugs may be purchased without a prescription directly from a pharmacist. The purchaser must be at least 18 years of age and must furnish suitable identification. All such transactions must be recorded by the dispensing pharmacist.

Prescribing physicians and dispensing pharmacists must be registered with the DEA, which also provides forms for the transfer of Schedule I and II substances and establishes criteria for the inventory and prescribing of controlled substances. State and local laws are often more stringent than federal law. In any given situation, the more stringent law applies.

MedWatch Reporting Form

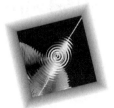

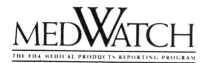

THE FDA MEDICAL PRODUCTS REPORTING PROGRAM

For **VOLUNTARY** reporting
by health professionals of adverse
events and product problems

Page _____ of _____

Form Approved: OMB No. 0910-0291 Expires: 12/31/94
See OMB statement on reverse

FDA Use Only **[DAVIS]**

Triage unit
sequence #

PLEASE TYPE OR USE BLACK INK

A. Patient information

1. Patient identifier

2. Age at time
of event:
or _____
Date
of birth:

In confidence

3. Sex
☐ female
☐ male

4. Weight
_____ lbs
or
_____ kgs

B. Adverse event or product problem

1. ☐ Adverse event   and/or   ☐ Product problem (e.g. defects/malfunctions)

2. Outcomes attributed to adverse event
(check all that apply)
☐ death _____ (mo day yr)
☐ life-threatening
☐ hospitalization – initial or prolonged
☐ disability
☐ congenital anomaly
☐ required intervention to prevent
permanent impairment/damage
☐ other: _____

3. Date of
event
(mo day yr)

4. Date of
this report
(mo day yr)

5. Describe event or problem

6. Relevant tests/laboratory data, including dates

7. Other relevant history, including preexisting medical conditions (e.g. allergies.
race. pregnancy. smoking and alcohol use. hepatic/renal dysfunction. etc.)

C. Suspect medication(s)

1. Name (give labeled strength & mfr/labeler, if known)
#1
#2

2. Dose, frequency & route used
#1
#2

3. Therapy dates (if unknown, give duration)
(from/to (or best estimate))
#1
#2

4. Diagnosis for use (indication)
#1
#2

5. Event abated after use
stopped or dose reduced
#1 ☐ yes ☐ no ☐ doesn't apply
#2 ☐ yes ☐ no ☐ doesn't apply

6. Lot # (if known)
#1
#2

7. Exp. date (if known)
#1
#2

8. Event reappeared after
reintroduction
#1 ☐ yes ☐ no ☐ doesn't apply
#2 ☐ yes ☐ no ☐ doesn't apply

9. NDC # (for product problems only)

10. Concomitant medical products and therapy dates (exclude treatment of event)

D. Suspect medical device

1. Brand name

2. Type of device

3. Manufacturer name & address

4. Operator of device
☐ health professional
☐ lay user/patient
☐ other: _____

5. Expiration date
(mo day yr)

6.
model # _____
catalog # _____
serial # _____
lot # _____
other # _____

7. If implanted, give date
(mo day yr)

8. If explanted, give date
(mo day yr)

9. Device available for evaluation?   (Do not send to FDA)
☐ yes   ☐ no   ☐ returned to manufacturer on _____ (mo day yr)

10. Concomitant medical products and therapy dates (exclude treatment of event)

E. Reporter (see confidentiality section on back)

1. Name, address & phone #

2. Health professional?
☐ yes ☐ no

3. Occupation

4. Also reported to
☐ manufacturer
☐ user facility
☐ distributor

5. If you do NOT want your identity disclosed to
the manufacturer, place an " X " in this box. ☐

FDA

Mail to: MEDWATCH   or FAX to:
5600 Fishers Lane   1-800-FDA-0178
Rockville, MD 20852-9787

FDA Form 3500 (6/93)   Submission of a report does not constitute an admission that medical personnel or the product caused or contributed to the event.

Recommended HIV Postexposure Follow-Up of Health Care Workers

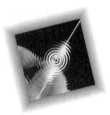

Time Post-exposure	Procedure and Comments
Less than 1 week	Informed consent should be obtained for a baseline HIV test. The legal implications of this test in terms of potential compensation claims should be explained. In Europe and in most states in the U.S., confidentiality of HIV test results is protected by law. The health care worker should be reassured of the confidentiality of test results at this point.
6 weeks	HIV test and physical examination. This marks the beginning of the period during which both acute infection and seroconversion are most likely to occur.
3 months	HIV test and physical examination. Testing at this point is required even if the 6-week test was negative, since seroconversion may have occurred in the interim.
6 months	HIV test and physical examination. It is unlikely that seroconversion will occur after this point, whether or not the health care worker has received post-exposure prophylaxis.
1 year	A final HIV test at 1 year may reassure health care workers who so far have had negative test results.

HIV, human immunodeficiency virus

Provisional Public Health Service Recommendations for Chemoprophylaxis After Occupational Exposure to HIV, by Type of Exposure and Source Material

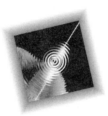

Type of Exposure	Source Material*	Antiretroviral Prophylaxis[†]	Antiretroviral Regimen[§]
Percutaneous	Blood[¶]		
	Highest risk	Recommend	ZDV plus 3TC plus IDV
	Increased risk	Recommend	ZDV plus 3TC, ± IDV**
	No increased risk	Offer	ZDV plus 3TC
	Fluid containing visible blood, other potentially infectious fluid[††], or tissue	Offer	ZDV plus 3TC
	Other body fluid (eg, urine)	Not offer	
Mucous membrane	Blood	Offer	ZDV plus 3TC, ± IDV**
	Fluid containing visible blood, other potentially infectious fluid[††], or tissue	Offer	ZDV, ±3TC
	Other body fluid (eg, urine)	Not offer	
Skin, increased risk[§§]	Blood	Offer	ZDV plus 3TC, ± IDV**
	Fluid containing visible blood, other potentially infectious fluid[††], or tissue	Offer	ZDV, ±3TC
	Other body fluid (eg, urine)	Not offer	

* Any exposure to concentrated HIV (eg, in a research laboratory or production facility) is treated as percutaneous exposure to blood with highest risk.

[†] *Recommend*—Postexposure prophylaxis (PEP) should be recommended to the exposed worker with counseling. *Offer*—PEP should be offered to the exposed worker with counseling. *Not offer*—PEP should not be offered because these are not occupational exposures to HIV (see *MMWR* 1990;39 [no.RR-1]:1).

[§] Regimens: zidovudine (ZDV), 200 mg three times a day; lamivudine (3TC), 150 mg two times a day; indinavir (IDV), 800 mg three times a day (if IDV is not available, saquinavir may be used, 600 mg three times a day). Prophylaxis is given for 4 weeks. For full prescribing information, see package inserts.

[¶] *Highest risk*—BOTH larger volume of blood (eg, deep injury with large diameter hollow needle previously in source patient's vein or artery, especially involving an injection of source patient's blood) AND blood containing a high titer of HIV (eg, source with acute retroviral illness or end-stage AIDS; viral load measurement may be considered, but its use in relation to PEP has not been evaluated). *Increased risk*—EITHER exposure to larger volume of blood OR blood with a high titer of HIV. *No increased risk*—NEITHER exposure to larger volume of blood NOR blood with a high titer of HIV (eg, solid suture needle injury from source patient with asymptomatic HIV infection).

** Possible toxicity of additional drug may not be warranted.

[††] Includes semen; vaginal secretions; cerebrospinal, synovial, pleural, peritoneal, pericardial, and amniotic fluids.

[§§] For skin, risk is increased for exposures involving a high titer of HIV, prolonged contact, an extensive area, or an area in which skin integrity is visibly compromised. For skin exposures without increased risk, the risk for drug toxicity outweighs the benefit of PEP.

Reprinted from *MMWR* 1996;45(no. 22):471.

A P P E N D I X   H

EPINet Postexposure Follow-Up Reporting Forms

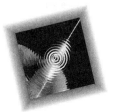

The Exposure Prevention Information Network (EPINet) forms that follow were developed to document elements of postexposure prophylaxis recommended by the Centers for Disease Control and Prevention (CDC) and to accommodate differences in follow-up protocols not to endorse any specific practices. If any of the following forms is photocopied so that the data appears both on the front and back of the page, the information cannot be detached or separated.

Postexposure Follow-Up

8/96

Date of Exposure:
month day year

EXPOSURE
PREVENTION
INFORMATION
NETWORK

Incident ID:

SOURCE PATIENT

1. Was the source patient identifiable?

☐ source known and tested   ☐ source known but not tested, reason: _____   ☐ source not known

2. Was the source patient positive for the pathogens below (even if tested before this exposure)?

PATHOGEN	TEST	RESULT			DATE DRAWN
Hepatitis B	HBsAg	☐ positive	☐ negative	☐ not tested	month day year
	HBeAg	☐ positive	☐ negative	☐ not tested	
	Anti HBs	☐ positive	☐ negative	☐ not tested	
	Anti HBc	☐ positive	☐ negative	☐ not tested	
Hepatitis C	Anti-HCV	☐ positive	☐ negative	☐ not tested	
	HCV-PCR	☐ positive	☐ negative	☐ not tested	
HIV	Anti-HIV	☐ positive	☐ negative	☐ not tested	
	#CD4 Cells	_____ count		☐ not tested	
	Antigen Load	_____ RNA copies/ml		☐ not tested	
	other				
Other					

3. If source patient was believed to be in high risk group for bloodborne pathogens, check all that apply:

☐ blood product recipient   ☐ elevated liver enzymes   ☐ sexual   ☐ dialysis
injection drug use   hemophilia   other, describe _____

4. If the source patient was HIV positive, had he been treated with any of the following before the exposure?

☐ Unknown   ☐ AZT   ☐ 3TC   ☐ ddC   ☐ IDV   ☐ other antiretroviral: _____

5. Additional source patient comments: _____

HEALTH CARE WORKER

1. Health care worker was seen by: ☐ Employee Health   ☐ Emergency Room   ☐ other, describe _____

2. Was the health care worker vaccinated against HBV before the exposure?   ☐ no   ☐ 1 dose   ☐ 2 doses   ☐ 3 doses

If yes, antibody level upon completion, if tested _____   Date antibodies tested: month year

3. Results of baseline tests:

PATHOGEN	TEST	RESULT			DATE DRAWN
Hepatitis B	HBsAg	☐ positive	☐ negative	☐ not tested	month day year
	HBeAg	☐ positive	☐ negative	☐ not tested	
	Anti HBs	☐ positive	☐ negative	☐ not tested	
	Anti HBc	☐ positive	☐ negative	☐ not tested	
Hepatitis C	Anti-HCV, EIA	☐ positive	☐ negative	☐ not tested	
	other assay, specify: _____	☐ positive	☐ negative	☐ not tested	
HIV	Anti-HIV	☐ positive	☐ negative	☐ not tested	
other	_____				
other	_____				

4. Check all post-exposure treatment/prophylaxis given to the health care worker and *fill in the dosage:*

TREATMENT	DOSE	DATE GIVEN	DURATION/COMMENTS
☐ IG	_____		
☐ HBIG	1_____ 2_____		
☐ HBV vaccine	1_____ 2_____ 3_____ Booster_____		
☐ AZT	_____		
☐ 3TC	_____		
☐ IDV	_____		
other, antiviral _____ other _____	_____		

5. Results of follow-up tests: (space is provided for repeated test results, however, testing protocols may vary in different institutions)

PATHOGEN	TEST		RESULT		DATE DRAWN		
	panel 1 HBsAg	☐ positive	☐ negative	☐ not tested	month	day	year
	Anti HBs	☐ positive	☐ negative	☐ not tested			
	Anti HBc	☐ positive	☐ negative	☐ not tested			
Hepatitis B	panel 2 HBsAg	☐ positive	☐ negative	☐ not tested			
	Anti HBs	☐ positive	☐ negative	☐ not tested			
	Anti HBc	☐ positive	☐ negative	☐ not tested			
	panel 3 HBsAg	☐ positive	☐ negative	☐ not tested			
	Anti HBs	☐ positive	☐ negative	☐ not tested			
	Anti HBc	☐ positive	☐ negative	☐ not tested			
Hepatitis C	Anti-HCV (test 1)	☐ positive	☐ negative	☐ not tested			
	Anti-HCV (test 2)	☐ positive	☐ negative	☐ not tested			
HIV	Anti-HIV (test 1)	☐ positive	☐ negative	☐ not tested			
	Anti-HIV (test 2)	☐ positive	☐ negative	☐ not tested			
	Anti-HIV (test 3)	☐ positive	☐ negative	☐ not tested			
	Anti-HIV (test 4)	☐ positive	☐ negative	☐ not tested			
other	_____	_____					
other	_____	_____					

6. Additional comments:

_____

_____

_____

EXPOSURE
PREVENTION
INFORMATION
NETWORK

Uniform Needlestick and Sharp Object Injury Report

6/96

Name: _____   Hospital ID: ☐☐☐

for office use only

1. ID: S ☐☐☐☐   **2. Date of injury:** ☐☐ ☐☐ ☐☐
(month / day / year)

3. Dept. where injury occurred: _____   **4. Home Dept.:** _____

5. Job Category: *(check one)*

1	M.D. *(attending/staff)*; specify specialty _____	10	clinical laboratory worker
2	M.D. *(intern/resident/fellow)*; specify specialty _____	11	technologist *(non-lab)*
3	medical student	12	dentist
4	nurse ____ specify ⟶	13	dental hygienist
5	nursing student	14	housekeeper
18	CNA	19	laundry worker
6	respiratory therapist/technician	20	security
7	surgery attendant	16	paramedic
8	other attendant	17	other student
9	phlebotomist/venipuncture/I.V. team	15	other, describe _____

nurse specify:
1 RN
2 LPN
3 NP
4 CRNA
5 midwife

6. Where did the injury occur? *(check one)*

1	patient room	9	dialysis facility *(hemodialysis and peritoneal dialysis)*
2	outside patient room *(hallway, nurses' station, etc.)*	10	procedure room *(x-ray, EMG, etc.)*
3	emergency department	11	clinical laboratories
4	intensive/critical care unit; specify type _____	12	autopsy/pathology
5	operating room	13	service/utility area *(laundry, central supply, loading dock, etc.)*
6	outpatient clinic/office	16	labor and delivery room
7	blood bank	17	home care
8	venipuncture center	14	other, describe _____

7. Was the source patient identifiable? *(check one)*

1 yes
2 no
3 unknown
4 not applicable

8. Was the injured worker the original user of the sharp item? *(check one)*

1 yes
2 no
3 unknown
4 not applicable

9. The sharp item was: *(check one)*

1 contaminated *(known exposure to patient or contaminated equipment)*
2 uncontaminated *(no known exposure to patient or contaminated equipment)*
3 unknown

10. For what purpose was the sharp item originally used: *(check one)*

1 unknown/not applicable
2 injection, intramuscular/subcutaneous, or other injection through the skin *(syringe)*
3 heparin or saline flush *(syringe)*
4 other injection into (or aspiration from) I.V. injection site or I.V. port *(syringe)*
5 to connect I.V. line *(intermittent I.V./piggyback/I.V. infusion/other I.V. line connection)*
6 to start I.V. or set up heparin lock *(I.V. catheter or Butterfly ™-type needle)*
16 to place an arterial/central line
7 to draw a venous blood sample ⎫
8 to draw an arterial blood sample ⎬ ———————⟶ if used to draw blood, was it a: 1 direct stick / 2 draw from a line
9 to obtain a body fluid or tissue sample *(urine/CSF/amniotic fluid/other fluid, biospy)*
10 fingerstick/heel stick
11 suturing
12 cutting
17 drilling
13 electrocautery
14 to contain a specimen or pharmaceutical *(glass items)*
15 other, describe _____

11. Did the injury occur: *(check one)*

1	before use of item *(item broke or slipped, assembling device, etc.)*
2	during use of item *(item slipped, patient jarred item, etc.)*
15	restraining patient
3	between steps of a multistep procedure *(between incremental injections, passing instruments, etc.)*
4	disassembling device or equipment
5	in preparation for reuse of reusable instrument *(sorting, disinfecting, sterilizing, etc.)*
6	while recapping a used needle
7	withdrawing a needle from rubber or other resistant material *(rubber stopper, I.V. port, etc.)*
16	device left on floor, table, bed, or other inappropriate place
8	other after use, before disposal *(in transit to trash, cleaning, sorting, etc.)*
9	from item left on or near disposal container
10	while putting the item into the disposal container
11	after disposal, stuck by item protruding from opening of disposal container
12	item pierced side of disposal container
13	after disposal, item protruded from trash bag or inappropriate waste container
14	other, describe _____

12. What device or item caused the injury?

(refer to list of items on attached page, enter item code here): [ ][ ] ➝ **If device defect was involved, specify manufacturer:**

If item is coded as "other" (29, 59, 79), then please describe the item: _____

13. If the item causing the injury was a needle, or sharp medical device, was it a "safety design" with a shielded, recessed, retractable, or blunted needle or blade?

1	yes
2	no/not applicable

14. Mark the location of the injury: ➝

15. Was the injury: *(check one)*

1	superficial *(little or no bleeding)*
2	moderate *(skin punctured, some bleeding)*
3	severe *(deep stick/cut, or profuse bleeding)*

16. If the injury was to the hands, did the sharp item penetrate: *(check one)*

1	single pair gloves
2	double pair gloves
3	no gloves

17. Was the injured worker: *(check one)*

1	right handed
2	left handed

18. Describe the circumstances leading to this injury: *(please note if a device malfunction was invovled)*

_____

_____

_____

_____

_____

_____

Costs: for office use only
(round to nearest dollar)

		lab charges, employee & source *(Hb, HIV, other tests)*
		treatment, prophylaxis *(HBIG, Hb vaccine, tetanus, AZT, other)*
		service charges *(Emerg. Dept., Empl. Health, other)*
		other costs *(Workers' Comp., surgery, other)*
		total

Is this incident OSHA reportable?
* Medical treatment (HBIG, Hepatitis vaccine, gamma globulin, AZT, etc.; not first aid, not tetanus)
* Restricted/lost work time; job transfer
* Illness/death

1	yes
2	no

If yes, enter:

		days away from work
		days restricted work activity

Does this incident meet the FDA medical device reporting criteria?

(yes if a device defect caused serious injury necessitating medical or surgical intervention, or death occurred within 10 work days of incident.)

1	yes
2	no

If yes, refer to EPINet manual for FDA reporting protocol.

E**XPOSURE**
P**REVENTION**
I**NFORMATION**
NETWORK

Uniform Blood and Body Fluid Exposure Report

6/96

Name: _____ Hospital ID: _____

for office use only

1. ID: B ☐☐☐☐

for office use only

2. Date of exposure: ☐ ☐ ☐

month　day　year

3. Dept. where exposure occurred: _____ **4. Home Dept.:** _____

5. Job Category: *(check one)*

1　M.D. *(attending/staff)*; specify specialty _____
2　M.D. *(intern/resident/fellow)*; specify specialty _____
3　medical student
4　nurse ——specify——➤　1 RN
5　nursing student　　　　　　2 LPN
18　CNA　　　　　　　　　　　3 NP
6　respiratory therapist　　　4 CRNA
7　surgery attendant　　　　5 midwife
8　other attendant
9　phlebotomist/venipuncture/I.V. team

10　clinical laboratory worker
11　technologist *(non-lab)*
12　dentist
13　dental hygienist
14　housekeeper
19　laundry worker
20　security
16　paramedic
17　other student
15　other, describe _____

6. Where did the exposure occur?　*(check one)*

1　patient room
2　outside patient room *(hallway, nurses' station, etc.)*
3　emergency department
4　intensive/critical care unit; specify type _____
5　operating room
6　outpatient clinic/office
7　blood bank
8　venipuncture center

9　dialysis facility *(hemodialysis and peritoneal dialysis)*
10　procedure room *(x-ray, EMG, etc.)*
11　clinical laboratories
12　autopsy/pathology
13　service/utility area *(laundry, central supply, loading dock, etc.)*
16　labor and delivery room
17　home care
14　other, describe _____

7. Was the source patient identifiable?　*(check one)*

1　yes
2　no
3　unknown
4　not applicable

8. Which body fluids were involved in the exposure?　*(check all that apply)*

☐ blood or blood products
☐ vomit
☐ sputum
☐ saliva
☐ CSF

☐ peritoneal fluid
☐ pleural fluid
☐ amniotic fluid
☐ urine
☐ other, describe _____

If the body fluid other than blood was visibly contaminated with blood, check here: ☐

9. Was the exposed part:　*(check all that apply)*

☐ intact skin
☐ non-intact skin
☐ eyes (conjunctiva)

☐ nose (mucosa)
☐ mouth (mucosa)
☐ other, describe _____

10. Did the blood or body fluid:　*(check all that apply)*

☐ touch unprotected skin
☐ touch skin between gap in protective garments
☐ soak through protective garment or barrier
☐ soak through clothing

11. Which items were worn at the time of the exposure?　*(check all that apply)*

☐ single pair latex/vinyl gloves
☐ double pair latex/vinyl gloves
☐ goggles
☐ eyeglasses
☐ eyeglasses with sideshields
☐ faceshield

☐ surgical mask
☐ surgical gown
☐ plastic apron
☐ lab coat, cloth
☐ lab coat, other _____
☐ other, describe _____

12. Was the exposure the result of: *(check one)*

1 | direct patient contact
2 | specimen container leaked/spilled
3 | specimen container broke
4 | I.V. tubing/bag/pump leaked/broke
10 | feeding/ventilator/other tube separated/leaked/splashed; specify tubing: _____
5 | other body fluid container spilled/leaked
6 | touched contaminated equipment/surface
7 | touched contaminated drapes/sheets/gowns, etc.
8 | unknown
9 | other, describe _____

If equipment failure, please specify: equipment type _____

manufacturer _____

13. For how long was the blood or body fluid in contact with your skin or mucous membranes?
(check one)

1 | less than 5 minutes
2 | 5-14 minutes
3 | 15 minutes to 1 hour
4 | more than 1 hour

14. Estimate the quantity of blood/body fluid that came in contact with your skin or mucous membranes: *(check one)*

1 | small amount *(up to 5 cc, or up to a teaspoon)*
2 | moderate amount *(up to 50 cc, or up to a quarter cup)*
3 | large amount *(more than 50 cc)*

15. Mark the size and location of the exposure:

Right

Left

Front

Back

16. Describe the circumstances leading to this exposure: (please note if equipment malfunction was involved)

_____

_____

_____

_____

_____

_____

Costs: for office use only
(round to nearest dollar)

lab charges, employee & source
(Hb, HIV, other tests)

treatment, prophylaxis
(HBIG, Hb vaccine, tetanus, AZT, other)

service charges
(Emerg. Dept., Empl. Health, other)

other costs
(Workers' Comp., surgery, other)

total

Is this incident OSHA reportable?

* Medical treatment (HBIG, Hepatitis vaccine, gamma globulin, AZT, etc.; not first aid, not tetanus)
* Restricted/lost work time; job transfer
* Illness/death

1 | yes
2 | no

If yes, enter:

_____ days away from work

_____ days restricted work activity

Does this incident meet the FDA medical device reporting criteria?

(yes if a device defect caused serious injury necessitating medical or surgical intervention, or death occurred within 10 work days of incident.)

1 | yes
2 | no

If yes, refer to EPINet manual for FDA reporting protocol.

Items Causing Needlestick and Sharp Object Injuries

3/96

NEEDLE
(for suture needle see "surgical instruments")

Item Codes

(1) disposable syringe *(includes standard syringes, insulin, tuberculin syringes)*
(2) prefilled cartridge syringe *(includes Tubex^{TM}/Carpuject^{TM}-type syringes)*
(3) blood gas syringe *(ABG)*
(4) syringe, other type
(5) needle on I.V. line *(includes piggybacks and I.V. line connectors)*
(6) winged steel needle I.V. set *(includes Butterfly^{TM}-type devices)*
(7) I.V. catheter *(stylet)*
(8) vacuum tube blood collection holder/needle *(includes VACUTAINER^{TM}-type devices)*
(9) spinal or epidural needle
(10) unattached hypodermic needle
(11) arterial catheter introducer needle
(12) central line catheter introducer needle
(13) drum catheter needle
(14) other vascular catheter needle *(cardiac, etc.)*
(15) other non-vascular catheter needle *(ophthalmology, etc.)*

(28) needle, not sure what kind
(29) other needle *(please describe device on the report form)*

SURGICAL INSTRUMENT OR OTHER SHARP ITEM
(for glass items see "glass")

(30) lancet *(finger or heel sticks)*
(31) suture needle
(32) scalpel, reusable (scalpel, disposable: code as 45)
(33) razor
(34) pipette *(plastic)*
(35) scissors
(36) electrocautery device
(37) bone cutter
(38) bone chip
(39) towel clip
(40) microtome blade
(41) trocar

(42) vacuum tube *(plastic)*
(43) specimen/test tube *(plastic)*
(44) fingernails/teeth
(45) scalpel, disposable
(46) retractors, skin/bone hooks
(47) staples/steel sutures
(48) wire *(suture/fixation/guide wire)*
(49) pin *(fixation/guide pin)*
(50) drill bit/bur
(51) pickups/forceps/hemostats/clamps

(58) sharp item, not sure what kind
(59) other sharp item *(please describe item on the report form)*

GLASS

(60) medication ampule
(61) medication vial *(small volume with rubber stopper)*
(62) medication/I.V. bottle *(large volume)*
(63) pipette *(glass)*
(64) vacuum tube *(glass)*
(65) specimen/test tube *(glass)*
(66) capillary tube
(67) glass slide

(78) glass item, not sure what kind
(79) other glass item *(please describe item on the report form)*

---

* Tubex^{TM} is a trademark of Wyeth Ayerst; Carpuject^{TM} is a trademark of Sanofi Winthrop; Butterfly^{TM} is a trademark of Abbott Laboratories; VACUTAINER^{TM} is a trademark of Becton Dickinson. Identification of these product categories does not imply involvement or endorsement of these specific brands.

A P P E N D I X I

Standards for Latex Allergy Precautions

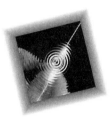

■ NURSING PRACTICE STANDARD

The nurse follows appropriate latex allergy precautions when caring for patients undergoing diagnostic tests and procedures. As allergy to latex products becomes more prevalent, both in the health care setting as well as the general environment, it becomes necessary for agencies to institute specific guidelines and protocols to maximize latex-free environments for patients and for health care personnel.

■ BACKGROUND INFORMATION

The rise in incidence of latex allergy may be attributed not only to increased use of latex products in patient care, especially since Standard Precautions have been mandated, but also to the ways raw latex is now collected and aged. Allergic reactions are caused by latex proteins retained in the finished products, which can then show great variations in latex allergen levels. Latex gloves and the powder from these gloves that becomes airborne produces the greatest environmental hazard exposure.

The Federal Drug Administration now requires that all medical devices containing natural rubber latex that may directly or indirectly contact the patient display the following statement: "THIS PRODUCT CONTAINS NATURAL RUBBER LATEX."
People at greatest risk include the following:

- Persons who frequently use or are exposed to latex products (eg, nurses, physicians, other health care workers, patients)
- Persons with spina bifida, spinal cord injury, or myelodysplasia
- Persons who have other allergies (eg, hay fever or fruit allergies)
- Persons with a chronic illness or a history of multiple surgeries
- Persons involved in the handling or manufacturing of latex
- Persons with atopic dermatitis or eczema
- Persons who have had intraoperative anaphylaxis for unknown reason

Increased exposure increases sensitivity to latex allergens.

■ SYMPTOMS OF LATEX ALLERGY

- Often begins with rash on hands (from gloves)
- Itchy, swollen eyes, runny nose, sneezing
- Asthma-like symptoms: chest tightness, wheezing, coughing, shortness of breath
- Anaphylactic shock (more rarely) is life-threatening. General hives, bronchospasm, hypotension, facial/laryngeal edema, tachycardia

■ LATEX ALLERGY PRECAUTIONS TO PROTECT THE PATIENT

Strategies and Protocols Include the Following:

- Identify allergic patients (history of problems related to condoms, latex gloves, balloons, toys, etc.); allergy testing may be desirable. Communicate and document data appropriately. Use signs and bracelets.
- Control latex in the environment by use of latex-free products, private room; don clean scrubs or uniform, cover, or gown.
- Avoid tissue contact with latex (wounds, mucous membranes, vaginal skin, etc.). PRACTICE PROPER HAND WASHING.

Note: Assembling and maintaining a cart with latex-free supplies and equipment may be desirable to facilitate safe patient care.

- Use latex-free products such as (list is not comprehensive):

Gloves	Stethoscopes
Endotracheal tubes	Temperature probe covers, tape, dressings,
Suction and wound drainage tubes and reservoir systems	"Ace" wraps
Catheters	Monitoring equipment and supplies (leads,
Blood pressure cuffs	pulse oximeter probes and cables)

Note: If latex-free blood pressure cuffs and stethoscopes are not available, shield the patient's arm with a stockinette and apply cuff over this. Small diameter (finger-sized) stockinette can be used to cover stethoscope tubing, leads, etc.

- Remove rubber stoppers from vials before withdrawing or reconstituting contents. Rinse syringes with sterile water or saline before use.
- Remove latex ports from IV tubing and replace with stopcocks or nonlatex plugs. Tape ports shut if no other alternative. Replace ports on IV bags with non-latex ports.
- Keep resuscitation equipment and emergency supplies and medications readily accessible at all times in the event that anaphylaxis occurs. (**Caution: Some resuscitation supplies and equipment may contain latex.**)
- Instruct the patient about latex-containig supplies—both medical and non-medical, which may pose problems (see lists).

THESE MEDICAL SUPPLY ITEMS FREQUENTLY CONTAIN LATEX (NOT ALL-INCLUSIVE):

Anesthesia equipment/ET tubes, airways
Bandaids/tapes

Bed protectors
Blood pressure tubing/cuffs
Bulb syringes
Catheters (many and varied types)
Dressings/elastic wraps
G-tubes/drains
IV access (Y-sites, tourniquets, adapters, etc.)
OR masks, hats, shoe covers
Oxygen masks/cannula/resuscitation devices
Suction equipment
Reflex hammers, syringes

THESE HOME/COMMUNITY ITEMS FREQUENTLY CONTAIN LATEX (NOT ALL-INCLUSIVE):

Balloons/toys/water toys and equipment
Art supplies (paint, glue, rubber bands, erasers, ink), kitchen gloves, appliance cords
Balls (tennis, koosh)
Carpet backing/rubber floors/cushions
Appliques (clothing); Spandex
Elastic in socks, underwear, etc.
Condoms/diaphragms
Crutch accessories (tips/grips)
Dental braces, chewing gum
Diapers/incontinence products
Feeding nipples/pacifiers
Handles on garden/sporting equipment
Tires, hoses

Note: If latex content is unknown, checking with the manufacturer or supplier before use is strongly advised.

The Spina Bifida Association of America publishes updated lists of products twice a year. Their address is:

Spina Bifida Association of America
4590 MacArthur Boulevard NW, Suite 250
Washington, DC 20007-4226
(800) 621-3141

■ LATEX ALLERGY PRECAUTIONS TO PROTECT *NURSES* AND OTHER HEALTH CARE *PERSONNEL*

Latex sensitivity is becoming a major health hazard to health care workers and workplace practices to reduce the incidence of exposure are absolutely necessary to maintain a safe environment for the caregivers.

- Use latex-free gloves whenever possible and keep exposure to latex at a minimum
- Advocate for and promote purchase of latex-free products that are of comparable function and quality.
- Practice frequent, proper hand washing.
- Observe all latex allergy precautions that apply to patients.

■ CLINICAL ALERT

Protocols for Management of an Allergic Reaction

- Maintain airway
- Administer oxygen
- Volume expansion (IV lactated Ringers or normal saline)
- Diphenhydramine
- Steroids
- Epinephrine
- Aminophylline

APPENDIX J

Websites of Interest to IV Nurses

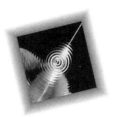

www.ins1.org
www.ons.org
www.aspen.org
www.nursingworld.org
www.nurseweek.com
www.wholenurse.com
www.springnet.com/top.htm
www.nih.gov/ninr/(research)
www.nursetutor.com
www.lib.uiowa.edu/hardin/md/nurs.html (Hardin Meta-Directory: Nursing Resources)
www.wwnurse.com
www.aone.org
www.cdc.gov/niosh/latexalt.html
www.latexallergyhelp.com
www.nursingcenter.com
www.cdc.gov
www.p4ps.com
www.paho.org
www.mederrors.com

Selected OSHA Guidelines to Enhance Safety in the Workplace

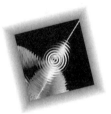

The Occupational Safety and Health Administration (OSHA) issued a revised Compliance Directive in November 1999 to meet part of its three-pronged plan to address the use of safer engineering controls in the healthcare workplace. The directive outlines, among other things, requirements for the adoption of sharps injury prevention devices, and will be used by OSHA compliance officers to establish uniform procedures for enforcing the bloodborne pathogen standard issued in December 1991. Recommendations for injury reporting and medical follow-up are reproduced below.

■ INJURY REPORTING AND MEDICAL FOLLOW-UP

Reporting of needlestick and sharps injuries is an essential component of an overall program to reduce occupational risk of needlestick injuries and bloodborne pathogen infections. Because such injuries also require urgent medical attention, protocols in place at health care organizations should also mandate procedures for timely medical evaluation and follow-up care of exposed workers.

It is likely that health care workers engaged in direct patient care and others providing certain support services may incur several needlestick or sharp object injuries during the course of their careers; however, up to 75% of these injuries are never reported. Cited reasons for failure to report include a belief that the risk of infection is low, concerns about confidentiality, or fears of reprisal and job discrimination. Also, the worker may not know that documentation of the injury is necessary to qualify for workers' compensation, or may not be aware of the urgency in providing postexposure preventive therapy immediately in order to enhance its effectiveness. Or finally, the worker may simply not know the proper procedure for reporting the injury.

For these reasons, workers must receive appropriate training and education on the need for prompt reporting of needlestick injuries and the procedures to follow when an incident occurs. They must be assured that confidentiality will be maintained during all reporting, counseling, and medical follow-up and should be made aware of the importance of prompt reporting so that, if needed, postexposure medical evaluation and treatment can begin immediately. Human immunodeficiency virus (HIV) postexposure prophylaxis, for example, is most effective if given within a few hours of the injury. Workers must also be assured that reporting of injuries will not result in disciplinary actions. Health care workers who are infected with bloodborne pathogens as a result of needlestick injuries on the job should be aware that if needlestick injuries are not reported, they are at risk of being left without workers' compensation coverage.

In the United States, hospitals are required to maintain records of health care workers' injuries and illnesses resulting from exposures to blood and body fluids. However, the criteria for defining cases for which records must be maintained vary from one health care facility to another. At the national level, criteria for recording of needlestick injuries have been established by the Occupational Safety and Health Administration (OSHA) under the Bloodborne Pathogen Standard of 1991. The Food and Drug Administration (FDA) also requires the reporting of certain needlestick injuries as part of the Safe Medical Device Act of 1990. At the state level, workers' compensation insurance carriers impose specific recordkeeping requirements related to compensable injuries and exposures. The result is a patchwork of requirements and policies that vary in recordkeeping methods and criteria for reporting and recording injuries.

At present, many hospitals have multiple recordkeeping systems in place for occupational exposures to bloodborne pathogens, including needlestick injuries. One system might be individual worker medical records for documenting exposures that require postexposure medical follow-up. Another might be a log of injuries to meet the OSHA requirement for documenting certain reportable injuries. Another might be focused recordkeeping of needlestick injuries and blood exposures for tracking the effectiveness of prevention efforts. Many of these systems may have redundant information and may not be practical for documenting and preventing exposures. Unfortunately, there is no national standard outlining the specific requirements for documenting, recording, and tracking all potentially hazardous needlestick injuries and other blood exposures.

The federal reporting requirements for needlestick and sharps injuries outlined here are mandated by law and must be incorporated into any system for recording such injuries. Even if the law does not require reporting of an incident, certain records must be kept for each exposure incident, including the route and circumstances of the exposure, and medical follow-up. These requirements also are included. Hospitals also should consult their specific state workers' compensation insurance carriers for additional reporting requirements, as well as other state mandates, such as requirements from state-approved OSHA plans. State-approved OSHA plans are listed, along with mailing addresses and telephone numbers in Box K–1.

■ OSHA REPORTING REQUIREMENTS

Under OSHA's reporting requirements for exposures to bloodborne pathogens, not all needlestick and sharp object injuries are required to be reported on the OSHA 200 Log of Occupational Illness and Injury; a determination must be made for each exposure incident.

Criteria for Reportable Incidents

A bloodborne pathogen-related injury or exposure (eg, needlestick, laceration, or splash) is to be reported on the OSHA 200 log if it meets one of the following criteria:

- The incident is work-related and involves loss of consciousness, transfer to another job, or restriction of work.

BOX K-1 Occupational Safety and Health Administration Regional Offices and State-Approved OSHA Plans

---

Region I (CT*, MA, ME, NH, RI, VT*)
JFK Federal Building, Room E 340
Boston, MA 02203
(617) 565-9860

Region II (NJ, NY*, PR*, VI*)
201 Varick Street, Room 670
New York, NY 10014
(212) 337-2378

Region III (DC, DE, MD*, PA, VA*, WV)
Gateway Building, Suite 2100
3535 Market Street
Philadelphia, PA 19104
(215) 596-1201

Region IV (AL, FL, GA, KY*, MS, NC*, SC*, TN*)
1375 Peachtree Street NE, Suite 587
Atlanta, GA 30367
(404) 347-3573

Region V (IL, IN*, MI*, MN*, OH, WI)
230 South Dearborn Street, Room 3244
Chicago, IL 60604
(312) 353-2220

Region VI (AR, LA, NM*, OK, TX)
525 Griffin Street, Room 602
Dallas, TX 75202
(214) 767-4731

Region VII (IA*, KS, MO, NE)
1100 Main Street, Suite 800
Kansas City, MO 64105
(816) 426-5861

Region VIII (CO, MT, ND, SD, UT*, WY*)
Federal Building, Suite 1690
1999 Broadway
Denver, CO
(303) 844-1600

Region IX (American Samoa, AZ*, CA*, Guam, HI*, NV*,
Trusts Territories of the Pacific)
71 Stevenson Street, 4th Floor
San Francisco, CA 94105
(415) 975-4310

Region X (AK*, ID, OR*, WA*)
1111 Third Avenue, Suite 715
Seattle, WA 98101-3212
(206) 535-5930

---

* These states and territories operate their own OSHA-approved job safety and health programs (Connecticut and New York plans cover public employees only). States with approved programs must have a standard that is identical to, or at least as effective as, the federal standard.

- The incident results in the administration or recommendation of medical treatment beyond first aid (eg, immune serum globulin, hepatitis B immune globulin, hepatitis B vaccine, zidovudine, or other prescription medications, regardless of the dosage).
- The incident results in the diagnosis of a seroconversion (reported as the nature or type of exposure) without revealing the employee's seroconversion status.

The employer is required to enter each reportable injury in the OSHA 200 log within six working days after information that the injury occurred is received. OSHA also requires specific information about each case, including number of workdays lost, number of days of restricted work activity, and date of death for fatalities. For each entry on the 200 log, OSHA also requires that an additional form (OSHA Form 101) be filled out providing a description of the incident or that a comparable workers' compensation report by compiled. OSHA will ask to see these forms during any worksite inspection. Additional information on OSHA reporting requirements can be found at OSHA's Internet site (http://www.osha.gov).

Maintaining Confidentiality

Because the OSHA 200 log is available to other employees and their representatives, concern has been expressed over possible violations of confidentiality of workers who may be HIV-positive. OSHA's position is that these events (eg, needlestick injuries, lacerations, etc.) are reported on the log as an injury and not as a seroconversion. This approach should allow the employer to record the case and provide access to other employees without revealing the seroconversion status of the affected worker.

Information About Exposures That Must be Documented

All workers who sustain needlestick injuries or other bloodborne pathogen exposures, regardless of whether the incident is reportable, must receive a confidential postexposure medical evaluation and follow-up immediately after the exposure incident. A mechanism must be established to document the route(s) of exposure and circumstances under which the incident occurred. This information can be used to focus efforts to reduce or eliminate incidents and exposure routes—by using safety devices, for example. Employers need this information to comply with OSHA's requirements that they have an exposure control plan in place.

Information to be Reported in the Employee's Health Record

OSHA's Bloodborne Pathogen Standard specifies that confidential employee medical records must be kept following an injury or exposure incident, including the following information:

- Evaluation of the exposure incident
- Collection and testing of the source individual's blood for hepatitis B virus (HBV), hepatitic C virus (HCV), and HIV serological status, if not already known
- Collection and testing of employee's blood for HBV, HCV, and HIV status
- Postexposure prophylaxis when medically indicated, according to U.S. Public Health Service recommendations in effect at the time of the exposure
- Counseling given
- Evaluation of any reported illnesses related to the exposure incident

Prompt reporting and recordkeeping further enables employers to understand the circumstances surrounding the exposure incident so that additional injuries can be prevented.

Other Data Reporting Considerations

OSHA's reporting requirements were designed to be uniform across many types of occupational hazards and settings, including manufacturing and construction. Consequently, many needlestick injuries do not meet the agency's criteria for reportable injuries. According to one report, fewer than 20% of bloodborne pathogen exposures, including needlestick injuries and mucocutaneous exposures, meet OSHA's criteria as reportable injuries.

At the state level, workers' compensation insurance carriers impose additional record-keeping requirements related to potentially compensable injuries or adverse exposures. Individual hospitals may also establish additional criteria for including or excluding exposure reports based on instituional infection control policies or legal liability considerations.

All states must have a bloodborne pathogen program, including reporting of needlestick injuries, that is at least as effective as the federal standard. States that operate their own OSHA-approved safety and health program are free to adopt more stringent requirements. Hospitals in these states should consult their state OSHA program.

■ SPECIAL REQUIREMENTS OF CALIFORNIA OSHA

In September 1998, the state OSHA-approved program in California was mandated by a state law to revise its bloodborne pathogen standard by August 1, 1999, to include a component for recording of exposure incidents in a sharps injury log, and the type and brand of the device involved in the injury (California Assembly Bill 1208). The law also mandates that the revised bloodborne pathogen standard must require employers to implement sharps injury prevention technology as an engineering control and that written exposure control plans include an effective procedure for identifying and selecting sharps injury prevention technology that is updated when necessary to reflect progress in implementation.

A temporary law was scheduled to be in place Jan. 15, 1999. (Additional information on this law is available at http://www.assembly.ca.gov.)

■ FDA REQUIREMENTS

The FDA's Medical Device Reporting (MDR) regulations, part of the Safe Medical Device Act of 1990, give the agency authority to require that manufacturers, distributors, and device users submit reports on certain types of medical device-related errors. A reportable event for a *device user facility* (eg, a hospital) is an event in which there is information that reasonably suggests that a device has or may have contributed to a death or serious injury. This includes events occurring as a result of failure, malfunction, improper or inadequate design, manufacture, labeling, or user error.

The device user facility is required to report the event to the device manufacturer and, in case of a death or serious injury, must also send a copy of the report of the FDA. Device user facilities include hospitals, nursing homes, ambulatory surgical facilities, and outpatient diagnostic or treatment facilities. Outpatient treatment facilities include home health agencies, ambulance providers, rescue services, and blood banks. Under nursing home services are included hospice care and rehabilitation services. Private physician and dental offices and private offices of health care practitioners are *not* considered to be device user facilities.

In addition to individual device reports, medical facilities must also submit semiannual reports to the FDA and maintain files related to reportable events for two years. Further, medical facilities must establish written procedures for reporting adverse medical device events that include (1) procedures for timely and effective identification and evaluation of events, (2) a standardized review process and procedure for determining whether events are reportable, (3) procedures to assure the timely submission of complete reports, and (4) mechanisms to assure compliance with documentation and recordkeeping requirements.

Reportable Needlestick Injuries

The FDA has issued a guidance document for determining when an event involving a needlestick injury is a reportable event. The FDA has concluded that an injury is reportable by the user facility if it involves a *malfunction* of the device that would likely cause or contribute to death or serious injury if it were to recur. Although user facilities are not required to report events that have not caused or contributed to serious injury or death, the FDA is encouraging health care practitioners to voluntarily report all medical device malfunctions and defective equipment under a program called MEDWatch.

Users, distributors, and manufacturers are exempt from reporting needlestick injuries that are due exclusively to user error and result in injuries that are not life threatening. Reports of deaths and life-threatening injuries due to user error or malfunctions must continue to be reported.

Copies of the regulations, guidance documents, forms, and instructions for MDR Reporting and MEDWatch are available from the FDA on the Internet (MDR Reporting: http://www.fda.gov/cdrh/mdr.html; MEDWatch: http://www.fda.gov/medwatch/report/hcp.htm).

Specific questions should be faxed to (301) 827-0039 or mailed to: Food and Drug Administration, Center for Devices and Radiological Health, Division of Surveillance Systems (HFZ-530), Medical Device Reporting (MDR) Inquiries, 1350 Piccard Drive, Rockville, MD 20850.

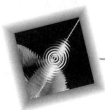

Answers to Questions

CHAPTER 1

1. C
2. A, B, C, D
3. A
4. B
5. B, C

CHAPTER 2

1. B
2. C
3. C
4. A
5. A
6. C
7. B
8. D
9. A, B, C
10. A, B, C

CHAPTER 3

1. D
2. A
3. A
4. A, B
5. B
6. D
7. A
8. D
9. D
10. C

CHAPTER 4

1. D
2. A
3. C
4. A, B, C, D
5. D
6. A, B, C
7. D

8. C
9. C

CHAPTER 5

1. B
2. A, B, C, D
3. C
4. A
5. D
6. A, B, C
7. C
8. D
9. D
10. A

CHAPTER 6

1. A, B, C, D
2. A, B, C
3. A, B
4. A, B
5. C
6. A, B
7. D
8. D
9. C
10. C

CHAPTER 7

1. A
2. D
3. A
4. A
5. A, B
6. A
7. A, B, C, D
8. A, B, C
9. A
10. B

CHAPTER 8

1. B
2. A
3. A
4. B, C
5. A
6. A
7. B
8. B
9. A, B
10. A

CHAPTER 9

1. A
2. A
3. D
4. B
5. D
6. A, B
7. D
8. D
9. D
10. B

CHAPTER 10

1. C
2. B
3. A
4. D
5. A, B
6. D
7. A, B, C, D
8. B
9. A
10. B

CHAPTER 11

1. D
2. A
3. D
4. A, B, C
5. A, C
6. C
7. D
8. A
9. D
10. B, C, D

CHAPTER 12

1. A
2. D
3. D
4. A
5. A
6. C, D
7. D
8. D
9. B
10. A

CHAPTER 13

1. B
2. B, C, D
3. A
4. B
5. B
6. D
7. A, B
8. D
9. B
10. B

CHAPTER 14

1. D
2. D
3. A
4. B
5. B
6. C
7. B
8. C
9. D
10. A

CHAPTER 15

1. A
2. A
3. B, C
4. D
5. D
6. D
7. A

8. B
9. C
10. A, B, C

CHAPTER 16

1. C
2. B
3. D
4. C
5. A
6. D
7. B
8. D
9. A
10. D

CHAPTER 17

1. A
2. C
3. A, B
4. A
5. B
6. C
7. A
8. B
9. C
10. B

CHAPTER 18

1. D
2. C
3. A, B, C, D
4. B
5. A, B, C
6. D
7. D
8. C
9. D
10. D

CHAPTER 19

1. B
2. D
3. A
4. C
5. D
6. C
7. B
8. D
9. C
10. B

CHAPTER 20

1. D
2. A
3. D

4. B
5. B
6. D
7. A
8. C
9. D
10. A

CHAPTER 21

1. A
2. B
3. D
4. B
5. D
6. A
7. C
8. A
9. C
10. D

CHAPTER 22

1. D
2. B
3. A, B
4. C
5. C
6. B
7. C
8. D
9. A
10. D

CHAPTER 23

1. A
2. C
3. D
4. A
5. B
6. A
7. A, B, C
8. C
9. B
10. D

Glossary

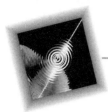

ABO system — a basic hereditary blood group system used to classify a person's blood group

Absorption — process by which medication moves from drug administration sites to vasculature

Acidosis — blood pH below normal (<7.35)

Active transport — the passage of a substance across a cell membrane by an energy-consuming process, permitting diffusion to occur

Adjuvant chemotherapy — the addition of drug therapy to surgery and/or radiation therapy to eradicate metastatic disease

Admixture — combination of two or more medications

Adsorption — attachment of one substance to the surface of another

Agglutination — clumping of red blood cells when incompatible bloods are mixed

Agglutinin — an antibody causing agglutination with its corresponding antigen

Alkalosis — blood pH above normal (>7.45)

Alkylating agents — agents that kill cells by cross-linking DNA strands (ie, disturbing the normal structure) in the DNA molecule

Alopecia — the loss of hair from the body and/or the scalp

Alpha (α)(1) — the level of statistical significance designating the probability of committing a type I error. Also known as the p value; (2) a reliability coefficient, such as Cronbach's alpha, to estimate internal consistency

Alternate site care — care that is delivered beyond the confines of an inpatient facility

Ambulatory infusion device — electronic infusion device specifically designed to be worn on the body to promote patient mobility and independence in the home or work environment

Analgesia — freedom from nociceptive stimuli; absence of pain

Analogue — a compound that resembles another in structure (eg, fluorouracil is an analogue of uracil)

Anorexia — absence or loss of appetite for food

Antibody — a substance present in the plasma that incites immunity and that can react with the specific antigen that caused its production

Antidiuretic hormone (ADH) — hormone secreted from a pituitary mechanism that causes the kidneys to conserve water

Anti-free-flow administration set — an IV administration device that stops when removed from the electronic infusion device, yet allows gravity flow when the user takes action

Antigen — an immunizing agent capable of inducing the body to form antibodies

Antimetabolites — anticancer drugs that substitute for or block the use of an essential metabolite

Antimicrobial — an agent that destroys or prevents development of microorganisms

Antimicrobial ointment — a semisolid preparation used to prevent the pathogenic action of microbes

Antineoplastic agent — a medication or treatment for cancer

Antitumor antibiotics — anticancer drugs that interfere with cellular production of DNA and/or RNA

Arterial pressure monitoring — monitoring of arterial pressure through an indwelling arterial catheter connected to an electronic monitor

Arteriovenous (AV) fistula — the surgical anastomosis of an artery and vein

Arteriovenous (AV) grafts — the insertion of a synthetic device connecting a vein and an artery

Aseptic technique — mechanism employed to reduce potential contamination

Assay determination — decision based upon an analysis and/or examination

Auscultation — process of listening to or for sounds in the body

Autologous — products or components of the same individual

Bacteria — microorganisms that may potentiate disease and infection

Benchmarking — comparing one's systems to others

Beta (β)(1) — statistical testing term referring to the probability of making a type II error; (2) the standardized regression coefficient in the regression equation indicating the relative weights of the independent variables

Biotransformation-metabolism — the enzymatic alteration of a drug molecule

Blood grouping — the testing of red blood cells to determine antigens present and absent

Body surface area — surface area of the body determined through use of a nomogram; important when calculating drug dosages

Bone marrow — the inner spongy tissue of a bone in which red blood cells, white blood cells, and platelets are formed

Cancer — the general name for more than 100 diseases in which abnormal cells grow out of control; a malignant tumor

Cannula — a hollow tube made of plastic or metal; used for accessing the vascular system

Catheter — a hollow tube made of plastic for accessing the vascular system

Cell kill — the number of cancer cells killed at a given dose by an antineoplastic drug

Cellular kinetics — study of mechanisms and rates of cellular changes

Chemical incompatibility — a change in the molecular structure or pharmacologic properties of a substance, which may or may not be visually observed

Chemotherapy — the chemical treatment for cancer patients with agents designed to kill cancer cells

Cognitive — behaviors that place primary emphasis on mental or intellectual processes

Cold agglutinin — a red blood cell agglutinin that acts at a relatively low temperature; part of a disease process caused by a transient infectious disease; may be idiopathic

Color coding — system developed by manufacturers that identifies products/medications by the use of a color system. These color code systems are not standardized and may vary with manufacturer.

Compartment syndrome — compression of circulation evidenced by impaired pulses, compromised circulation, and pain

Compatibility — capacity for being mixed and administered without undergoing undesirable chemical and/or physical changes or loss of therapeutic action

Compatibility test — all tests performed on donors and recipients to determine compatibility of blood; also known as *cross matching*

Complement — a group of proteins in normal blood serum and plasma that, in combination with antibodies, cause the destruction of particular antigens

Contamination — introduction of pathogens or infectious material from one source to another

Corrective action — a defined plan to eliminate deficiencies

Cross-contamination — movement of pathogens from one source to another

Curative — healing or corrective

Cutdown — surgical procedure for exposure and catheterization of a vein

Delayed reaction — in relation to blood transfusions, adverse effect occurring after 48 hours and up to 180 days after the transfusion

Delivery system — product that facilitates administration of drug(s); can be integral or have component parts. Delivery systems encompass all products used, from the solution container down to the cannula.

Dermatomes — segmental distribution of the spinal nerves. Dermatomes are labeled according to their exit point on the spinal cord. The spinal canal has 31 dermatomes. Dermatome pathways are not defined or determined through dissection, but by observation of patients with spinal cord injuries for the resultant neurologic effects.

Diffusion — passage of molecules of one substance between the molecules of another to form a mixture of the two

Disinfectant — an agent that eliminates all microorganisms except spores; generally used on inanimate objects

Distal — furthest from the heart; furthest from point of attachment; below previous site of catheterization

Distention — expansion due to pressure within

Document — a written or printed record that contains original, official, or legal information

Documentation — a recording in written or printed form containing original, official, or legal information

Dome — a plastic component used in hemodynamic monitoring

Dose-limiting toxicity — the degree of toxicity that dictates the maximum amount of drug that safely can be administered

Drug-nutrient interaction — an event that occurs when nutrient availability is altered by a medication or when a drug effect is altered, or an adverse reaction caused by the intake of nutrients

Ecchymoses — bruising resulting from escape of blood from injured vessels

Electronic infusion device — an electronic instrument that regulates the flow rate of the prescribed therapy; often referred to as an EID

Embolus — a blood clot or other foreign substance that is carried in the blood stream; has the potential to impede and/or obstruct circulation

Enteral nutrition — nutrition provided via the gastrointestinal tract

Epidemiology — the division of medical science concerned with defining and explaining the interrelationships of the host, agent, and environment in causing disease

Epidural — a potential space that is part of the spinal canal outside the dura mater. This space contains a network of large and thin-walled veins as well as fat that is proportional in volume to a person's body fat.

Epithelialized — the growth of epithelial cells over a wound or over and around a catheter site

Erythema — redness

Extravasation — inadvertent escape of a solution or medication (usually a vesicant) into surrounding tissue

Filter — a porous device used to prevent the passage of undesired substances

Filtration — process of passing fluid through a filter using pressure

Free-flow — nonregulated, inadvertent administration of fluid

Fungi — vegetable cellular organisms that subsist on organic matter

Gram negative bacteria — organisms that remain unstained by Gram's method, *including Klebsiella, Escherichia coli, Pseudomonas, Serratia,* etc.; associated with infusate contamination and arterial catheters

Gram positive bacteria — organisms holding the dye after being stained by Gram's method, including *Staphylococcus aureus, S, epidermidis,* and others; associated with venous catheter contamination

Grounded theory — theory that is constructed from theoretical propositions based on data obtained in the real world

Hematocrit — an expression of the volume of red cells per unit of circulating blood

Hematogenous — produced by or derived from the blood; disseminated through the bloodstream or via circulation

Hemodynamic pressure monitoring — the measurement of pulmonary artery pressure, arterial pressure, cardiac output, and so forth, via an electronic monitor and internally placed catheter

Hemoglobin — the iron-containing pigment of red blood cells; functions primarily in transporting oxygen from the lungs to the body tissues

Hemolysis — rupture of the red blood cell membrane causing the release of hemoglobin

Hemorrhage — abnormal discharge of blood, either external or internal

Hemostasis — cessation of the flow of blood through a port or vessel

HLA system — human leukocyte antigens; a complex array of genes that are involved in immune system regulation and cell differentiation

Homeostasis — ability to restore equilibrium under stress

Hypercalcemia — serum calcium concentrations above normal levels

Hyperkalemia — excess of potassium in the blood

Hypertonic — solution more concentrated than that with which it is compared; a fluid having a concentration greater than the normal tonicity of plasma

Hyperuricemia — uric acid blood concentrations above normal levels

Hypokalemia — low potassium concentration in the blood

Hypotonic — solution less concentrated than that with which it is compared; a fluid having a concentration less than the normal tonicity of plasma

IgA — immunoglobulin A; a class of immunoglobulins in body secretions

IgG — immunoglobulin G; a class of immunoglobulins or circulating antibodies in the blood that frequently causes sensitization

IgM — immunoglobulin M; a class of immunoglobulins or circulating antibodies in the blood that is capable of binding complement

Immediate reaction — in blood transfusions, an adverse effect occurring immediately or up to 48 hours after the transfusion

Immunocompromised — decreased resistance to disease

Immunoglobulin — a protein with antibody activity

Immunohematology — the study of blood and blood reactions

Implanted port or pump — vascular access device placed totally beneath the skin surface by surgical procedure

Incident — an unusual occurrence that requires documentation and action because of potential or implied consequences

Incompatible — incapable of being mixed or used simultaneously without undergoing chemical or physical changes or producing undesirable effects

Infection — invasion of the body by living microorganisms

Infiltration — the inadvertent administration of a nonvesicant solution or medication into surrounding tissues

Infusate — parenteral solution administered into the vascular system

Integumentary — cutaneous; dermal

Intermittent intravenous therapy — IV therapy administered at prescribed intervals with periods of infusion cessation

Interval variables — consisting of an ordered set of categories if categories form a set of intervals that are all exactly the same

Intraosseous — within the cavity of a bone that is filled with marrow

Intrathecal — a space that contains cerebral spinal fluid and bathes the spinal cord. The intrathecal space runs parallel to the epidural space. The two spaces are separated by the dura mater.

Intrinsic contamination — contamination during product manufacture

Isolation — the separation of potentially infectious persons and/or materials

Isotonic — solution having the same concentration as that with which it is compared (ie, plasma)

Laminar flow hood — a contained work area in which the air flow within the area moves with uniform velocity along parallel flow lines with a minimum of eddies

Latex injection port — a resealable rubber cap designed to accommodate needles for administration of solutions into the vascular system

Leukopenia — total number of leukocytes in the circulating blood less than normal, the lower limit of which generally is regarded as $5000/\mu L$

Lumen — the interior space of a tubular structure, such as a blood vessel or cannula

Lymphedema — swelling of an extremity caused by obstruction of the lymphatic vessel(s)

Malignancy — uncontrolled growth and dissemination of a neoplasm

Malnutrition — any disorder of nutritional status including those resulting from a deficient intake of nutrients, impaired nutrient metabolism, or overnutrition

Medical act — procedure performed by a licensed physician

mEq — the measure of the chemical-combining power of an ion with hydrogen

Metastasis — the spread of cancer to sites distant from the site of origin

Microabrasion — break in skin integrity, which may predispose the patient to infection

Microaggregate — microscopic collection of particles, such as platelets, leukocytes, and fibrin, that occurs in stored blood

Microaggregate blood filter — filter that removes potentially harmful microaggregates and reduces nonhemolytic febrile reactions

Microorganisms — extremely minute living matter which can only be seen with the aid of a microscope

Midline — peripherally inserted catheter with tip terminating in the proximal portion of the extremity, usually 6 inches in length

Monoclonal antibody — antibody produced by a clone of cells derived from a single cell in large quantities for use against a specific antigen

Morbidity — number of infected persons or cases of infection in relation to a specific population

Mortality — ratio of number of deaths in a population to number of individuals in that population

Multiple-dose vial — medication bottle that is hermetically sealed with a rubber stopper and designed to be entered more than one time

Nadir — the lowest level; in chemotherapy, the nadir is the lowest level to which the blood count drops in response to an antineoplastic agent.

Needle — a slender, pointed, hollow metal device

Neoplasm — a new growth or tumor, either benign or malignant

Nitrosoureas — anticancer drugs that produce metabolites that attack DNA in a manner analogous to alkylating agents

Nominal variables — names of categories

Nonpermeable — able to maintain integrity

Nonvesicant — intravenous medications, including, but not limited to, medications administered for cancer; these medications generally do not cause damage or sloughing of tissue

Nutrient — proteins, carbohydrates, lipids, vitamins, minerals, trace elements, and water

Nutritional assessment — a comprehensive evaluation to define nutritional status; includes medical history, dietary history, physical examination, anthropometric measurements, and laboratory data

Nutritional screening — the process of identifying characteristics known to be associated with nutrition problems, particularly in individuals who are at risk for malnutrition or who are malnourished

Nutritional support — provision of specially formulated and/or delivered parenteral or enteral nutrients to maintain or restore optimal nutrition status

Occlusion — a blockage; may result from precipitation or clot formation

Oncology — the study of tumors

Oncotic — within the tissue; tissue pressure

Opiate receptor sites — cells that receive only one particular kind of drug. These are located in the dorsal horn of the spinal cord and the periaquaductal grey region of the brain. The discovery of spinal opiate receptors in 1973 led to the development of selective spinal opiate analgesia.

Opioids — narcotics that stimulate the opiate receptor site to produce analgesia

Ordinal variables — sets of ordered categories

Osmolarity — number of solutes contained in solution measured in milliosmoles per liter

Outcome — the interpretation of documented results; and educational goal

Palliative — treatment that may be provided for comfort and/or temporary relief of symptoms, but that does not cure

Palpable cord — a vein that is rigid and hard to the touch

Palpation — examination by touch

Parenteral — denoting any route other than the alimentary canal, such as intravenous

Parenteral nutrition — nutrients that are administered intravenously, comprising carbohydrates, proteins, and/or fats, and additives, such as electrolytes, vitamins, and trace elements

Paresthesia — abnormal spontaneous sensations (eg, burning, prickling, tingling, or tickling without physical stimulus)

Particulate matter — relating to or composed of fine particles

Pathogens — disease-producing microorganisms

PCA — patient-controlled analgesia

Percutaneous puncture — puncture performed through the skin

Peripheral — pertains to veins of the extremities, scalp, and external jugular; not central

Peripheral neuropathy — dysfunction of postganglionic nerves, ranging from paresthesia to paralysis

Peristalsis — progressive wave-like movement that occurs involuntarily

Phlebitis — inflammation of a vein; may be accompanied by pain, erythema, edema, streak formation, and/or palpable cord; rated by a standard scale (see phlebitis topic); a possible precursor to sepsis

Phlebotomy — withdrawal of blood from a vein

Physical incompatibility — an undesirable change that is visually observed

Plant alkyloids — anticancer drugs derived from plants, such as the periwinkle (vincristine and vinblastine) in the vinca family

Port — port of entry

Positive pressure — maintaining a constant, even force within a lumen to prevent reflux of blood; achieved while injecting by clamping or withdrawing needle from cannula

Postinfusion phlebitis — inflammation of a vein occurring after cannula removal

Pounds per square inch (psi) — a measurement of pressure; psi equals 50 mm Hg or 68 cm H_2O.

Preservative-free — containing no added substance capable of inhibiting bacterial contamination

Priming — initial filling of the administration set with infusate

Process — actual performance and observation of performance based on compliance with policies, procedures, and professional standards

Product integrity — intact, uncompromised product; condition suitable for intended use

Proximal — nearest to the heart; closest to point of attachment; above previous site of cannulation

Pruritis — itching

Psychomotor — behaviors that place primary emphasis on the various degrees of physical skills and dexterity as they relate to the thought process

Purpura — condition in which spontaneous bleeding occurs in subcutaneous tissue resulting in purple patches visible on the skin

Purulent — containing or producing pus

Push — direct injection of a medication into a vein or access device

Quality indicator — a systematic process for monitoring, evaluating, and problem-solving

Radiopaque — ability to be detected by radiography

Ratio variables — having all features of interval variables but adding an absolute zero point, indicating absence of a point being measured

Rh system — a blood group system denoting the presence or absence of the D (Rh) red blood cell antigen

Risk management — process that centers on identification, analysis, treatment, and evaluation of real and potential hazards

Roller bandage — a roll of gauze or other material used for protecting an injured part, for immobilizing a limb, for keeping dressings in place, etc.

Sclerotic — fibrous thickening of the wall of the vein resulting in decreased lumen size. On palpation, usually feels hard to the touch.

Semi-quantitative culture technique — a laboratory protocol used for isolating and identifying microorganisms

Sensitization — the initial exposure of an individual to a specific antigen that results in an immune response

Sepsis — infectious microorganisms or their toxins in the blood stream

Septum — a wall dividing two or more cavities

Single-use vial — medication bottle intended for one-time use that is hermetically sealed with a rubber stopper

Skin-cannula junction — point at which the cannula enters the skin

Spike — insertion of the administration set into the solution container

Statistics — the science of collecting, classifying, and interpreting information based on the numbers of things

Stomatitis — sores on the inside of the mouth

Structure — describes the elements on which a program is based. Elements may include resources such as federal and state laws, professional standards, position descriptions, patient rights, policies and procedures, documentation forms, quality controls, corrective action programs, etc.

Stylet — a rigid metal object within a catheter designed to facilitate insertion

Surfactant — material whose properties reduce the surface tension of fluid

Surveillance — the active, systematic, ongoing observation of the occurrence and distribution of disease within a population and of the events or conditions that increase or decrease the risk of such disease occurrence

Sympathetic — part of the autonomic nervous system responsible for the fight-or-flight response. The sympathetic system is dominant when a person experiences pain. The effects on the body are from a release of norepinephrine in the body, resulting in increased heart rate, blood pressure, respiration.

Systemic — pertaining to the whole body rather than one of its parts

Tamper-proof — impossible to alter

Thrombocytopenia — decrease in thrombocyte or platelet count

Thrombolytic agent — a pharmacologic agent capable of dissolving blood clots

Thrombophlebitis — inflammation of the vein with clot formation

Thrombosis — formation of a blood clot within a blood vessel

Total nutrient admixture — parenteral nutrition formulation containing carbohydrates, amino acids, lipid, vitamins, minerals, trace elements, water, and other additives in a single container

Trace elements — minute amounts of essential elements present in the body

Transfusion reaction — any adverse effect to the

transfusion of whole blood or its components or derivatives

Transitional feeding — progression from one mode of feeding to another, while continuously administering estimated nutrient requirements

Transparent semipermeable membrane (TSM) — a sterile dressing that allows visualization, repels water, and allows air to permeate it

Trendelenburg — a position in which the head is lower than the feet; used to increase venous distention

Tunneled catheter — a central catheter designed to have a portion lie within a subcutaneous passage before exiting the body

Valsalva maneuver — the process of making a forceful attempt at expiration with the mouth, nostrils, and glottis closed

Vascular access — means of approaching or entering the vascular system

Vascular access devices — catheters placed directly into the venous system for infusion therapy and/or phlebotomy

Venipuncture — puncture of a vein for any purpose

Vesicant — caustic intravenous medication that causes blisters and tissue injury when it escapes into the surrounding tissue(s)

Volumetric — relating to measurement of a substance by its volume

I N D E X

System Requirements

Any hardware (either PC or MAC) with the following options:
CD-ROM drive
Internet Browser (ie, Internet Explorer or Netscape)

Simple Installation Guidelines

PC with Windows software
Insert CD-ROM into CD-ROM drive
CD Autoplay will automatically open the disk

MAC
Insert CD-ROM into CD-ROM drive
Drag the web page file named "index.htm" from the CD to the browser program

Plumer's Principles & Practice of Intravenous Therapy, 7E CD-ROM

Program Features

- Browser based – with EASY PC AUTOPLAY installation capability – just turn on your computer and insert the CD-ROM into the CD-ROM drive. It opens automatically on your PC !!!!
- Easy access to more than 140 intravenous drug monographs – using either generic or trade drug names: go to Generic Name Lookup or Trade Name Lookup; click on desired letter on the alphabet selection bar and then click on desired drug name from the drug index screen
- Print out complete drug monographs quickly! Just click on "File" on your toolbar, then select "Print". Your printer will print the drug monograph that appears on your screen.
- Unique option to CUSTOMIZE and print out Drug-specific teaching points – just click on the blue Drug-specific teaching points heading within any drug monograph. Now you can type in your patient's name and the indication for which the drug was prescribed before printing out your customized patient teaching handout.

Browser-Based Functions

To navigate: use your browser toolbar to move forward (click on forward arrow) or backward (click on backward arrow)
To print screen: click on File (on browser toolbar) then click on Print

Accessing and Using CD-ROM Contents

Drug Monographs: Two Ways to Access

- *Generic Name Lookup* – click on letter from Alphabet selection bar; click on desired Generic Name

- *Trade Name Lookup* – click on letter from Alphabet selection bar; click on desired Trade Name

- *Technical Support* – 1-800-638-3030